Scientific and Technical Publication No. 622

Health in the Americas

Americas

2007 VOLUME I–REGIONAL

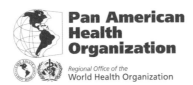

Pan American Health Organization

Regional Office of the
World Health Organization

PAN AMERICAN HEALTH ORGANIZATION
Pan American Sanitary Bureau, Regional Office of the
WORLD HEALTH ORGANIZATION
525 Twenty-third Street, N.W.
Washington, D.C. 20037, U.S.A.

2007

Also published in Spanish (2007), as:
Salud en las Américas, 2007
Publicación Científica y Técnica No. 622
ISBN 978 92 75 31622 8 (Obra completa, dos volúmenes)
ISBN 978 92 75 31626 0 (Volumen I–Regional)

PAHO Library Cataloguing-in-Publication Data

Pan American Health Organization
   Health in the Americas: 2007
Washington, D.C.: PAHO, © 2007—2v.
(PAHO Scientific and Technical Publication No. 622)

ISBN 978 92 75 11622 9 (Two volume set)
ISBN 978 92 75 11626 1 (Volume I–Regional)

I. Title   II. (Series)
III. Author

1. HEALTH STATUS INDICATORS
2. PUBLIC HEALTH ESSENTIAL FUNCTIONS
4. EQUITY IN HEALTH CONDITIONS
4. HEALTH CARE REFORM
5. SUSTAINABLE DEVELOPMENT
6. AMERICAS

NLM WA 110

The Pan American Health Organization welcomes requests for permission to reproduce or translate its publications, in part or in full. Applications and inquiries should be addressed to the Publications Area, Pan American Health Organization, Washington, D.C., U.S.A., which will be glad to provide the latest information on any changes made to the text, plans for new editions, and reprints and translations already available.

CONTENTS

See page xiii for the list of figures and tables.

LIST OF FIGURES AND TABLES

1. HEALTH IN THE CONTEXT OF DEVELOPMENT

2. HEALTH CONDITIONS AND TRENDS

3. SUSTAINABLE DEVELOPMENT AND ENVIRONMENTAL HEALTH

4. PUBLIC POLICIES AND HEALTH SYSTEMS AND SERVICES

5. HEALTH AND INTERNATIONAL COOPERATION

PREFACE

The Secretariat of the Pan American Health Organization has a constitutional responsibility to report to the Pan American Sanitary Conference on health conditions and trends in the Region. Such is the principal purpose of this 2007 edition of *Health in the Americas*. It offers an updated, comprehensive presentation of the health situation throughout the hemisphere generally and specifically in the 46 countries and territories of the Americas, and it describes and analyzes the progress, constraints, and challenges of PAHO Member States in their efforts to improve the health of the peoples of the Region.

As a health agency, our core discipline is epidemiology, which enables us to measure, define, and compare health problems and conditions and their distribution from the perspectives of population, geography, and time. This publication addresses the issue of health as a human right, taking into account both the individual and community contexts, and examines various critical determinants of health, including those of a biological, social, cultural, economic, and political nature. That examination reveals the existence of gaps, disparities, and inequities that persist in our Region, especially those related to access to basic services, health, nutrition, housing, and adequate living conditions as well as to the lack of opportunities for human development—all of which contribute to the greater vulnerability to diseases and health risks of some population groups.

Therefore, in addition to the Secretariat's institutionally specific remit to describe and analyze health problems and the response of the health sector to those problems, we have chosen to frame our analysis in the context of the universal commitment to the Millennium Development Goals of reducing hunger and poverty, promoting gender equity in opportunities for education, preventing and controlling diseases, managing and furthering cooperation among countries, and creating and strengthening subregional and intersectoral partnerships between governments and civil society—as necessary conditions to achieve better health for the peoples of the Americas.

Production of this publication has been a major and complex undertaking of more than 500 of the Secretariat's staff members. In the course of their work, they have consulted countless sources, both official and unofficial, to compile this compendium of information; consequently, some discrepancies in the presentation of data may have occurred. It bears noting, moreover, that the quality of information from the countries varies considerably and that it was impossible to obtain from some of them within-country disaggregations of data that would enable measurement of disparities in the health status of specific population groups. Nonetheless, this regional panorama expresses our commitment to work with the countries to address the unfinished agenda of unnecessary, preventable deaths of mothers, children, and other vulnerable population groups; to continue and renew efforts to sustain achievements in health, such as the elimination of diseases preventable by immunization; and to tackle ongoing and future challenges such as, among others, HIV/AIDS, multiresistant tuberculosis, juvenile violence, and new forms of bioterrorism.

In our determination to add value to the information we provide our readers, this edition of *Health in the Americas* offers some new features such as individual highlights of each country's efforts to deal with a specific national health problem, and several other features described in the note to our readers (see next page). And, in our continuing attempts to broaden the reach of our information and to capitalize on changing technologies for the benefit of our readers, we are publishing this edition of *Health in the Americas* in print, online, and other digital platforms.

Along with the description and analysis of regional health conditions, this edition provides the perspectives of 10 internationally renowned experts regarding the "Health Agenda for the Americas, 2008-2017," an initiative of the countries of the Region launched on the occasion of the XXXVII General Assembly of the Organization of American States (Panama City, 3 June 2007), the aim of which is to pursue over the coming decade an integrated, collective enterprise to attain the health goals of the Region.

In closing, we aver that this latest in a series of 14 editions of our flagship publication gathers facts and presents intelligence with regard to health in the Americas, by providing analysis, perspectives, and context as accurately, fairly, and authoritatively as possible. We hope that our readers will bear in mind that behind every number and every statistic in this publication is the life of a girl, a boy, a woman, or a man living in some corner of the Region. We further hope that the 2012 edition of the publication will bring news of the countries' great progress in their common covenant to attain better health and longer, fuller, more fruitful lives for all the peoples of the Americas, especially those who thus far have been excluded from the benefits of development.

Mirta Roses Periago
Director

NOTE TO OUR READERS

This edition of *Health in the Americas* introduces a number of changes to previous editions.

The Regional Volume includes an opening chapter that provides an overview of health in terms of the Millennium Development Goals; of the health status continuum—the unfinished agenda, the protection of health gains, and the confrontation of emerging threats; and of the national and international health sector response to that health status. Also added is a final chapter that contemplates a vision of the future of public health in the Region in the context of the Health Agenda for the Americas, 2008-2017, with commentaries from a number of distinguished international experts. Each of the intervening chapters commences with an introductory summary, which is set off from the main text with a different format. Color is used throughout the volume to assure the clarity of graphic material. Finally, as one of the main purposes of the series *Health in the Americas* is to trace regional trends in health conditions and health systems over time, complementing this edition are quotations from the Directors of the Organization—from Hugh S. Cumming in the 1920s to Mirta Roses Periago in the 21st century—that are germane to the subjects of the various chapters.

The Country Volume presents maps of each country and territory, as well as short notices that highlight a specific health challenge and the response of the national health sector to that challenge.

Throughout both volumes, text boxes are introduced to provide additional material; figures and tables are inserted as close as possible to their in-text mention; and bibliographic references are included.

We hope that these editorial enhancements will serve both to interest and to enlighten you, our readers.

CONTRIBUTORS

COUNTRY VOLUME

Anguilla: Serene Carter-Davis (Coordinator), Byron Crape, Margaret Hazlewood, Bonnie Richardson-Lake, Thomas Yerg • **Antigua and Barbuda:** Rhonda Sealey-Thomas (Coordinator), Byron Crape, Margaret Hazlewood, James Knigth, Thomas Yerg • **Argentina:** Enrique Vázquez (Coordinator), José Luis Castro, Hugo Cohen, Luis Roberto Escoto, Carla Figliolo, María Angélica Flores, Salvador García, Caty Iannello, José Antonio Pagés, Celso Rodríguez, Luis Eliseo Velásquez, Marcelo Vila, Claudia Vivas • **Aruba:** Alejandro López (Coordinator), Gregory Fung-a-Fat, Renato Gusmao, Sharline Kolman-Weber, Patricia L. Ruiz, Thomas Yerg • **Bahamas:** Yitades Gebre (Coordinator), Charlene Bain, Byron Crape, Merceline Dahl- Regis, Camille Deleveaux, Pearl McMillan, Linda Rae-Campbell, Thomas Yerg • **Barbados:** Pascal Frison (Coordinator), Veta Brown, Reeshemah Cheltenham Niles, Samuel Deane, César Gattini, Alejandro Giusti, Margaret Hazlewood, Carol Boyd-Scobie, John Silvi, Thomas Yerg • **Belize:** Guillermo Troya (Coordinator), Diana Beverly-Barnett, Emir Castaneda, Englebert Emmanuel, Margaret Hazlewood, Kathleen Israel, Sandra Jones, Ricardo Luján, Rony Maza, Nancy Naj, John Silvi, Lorraine Thompson, Thomas Yerg • **Bermuda:** Jacqueline Gernay (Coordinator), J. Cann, E. Casey, Janice Chang, Byron Crape, Ernest Pate, Marion Pottinger, John Silvi, Ana Treasure, Godfrey Xuereb, Thomas Yerg • **Bolivia:** Carlos Ayala (Coordinator), Dora Caballero, María del Carmen Daroca, Christian Darras, Percy Halkyer, Susana Hannover Saavedra, Henry Hernández, Martha Mejía, Juan Pablo Protto, Olivier Ronveaux, Diddie Schaaf, Ivelise Segovia, Marco F. Suárez, Jorge Terán • **Brazil:** José Antonio Escamilla (Coordinator), Zuleica Albuquerque, Paola Barbosa Marchesini, Roberto Becker, Maria Lúcia Carneiro, Luciana de Deus Chagas, Mauro Rosa Elkhoury, Rubén Figueroa, James Fitzgerald, Alejandro Giusti, Diego González, Adriana Maria P. Marques, Roberto Montoya, Marcia Moreira, José Paranaguá de Santana, João Baptista Risi Junior, Luis Fernando Rocabado, Rodolfo Rodriguez, Patricia L. Ruiz, Celsa Sampson, Rosa Maria Silvestre, Orenzio Soler, Valeska Stempliuk, Julio Manuel Suárez, Horacio Toro, Cristiana Toscazo, Enrique Vázquez, Matias Villatoro, Zaida Yadón • **British Virgin Islands:** Irad Potter (Coordinator), Byron Crape, Ronald Georges, Margaret Hazlewood, Tracia Smith-Jones, Thomas Yerg, Fernando Zacarías • **Canada:** Nick Previsich (Coordinator), Mara Brotman, Stephanie Blondin, Byron Crape, Kate Dickson, Jennifer Rae, John Silvi, Thomas Yerg • **Cayman Islands:** Jacqueline Garnay (Coordinator), E. Casey, Janice Chang, Margaret Hazlewood, Kiran Kumar, Timothy McLaughlin-Munroe, Ernest Pate, Marion Pottinger, Linda Rae-Campbell, Ana Treasure, Godfrey Xuereb, Thomas Yerg • **Chile:** Alejandro Giusti (Coordinator), Oscar Arteaga, Paula Bedregal, Paula Margozzini, Juan Manuel Sotelo • **Colombia:** Roberto Sempértegui Ontaneda (Coordinator), Pier Paolo Balladeli, Sergio Calderón, Patricia de Segurado, Jose Pablo Escobar, Bertha Gómez, Susana Helfer-Vogel, María Cristina Latorre, Juan Guillermo Orozco, Magda Palacio, Rafael Pardo, Desiree Pastor, José Ruales, Isabel Cristina Ruiz, Martha Idalí Saboya • **Costa Rica:** Humberto Montiel Paredes (Coordinator), Rosa María Borrell, Xinia Bustamante, Miryan Cruz, Catty Cuellar, Roberto Del Águila, Gerardo Galvis, Leonardo Hernández, Wilmer Marquito, Sandra Murillo, Shirley Quesada, Mayra Rodríguez, Carlos Samayoa, Javier Santacruz • **Cuba:** José Gómez (Coordinator), Adolfo Álvarez Blanco, Osvaldo Castro, Antonio González Fernández, Idalis González Polanco, Lea Guido, Gilda Marquina, Néstor Marimón Torres, Rolando Miyar, Gabriel Montalvo, Mario Pichardo, Daniel Purcallas, Ana María Sánchez Calero, Maritza Sosa, Rosa María Torres Vidal • **Dominica:** David Johnson (Coordinator), Byron Crape, Margaret Hazlewood, Paul Ricketts, Thomas Yerg • **Dominican Republic:** Celia Riera (Coordinator), Gerardo Alfaro, F. Rosario Cabrera, Pedro Luis Castellanos, Dalia Castillo, Maria Antonieta González, Rosario Guzmán, Cecilia Michel, Raúl Montesano, Carlos Morales Castillo, Cristina Nogueira, Oscar Suriel, Selma Zapata • **Ecuador:** Miguel Machuca (Coordinator), Víctor Aráuz, Caroline Chang, Luis Codina, Delmin Cury, Jean Marc Gabastou, Carlos Roberto Garzón, Edmundo Granda, Irene Leal, Jorge Luis Prosperi, Ana Quan, Rocío Rojas, Ángel Valencia, Diego Victoria • **El Salvador:** Gerardo de Cosío (Coordinator), Julio Armero Guardado, Eduardo Guerrero, Lucio Isaí Sermeño Hernández • **French Guiana, Guadeloupe and Martinique:** Henrietta Chamouillet (Coordinator), Chloé Chiltz, Thierry Cardozo, Jean-Pierre Diouf, Pascal Frison, Alejandro Giusti, Claire Lietard, Sylvie Merle, Michelle Ooms, Georges Para, Annick Vezolles, Fernando Zacarías • **Grenada:** Gabriel Clements (Coordinator), Carlene Radix, Tessa Stroude • **Guatemala:** Enrique Gil Bellorin (Coordinator), Fernando Amado, Rosario Castro, Isabel Enriquez, América de Fernández, Maggie Fischer, Daniel Frade, Federico Hernández, Jaime Juárez, Hilda Leal, Joaquín Molina, Rodrigo Rodríguez, Juanita de Rodríguez • **Guyana:** Tephany Griffith (Coordinator), Enias Baganizi, Keith Burrowes, Byron Crape, Debra Francis, Hedwig Goede, Margaret Hazlewood, Kathleen Israel, Tamara Mancero, Teofilo Monteiro, Renee Franklin Peroune, Vaulda Quamina-Griffith, Luis Seoane, Bernadette Theodore-Gandi, Luis Valdes, Thomas Yerg • **Haiti:** Michelle Ooms (Coordinator), Philippe Emmanuel Allouard, Gabriel Bidegain, Jean-Philippe Breux, Beatrice Bonnevaux, Vivianne Cayemites, Henriette Chamouillet, Philippe Doo-Kingue, Hélène Duplan-Prudhon, Karoline Fonck, Pascal Frison, Neyde Gloria Garrido, Alejandro Giusti, Carlos Gril, María Guevara, Marie-Charleine Hecdivert, Donna Isidor, Vely Jean-François, Siullin Clara Joa, Johann Julmiste, François Lacapère, Elsie Lafosse, Gerald Lerebours, Roc Magloire, Frantz Metellus, Christian Morales, José Moya, Françoise Ponticq, Jacques Hendry Rousseau, Patricia L. Ruiz, Malhi Cho Samaniego, Elisabeth Verluyten, Thomas Yerg, Fernando Zacarías • **Honduras:** Guillermo Guibovich (Coordinator), José Fiusa Lima, Raquel Fernández Pacheco, Lillian Reneau-Vernon • **Jamaica:** Jacqueline Garnay (Coordinator), Roberto Becker, E. Casey, Janice Chang, Jacqueline Duncan, Sydney Edwin, Denise Eldemire–Shearer, Donna Fraser, Andriene Grant, Margaret Hazlewood, Erica Hedmann, Maureen Irons-Morgan, Everton G. Kidd, Peter Knight, Karen Lewis Bell, Andre McNab, Valerie Nam, Ernest Pate, Marion Pottinger, Lundie Richards, Ana Treasure, Earl Wright, Godfrey Xuereb, Thomas Yerg • **Mexico:** José Moya (Coordinator), Gustavo Bergonzoli, Angel Betanzos, Verónica Carrión, Luis Castellanos, Jacobo Finkelman, Guilherme Franco Netto, Sergio Garay, Ivonne Orejel, Juan de Dios Reyes • **Montserrat:** Pascal Frison (Coordinator), Byron Crape, Lyndell Creer, Alejandro Giusti, Dorothea Hanzel, Margaret Hazlewood, Thomas

Yerg, Fernando Zacarías • **Netherlands Antilles:** Renato Gusmao (Coordinator), Sonja Caffe, Byron Crape, Izzy Gerstenbluth, Thomas Yerg • **Nicaragua:** Marianela Corriols (Coordinator), Reynaldo Aguilar, Sylvain Aldighieri, Mario Cruz, Maria A Gomes, Socorro Gross, Silvia Narváez, Eduardo Ortiz, Cristina Pedreira • **Panama:** Guadalupe Verdejo (Coordinator), Jorge Jenkins, Percy Minaya, Jorge Rodríguez, José Luis San Martín, Ángel Valencia, Gustavo Vargas • **Paraguay:** Marcia G. Moreira (Coordinator), Maria Almirón, Gladys Antonieta de Arias, Javier Espíndola, Julio Galeano, Gladys Cecilia Ghisays, Epifania Gómez, Bernardo Sánchez, Isabel Sánchez, Carmen Rosa Serrano, Sonia Tavares, Javier Uribe • **Peru:** Fernando Gonzáles Ramírez (Coordinator), Maria Edith Baca, Gaby Caro, Rigoberto Centeno, Miryan Cruz, Miguel Dávila, Adrián Díaz, Luis Gutiérrez, Mario Martínez, Mónica Padilla, Manuel Peña, Germán Perdomo, Homero Silva, Hugo Tamayo, Washington Toledo, Mario Valcárcel, Gladys Zarate • **Puerto Rico:** Raúl Castellanos (Coordinator), Dalidia Colón, Byron Crape, Raúl Figueroa Rodríguez, Patricia L. Ruiz, Migdalia Vázquez González, Thomas Yerg • **Saint Kitts and Nevis:** Patrick Martin (Coordinator), Andrew Skerritt , Thomas Yerg • **Saint Lucia:** Pascal Frison (Coordinator), Adelaide Alexander, Dwight Calixto, Xista Edmund, Margaret Hazlewood, Alinda Jaime, Kerry Joseph • **Saint Vincent and the Grenadines:** Roger Duncan (Coordinator), Severlina Cupid, Kari da Silva, Anne de Roche, Sandra Grante, Margaret Hazlewood, Nykieska Jackson, Thomas St Clare, Anneke Wilson • **Suriname:** Elwine VanKanten (Coordinator), Roberto Becker, Gustavo Bretas, Byron Crape, Alma Catharina Cuellar, Margaret Hazlewood, Stephen Simon, Thomas Yerg • **Trinidad and Tobago:** Gina Watson (Coordinator), Roberto Becker, Carol Boyd-Scobie, Alma Catharina Cuellar, Byron Crape, Marilyn Entwistle, Margaret Hazlewood, James Hospedales, Leah-Mari Richards, John Silvi, Avril Siung-Chang, Thomas Yerg • **Turks and Caicos Islands:** Yitades Gebre (Coordinator), Tashema A. Bholanath, Cheryl Ann Jones, Jackurlyn Sutton, Rufus W. Swing, Thomas Yerg • **United States of America:** MaryLou Valdéz (Coordinator), Mark A. Abdoo, Roberto Becker, Byron Crape, Alicia Díaz, Ruth Katz, Ch'uya H. Lane, Sam Notzon, Thomas Yerg • **Uruguay:** Alejandro Gherardi (Coordinator), Mónica Col, Alejandro Giusti, Elizabeth Jurado, Patricia L. Ruiz, Roberto Salvatella, Enrique Vázquez • **Venezuela:** Alejandro López Inzaurralde (Coordinator), Oswaldo Barrezueta Cobo, Renato Gusmao, Natasha Herrera, Marcelo Korc, Miguel Malo Serrano, Soledad Pérez Évora • **United States-Mexico Border Area:** Kam Suan Mung (Coordinator), Lorely Ambriz, Maria Teresa Cerqueira, Byron Crape, Sally Edwards, Luis Gutiérrez, Piedad Huerta, Guillermo Mendoza, Rosalba Ruiz, Patricia L. Ruiz, Thomas Yerg.

REGIONAL VOLUME

Overview: Judith Navarro (Coordinator), Byron Crape, Anabel Cruz, Andrea DiPaola, Oscar Mujica, Alfonso Ruiz, Patricia L. Ruiz, John Silvi, Fernando Zacarías • **Chapter 1:** Sofíaleticia Morales (Coordinator), Marco Akerman, Alfredo Calvo, Rafael Flores, Saúl Franco, Guilherme Franco Netto, Alejandro Giusti, Elsa Gómez, Jorge Iván González, Antonio Hernández, Lilia Jara, Fernando Lolas, Jesús López Macedo, Enrique Loyola, Rocío Rojas, Maria Helena Romero, Patricia L. Ruiz, Rubén Suárez, Cristina Torres, Javier Vázquez • **Chapter 2:** Gabriela Fernández (Coordinator), Raimond Armengol, Steven Ault, Alberto Barceló, Roberto Becker, Yehuda Benguigui, Keith Carter, Carlos Castillo Solórzano, Carolina Danovaro, Mirta del Granado, Amalia del Riego, Chris Drasbek, John Ehrenberg, Rainier Escalada, Saskia Estupiñán, Daniela Fernandes da Silva, Ricardo Fescina, Érika García, Andrea Gerger, Alejandro Giusti, Thomas Harkins, James Hospedales, Ithzak Levav, Marlo Libel, Silvana Luciani, Chessa Lutter, Miguel Machuca, Matilde Maddaleno, Sara Marques, Christina Marsigli, Rafael Mazín, Oscar Mujica, Monica Palak, Marta Peláez, Pilar Ramon-Pardo, Jorge Rodríguez, Rocío Rojas, Alba María Ropero, Roberto Salvatella, Roxane Salvatierra, Celsa Sampson, José Luis Sanmartin, Cristina Schneider, Juan Carlos Silva, John Silvi, Cristina Torres Parodi, Ciro Ugarte, Armando Vásquez, Enrique Vega • **Chapter 3:** Samuel Henao, Enrique Loyola y Cristina Schneider (Coordinators), Adriana Blanco, María Teresa Cerqueira, Alberto Concha-Eastman, Vera Luiza Da Costa Siva, Diego Daza, Hernan Delgado, Luiz A. Galvão, Genaro García, Diego González, Eduardo Guerrero, Josefa Ippolito-Shepherd, Fernando Leanes, Jorge López, Mildred Maisonet, Maristela Monteiro, Sofíaleticia Morales, José Naranjo, Mireya Palmieri, Mauricio Pardón, Enrique Pérez, Emilio Ramírez, Marilyn Rice, Eugenia Rodrigues, Celso Rodríguez, Alfonso Ruiz, Henry Salas, Rosa Sandoval, Víctor Saravia, Kerstin Schotte, Heather Selin, Homero Silva, Luz Maritza Tennassee, Ricardo Torres • **Chapter 4:** Cristina Puentes-Markides (Coordinator), Gisele Almeida, Jorge Bermúdez, Jaume Canela Soler, Regina Castro, María de los Angeles Cortés, José Ramiro Cruz, Rafael Flores, Amparo Gordillo Tobar, Pablo Jiménez, Eduardo Levcovitz, Ramón Martínez, Carme Nebot, Abel Packer, Daniel Purcallas, Priscilla Rivas-Loria, Patricia L. Ruiz, Rubén Suárez Berenguela, América Valdés, Fernando Zacarías • **Chapter 5:** Rebecca de los Ríos y Hugo Prado (Coordinators), Carlos Arosquipa, Alfredo Calvo, Mariela Canepa, Paul Mertens, Patricia L. Ruiz, Ciro Ugarte, Fernando Zacarías • **Chapter 6:** Judith Navarro (Coordinator), George A.O. Alleyne, Stephen Blount, Paulo Buss, Nils Kastberg, Gustavo Kourí, Jay McAuliffe, Sylvie Stachenko, Muthu Subramanian, Ricardo Uauy, Marijke Velzeboer-Salcedo.

Inter Programmatic Working Group for Health in the Americas 2007: Fernando Zacarías (Coordinator), Patricia L. Ruiz (Technical Secretary), Gustavo Bergonzoli, Carlos Castillo Solórzano, Anabel Cruz, Gerardo de Cosio, Amalia del Riego, Ricardo Fescina, Samuel Henao, Branka Legetic, Eduardo Levcovitz, Marlo Libel, Chessa Lutter, Miguel Machuca, Mildred Maisonet, Humberto Montiel, Hernán Montenegro, Sofíaleticia Morales, Oscar Mujica, Judith Navarro, Armando Peruga, Cristina Puentes-Markides, Alba María Ropero, Alfonso Ruiz, Cristina Schneider, Javier Uribe, Enrique Vázquez, Gina Watson.

Editing and production: Anabel Cruz (Coordinator), Leslie Buechele, Patricia De los Ríos, Andrea DiPaola, Mariesther Fernández, Judith Navarro, Roberta Okey, Lucila Pacheco, Cecilia Parker, Alfonso Ruiz, Haydée Valero • **Promotion:** José Carnevali, Daniel Epstein, Mylena Pinzón, Evelyn Rodríguez, Eleana Villanueva • **Graphic Design:** Gilles Collete, Guenther Grill, Ajibola Oyeleye • **Web site:** Marcelo D'Agostino, Erico Pérez-Neto.

General Coordinator: Fernando Zacarías • **Technical Coordinator:** Patricia L. Ruiz.

We would like to thank the personnel of the ministries of health and other governmental institutions, international agencies, nongovernmental organizations, and other entities for so generously supplying the data and information used for this publication. In spite of the fact that great efforts have been made to include all contributors, we apologize for any possible errors or omissions that may have occurred.

AN OVERVIEW
OF REGIONAL HEALTH

Since the inception of the Pan American Health Organization in 1902, the governments of the Americas have jointly addressed their concerns regarding health and the environment, committing to collective action and defining strategies to respond to emerging challenges. From the beginning, the collection, analysis, and dissemination of health information has been a primary function of the Organization. Starting in 1924, health conditions and trends reported by countries were a main feature of annual reports of the Director. In 1954, the Secretariat of PAHO produced the first separate report on health conditions in the Americas, thus launching an uninterrupted quadrennial, now quinquennial, publication of information on health in the Region.

This 2007 edition of *Health in the Americas* presents a broad picture of the regional situation and that of all the countries with regard to health and human development; specific disease conditions and risk factors; environmental health, and the evolution of health systems and services. In addition, it considers and discusses progress made regarding the global commitment, expressed in the United Nations Millennium Development Goals (MDGs), to tackle extreme poverty, hunger, disease, lack of water and sanitation, inadequate housing, and social exclusion and to promote gender equality, education, and environmental sustainability. That expression of countries' collective commitment to social equity informs the text throughout this publication.

HEALTH IN THE CONTEXT OF DEVELOPMENT

In the Region of the Americas, human development and health have advanced over the past quarter-century, as shown by selected indicators in Table 1. Population growth has slowed, dropping in 2006 to a rate of 1.2% per year—ranging from 0.4% in the non-Latin Caribbean to 2% in Central America. Urbanization has expanded from 68.6% in 1980 to 78.9% in 2006. Coverage of basic services is on the increase for the

TABLE 1. Improvements in health and development in the Americas, selected indicators, 1980–2010.

Indicator[1]	1980–1985	1990–1995	2005–2010
Life expectancy at birth (years)	68.8	71.1	74.9
Total fertility rate (children/woman)	3.1	2.6	2.6
Infant mortality (per 1,000 live births)	37.8	22.5	16.5
Urban population (%)	68.6	72.8	79.1
Indicator[2]	**1980–1984**	**1990–1994**	**2000–2004**
Mortality from communicable diseases (rate/100,000 inhabitants)	109	62.8	55.9
Mortality from diseases of the circulatory system (rate/100,000 inhabitants)	280	256.2	229.2
Indicator[3]	**1980**	**1990**	**2005**
Literacy rate (%)	88	87.6	93.8
Immunization coverage (%): DPT3	45	76.8	93
Immunization coverage (%): Measles	48	82.5	93
Access to drinking water (%)	76	80	93
Access to sanitation services (%)	59	66	84
Nurses per 10,000 inhabitants	23.1	37.9	30

Sources:

[1]United Nations, Department of Economic and Social Affairs, Population Division (2005). World Population Prospects: The 2004 Revision. CD-ROM Edition Extended Dataset. U.N. Publications Sales No. 05.XIII.12.

[2]PAHO/Health Analysis and Statistics Unit (HA). Mortality Database System. 2004.

[3]PAHO, *Health Situation in the Americas: Basic Indicators, 2006*. Washington, D.C.; *Health Conditions in the Americas, 1994 Edition* and UNESCO for 1985–1994; PAHO, Evaluación Regional de Agua y Saneamiento, Washington, D.C. 2000; and http://stats.uis.unesco.org/unesco/TableViewer/tableView.aspx?ReportID=201.

most part, although less so in rural areas: the general population has better access to education, water and sanitation services, primary health care, cost-effective technologies, and immunizations. This increased coverage has enabled measurable progress toward preventing and controlling numerous communicable diseases that heretofore represented a significant burden. At the same time, life expectancy at birth has increased by an average of six years, and the incidence of infant mortality has decreased by one-half (*1*). The slowing of population growth, the lengthening of life spans, and the stemming of deaths from communicable diseases and perinatal conditions are among the foremost advances in health in the Region.

Notwithstanding these important gains in regional health, many major challenges remain: communicable diseases such as HIV/AIDS, malaria, and tuberculosis; various chronic noncommunicable diseases and conditions such as obesity, hypertension, cardiovascular diseases, diabetes, and cancer; and accidents and violence. Those health problems, in turn, stem from risk factors related to various demographic, social, and economic shifts in the Americas, including the aging of the population; changes in diet and physical activity as well as the consumption of tobacco, alcohol, and drugs; and the deterioration of social structures and supports.

The Millennium Development Goals set markers of progress in terms of human development and, at the same time, are indicators of the effectiveness of health systems. Having brought investment in people's health to the core of the global development agenda, the MDGs afford new opportunities for the health sector and health organizations to gain wide support for the health agenda.

The greatest share of health problems is attributable to broad social determinants—the "causes behind the causes" of ill-health: poverty, malnutrition, unemployment, lack of access to education and health services, the social exclusion of certain population groups, among others. These social determinants are analyzed in depth in Chapter 1 of this publication, "Health in the Context of Development," which covers the economic, political, social, and environmental contexts of health. Some of the salient factors impacting on health in the Americas are presented summarily in the paragraphs that follow.

Demographics. The Region of the Americas continues to experience three major demographic shifts: population growth, urbanization, and aging. Since 1950, the regional population has almost tripled, reaching 900.6 million inhabitants in 2006, according to the latest United Nations population revision (*2*). Under a mid-fertility variant scenario, this population is projected

FIGURE 1. Total population trends and projections by main geographic subregion, Region of the Americas, 1950–2050.

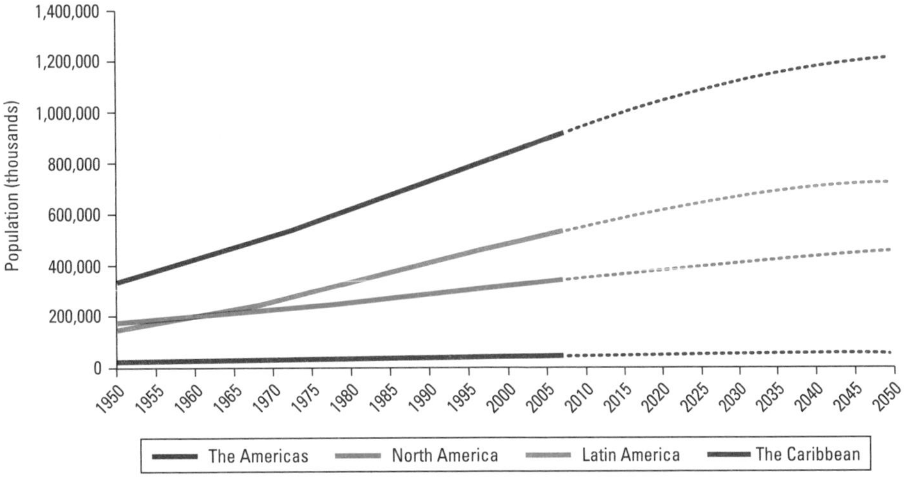

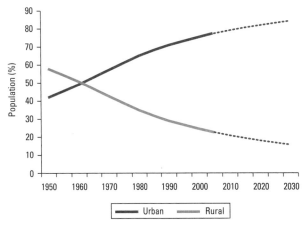

Source: United Nations Population Division. World Population Prospects: The 2006 Revision. New York. 2007.

to surpass the mark of 1 billion people, more than 600 million of them in Latin America and the Caribbean, in 2016 (Figure 1).

Social and economic disadvantages in rural areas and smaller population centers have led people, both worldwide and in the Americas, to migrate toward urban areas in search of employment and better living conditions, and urbanization is indeed a prominent feature of regional demographic change. Considerable differences exist among subregions, however: the urban population in the non-Latin Caribbean is 46.3%; in Central America, 54.8%; in the Latin Caribbean, 67.4%; in the Andean Area, 75.8%; in North America, 81%; and in the Southern Cone, 86.8%. Nearly 20% of the total population is now concentrated in only 20 of the Region's largest cities. In Latin America and the Caribbean, migration has spawned large, sprawling cities with marginalized areas that breed poverty, unemployment, violence, insecurity, pollution, and poorly distributed basic services. Since 1950, when rural population represented 58% of the total population, urban population has been growing, reaching 77.4% in 2005. If that trend persists unaltered, in 2030 the urban population in Latin America and the Caribbean is projected to reach almost 85%, as shown in Figure 2 (2).

The two population groups with the fastest growth in the Americas are the 60 and older and the 80 and older age groups. In North America, where the population-aging process began earlier, people 60 years of age and older went from representing 12.4% of the total population in 1950 to 16.7% in 2005; it is projected that this population group will increase to 20.1% of the total population in 2015 and to 27.3% in 2050. In Latin America and the Caribbean, on the other hand, the 60 and older age group comprised 5.6% of the 1950 population, increasing to 9.0% in 2005; it is projected to reach 11.3% of the total population in 2015 and

24.3% in 2050. The proportion of the total population represented by the 80 and older age group jumped from 1.1% in 1950 to 3.5% in 2005 in North America (and is projected to reach 3.7% in 2015), and from 0.4% to 1.2% in Latin America and the Caribbean (projected to increase to 1.7% in 2015). As the population ages, the ratio of productive adults to elderly individuals shrinks, as does potential funding of support for the elderly (Figure 3).

Economic growth, income, and employment. The Region's economy has undergone a series of shifts from low to high growth rates. After a period of declining growth and persistent

FIGURE 2. Urban and rural population trends and projections in Latin America and the Caribbean, 1950–2030.

Source: United Nations Population Division. World Population Prospects: The 2006 Revision. New York. 2007.

3

The Millennium Development Goals

GOAL 1. ERADICATE EXTREME POVERTY AND HUNGER

TARGET: HALVE, BETWEEN 1990 AND 2015, THE PROPORTION OF PEOPLE WHOSE INCOME IS LESS THAN US$ 1 A DAY.

Population living in extreme poverty (%), in Latin America and the Caribbean, 2005.

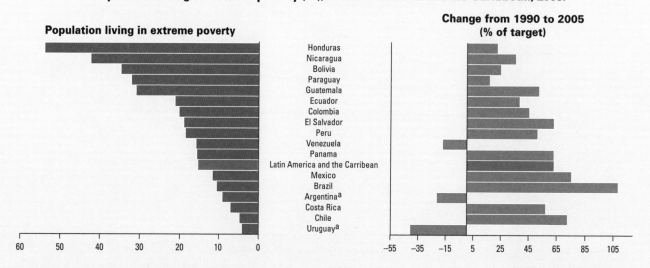

TARGET: HALVE, BETWEEN 1990 AND 2015, THE PROPORTION OF PEOPLE WHO SUFFER FROM HUNGER.

Underweight children under 5 years of age (%), in Latin America and the Caribbean, 1995–2003.

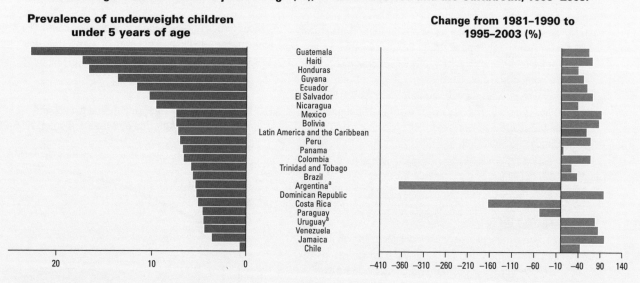

[a] Numbers refer to urban areas.

Note: The absence of bars means no change.

Sources: Economic Commission for Latin America and the Caribbean (ECLAC). The Millennium Development Goals: A Latin American and Caribbean Perspective. Produced in collaboration with the Pan American Health Organization; International Labor Organization; Food and Agricultural Organization of the United Nations; United Nations Educational, Scientific, and Cultural Organization; United Nations Development Program; United Nations Environment Program; United Nations Children's Fund; United Nations Population Fund; World Food Program; United Nations Human Settlements Program; United Nations Development Fund for Women. Santiago, Chile: ECLAC; 2005.

United Nations Statistical Division online database: http://millenniumindicators.un.org/unsd/mispa/mi_goals.aspx; and ECLAC Statistics and Economic Projections Division online database: http://websie.eclac.cl/sisgen/ConsultaIntegrada.asp?idAplicacion=1.

in Latin America and the Caribbean

GOAL 2. ACHIEVE UNIVERSAL PRIMARY EDUCATION

TARGET: ENSURE THAT, BY 2015, ALL CHILDREN EVERYWHERE, BOYS AND GIRLS ALIKE, WILL BE ABLE TO COMPLETE A FULL COURSE OF PRIMARY SCHOOLING.

Net enrollment in primary education (%), in Latin America and the Caribbean, 2004.

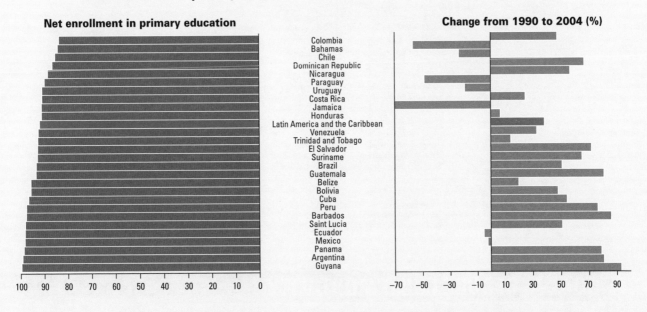

Youth literacy rate (%), in Latin America and the Caribbean, 2000/2004.

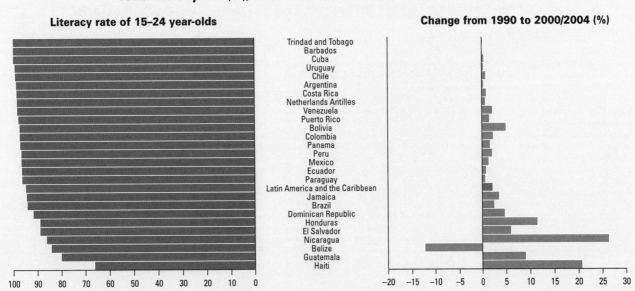

GOAL 3. PROMOTE GENDER EQUALITY AND EMPOWER WOMEN

TARGET: ELIMINATE GENDER DISPARITY IN PRIMARY AND SECONDARY EDUCATION, PREFERABLY BY 2005, AND IN ALL LEVELS OF EDUCATION NO LATER THAN 2015.

Share (%) of women in nonagricultural wage employment in Latin America and the Caribbean, 2001.

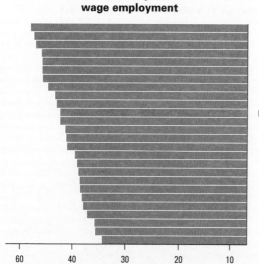

Women in nonagricultural wage employment

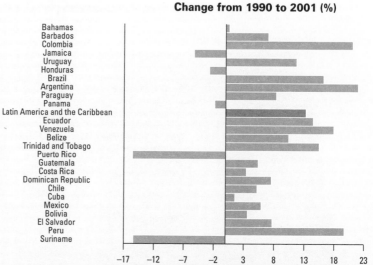

Change from 1990 to 2001 (%)

GOAL 4. REDUCE CHILD MORTALITY

TARGET: REDUCE BY TWO-THIRDS, BETWEEN 1990 AND 2015, THE UNDER-5 MORTALITY RATE.

Under-5 mortality rate per 1,000 live births, in Latin America and the Caribbean, 2003.

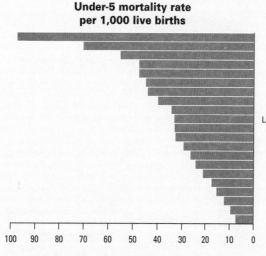

Under-5 mortality rate per 1,000 live births

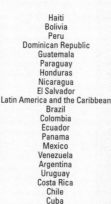

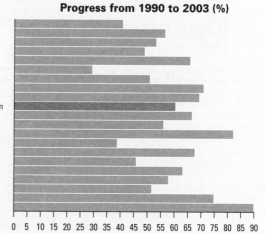

Progress from 1990 to 2003 (%)

Note: The absence of bars means no change.

Sources: Economic Commission for Latin America and the Caribbean (ECLAC). The Millennium Development Goals: A Latin American and Caribbean Perspective. Produced in collaboration with the Pan American Health Organization; International Labor Organization; Food and Agricultural Organization of the United Nations; United Nations Educational, Scientific, and Cultural Organization; United Nations Development Program; United Nations Environment Program; United Nations Children's Fund:; United Nations Population Fund; World Food Program; United Nations Human Settlements Program; United Nations Development Fund for Women. Santiago, Chile: ECLAC; 2005.

United Nations Statistical Division online database: http://millenniumindicators.un.org/unsd/mispa/mi_goals.aspx; and ECLAC Statistics and Economic Projections Division online database: http://websie.eclac.cl/sisgen/ConsultaIntegrada.asp?idAplicacion=1.

GOAL 5. IMPROVE MATERNAL HEALTH

TARGET: REDUCE BY THREE-QUARTERS, BETWEEN 1990 AND 2015, THE MATERNAL MORTALITY RATE.

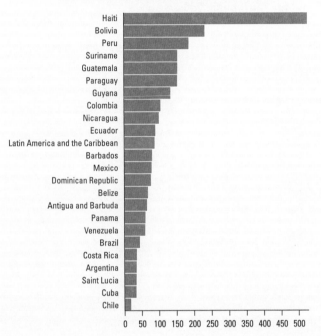

Maternal mortality rate per 100,000 live births, Latin America and the Caribbean, 2000.

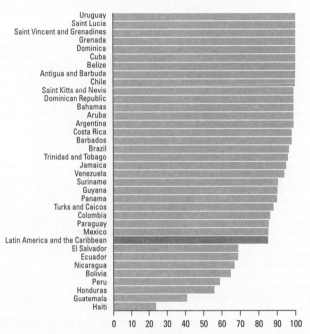

Proportion (%) of deliveries attended by skilled health personnel, Latin America and the Caribbean, 2000.

GOAL 6. COMBAT HIV/AIDS, MALARIA, AND OTHER DISEASES

TARGET: HAVE HALTED, BY 2015, AND BEGUN TO REVERSE THE SPREAD OF HIV/AIDS.

HIV/AIDS prevalence rate (%) among 15–49 year-olds, in Latin America and the Caribbean, 2005.

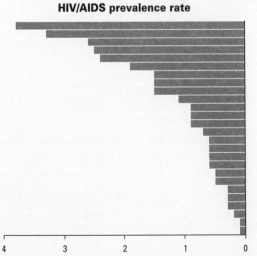

HIV/AIDS prevalence rate

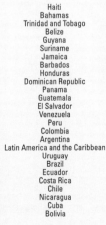

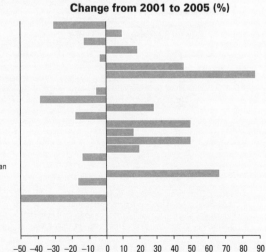

Change from 2001 to 2005 (%)

7

GOAL 7. ENSURE ENVIRONMENTAL SUSTAINABILITY

TARGET: HALVE, BY 2015, THE PROPORTION OF PEOPLE WITHOUT SUSTAINABLE ACCESS TO SAFE DRINKING WATER AND BASIC SANITATION.

Proportion of the rural population with sustainable access to an improved water source (%), in Latin America and the Caribbean, 2004.

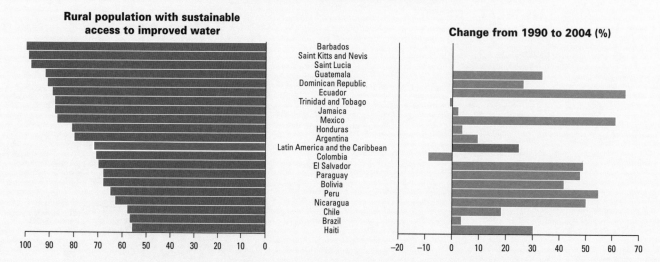

Proportion of the urban population with improved sanitation services (%), in Latin America and the Caribbean, 2004.

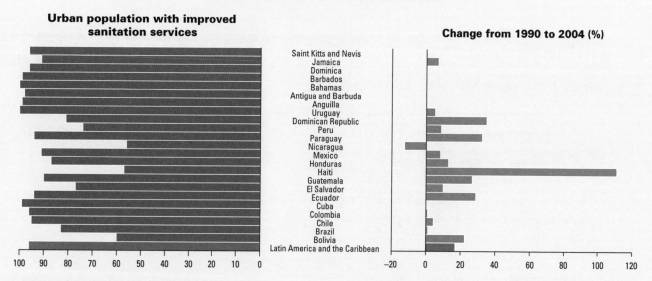

Note: The absence of bars means no change.

Sources: Economic Commission for Latin America and the Caribbean (ECLAC). The Millennium Development Goals: A Latin American and Caribbean Perspective. Produced in collaboration with the Pan American Health Organization; International Labor Organization; Food and Agricultural Organization of the United Nations; United Nations Educational, Scientific, and Cultural Organization; United Nations Development Program; United Nations Environment Program; United Nations Children's Fund; United Nations Population Fund; World Food Program; United Nations Human Settlements Program; United Nations Development Fund for Women. Santiago, Chile: ECLAC; 2005.

United Nations Statistical Division online database: http://millenniumindicators.un.org/unsd/mispa/mi_goals.aspx; and ECLAC Statistics and Economic Projections Division online database: http://websie.eclac.cl/sisgen/ConsultaIntegrada.asp?idAplicacion=1.

GOAL 8. DEVELOP A GLOBAL PARTNERSHIP FOR DEVELOPMENT

TARGET: IN COOPERATION WITH DEVELOPING COUNTRIES, DEVELOP AND IMPLEMENT STRATEGIES FOR DECENT AND PRODUCTIVE WORK FOR YOUTH.

Unemployment rate (%) of young people aged 15–24 years, both sexes, in Latin America and the Caribbean, 2001.

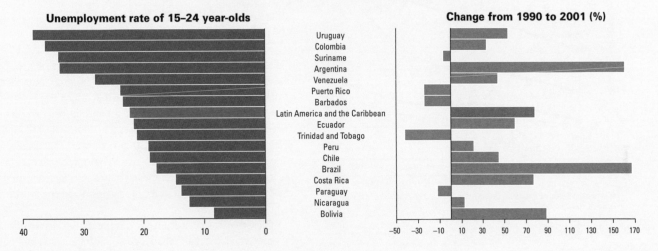

Health at the Core of Development

The Millennium Development Goals reflect the outcomes of decades of consensus-building within the United Nations system and of numerous global gatherings, starting with the International Conference on Primary Health Care in 1978 and including the World Summit for Children in 1990. Through the Millennium Declaration adopted by 189 countries in 2000 and the outcomes of the International Conference on Financing of Development in 2002, the world community reconfirmed agreements reached at earlier United Nations summits and reinforced them through the 2015 target date. The key challenge of the MDGs is not technical but political: never before had the community of nations set for itself such a focused common agenda, calling on governments, civil society, the private sector, and international organizations to give priority to poverty reduction and to redress inequalities in access to key determinants of development. The Millennium Declaration gives a new sense of urgency and provides a framework that transcends individual sectors; now, within the context of the MDGs, education, health, and the environment are understood, together as an indivisible package, as prime investment areas for poverty reduction and human development. At the same time, because three of the eight MDGs refer explicitly to health and all of them relate in some measure to health, the world community has made clear its collective recognition of the crucial role of health at the center of economic and social development.

FIGURE 3. Trends and projections in aging, North America and Latin America and the Caribbean, 1950–2050.

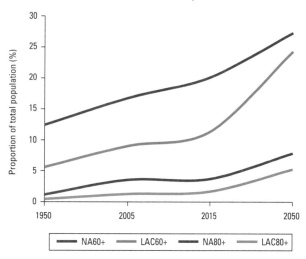

Source: United Nations Population Division. World Population Prospects: The 2006 Revision. New York. 2007.

downturns in the 1980s, the countries began to experience sluggish growth—averaging around 1.4% per year in the 1990s. Between 2000 and 2003, another crisis produced a new decline in economic growth. Growth resumed in 2004, however, reaching a regional average of 6%; in 2005, around 4%; and in 2006, a projected 3–5.5% increase in most of the countries.

Although advances have been scored in poverty reduction in recent years, in 2005 40.6% of the population of the Americas (almost 213 million persons) continued to live in poverty and 16.8% (88 million persons) in extreme poverty; furthermore, despite overall regional economic growth, the gap in wealth between the richest and the poorest countries, far from narrowing, widened between the late 1970s and the early 2000s—a trend that, if current conditions persist, is projected to continue (3).

Unemployment precludes subscription in the social security system and, consequently, limits access to health care. Informal employment and child labor further complicate the situation. As regards women, their entry into the paid labor force over the past two decades, while augmenting family income and purchasing power, has overburdened many of them, as women continue to be the principal homemaker—a role that, paradoxically, is increasingly neglected; yet even when they hold jobs traditionally held by men, women tend to be paid less. As for the younger generation, the eighth MDG—the aim of which is to forge a global partnership for development—targets the promotion of decent and productive work for youth, whose unemployment rates in Latin America and the Caribbean have worsened since 1995.

Education. In the Americas, progress in education has been significant over the past quarter-century, as measured by the re-

gional literacy rate, which has increased from 88% in the 1980s to around 94% in 2006. Notwithstanding, educational progress has not been uniform across all population groups: women still have lower literacy rates than men; rural residents have lower rates than their urban counterparts; and the poor are less literate than the rich. Still, access to education is improving throughout Latin America and the Caribbean, as indicated by the increase in net enrollment in primary education for boys and girls alike, from 86% in 1990 to 95% in 2004.

Environment. Historically, human health has been shaped by the interaction of diverse environmental, biological, economic, social, political, and cultural determinants, which can result in unsatisfactory living conditions, environmental risks and hazards, lifestyle and behavioral changes and, ultimately, in illness, disability, and death. A 2004 WHO report found that, of the 102 major diseases, 85 were partially caused by exposure to environmental risks and that environmental causes contributed to about one-fourth of disability-adjusted life years lost and one-fourth of associated deaths (4).

In the Americas, socioeconomic deterioration—characterized by poverty, rapid urbanization, and social fragmentation—has contributed to greater inequalities and unhealthier environments, particularly affecting rural agricultural and traditional indigenous populations. Other environmental inequalities are observed in marginal urban areas where housing conditions and access to drinking water and sanitation are poor and people are more exposed to noise, chemical contamination, and violence. These conditions are worsening in some countries; for instance, 60% of the urban population in Haiti had access to drinking water in 1990, whereas by 2004 only 58% did. Chapter 3 discusses these environmental issues in detail.

In addition, violence resulting from unhealthy social environments in marginal urban areas is taking a deadly toll. Official registries show that in the last 10 years 110,000–120,000 homicides and 55,000–58,000 suicides occurred in the Region (5). Governments and the health sector in a number of Latin American countries are growing increasingly concerned about juvenile violence, which is leading to the formation of gangs that conduct such transnational operations as kidnapping, human trafficking, and weapon and drug smuggling.

Urban growth results in increased needs for transportation, which in turn leads to greater risks of injuries and more air pollution. Every year in the Americas an estimated 130,000 people die, more than 1.2 million suffer injuries, and hundreds of thousands become disabled as a result of traffic-related injuries. Low-income countries in Latin America are more affected because of the use of poorly maintained vehicles, the wide variety of public road users (pedestrians, cyclists, and motorcyclists), less safety education, and lack of adequate regulations (Chapter 3).

Urban air pollution, intensified by rapid urbanization and industrialization and the associated increase in fossil fuel use and carbon dioxide emissions, also affects human health and is reported to contribute to climate change and global warming. The 2001 report of the United Nations Intergovernmental Panel on Climate Change (IPCC) showed that over the course of the 20th century the global temperature had increased 0.2–0.6° Centigrade and that the sea level had risen 10–20 cm. The IPCC projected a global warming of 1.4–5.8°C by 2100. As a result, along with other regions of the world, the Americas will experience periods of intense precipitation, hurricanes, and flooding that will severely affect human health and well-being. Four countries of the Americas are among the world's largest carbon-dioxide emitters: the United States, Canada, Brazil, and Mexico (6). The 2007 report of the IPCC confirmed that human activity is warming the planet at a potentially disastrous and irreversible rate (7).

Globalization. The world's increasing connectivity, integration, and interdependence in the economic, social, technological, cultural, political, and ecological spheres—a process generally referred to as "globalization"—is one of the greatest challenges confronting the health sector. The world's changing economic and social structures are imposing competitive conditions and raising the risk of economic crises. Countries, institutions, and individuals are having to adapt to these changes to assure their place in the local and global scenarios. At the same time, globalization is creating opportunities that transcend national borders. In the Americas, this phenomenon has resulted in connectivity and collaboration among countries, as expressed in various international summits to advance the human condition throughout the hemisphere, and in the formation of subregional economic blocs (Chapter 1).

Science and technology. Scientific and technological advances, industrialization, socioeconomic development, improved communication, better hygiene and increased food intake have contributed to increasing life expectancy and reducing mortality rates throughout the world. In the last 50 years many technological developments have led to new diagnostic and therapeutic possibilities in medicine, such as imaging technologies, materials for internal or external prosthesis, laser technology and biosensors. Vaccine research has produced numerous successes, among them vaccines for hepatitis B and *Haemophilus influenzae* type B as well as ongoing development of vaccines for cholera, malaria, tuberculosis, and HIV/AIDS. Many state-of-the-art technologies—such as genetic engineering, microsurgery, and custom-designed drugs—are becoming increasingly available. As a result of breakthroughs in DNA technology, specific, highly sensitive diagnostic tests have been developed for field use in tropical countries, giving rise to more precise surveillance and tracking of microorganisms and diseases. Transgenic animals are being bred to produce drugs, vaccines, hormones, and other substances of value to the pharmaceutical industry; transgenic pigs have been bred as a source of organs and tissues for transplantation, raising concerns about the possibility of the transmission of viruses or other pathogens to

"There is in our societies a persistently high degree of stigma and discrimination. This, coupled with a lack of true political participation in each country's development plans, makes the situation unsustainable. The permanent denial of fundamental rights has led to the marginalization of the indigenous population, leading to alarming poverty rates, lack of land, low earnings, high unemployment, high rates of illiteracy especially among women, high rates of school dropouts, and an epidemiological profile with high rates of illnesses and premature death where preventable causes are predominant. The communities and municipalities with the highest percentage of indigenous population are those furthest from the goals set by the Millennium Declaration."

Mirta Roses, 2006

humans. The introduction of gene manipulation techniques has also led to bigger crop yields and better food quality, by providing resistance to pests and weeds; however, concerns that engineered organisms in nature might alter native ecosystems or even harm people's health is resulting in demands for ethical standards for genomics, cloning, and genetic engineering.

Regional health information systems have improved significantly in recent years. Although the collection of comprehensive information about priority diseases in different geographic, demographic, and social segments of a community is difficult even in developed countries, virtually enabled advances, such as geographic information systems and collaborative work methods, are reducing the cost and improving the quality of health information.

Today the scientific and public health communities confront the challenge of making the benefits of science and technology available to the maximum number of people so as to improve, equitably, the quality of their lives. Currently, Latin America and the Caribbean trail more developed countries in the numbers of scientific and technological programs. Research productivity in the region is still low compared to developed countries, as expressed in the fact that only 3% of the 1.1 million scientific papers included in MEDLINE during the period 2000–2003 were authored by Latin American and Caribbean investigators (8).

One of the main constraints to the advancement of science and technology has been the low allocation of resources towards that end. As a percentage of GDP, the allocation for research and development in Latin America and the Caribbean was 0.5% in 1990 and rose to 0.6% in 2002, while in the United States the comparable allocation was about 2.6%, a proportion that remained constant throughout the period 1990–2002. Moreover, Latin America and the Caribbean have 0.7 investigators per 1,000 population as compared to the international benchmark of 6–10 per 1,000 (9).

TACKLING THE UNFINISHED AGENDA

Almost three decades have passed since the signing of the Declaration of Alma-Ata at the International Conference on Primary Health Care (Alma-Ata, Kazakhstan, September 1978), and in the Americas much progress has been made towards realizing the agenda it set forth (for more in that regard, see the section below on "Protecting Health Gains"). The countries of the Region have placed primary health care policies and programs at the center of their national health systems so as to meet the goal of health for all. The number of people living in extreme poverty (less than $1 a day) fell by about 3 million from 1990 to 2005. The Region is close to achieving universal primary education—some 97% of children are completing primary school, although regional averages disguise the situation in countries that lag behind. The youth illiteracy rate has fallen by 12% in 30 years. And life expectancy is nearly 20 years longer, on average, than it was 50 years ago (*10*).

Notwithstanding, work towards realization of the primary health care agenda remained unfinished at the start of the new millennium: in some countries and in many within-country areas, diseases and conditions have persisted that hamper attainment of health for all. Despite the availability of cost-effective solutions and simple interventions, a scenario of disparities prevails in which a "tyranny of averages"—that is, excessive reference to the middle value—hides the continuing presence of priority health problems. In many countries and within-country areas, the "unfinished agenda" means the persistence of problems resolved elsewhere, including:

- Extreme poverty and hunger
- High mortality in children under 5
- Lack of improvement in maternal health
- Inadequate prevention and control of HIV/AIDS, tuberculosis, and malaria
- Limited access to essential drugs
- Insufficient access to water and sanitation
- Barriers to improving health of indigenous people
- Neglected diseases in neglected populations

Addressing inequities. The benefits of improvements in regional social and health indicators have not reached all groups and populations alike, resulting in inequitable disparities in morbidity, mortality, and access to health services. Income, ethnicity, and education continue to matter. In many of the countries in the Region, health conditions remain unacceptably—and unnecessarily—poor. Poor health translates into grief, misery, stalled economic growth, and thwarted efforts to reduce poverty. Those most hurt are children in low-income countries, women, indigenous people, the uneducated, rural dwellers, migrant workers, sex workers, street children, and the elderly. Geography also matters:

the situation with regard to mortality rates in Central America and the Latin Caribbean in 2005, for instance, is closer to the regional average of the early 1980s. These inequities in health are expressed as large disparities in health status, differential access to health care, and disproportionate exposure to health risks—unsafe water and sanitation, malnourishment, pollution, and exposure to climatic and geographic threats.

Health inequities in the Americas are extensive and profound, as expressed in countless examples, including among others:

- The greatest share of maternal mortality takes place in the poorest countries of Latin America and the Caribbean.
- Life expectancy at birth ranges from a minimum of 68.8 years in Central America to a maximum of 77.9 years in North America (2005).
- Differences in life expectancy among countries are even more dramatic, particularly the gap between the richest and the poorest, which has widened to nearly 20 years.
- Although women have a life expectancy at birth that is on average six years greater than that of men, the social status of many women compromises the quality of their lives.
- The differential distribution of newly emerging health threats and their risk factors have further exacerbated health inequalities in the countries.
- Some 218 million people are without protection against disease risk because they lack social security coverage in health; and 100 million are without access to health services due to geographic location, economic barriers, or the lack of health service facilities near their homes or workplaces.

The status of women. One of the main constraints to completing the primary health care agenda is the status of women. While women represent over two-fifths of the labor force in Latin America and the Caribbean, their economic advancement is curtailed because they have difficulty securing paid jobs, earn less, are kept out of some occupations, and work disproportionately in the informal sector. Thus, despite the international community's commitment to gender equality, the lives of millions of women and girls throughout the Region are compromised by discrimination, disempowerment, poverty, and violence. Attainment of the third MDG—promoting gender equality and empowering women—will reap the "double dividend" of bettering the lives of both women and children (*11*).

The status of ethnic groups. In the Americas today, between 45 and 50 million people belong to more than 400 unique ethnic groups—around 7% of the regional population; 40% of the rural population in Latin America and the Caribbean; and over 40% of the total population in Peru, Guatemala, Bolivia, and Ecuador. The incidence of poverty is higher among indigenous groups in the Americas, and they experience higher levels of illiteracy, greater unemployment, and less access to health care services—including vaccination against preventable diseases. They suffer disproportionate rates of maternal and infant mortality, malnutrition, and infectious diseases (*12*). "In Mexico, there are an estimated 96.3 doctors per 100,000 people nationally, but only 13.8 per 100,000 in areas where indigenous people make up 40% or more of the population" (*13*). One of the principal problems for indigenous people is the lack of official documentation. In any country, birth registration is important because it gives an individual an official identity as a member of society and may be needed for access to services later in life. Latin America and the Caribbean have among the highest rates of birth registration in the developing world: 92% in urban areas and 80% in rural areas. But indigenous children are less likely to be registered at birth: "in the Amazonian region of Ecuador only 21% of under-fives have a birth certificate, compared with the national average of 89% . . . [and] more than 85% of Bolivians living in rural indigenous communities lack the official documentation that would allow them to inherit land, register their children in school, or vote" (*14*).

Infant and child health. Despite significant improvements in child survival in the Americas since the "health for all" initiative was launched in 1978, a profound inequality in its attainment has persisted unabated. The distribution of the risk of dying before age 5, as reflected by child mortality rates, in the population of the Americas—ranked from poorest to richest according to their country's national gross income per capita (purchasing power parity-adjusted)—shows an inequality concentration index of –0.3, which means that the poorest 20% (quintile) of the regional population concentrates almost 40% of the total number of child deaths, whereas the richest 20% accounts for only 8% of child deaths (Figure 4).

The Region of the Americas has made huge progress in reducing infant and child mortality rates. Notwithstanding the achievements in reducing mortality in the very young, differences in child mortality continue to prevail among countries as well as within them. In countries with high child mortality rates (e.g., Bolivia, Peru, Guatemala, and Brazil) but also in others with relatively low rates (e.g., Colombia and Belize), significant internal inequalities persist. Three of the many critical determinants of health inequalities among infants and children are ethnic group, geographic location, and education. In Bolivia, Ecuador, Guatemala, Mexico, and Panama, which have collected information on ethnic group and mother's area of residence (i.e., urban vs. rural), infant mortality rates are consistently higher among rural indigenous populations than among their non-indigenous rural peers as well as among urban indigenous populations (see Chapter 2). Similarly, an analysis of inequalities in mortality of children under 5 in relation to maternal education in Bolivia, Brazil, Colombia, the Dominican Republic, Guatemala, Haiti, and

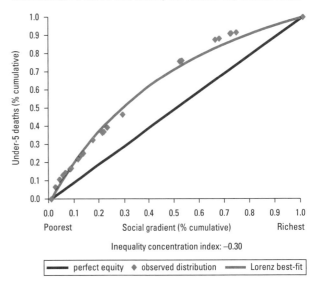

FIGURE 4. Inequalities in child survival: under-5 mortality concentration curve and index, the Americas, around 2005.

Inequality concentration index: –0.30

perfect equity ◆ observed distribution Lorenz best-fit

Source: Pan American Health Organization. Health Situation in the Americas. Basic Indicators 2006.

Peru indicates that child mortality level and mother's educational level are inversely related; moreover, the same analysis shows that, although overall mortality dropped greatly between the late 1980s and the early years of the present century, the size of the mortality gaps among the educational segments remained practically unchanged (*15*).

What are the constraints that must be overcome to achieve the fourth MDG—that is, to reduce child mortality by two-thirds? Principal among them are the lack of safe water to drink, exposure to disease-bearing mosquitoes, lack of immunization, and poor nutrition. The great majority of childhood deaths could be prevented with the proven technologies of the child survival revolution—breastfeeding, vaccinations against the main childhood diseases, clean water sources, oral rehydration therapy, and bed nets to prevent malaria. In fact, the interventions needed to prevent and treat the causes of death in children that could lead to a two-thirds reduction in child mortality are available, "but they are not being delivered to the mothers and children who need them" (*16*).

The children most at risk are those in the poorest countries and in the most deprived communities within countries; those who are discriminated against because of gender, race, or ethnicity; those affected by HIV/AIDS; those lacking good nutrition; those who have been orphaned, many as a result of AIDS, and end up responsible for themselves and often for their siblings; those subjected to violence, abuse, or exploitation; those who have to work for a living; and, in general, those who lack access to essential goods and services. For instance, in Latin America and the Caribbean in 2003, of all children under age 18, 6.2% were orphans; and, during the period 1999–2004, 8% of females and 11% of males in the 5–14 year age group were involved in child labor. The persistence of inequalities in health are further confirmed by the ranking of perinatal disorders and malnutrition among the 10 leading causes of death in several Latin American countries and in subnational areas of others—information that reflects a high proportion of childhood deaths, as most occur in the first years of life.

Maternal health. Many public health scholars consider that, in addition to life expectancy, a country's health status can best be judged by its maternal survival "marker": "if the maternal mortality rate drops, it can be assumed that a population's other health problems are also improving; if, on the other hand, maternal mortality remains the same, other attempts to improve the population's health will ultimately have little effect on its wellbeing" (*17*). Each year, more than 22,000 women in Latin America and the Caribbean die from complications of pregnancy and childbirth. Most of those deaths would be preventable if appropriate interventions and care were available throughout pregnancy, childbirth, and the postnatal period (*18*). And, although maternal mortality has declined significantly in the Region in recent decades, in five countries the maternal mortality rate exceeds the rate registered 60 years ago in the United States. The Americas still had a rate of 70 deaths per 100,000 live births in 2006, and if only Latin America and the Caribbean are considered the rate rises to 91.1, with Haiti registering the highest rate at 523 and Chile the lowest at 17.3 (*1*). Figure 5 reflects the magnitude of the inequality in maternal mortality in the Americas: the poorest 20% of the regional population concentrates 50% of the maternal deaths, whereas the richest quintile only accounts for 5% of those deaths (inequality concentration index = –0.43). Pregnancies among adolescents, for the most part unplanned, have reached 20% of total pregnancies in many countries, a situation implying evident challenges for those future mothers and their children.

As expressed in the fifth MDG, the world community has committed to reducing maternal mortality by three quarters. Toward that end, the Regional Strategy for Maternal Mortality and Morbidity Reduction in the Americas is founded on firm convictions:

Maternal death is preventable; effective interventions are known; and investment in safe motherhood will not only reduce maternal and infant death and disability, but will also contribute to improved health, quality of life, and equity for women, their families, and communities. Safe motherhood interventions are among the most cost-effective in the health sector, particularly at the primary care level (*19*).

Persistent inequalities in access to health services and resources are at the core of child and maternal survival in the Amer-

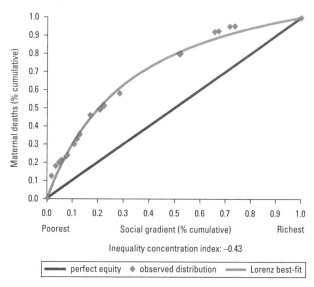

FIGURE 5. Inequalities in maternal health: maternal mortality concentration curve and index, the Americas, around 2005.

Inequality concentration index: –0.43

— perfect equity ◆ observed distribution — Lorenz best-fit

Source: Pan American Health Organization. Health Situation in the Americas. Basic Indicators 2006.

icas (Figure 6). Paramount health indicators such as availability of physicians per population, proportion of deliveries attended by skilled personnel, low birthweight prevalence, and public health expenditure as a proportion of the gross domestic product are unequally distributed along the income quintiles of the Region's population, where the more socioeconomically disadvantaged are the ones with disproportionately higher health risks. It bears noting, however, that the percentage of births attended by skilled health personnel in the Americas compares favorably with the rest of the world: in 2004, seven of eight deliveries in the Americas were attended by skilled personnel.

Nutrition. An important indicator of a country's nutritional status is the proportion of newborns with low birthweight—i.e., <2,500 g. Birthweight largely depends on the nutritional status of the mother during pregnancy and prior to conception. In that regard, birthweight also becomes an indirect indicator for evaluating maternal nutrition and, up to a point, for predicting the future development of the child.

Of the two forms of child growth failure, length and weight, that of length—or stunting—is three to six times more prevalent in Latin America and the Caribbean. Since underweight can be reversed but stunting is permanent, children with stunted growth are at risk of becoming overweight, thereby putting them at an increased risk of developing chronic diseases in adulthood. It is in the first two years of life both when stunting can occur and when efforts to prevent it through good nutrition are most op-

FIGURE 6. Inequalities in health services resources and access, by income quintiles, the Americas, around 2005.

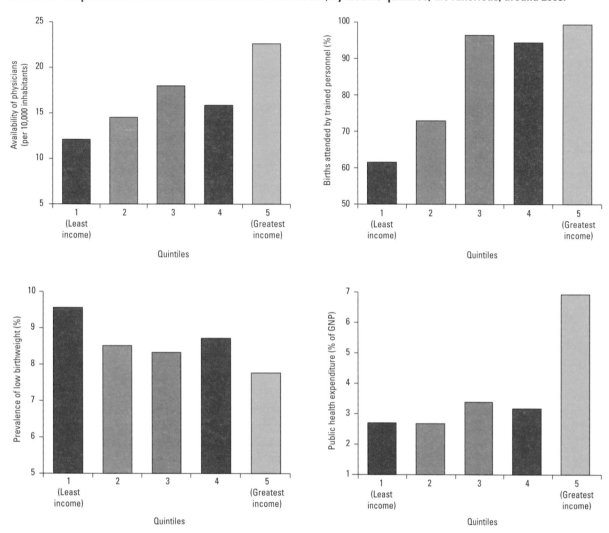

Source: Pan American Health Organization. Health Situation in the Americas. Basic Indicators 2006.

portune. In general, the trend data show very slowly declining prevalence of stunting. Brazil is the country with the most significant reduction, 60% in 10 years, followed by Colombia and the Dominican Republic, with declines of slightly more than 40% during roughly the same period. Notwithstanding, it is troubling that, as of 2000, the growth of one in every two children in Guatemala and one in every three children in Bolivia, Honduras, and Peru was stunted (Chapter 2).

Preventing and controlling local endemic diseases. Despite a reduction in its incidence, **malaria**, a disease that is preventable, continues to constitute a significant public health problem. More than one million people—most of them children under 5—die each year from the disease, and in the Americas

malaria is the cause of 0.4% of deaths among children under 5 (*20*). Malaria transmission still occurs in 21 countries of the Americas, and an estimated 250 million people live in zones at risk for transmission, 40 million of which reside in moderate- and high-risk areas. Of the approximately one million cases reported annually, three-fourths are caused by the principal parasite, *Plasmodium vivax* (*21*).

In recent years, **dengue** has been on the rise, increasing from almost 400,000 cases in 1984 to over 430,000 cases in 2005 (*1*). Carried by the *Aedes aegypti* mosquito, dengue flourishes in areas with poor sanitation and high precipitation; there is no vaccine or cure for the disease, and people can best deal with it by keeping their homes free of breeding places for the mosquito. In January 2007, Paraguay declared an epidemiological alert as new

"Hypertension, or high blood pressure, is a silent but dangerous disease affecting an estimated 140 million men and women of all ethnic backgrounds in the Americas."

Mirta Roses, 2003

cases of dengue began to emerge; by early February some 9,000 cases had been reported, including 40 cases of dengue hemorrhagic fever, prompting the declaration of a national emergency. As a result, health authorities in Paraguay, Argentina, Brazil, and Bolivia stepped up prevention in border areas, including intensified surveillance and control measures.

An ongoing health priority throughout the Americas, **tuberculosis** afflicts over 350,000 people, and 50,000 die of the disease every year. The regional disease rate was 26.8 per 100,000 in 2004, with Latin Caribbean and Andean Area countries reporting rates as high as 61.5 and 55.5 per 100,000, respectively. This situation is aggravated by TB/HIV coinfection and the resistance of tuberculosis to multidrug therapy, which jeopardizes attempts to control the disease throughout the Region.

The so-called **neglected tropical diseases**—which can cause excruciating pain, disfigurement, and disability—vary in distribution, but are directly associated with poverty, malnutrition, lack of schooling, and unemployment. Their burden is substantial among the 568 million people living in Latin America and the Caribbean, where the estimated currently infected populations (and, where relevant, the percentage of the total population in 2005) are, respectively:

Chagas' disease: 18 million (3.2%)
Trichuriasis: 99 million (17.6%)
Ascariasis: 82 million (14.6%)
Schistosomiasis: 3 million cases in Brazil (1.6% of the country's total population)
Leprosy: 86,652 cases
Hookworm infection: 34 million (6%)
Leishmaniasis: 60,000 cases of the cutaneous form of the disease were reported in Brazil in 2003, and 3,500 cases of the visceral form in 2004
Onchocercosis: 63 new cases reported in 2004 from Colombia, Ecuador, Mexico and Guatemala combined (0.3%)
Lymphatic filariasis: 720,000 cases, principally in Haiti (8.4% of the country's total population)
Trachoma: of 150,000 cases examined in Brazil in 2004, 10,000 were found to be positive.

Lack of routine epidemiological surveillance and data collection for the neglected diseases in almost all countries in Latin America and the Caribbean make it very difficult to accurately estimate disease burden, with the exception of leprosy (22).

Safe water and basic sanitation. Availability of drinking water has improved in the Americas since 1990, but that improvement has not grown at an even pace throughout the hemisphere. By 2002, 93% of the population in the Americas used improved sources of drinking water, while coverage in the North American region (the United States and Canada) was 100%, in Central America was 83%, and within that subregion, in Guatemala the proportion of the population using improved sources of drinking water was only 75%. The differences are greater between urban and rural populations. In Brazil, for example, the proportion of the urban population using improved sources of drinking water reaches 96%, while the rural population having service is only 58%. Basic sanitation services reach even less of the regional population, 84%, and in addition to the marked differences between urban and rural access, the total (urban and rural) coverage in Central America and the Latin Caribbean is much lower relative to other subregions—63% and 66%, respectively (Figure 7). The situation is critical in rural areas of a few countries like Guatemala, Belize, Haiti, and Bolivia, where coverage of improved sanitation facilities in rural areas is between 17 and 23%. The relationship between coverage of water and sanitation services and levels of health and human development is described in Chapter 3. Among other examples of that relationship, the regional child mortality rate due to diarrheal diseases was 3.7% and as high as 7.8% in the Andean subregion in 2000–2005.

In summary, while great advances are underway in science and technology, not all of humankind is benefiting from them. A gap still exists between the targeted (2015) and recent (2005) rates of reduction in child mortality, while within each country there are further gaps in the rates. Although progress has been extraordinary—diseases have been eradicated or eliminated and the public health infrastructure has been strengthened—it has been uneven. Some countries still have a significant proportion of their populations living in districts where vaccination coverage remains below 95%. Sporadic outbreaks of diphtheria and pertussis still occur because of an accumulation of susceptibles missed by routine national programs. This accumulation also puts countries at risk for large measles outbreaks when importations of the measles virus occur, as recently happened in Venezuela (2001–2002), Colombia (2002), and Mexico (2003–2004). Thus, although progress has been scored toward attainment of the goal of health for all, the agenda remains unfinished.

PROTECTING HEALTH GAINS

Improvements in human health in the Americas for over a century have been profound, extensive, and unprecedented.

After 1840, the upward trend in life spans proceeded at a surprisingly sustained and uniform rate of increase of 2.5 years

FIGURE 7. Proportion of the total, urban, and rural populations using improved sanitation facilities, Region of the Americas, main subregions, and large countries, 2002.

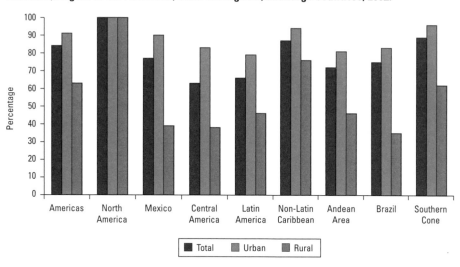

Source: Pan American Health Organization. Health Situation in the Americas. Basic Indicators 2006.

per decade for the next 160 years. . . . Even though life expectancy in high-income countries exceeds that in developing regions, convergence is notable. In 1910, for example, a male born in the United States could expect to live 49 years, but had he been born in Chile, his life expectancy would have been only 29 years. By the late 1990s, in contrast, U.S. life expectancy had reached 73 years and that of Chile had reached 72 years (*23*).

And gains have continued since the 1990s. Infant and child mortality have fallen significantly: the under-5 mortality rate decreased from 54 per 1,000 live births in 1990 to 25 per 1,000 live births in 2005—a 54% drop. The infant mortality rate decreased from 42 to 19 per 1,000 live births (from 2001 to 2005, depending on the country). Diseases that at one time could wipe out entire populations and leave survivors disfigured and crippled—smallpox, poliomyelitis, measles, and tuberculosis—no longer do. Life expectancy has lengthened from 56 years of age in 1960 to almost 75 years in 2006.

These gains can be attributed to a mosaic of variables, among them: changing demographics, improved economic productivity, greater urbanization, with more access to health services; increased food supplies; advances in medical science; more and better sanitation services; strengthened institutions, especially technical progress in the application of simple treatments such as oral rehydration therapy, preventive care such as better hygiene and vaccination, innovative treatment methods for some communicable diseases, such as the directly observed treatment strategy (DOTS); institutional and managerial innovations in

public health services, training and epidemiological surveillance; increases in financing of health interventions; social security; greater agricultural productivity, infrastructure, education; and social changes such as improvements in the status of women. As countries have taken advantage of technical advances, they have experienced proportionately significant progress in health.

Certainly, one of the major reasons for the breathtaking improvements in child survival in the Americas is the success of national immunization programs (for an in-depth analysis of the situation with regard to immunizable diseases, see Chapter 2). Of all the regions of the world, the Americas was the first to eradicate smallpox and poliomyelitis and to eliminate measles and neonatal tetanus by attaining high levels of immunization coverage. Thanks to those efforts, the peoples of the Americas now live free of indigenous polio and measles; neonatal tetanus, diphtheria, and pertussis have been well controlled; protection coverage against rubella has increased significantly, and new vaccines, have been added to national immunization programs and their application has been sustained. Countries' efforts to reduce child and infant mortality rates have resulted in avoiding the deaths of millions of children. The focus now is on sustaining immunization achievements and reaching the people who have not benefited from existing and new vaccines.

To protect the gains achieved, countries will have to persist in their efforts to extend the coverage rates of their national immunization programs. Health gains are not necessarily cumulative and permanent. Their underlying causes must be managed and maintained. Otherwise, the progress that has been achieved in health can stop and even reverse. Outbreaks of diseases preventable by

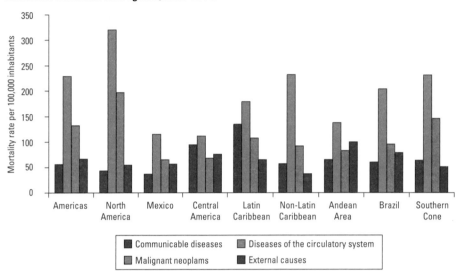

FIGURE 8. Estimated mortality rates due to broad groups of diseases, Region of the Americas and main subregions, 2002–2004.

Source: Pan American Health Organization. Health Situation in the Americas. Basic Indicators 2006.

immunization have occurred in some countries due to reduced vaccination coverage. Economic crises can result in malnutrition among the general population. Furthermore, sustained health progress can be threatened with reductions in investments in health, natural disasters, war, violence, and other forms of social unrest, and the emergence of new diseases and risks. The focus must be on the strengthening of national institutions that will ensure that accomplishments in health in the Americas continue and are scaled to the entire Region. To protect the gains attained, it will be necessary to:

• Strengthen and expand vaccination programs
• Sustain DOTS for tuberculosis
• Provide safe blood
• Ensure food security and food safety
• Keep free from foot-and-mouth disease
• Mitigate the impact of emergencies and disasters
• Produce core health data
• Improve epidemiological surveillance systems
• Monitor and analyze health inequities
• Share health data, information, and knowledge

CONFRONTING EMERGING CHALLENGES

The epidemiological profile in the Americas has undergone significant changes in recent decades as many of the old public health problems have been solved, while new ones emerge and old ones reemerge. Over the next 10 years, deaths from chronic

diseases will increase by 17% and, most alarmingly, deaths from diabetes will increase by over 80% (*24*). The projected increase in the burden of chronic diseases is attributable to aging of the population as well as to unhealthy behavior and choices that individuals and whole communities make related to poor nutrition, overweight and obesity, tobacco and alcohol. As described in Chapter 2 of this publication, in almost all countries, chronic degenerative diseases have replaced communicable diseases as leading causes of illness, disability, and death, except in Haiti where communicable diseases remain the leading cause of mortality with a total estimated rate of 351.2 per 100,000, followed by diseases of the circulatory system with a mortality rate of 227.9 per 100,000 (*25*). Diseases of the circulatory system, malignant neoplasms, chronic respiratory diseases, and diabetes have become the leading causes of death, along with external causes such as accidents, homicides, and other sources of violence (Figure 8).

An analysis of the disease burden in the Americas in 2006 indicates that the leading causes of death that have the greatest effect on years of life lost in males are diabetes, AIDS, and homicides; their effects, however, occur in different age groups, with homicides being a fundamental problem of young adults and adults; AIDS of adults; and diabetes of persons ≥50 years of age. The disease burden in females shows a different pattern: the leading causes are diabetes, AIDS, and lung cancer, with diabetes mainly affecting women over 45 years of age; AIDS, young women; and lung cancer, associated with a new pattern of tobacco consumption among females, women over 45 years of age. External causes—especially homicides and motor vehicle accidents—and HIV/AIDS lead to many more male than female deaths, primarily in young people, and are thus the principal reason why life expectancy has increased more in women than in men, an increase of as much as five to eight years in several countries (26).

During the past decade, and in good measure due to the growing permeability of transnational borders, diseases once thought to have been brought under control—such as tuberculosis, malaria, dengue, plague, yellow fever—have been reappearing, while relatively new communicable diseases—such as HIV/AIDS, SARS, and more recently, West Nile fever and the new variant of avian influenza (H5N1)—are emerging as major health threats.

After the bioterrorism-related anthrax cases reported in several cities of the United States during 2001, those threats were expected to continue, challenging national surveillance and response systems. Early detection of a bioterrorist attack is crucial to decrease illnesses and deaths, especially in the event of a covert attack with a biologic agent. Better knowledge of the geographic distribution, incidence, and epidemiological characteristics of potential bioterrorism endemic agents, particularly zoonoses, is needed to initiate investigations of a suspected outbreak or terrorism attack.

Concern about health threats from excessive antibiotic use is increasing in the Americas, particularly in those countries of Latin America where antibiotics are available to the public without medical prescription. Excessive use of antibiotics among outpatients has contributed to the emergence and spread of antibiotic-resistant bacteria in many communities; important common pathogens such as *Mycobacterium tuberculosis, Escherichia coli, Salmonella* spp., *Staphylococcus aureus*, and *Streptococcus pneumoniae* have developed resistance to common antibacterial drugs, complicating treatment for the diseases they cause. On the other hand, antimicrobial-resistant foodborne infections caused by improper use of antibiotics in animal production have contributed to the resistance of *Salmonella* spp. and *Campylobacter jejuni*. While new biological markers and DNA microarray technologies are being developed, the challenge going forward will be to devise simple, computerized diagnostic technology that permits rapid identification of antimicrobial resistance soon after the onset of symptoms (27). While the use of new antimicrobial agents and the improved use of currently available antimicrobial drugs will become standard practice in high-income countries, resulting in good treatment and rare complications, proper treatment of antimicrobial-resistant infections will not be available to the poor, thus perpetuating health inequities. Such is already the case with the HIV/AIDS epidemic, which—despite good coverage in the Americas of antiretroviral drugs—is expected to expand among poorer groups of population (27).

Aging of the population. In most countries of the Americas, the population is aging due to longer life expectancies and declining or stabilizing fertility rates. In the last 25 years, life expectancy at birth in the Americas has increased by 17 years, and the average life expectancy exceeds 70 years—with a seven year difference in the average between North America and Latin America and the Caribbean. Of the Latin American and Caribbean population born today, 78.6% will live longer than 60 years and four out of 10 will live beyond 80 years. Older people place greater demands on health services, because they require more frequent and comprehensive care and need services related to the treatment of chronic diseases and disabilities. The assessment of health policies and of the performance of health services for the elderly should target increasing the years of life free of disability after age 60 (28).

Unhealthy lifestyles, risky behaviors, and noncommunicable diseases. One of the biggest culprits in the increase in noncommunicable diseases is unhealthy lifestyles. The nutritional habits of the population of the Americas are changing: increasingly, people are consuming fewer fruits, vegetables, legumes, whole grains, and cereals and more processed foods, milk, refined cereals, meats, and sugar. Poor nutrition is further complicated by deficiencies of micronutrients—iodine, vitamin A, iron, zinc, and folate. At the same time, 30-60% of the population in the Americas do not achieve the minimum recommended levels of physical activity. The occupational shift from manual labor and agriculture to the service sector in most of the Region means that physical activity is generally on the decline. That decline has been aggravated by increased urbanization, motorized transportation, and the introduction of labor-saving devices and computers in the home. This coupling of poor diets and sedentary lifestyles is leading to an epidemic of noncommunicable diseases among adults (see Chapter 2). According to WHO, of the 6.2 million deaths estimated to have occurred in the Region in 2005, more than three-fourths were related to chronic diseases, and over the next 10 years 53 million people will die from a chronic disease. At least 80% of premature heart disease, stroke, and type 2 diabetes, and 40% of cancer in the Americas could be prevented through healthy diet, regular physical activity, and avoidance of tobacco products; chronic disease death rates could drop an estimated 2% per year over the next 10 years, saving almost 5 million lives (24). A recent study of more than 3,000 young people from 26 developing countries—including Argentina, Brazil, the Dominican Republic, Honduras, Mexico, and Peru—singled out "developing a healthy lifestyle" as one of the five pivotal phases of life that can impact the future of youth: "It has been estimated that nearly two-thirds of premature deaths and one-third of the total disease burden of adults can be associated with conditions or behavior begun in youth" (29). Again, those conditions or behaviors, many of them interrelated, include smoking, heavy alcohol consumption, drug use, traffic accidents, unsafe sex, violence, sedentary lifestyles, and poor nutrition. Unless those trends reverse, the impact on health in the future will be huge, and the demand for health services overwhelming.

"Despite significant ongoing efforts to expand and improve maternal health services in the Region, including the introduction in recent years of insurance to cover the cost of mother and child care, maternal mortality ratios have changed only slightly in the past decade."

Mirta Roses, 2004

Overweight and obesity. Changes in consumption patterns along with lower levels of physical activity are linked with increased prevalence of overweight (body mass index equal to or greater than 25 and less than 30 kg/m^2) and obesity (body mass index equal to or greater than 30 kg/m^2). Surveys conducted in Latin American and Caribbean countries in 2002 found that 50–60% of adults and 7–12% of children under 5 years of age were overweight or obese. In Argentina, Colombia, Mexico, Paraguay, Peru, and Uruguay, more than half of the population is overweight and more than 15% obese. Even more disturbing, the trend is growing among the Region's children: in Chile, Mexico, and Peru, an alarming one in four 4–10 year olds is overweight. Between now and 2015, the prevalence of overweight in the Americas is expected to increase in both men and women. In the United States, 64% of adults are overweight and 30.5% are obese. Canada trails somewhat behind the United States, with 50% of adults overweight and 13.4% obese (*30*).

Diabetes. As of 2006, an estimated 35 million persons were diabetic in the Americas—a number that is projected to increase to 64 million by 2025. The projected increase in the prevalence of diabetes parallels the increase in the prevalence of obesity, a leading risk factor for diabetes. It is estimated that in 2003, diabetes was associated with 300,000 deaths in Latin America and the Caribbean. For women of all ages in almost all countries of the Americas, diabetes is among the three leading causes of death. Prevalence rates are highest in the adult population of the Caribbean: prevalence of diabetes ranges from 18% in Jamaica and 17% in Barbados to an estimated 8% in South America and 6% in Central America (*31*). The total societal cost of diabetes in Latin America and the Caribbean is estimated to be US $65 billion.

Tobacco. WHO has estimated that tobacco is the second cause of preventable deaths, after high blood pressure, and responsible for 900,000 deaths every year in the Americas (see Chapter 3). If current trends continue, tobacco will result in the deaths of over 1 billion people in the 21st century. In 2006, over 20% of youth 13–15 years of age in the Americas had used tobacco, the highest prevalence in the world for that age group (*32*); more than 70% of smokers in the Region started using tobacco before age 18. In 2000, the prevalence of smoking among youth 13–15 years of age ranged from 14–21% in the Caribbean countries to 40% in the Southern Cone. In the United States and Canada, almost one-quarter of youth used tobacco. Tobacco use is estimated to currently cause one million deaths every year in the Americas, with the Southern Cone having the highest mortality rate due to smoking tobacco. An estimated one-third of heart disease and cancer deaths in the Region are attributed to tobacco use. Increasingly concentrated in poorer countries and among the poor within them, tobacco is associated with chronic obstructive pulmonary disease, cancer, and heart disease; contributes significantly to asthma and deaths from tuberculosis; and is projected to cause an exponential increase in deaths—6.4 million people a year by 2015, 50% more than HIV/AIDS.

Alcoholism. For its part, alcoholism has been shown to be the leading risk factor, among 27 different such factors, for the burden of disease in the Americas (Chapter 3). Intoxication, alcohol dependency, and biological damage due to the consumption of alcohol can cause long-term health and social consequences. "Alcohol-related diseases account for about 4% of global disability-adjusted life years (DALYs) each year and for 8.8% in Latin America and the Caribbean" (*33*).

Malignant neoplasms. Malignant neoplasms are responsible for one-fifth of all chronic disease mortality in the Americas, accounting for an estimated 459,000 deaths in 2002. This represents an increase in cancer deaths of one-third since 1990. Lung and colon cancer are included in the 10 leading causes of death in many countries of the Americas. Prostate, breast, and uterine cancers are also major causes of death in several countries of Latin America. In North America, lymphatic tissue neoplasm is one of the 10 leading causes of death in the general population and among the top five among 5–24 year olds (*26*).

Diseases of the circulatory system. Circulatory system diseases combined represent approximately 20% of all deaths in the Americas, the highest proportion of leading causes of death in all countries of the Region. Within that group, ischemic heart disease and cerebrovascular disease deaths figure most prominently. Hypertensive diseases and heart failure also stand out as major causes of death; 8–30% of the population in the Americas have hypertension, a strong independent risk factor for heart disease and stroke. Mexico, which has conducted risk-factor surveys, has experienced an increase in the prevalence of hypertension from 26% in 1993 to 30% in 2000 (*26*). These diseases always appear among the five or 10 principal causes of death for the general population (both sexes).

Mental health problems. Mental health problems impact both the young and the old in the Region, albeit in different forms. For the year 2000 suicide, the most reliable indicator of

TABLE 2. Projection of Alzheimer's disease prevalence (in millions), in Latin America and the Caribbean, in North America, and worldwide, in 2006 and 2050, by stage of disease.

| | Prevalence (in millions) | | | | | |
| | 2006 | | | 2050 | | |
	Overall	Early stage	Late stage	Overall	Early stage	Late stage
Latin America and the Caribbean	2.03	1.14	0.89	10.85	5.99	4.86
North America	3.10	1.73	1.37	8.85	4.84	4.01
Worldwide	26.55	14.99	11.56	106.23	58.75	47.48

Source: Ron Brookmeyer, Elizabeth Johnson, Kathryn Ziegler-Graham, and H. Michael Arrighi, "Forecasting the Global Burden of Alzheimer's Disease," Johns Hopkins University Department of Biostatistics Working Paper 130, 2007.

mental health problems, was the third leading cause of death among 10–19 year olds and the eighth leading cause of death among 20–59 year olds in the Americas overall. Alzheimer's disease and cerebrovascular dementia was the 10th leading cause of death for the entire population of the Americas and ranked eighth for persons 60 years and older. Alzheimer's disease and cerebrovascular dementia was one of the leading causes of death in Canada, Chile, Cuba, Puerto Rico, the United States, and Uruguay. The prevalence of Alzheimer's disease in the Americas—estimated at 2.0 million cases in Latin America and 3.1 million cases in North America—is expected to increase as countries' populations age. More than 26 million people worldwide have Alzheimer's disease, a number expected to quadruple to over 106 million by 2050, including almost 9 million in North America and almost 11 million in Latin America and the Caribbean (Table 2).

Road traffic injuries and deaths. In 2002 the Americas registered approximately 374,000 deaths due to road traffic accidents, and every year many hundreds of thousands suffer injuries and disabilities due to these accidents (Chapter 3). Road traffic injuries ranked as the ninth leading cause of death for the Region overall for 2002. For the same year, low- and middle-income countries in the Americas had road traffic injury mortality rates of 16 deaths per 100,000 population, and high-income countries experienced 15 deaths per 100,000 population (*34*).

Violence. In 2002 the Region of the Americas registered approximately 384,000 homicides and 179,000 suicides (Chapter 3). In countries where motor vehicle accidents is not the first leading cause of death among adolescent and young adult males, homicide is. Homicide rates per 100,000 population exceed very high or critical levels in a number of countries, notably Brazil (28), Venezuela (35), Jamaica (44), El Salvador (45), Guatemala (50), Honduras (55), and Colombia (65). The number of violent crimes is increasing throughout the Region, compromising health

TABLE 3. Percentage of women reporting having experienced violence, five countries in the Americas, 2000–2005.

	Physical violence	Sexual violence
Bolivia	53	12
Peru	42	10
Colombia	39	12
Ecuador	31	12
Haiti	29	17

Source: National Demographic and Health Surveys for Bolivia (2003), Peru (2000), Colombia (2005), Ecuador (2004), and Haiti (2000).

conditions and overburdening health services. Approximately one in three women in Latin America and the Caribbean has been a victim of sexual, physical, or psychological violence at the hands of domestic partners (Table 3). Violence against women not only exacts an enormous public health toll, it impedes social and economic development by preventing its victims from contributing fully to their communities.

Emerging threats. The international spread of infectious diseases poses problems for global health security, in large measure due to factors related to today's interconnected and interdependent world. Among other factors raising the risk of spread of these threats are population movements, through tourism, migration, or as a result of disasters; growth of international trade in food and biological products; social and environmental changes linked with urbanization, deforestation, and alterations in climate; and changes in methods of food processing, distribution, and consumer habits. These factors once again demonstrate that infectious disease events in one country or region are potentially a concern for the entire world (*35*). Another concern is the possibility of outbreaks resulting from intentional or accidental release of biological agents. Both epidemics that might occur naturally and those due to the release of biological agents present a threat to

"*Every year in Latin America and the Caribbean some 200,000 people are diagnosed with tuberculosis, and an estimated 50,000 or more die as a result of the disease. Yet tuberculosis is curable; these deaths are preventable. Only with strong and active community participation can we improve the detection of cases and increase the number of people who can be cured. Tuberculosis can affect everyone, without regard to age, sex, race or social status; but poor and neglected populations are particularly vulnerable to the disease.*"

Mirta Roses, 2004

global health security. Moreover, because of the impact that problems such as SARS, avian influenza, food contamination, and antibiotic resistance to pesticides can have on a nation's and the international community's economy and security, their surveillance must now encompass many new areas and agents (*36*).

What is new [about the international spread of diseases] is: (1) the broader scope of identified 'emerging' or 'reemerging' diseases; (2) the extent of globalizing factors that unleash them; (3) the intrusion of new actors in the arena of public health surveillance, bringing in economic or security concerns; (4) the blurred limits between potential hazards of deliberate and natural outbreaks; and (5) the ever-increasing demand from the public and press agencies for real-time information.... At the international level, it is not enough to acknowledge the global threat of emerging or reemerging diseases and to focus on a strategy based on externally driven surveillance and response. With equal urgency, preparedness for future epidemics has to comprise a parallel overhaul of health systems, including the essential issues of human resources development, governance, and equity in access to care (*37*).

HIV/AIDS. After sub-Saharan Africa, the Caribbean is the second subregion in the world most affected by HIV/AIDS. An estimated 1.2% of the Caribbean population, one quarter of a million people, was living with HIV in 2006. The Caribbean's largely heterosexual epidemics occur in the context of harsh gender inequalities and are being fuelled by a thriving sex industry: half of the people infected are women, and young women are 2.5 times more prone to be infected than young men. Nearly three-quarters of them are in the Dominican Republic and Haiti, but HIV prevalence is high throughout the subregion: 1%–2% in Barbados, the Dominican Republic, and Jamaica; 2%–4% in the Bahamas, Haiti, and Trinidad and Tobago. North America had an estimated prevalence of 0.8% or 1.4 million persons and Latin America 0.5% or 1.7 million persons. Despite prevention campaigns to reduce the risk of HIV infection, advances in treatment, and expanded treatment coverage to extend the lives of persons living with AIDS, the HIV/AIDS pandemic continues to be one of the Region's leading public health challenges.

From 1981 to 2005, more than 1.7 million persons with AIDS were officially reported in the Americas, with 38,000 of these cases younger than 15 years of age. The percentage of females with AIDS reported in the Americas increased from 6% of all prevalent AIDS cases in 1994 to approximately 31% in 2005, with this general trend repeated in all subregions. Although the number of persons living with AIDS continues to slowly increase in the Americas, the best estimate of the number of deaths due to AIDS in the Caribbean has declined from 2004 to 2006, thanks in good measure to the advent of improved treatment and expanded coverage of treatment. Many Latin American countries have also shown a decline in the number of AIDS deaths over the past decade. For the period 2003-2005, however, the number of AIDS deaths increased from 53,000 to 65,000, which means that on average 200 people die from HIV/AIDS every day in Latin America and the Caribbean. HIV/AIDS antiretroviral treatment coverage goals for the Americas—as part of the regional commitment to WHO's "3 × 5" initiative to treat 3 million people by the end of 2005—had been surpassed by 13% by the target deadline. It is estimated that in June 2006 three-quarters of persons needing antiretroviral treatment for HIV/AIDS in the Americas were receiving that treatment—the highest coverage in the developing world. During 2006, according to reports from 28 countries in the Americas, more than 1 million people were tested for HIV/AIDS, and access to counseling, testing, and prevention of mother-to-child transmission also increased substantially (*38–41*).

Pandemic influenza. Since the influenza pandemic of 1918, which killed tens of millions of people worldwide, many prevention and control measures have been taken to reduce the likelihood of similar or worse pandemics, including implementing influenza surveillance, developing vaccines and antiviral drugs, and taking preventive actions such as the recent rapid destruction of 1.5 million poultry in Hong Kong to control the spread of avian influenza. Worldwide disaster and emergency surveillance and preparation for pandemic influenza, especially the highly mutational, highly pathogenic avian influenza subtype H5N1, is ongoing. To date, avian influenza subtypes are primarily limited to the spread from bird to bird, occasionally jumping to and sickening a human host. No sustained human-to-human spread of this influenza has yet been identified; however, serious concern exists that a dangerously pathogenic strain of this influenza will mutate or acquire other viral genes, allowing it to easily pass from human-to-human. Certainly, avian influenza, only the latest serious influenza threat, will not be the last (*42–45*).

RESPONDING TO THE POPULATION'S HEALTH NEEDS

Meeting the pending health needs, sustaining the health gains, and confronting the emerging health challenges described in the foregoing pages will require strong public sector governance, equitable delivery of services, sufficient financing of the health system, a critical mass of well-prepared health workers, coordination among the various social sectors, and a robust pro-health alliance among countries and the international community. Chapter 4—"Public Policies and Health Systems and Services"—analyzes in depth health systems, financing of health care, health legislation, human resources, essential public health functions, health technologies, scientific health information, and the renewal of primary health care. And Chapter 5—"Health and International Cooperation in the Americas"—presents information on official development assistance, public-private partnerships, technical cooperation among developing countries, and regional integration processes.

Governance. In some countries, advances that had accrued from democratization processes that began in the 1980s and became further entrenched in the 1990s have been compromised by recent political, social, economic, and institutional crises—not least of which has been widespread corruption. Those crises have tarnished the image and credibility of public institutions and of the political class in general and, in so doing, have contributed to increasing social unrest, violence, and insecurity. In some countries, the promises of self-determination, the return of power to people and communities, and effective citizen participation have gone unfulfilled. In others, where decision-making power has been incompletely transferred from the national to the subnational level, local institutional capacities have not been adequately developed. Giving public agencies greater managerial autonomy has not always resulted in better, more efficient services. While much has been said about the need to increase donor assistance and transfer technological solutions for health in the developing world, recipient countries have a stake in, and must be held accountable for, developing the institutions that can implement health programs and technology.

Improving public health in the countries of the Americas takes strong states, strong public health systems, and adequate infrastructure. Growing demands on the health care system are triggering greater competition for limited resources. Anticipating and responding adequately to the many epidemiological, technological, and organizational challenges to health, social security, and surveillance systems will require ever-better governance and management of those systems. Although health sector reform and modernization of the State, widely promoted in the 1990s, yielded some benefits and facilitated the involvement of new actors in the sector, particularly the private sector, reform focused primarily on financial and organizational aspects, relegating critical public health issues to the sidelines. As a result, the role of government in key areas weakened, as did the capability of ministries of health to exercise their steering role and perform essential public health functions. Now regulation of the sector, taking into consideration both its public and private components, poses a major challenge. Meeting that challenge will require that the two biggest health infrastructure constraints—segmentation and fragmentation—be addressed (see Chapter 4).

The division of the health system into subcomponents that "specialize" in different population groups—or its **segmentation**—generally takes the forms, both for provision and insurance, of: (1) a public subsystem oriented toward the poor; (2) a social security subsystem that covers formal workers and their dependents; and (3) a for-profit private subsystem used mainly by the wealthiest segments of the population. By imposing conditions on access to the latter two subsystems that can only be met by those groups that are socially, occupationally, and financially well placed, segmentation prevents or complicates the implementation of cost-effective health care interventions and makes it harder to reach some population groups, thereby consolidating and entrenching inequities that especially affect the poor, the formally unemployed, the indigenous, and women. Changes in the labor market, particularly growth of the informal economy, have aggravated this situation. Ethnic origin is a factor limiting health-system access: in at least five countries in the Region—Bolivia, Ecuador, Guatemala, Paraguay, and Peru—belonging to an indigenous group or speaking only an indigenous language constitutes a barrier. And, since access to health systems is linked to formal-sector employment, women experience greater exclusion than men: because of their domestic duties, over half of all women in the Region are not gainfully employed, and, when they are, they are more likely than men to work in the informal sector and in part-time occupations that are not usually covered by social security; moreover, although over 30% of households in the Region are headed by women, women are often dependents who, along with their children, rely heavily on the person who has health coverage being employed and remaining in the household (26).

Where there is **fragmentation** of services in the health sector—that is, when the different subsystems do not operate in a coordinated, synergistic way, but tend instead to ignore and even compete with each other—a centering of health service delivery in hospitals and on individual care tends to result, to the detriment of public health services. Fragmentation hinders implementation of cost-effective interventions; makes it difficult to standardize the quality, content, cost, and application of health measures; raises their cost; and encourages inefficient use of resources within the system. Such inefficiency is exemplified by the coexistence of low hospital occupancy rates in the social security subsystem and high percentages of unmet demand for services in the public subsystems of Bolivia, the Dominican Republic, Ecuador, El Salvador, Guatemala, Honduras, and Paraguay. In some countries—among them, Bolivia, Honduras, Guatemala, and Ecuador—the fragmentation of services has a territorial dimension, where deficient referral and counter-referral mechanisms in rural areas severely constrain health care delivery (*26*).

Provision of and access to health services. In many countries, the gap between those who can and those who cannot access health care is widening. The reasons for that growing inequity, and the resultant profound adverse consequences for the population's health, are many: the downside of globalization, poverty, the loss of employment, lowered incomes, and great disparities in income distribution, all of which can lead to impoverished living conditions, social fragmentation, and high vulnerability. Although many of the countries have undertaken pro-poor health-related interventions, such interventions do not always reach those most in need; to the contrary, they often favor and extend the health gap between the rich and the poor. Research published in the 2004 *World Development Report* showed that in the 21 countries studied, the highest income quintile received, on average, 25% of government health service expenditure compared with only 15% among the lowest quintile (*46*).

Notwithstanding persistent gaps in health care access in the Region, some countries have made notable progress in their quest for equitable delivery of health services through pro-poor interventions. Among outstanding examples of these success stories are:

- **Colombia** created and financed an equity fund that increased health insurance coverage for the poor and lowered financial barriers to the use of services. "While insurance coverage among those in the highest income quintile increased modestly with the reform, from 60% in 1993 to 81% in 2003, insurance coverage among the poorest quintile of income increased from 9% in 1993 to 48% in 2003" (*47*).
- **Mexico** provided direct cash transfers to poor families so that they could use those funds to pay for health services; by 2003, almost 60% of the people reached by this program belonged to the poorest 20% of Mexico's population and 80% of the beneficiaries were in the poorest 40% of the country's population (*48*).
- **Honduras, Peru,** and **Nicaragua,** set up "social funds" to encourage communities and local institutions, especially in poorer areas in those countries, to take the lead in identifying and carrying out small-scale investments in health clinics and water and sanitation systems. "These poverty-targeted investments tend to increase the utilization of health services, especially maternal and child health, and translate

into improved health incomes including significant reductions in infant and child mortality" (*49*).

Financing. Serious deficiencies in health system financing persist: some countries have extremely low health expenditures, while others are excessively dependent on external resources and thus highly vulnerable. In many countries, out-of-pocket spending has greatly increased, with the consequent regressive effect that the poorest are the most affected. The amount and distribution of public health expenditure are critical factors in the equity/inequity that characterize health systems. Where highly segmented health systems prevail—most countries in Central America (El Salvador, Guatemala, Honduras, Nicaragua) and in the Andean Area (Bolivia, Ecuador, Peru, Venezuela)—public sector health funding is generally low and public sector coverage therefore limited, while private expenditure is high and covers mostly private individuals. In those countries, where a large percentage of the population is poor, serious inequities in health care access result from low public sector spending on health and high out-of-pocket expenditure, which is proportionately higher in the poorer of those countries (*26*).

Around 2005, national health expenditure for all countries in Latin America and the Caribbean accounted for approximately 7% of the region's gross domestic product or an annual expenditure of approximately US$500 per capita (Chapter 4). Approximately 45% of this expenditure corresponded to public spending on health—on services by ministries of health, other central government and local government institutions, and through compulsory contributions to privately run health funds or social security institutions. The remaining 55% corresponded to private expenditure, including direct out-of-pocket expenditure to purchase health goods and services and to cover health services consumed through private health insurance plans or pre-paid health care plans. Notably, because women have more need to use health services, their out-of-pocket health expenditures tend to be higher than men's—a gender-based inequity that looms even larger when considering that women's incomes average only about 70% of those of men.

In addition to the amount of public sector spending on health, its distribution among the poorest groups in a population (generally referred to as its "progressiveness") is a critical factor in those groups' access to health services. Out-of-pocket spending by the poorest households is lower in countries where the distribution of public spending is tilted toward low-income groups; Chile, Costa Rica, and Uruguay distribute about 30% of public spending among the lowest-income population. Inversely, where distribution of public spending disregards the greater needs of the poor, the poor have to pay more for access; in Ecuador and Guatemala just over 12% of public health expenditure goes to the first income quintile (the poorest), while the fifth quintile (the richest) receives over 30%; Peru distributes public spending across all income groups alike. Chile, Costa Rica, and Uruguay have national health insurance systems, while Ecuador, Guatemala, and Peru have highly segmented health systems (*26*).

Health workers. It stands to reason that the greater the number of health workers available to a population the greater their influence will be on its level of health. A clear case in point is the relationship between adequate numbers of health care providers and reductions in maternal and infant mortality: as the availability of health workers increases, the rates of mortality decrease. The inverse occurs in countries with a low density of health workers: the rate of mortality among children under 5 increases; the maternal mortality rate increases; and the proportion of deliveries handled by qualified personnel decreases (*50*).

In 2005, an estimated 21.7 million people comprised the full-time health workforce in the Americas. Many of the countries in the Region have a critical shortage of health workers, and that shortage is expected to grow more acute with the projected growth in population, the aging of the health workforce, and the ever-increasing burden of disease. In less-developed countries, competition for limited human resources and the international migration of health workers are expected to further destabilize the workforce; already, 72% of the countries of the Region have experienced a loss due to migration.

Serious imbalances persist in the distribution of health workers in the Region, both within countries and from country to country. The optimal (density) ratio of physicians and nurses to inhabitants is 25:10,000. In 11 countries that ratio is greater than 50, which translates into 30% of the population in the hemisphere having 73% of all physicians and nurses. In 15 countries the density ratio is below 25, which translates into 20% of the regional population having 6% of the human resources in health; 128,000 more physicians and nurses would need to be added to the workforce to reach the optimal ratio. Women make up almost 70% of the health work force, and yet they also represent a disproportionately high percentage of unemployed health workers, which averaged 6.2% in a sample of 13 countries. The within-country distribution of health workers is greatly uneven, with urban areas having from 8 to 10 times more physicians than rural areas. At the regional level, while in North America there are three nurses for every one physician, in Latin America and the Caribbean there are three physicians for every nurse (*51*).

Intersectoral engagement. Many advances in health conditions over the past decades have been the result of collaboration between the health sector and other social sectors: water supply and sanitation and the environment in general, education, labor, agriculture, and transportation, to name a few. The potential of the synergies of intersectoral collaboration was recognized in the 1978 Declaration of Alma-Ata. Decades later, in 2000, the multi-

> *The countries have made a tremendous effort to interrupt the mother-to-child transmission of HIV/AIDS. Likewise, spread of the disease by blood transfusions has halted. Access to treatment has improved significantly: the Americas was the first region in the world to negotiate a reduction of the price of antiretrovirals. But the regional situation is uneven, and in some countries less than 30% of those who need treatment are receiving it.*
>
> Mirta Roses, 2006

sectoral approach drove elaboration of the Millennium Development Goals, which, as has been seen, propose to integrate action to reduce poverty and hunger and promote education, women's empowerment, health, environment, and global partnerships to further those goals.

International involvement. The international architecture of development assistance for health—the cooperation of multilateral organizations, bilateral assistance, and private philanthropic aid—has undergone radical change over the past decade: "new multilateral organizations, initiatives, and foundations have assumed a prominent role in financing health, nutrition, and population activities, among them the Global Fund to Fight AIDS, Tuberculosis, and Malaria; the Global Alliance for Vaccines and Immunization (GAVI); the Global Alliance for Improved Nutrition (GAIN); and the Bill and Melinda Gates Foundation" (*52*). While the actors have proliferated, the debate regarding the most desirable investment of international cooperation in health goes unresolved (Chapter 5).

The challenges of persisting inequities and unsolved health problems are being confronted by concerted intersectoral national and international efforts as well as through the opportunities afforded by initiatives such as the Millennium Development Goals and renewal of the primary health care movement. The prospects for improving health in the Region are addressed in Chapter 6 by a group of internationally renowned experts who offer their comments on the "Health Agenda for the Americas, 2008–2017," which has been adopted by the governments of the Region, and provide advice to policymakers regarding how to implement each of its eight areas of action.

* * *

In summary, the current health status of the peoples of the Americas is a reflection of interactions and changes in the size, composition, distribution, and behavior of the population; the dynamic and continuing shifts in the nature, incidence, and burden of disease; and, to a large extent, the ongoing and often dramatic turns in the political, social, economic, and physical environment in which individuals, communities, nations, and the Region as a whole are developing.

References

1. Pan American Health Organization. Health Situation in the Americas: Basic Indicators, 2006. Washington, D.C.: PAHO; 2006.

2. United Nations Secretariat. Population Division of the Department of Economic and Social Affairs. World Population Prospects: The 2006 Revision. New York: United Nations; 2007.

3. United Nations Secretariat. Population Division of the Department of Economic and Social Affairs. World Urbanization Prospects: The 2005 Revision. New York: United Nations; 2006.

4. Prüss-Üstün A, Corvalán C. Preventing disease through healthy environments. Geneva: WHO; 2006.

5. Pan American Health Organization. Health Situation in the Americas. Basic Indicators Annual Publication from 1996–2005. Washington, D.C.: PAHO; 2005.

6. United Nations. Department of Public Information. Intergovernmental Panel on Climate Change 2001 Report: Global Climate Change. New York, 2002. Available from: http://www.un.org/News

7. Intergovernmental Panel on Climate Change. Available from: http://www.ipcc.ch.

8. Roses Periago M. Health inequalities in the Americas: Addressing their social determinants to sustain governance. Special presentation at Harvard University, April, 2005.

9. Cehelsky M. Building science, technology, and innovation capacity: Latin America and the Caribbean. American Association for the Advancement of Science. 32nd Annual AAAS Forum on Science and Technology Policy, Washington, D.C., May, 2007.

10. World Bank. World Development Indicators 2006. Washington, D.C., 2006.

11. United Nations Children's Fund. The State of the World's Children 2007: Women and Children—The Double Dividend of Gender Equality. New York, 2006, p. 82.

12. Pan American Health Organization. Health of the Indigenous Peoples of the Americas. Document CD47/13. Presented to the 47th Directing Council Meeting, Washington, D.C., 25–29 September 2006.

13. United Nations Children's Fund. The State of the World's Children 2006. Excluded and Invisible. New York, 2005, p. 25.

14. Ibid, p. 69.

15. Economic Commission for Latin America and the Caribbean. The Millennium Development Goals: A Latin American and Caribbean Perspective. Santiago: ECLAC; 2005.

16. Jones G, Steketee RW, Black RE, Bhutta ZA, Morris SS, and the Bellagio Child Survival Study Group. How many deaths can we prevent this year? Lancet. 2003;362:65.

17. Garrett L. The Challenge of Global Health. Foreign Affairs. January/February 2007, p. 32.

18. Pan American Health Organization. Maternal and Neonatal Health Annual Report. Washington, D.C., October 2005–September 2006, p. 4.

19. Pan American Health Organization. Regional Strategy for Maternal Mortality and Morbidity Reduction, 26th Pan American Sanitary Conference, Washington, D.C., 2002.

20. World Health Organization. World Health Statistics. Geneva: WHO; 2006.

21. Pan American Health Organization. PAHO database. Washington, D.C., 2006.

22. Pan American Health Organization. Regional Strategic Plan Framework, 2006-2015. Washington, D.C., 2007.

23. World Bank. Priorities in Health. Disease Control Priorities Project. Washington, D.C., 2006, pp. 3–4.

24. World Health Organization. Facing the Facts: the Impact of Chronic Disease in the Americas. Geneva: WHO; 2005.

25. Pan American Health Organization, Basic Indicators 2006.

26. Pan American Health Organization. Health Situation and Trends in the Americas. Document presented at the PAHO Annual Managers Meeting, Airlie, Virginia, 14–19 October 2006.

27. Dunne WM Jr, Pinckard JK, Hooper LV. Clinical microbiology in the year 2025. J Clin Microbiol. 2002;40:3889–93.

28. Pan American Health Organization, Governance and Policies Unit. Salud del Adulto Mayor. Washington, D.C., 2003.

29. World Bank. World Development Report 2007: Development and the Next Generation. Washington, D.C., 2006, pp. 123–124.

30. Eberwine D. Globesity: the crisis of growing proportions. Perspect Health. 2002;7(3).

31. Education is the key in treating diabetes. Posted on 18 December 2006. Available from: http://www.presstelegram.com.

32. World Health Organization. World Health Statistics 2006. Geneva, 2006, p. 11.

33. World Bank. Priorities in Health. Disease Control Priorities Project. Washington, D.C., 2006, p. 120.

34. Pan American Health Organization. Mortality database. Washington, D.C., 2002.

35. World Health Organization. Fifty-fourth World Health Assembly Resolution Provisional agenda item 13.3. Global health security–epidemic alert and response, 2 April 2001.

36. Calain P. Exploring the international arena of global public health surveillance. Health Policy and Planning 2007; 22: 9–10.

37. Calain P. From the field side of the binoculars: a different view on global public health surveillance. Health Policy and Planning 2007; 22:19.

38. UNAIDS, UNFPA, and UNIFEM. Women and HIV/AIDS: Confronting the Crisis. New York, 2004.

39. UNAIDS/WHO. AIDS Epidemic Update. Geneva, December 2006.

40. Pan American Health Organization. 2006 Annual Report of the Director. Washington, D.C., 2006, p. 18.

41. Pan American Health Organization. Press release (Internet version): Día Mundial del SIDA 2006: Los Números no Dejan Lugar a Dudas. 1 December 2006.

42. Zamiska N. Risk of Bird-Flu Pandemic Seen as "Permanent Threat". The Wall Street Journal. 16 January 2007, p. A12.

43. United Nations. World Economic Situation and Prospects, 2006. New York. 2006.

44. The Economist. Pandemic Influenza: One Step Closer. 18 November 2006, p. 85.

45. United States National Institutes of Health. News in Health. Washington, D.C., December 2006, pp. 1–2.

46. World Bank. World Development Report 2004, Washington, D.C., 2004.

47. Escobar ML. Health Sector Reform in Colombia. World Bank Institute. Reaching the Poor with Health Services. Washington, D.C., 2005, pp. 6–22.

48. Coady DP, Filmer DP, Gwatkin DR. PROGRESA for Progress. World Bank Institute. Reaching the Poor with Health Services. Washington, D.C., 2005, pp. 10–12.

49. Rawlings LP. Do Social Funds Reach the Poor? World Bank Institute. Reaching the Poor with Health Services. Washington, D.C., 2005, pp. 13–35.

50. Pan American Health Organization. Informe sobre la situación de los recursos humanos en salud. Washington, D.C., 2006.

51. Pan American Health Organization. Annual Report of the Director, 2006. Washington, D.C., 2006, pp. 8–9.

52. World Bank. Healthy Development: The World Bank Strategy for Health, Nutrition, and Population Results. Washington, D.C., April 2007, p. 11.

Chapter 1
HEALTH IN THE CONTEXT OF DEVELOPMENT

At the dawn of the new millennium, 189 countries committed themselves to reducing poverty by 2015. To that end, they set eight Millennium Development Goals (MDGs), all of which relate in some measure to health. Their commitment underscores a growing recognition that economic growth, the distribution of income, and investment in human capital have a huge impact on peoples' quality of life and on their health. At the same time, a realization of the social determinants of health is fuelling greater emphasis on collaboration among all social sectors to improve the population's health and on the international recognition of human rights.

One of the principal indicators of development, and of health, is life expectancy. The inhabitants of more developed countries tend to live longer than their counterparts in developing countries. National averages, moreover, tend to mask disparities within countries, whose more vulnerable groups tend to have shorter lives. The population's collective years of life lost translate, in turn, into lowered national productivity.

Despite a reduction in the rates of poverty in Latin America and the Caribbean as a result of economic growth that began in the 1990s (as measured by gross national product), that reduction has not been sufficient to counter the increase in poverty that had occurred in previous decades. In addition, no measurable improvements have been registered in indicators of the distribution of income in the region, which continues to show vast inequalities, as discernible from a comparison between the richest and the poorest quintiles of the population in most countries.

In the past couple of decades, the governments of Latin America and the Caribbean have significantly increased public funding for social sectors. In general, however, a disproportionate amount of that funding has gone to social security/social welfare and education, with lesser portions targeting health and housing. Governments also have embarked on various forms of collaboration, as expressed in many international summits designed to advance the human condition throughout the Hemisphere.

Among the social determinants of inequity, the greatest is poverty—defined for Latin America as insufficient income to meet basic needs. Such poverty results, in large measure, from low levels of growth, low productivity, limited development of human capital, and ineffective economic and social policies. Both the rates of poverty and the absolute number of poor people in Latin America and the Caribbean have been dropping in the past several years, but within the region, and within countries, huge disparities persist.

Efforts to reduce hunger and malnutrition, likewise targeted in the MDGs, have also scored gains in Latin America and the Caribbean, but progress is uneven throughout the region, with certain areas actually experiencing upticks in both the numbers and prevalence rates of the undernourished.

Employment is a basic determinant of health from many different angles—access to labor markets, income, and working conditions—and sustained employment is critical to countries' ability to reduce poverty. The unemployment rate has been rising in Latin America and the Caribbean in recent years, during which time informal employment has increased as a share of overall employment. Youth unemployment also is increasing, and that of women is much higher than men.

The reciprocal relation between health and education is clear and explains the MDG focus on universal primary education as a principal strategy for reducing poverty. The Americas is on pace to achieve the goal of 100% completion of primary school by 2015, having already attained coverage higher than 97%.

For the most part, inequitable health conditions—that is, those that are unnecessary, unjust, and remediable—reflect an unfair distribution of the social determinants of health. While the "average" health status in Latin America and the Caribbean is relatively good, great disparities across an array of indicators—such as in infant mortality, child mortality, proportion of births attended by skilled personnel, maternal mortality—exist among and within countries. These and other inequities—such as differential rates of infectious diseases, chronic diseases, access to health care services—disproportionately afflict women, ethnic and racial groups.

The environment is yet another major determinant of health. Latin America and the Caribbean have the highest urbanization level in the developing world, with more than three in every four persons living in cities. While urban areas generally offer advantages over rural areas in terms of access to social services, employment, and the like, many of the cities in the region have grown beyond their capacity to provide adequate services. Access to water and sanitation, although having improved significantly over the past several decades, continues to be inequitable in that coverage is greater in urban than in rural areas. Among other environmental challenges are air pollution, shrinking forests and land degradation, degraded coasts and polluted seas, and the looming global impact of climate change.

THE ECONOMIC AND POLITICAL CONTEXT

Life Expectancy

Life expectancy has traditionally been recognized as a key indicator of a country's development, while the life expectancy index reflects the overall health of a population. In examining these indicators, it is necessary to consider not only national averages and possible similarities between the countries of the Americas, but differences within countries as well, in order to be able to identify inequities affecting the most vulnerable groups.

Figure 1 shows the evolution of life expectancy at birth in the United States since 1930 and in Latin America and the Caribbean since 1950–1955. In 2005, life expectancy in Bolivia, Guatemala, and Haiti reached the levels seen in the United States more than 60 years ago. That same year, life expectancy in Brazil, Nicaragua, and Peru was similar to the level attained in the United States in the 1950s.

The difference between life expectancy in Latin America and the Caribbean and that in the United States and Canada is decreasing. While the gap was 10 years in the mid-1960s (57 years in Latin America and the Caribbean and 67 years in the United States and Canada), in 2000–2005, it narrowed to 6 years (71 and 77, respectively). Despite this convergence, there are significant country-to-country differences in Latin America and the Caribbean—for example, life expectancy in Haiti is 59.7 years, in Costa Rica it is 77.7 years.

Figure 2 shows the life expectancy index for a selected set of countries. The index has been pegged to life expectancy in the Netherlands, a country that has the longest-living population and the highest life expectancy rates in the world. The index shows that Chile, Costa Rica, Cuba, and Panama have the best health

FIGURE 1. Life expectancy at birth in the United States (1930–2005) and in Latin America and the Caribbean (1950–2005) and life expectancy at birth in selected Latin American and Caribbean countries (2000–2005) in relationship to the United States.

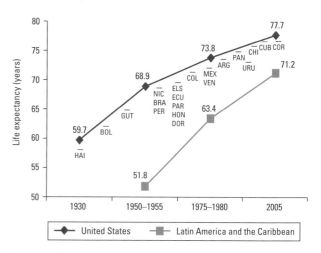

Source: Pan American Health Organization, Area of Health Systems Strengthening, Health Policies and Systems Unit, 2006.

conditions in Latin America, with survival rates over 0.90, which is close to the maximum potential observed. The potential survival rate for Haiti is just 0.73.

Economic Growth and Inequality

An analysis of data on economic growth, poverty, and inequality in income distribution in Latin America and the Caribbean

FIGURE 2. Life expectancy index, selected Latin American and Caribbean countries, 2000–2005.

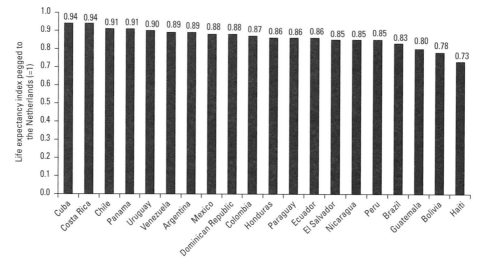

Source: Pan American Health Organization, Area of Health Systems Strengthening, Health Policies and Systems Unit, 2006.

TABLE 1. Changes in gross domestic product for Latin America and the Caribbean, Latin America, the Caribbean, and countries in the region, 2000–2006.

Country/region	2000	2002	2003	2004	2005	2006[a]
Antigua and Barbuda	1.5	2.5	5.2	7.2	4.6	11.0
Argentina	−0.8	−10.9	8.8	9.0	9.2	8.5
Bahamas	1.9	2.3	1.4	1.8	2.7	4.0
Barbados	2.2	0.5	1.9	4.8	3.9	3.9
Belize	12.9	5.1	9.3	4.6	3.5	2.7
Bolivia	2.5	2.5	2.9	3.9	4.1	4.5
Brazil	4.4	1.9	0.5	4.9	2.3	2.8
Chile	4.5	2.2	3.9	6.2	6.3	4.4
Colombia	2.9	1.9	3.9	4.9	5.2	6.0
Costa Rica	1.8	2.9	6.4	4.1	5.9	6.8
Cuba	6.1	1.5	2.9	4.5	...	...
Cuba[b]	...	1.8	3.8	5.4	11.8	12.5
Dominica	0.6	−4.2	2.2	6.3	3.3	4.0
Dominican Republic	7.9	5.0	−0.4	2.7	9.2	10.0
Ecuador	2.8	4.2	3.6	7.9	4.7	4.8
El Salvador	2.2	2.3	2.3	1.8	2.8	3.8
Grenada	7.0	1.5	7.5	−7.4	13.2	7.0
Guatemala	3.6	2.2	2.1	2.8	3.2	4.6
Guyana	−1.4	1.1	−0.7	1.6	−3.0	1.3
Haiti	0.9	−0.3	0.4	−3.5	1.8	2.5
Honduras	5.7	2.7	3.5	5.0	4.1	5.6
Jamaica	0.7	1.1	2.3	0.9	1.4	2.6
Mexico	6.6	0.8	1.4	4.2	3.0	4.8
Nicaragua	4.1	0.8	2.5	5.1	4.0	3.7
Panama	2.7	2.2	4.2	7.5	6.9	7.5
Paraguay	−3.3	...	3.8	4.1	2.9	4.0
Peru	3.0	5.2	3.9	5.2	6.4	7.2
Saint Kitts and Nevis	4.3	1.1	0.5	7.6	5.0	5.0
Saint Vincent and the Grenadines	1.8	3.7	3.2	6.2	1.5	4.0
Saint Lucia	−0.2	3.1	4.1	5.6	7.7	7.0
Suriname	4.0	1.9	6.1	7.7	5.7	6.4
Trinidad and Tobago	6.9	6.9	12.6	6.4	8.9	12.0
Uruguay	−1.4	−11.0	2.2	11.8	6.6	7.5
Venezuela	3.7	−8.9	−7.7	17.9	9.3	10.0
Latin America and the Caribbean[c,d]	**3.9**	**−0.8**	**2.0**	**5.9**	**4.5**	**5.3**
Latin America[c]	**4.0**	**−0.8**	**1.9**	**6.0**	**4.5**	**5.3**
Caribbean[d]	**3.4**	**3.3**	**5.8**	**3.8**	**4.9**	**6.8**

[a]Preliminary figures.
[b]Data provided by the Oficina Nacional de Estadísticas de Cuba, which are being evaluated by ECLAC.
[c]Does not include Cuba.
[d]Barbados, Dominica, Guyana, and Jamaica GDPs are expressed in factor costs.
Source: ECLAC. Statistical Yearbook for Latin America and the Caribbean, 2006, p. 85.

suggests that poverty reduction during the economic recovery that began in the early 1990s has not been able to offset the growth in poverty in the 1980s. Nor has income distribution changed significantly, remaining as unequal in the 1990s as in the 1980s. This confirms the hypothesis that the rewards of economic growth are not distributed equally among different population strata. In times of economic recession, poverty has grown quickly while in periods of economic growth, poverty has declined very slowly.

During the 1980s, the so-called "lost decade," per capita income in Latin American and Caribbean countries as a whole fell by an annual average of 0.7%. In 1990, average per capita income

was approximately US$ 3,300, almost 10% lower than at the start of the 1980s (US$ 3,500). The economic recovery in the 1990s made for significant growth in per capita income, which was US$ 3,800 in 2001, for a 15% increase over 1990.

Since 2000, annual growth in GDP in Latin America and the Caribbean underwent major changes, with significant differences from country to country and variations from one year to the next (Table 1).

In 2000, average growth in Latin American and Caribbean countries was 3.9%, with extremes ranging from −3.3% (Paraguay) to 12.9% (Belize); Argentina, Guyana, and Uruguay showed

"When living conditions improve, as a result of either preventive or curative activities, they promote well-being and, consequently, productivity. In either case the funds assigned to health are an investment; the more prevalent the problem the greater the return it gives."

Abraham Horwitz, 1964

signs of slowing growth. Between 2000 and 2002, many of the countries suffered a sharp slowdown in growth associated with serious problems in South America and Mexico. Argentina, Uruguay, and Venezuela saw their growth shrink by close to 10% or more in that period and faced serious economic difficulties, such as the temporary closure of banks, suspension of payments, and widespread unemployment. Thanks to a series of measures designed to curb inflation and to halt the flight of capital and investments, however, the economy was reactivated between 2003 and 2004, when average growth in Latin America and the Caribbean climbed to 5.9%. The countries that grew the fastest were the ones that had most suffered during the crisis, which experienced rates averaging close to 9% or more. In 2005, average growth in Latin America and the Caribbean was 4.5%. That year, close to one-third of the countries experienced growth of more than 6%, which surpassed the per capita gross national income (GNI)[1] levels seen before the 2002 crisis.

In 2000–2005, the level of wealth in the countries of the Americas, measured by their GNI, also shows uneven advances. By the end of the period, the average weighted GNI for the Americas was about US$ 19,500 (value adjusted by purchasing power parity or ppp), which ranks it among the regions with the highest income in the world. However, there are major differences from subregion to subregion: Central America (US$ 5,687), the Andean area (US$ 5,300), the Latin Caribbean (US$ 6,528), and the English-speaking Caribbean (US$ 7,410) present levels that are below the Latin American and Caribbean general average (US$ 8,771). The Southern Cone (US$ 10,042) and North America (US$ 37,085), on the other hand, are higher. Wide gaps also exist between countries, with GNI values ranging from US$ 1,840 in Haiti to US$ 41,950 in the United States (Table 2).

Figure 3 shows the per capita gross national income for selected countries of the Americas and allows comparisons to be made between groups of countries. According to 2005 GNI levels and the weighted average for each group of countries, the income of the countries in the wealthiest quintile (US$ 22,288) was seven times higher than that in the lowest quintile (US$ 3,218). In ad-

dition, the GNI in three of the groups, totaling 20 countries, falls below the Latin American and the Caribbean average.

Growth in GDP and GNI rates, partly owing to their variability, has not translated into significant improvements in poverty rates or income distribution in Latin America and the Caribbean.

Income distribution is generally measured by the Gini coefficient, which uses a value of 0 for greatest equality and a value of 1 for greatest inequality. Latin America and the Caribbean continues to be the region with the greatest inequality in income distribution in the world, except for sub-Saharan Africa (see Figure 4).

Another way to measure income distribution is by using the ratio between the income of the 20% wealthiest population and the 20% poorest. In the Americas as a whole, the ratio of the income of the wealthiest 20% to the poorest 20% is close to 20. Some countries have less economic inequality, with a ratio under 10 (Canada, Jamaica, Nicaragua, the United States); conversely, some have a ratio higher than 25 (Bolivia, Colombia, Haiti and Paraguay), as shown in Figure 5. Both measures reflect significant inequalities between countries in the Americas.

Inequality in Latin America and the Caribbean also is expressed in terms of access to good quality drinking water, sanitation, schooling, and health care; a respect for property rights; and political representation. Large inequalities also exist with regard to the power and influence exercised by individuals and, in many countries, in the administration of justice. Inequalities in consumption—which can be measured more accurately—also are higher in Latin America than elsewhere in the world, although the differences are not as sharp as those for income inequalities (1).

Trends in Social Spending

As part of public policy adjustments, to compensate for some of the population's economic difficulties (some of which worsened after structural reforms were put in place), and to provide effective redistribution of wealth, Latin American and Caribbean governments substantially increased the public funds devoted to social spending. Between the start of the 1990s and 2003, social spending experienced a sustained increase in most countries. Social spending as a percentage of GDP rose from 12.8% to 15.1%, representing an increase of 39% in per capita spending in real terms (2).

The Economic Commission for Latin America and the Caribbean (ECLAC) estimates that public sector per capita social spending in the 21 countries for which data are available for the 2002–2003 was US$ 610 (US$ 170 more than in 1990–1991 in constant 2002 dollars). In this period, there were significant differences between the countries, ranging from a minimum of US$ 68 (Nicaragua) to a maximum of US$ 1,284 (Argentina). Table 3 shows the wide variation seen from country to country when investments in social spending as percentages of GDP are compared—from a minimum of 5.5% (Trinidad and Tobago) to a maximum of 29.3% (Cuba).

---

[1]Previously called per capita gross national product (GNP), this indicator measures the total output of goods and services for final use produced by residents and non-residents, regardless of the allocation to domestic and foreign claims, in relation to population size.

TABLE 2. Per capita gross national income (in ppp-adjusted $), countries of the Americas, 2000–2005.

Country	2000	2001	2002	2003	2004	2005
Antigua and Barbuda	9,200	9,190	9,520	9,730	11,100	11,700
Argentina	11,930	11,570	10,380	11,410	12,530	13,920
Bahamas	16,200	16,000	16,140	. . .	16,350	. . .
Barbados	14,840	14,810	14,660	15,060	15,060	. . .
Belize	5,470	5,700	5,850	6,320	6,550	6,740
Bolivia	2,330	2,380	2,430	2,490	2,600	2,740
Brazil	7,150	7,310	7,480	7,510	7,940	8,230
Canada	27,180	28,070	29,170	30,040	30,760	32,220
Chile	8,850	9,200	9,440	9,810	10,610	11,470
Colombia	5,940	6,060	6,160	6,410	6,940	7,420
Costa Rica	8,190	8,340	8,560	9,140	9,220	9,680
Dominica	5,230	5,160	4,970	5,020	5,290	5,560
Dominican Republic	5,830	6,060	6,310	6,310	6,860	7,150
Ecuador	3,050	3,240	3,350	3,440	3,770	4,070
El Salvador	4,610	4,730	4,820	4,910	4,890	5,120
Grenada	6,900	6,630	6,600	7,030	7,050	7,260
Guatemala	3,910	3,990	4,040	4,090	4,260	4,410
Guyana	3,750	3,950	3,950	3,980	4,240	4,230
Haiti	1,760	1,740	1,730	1,730	1,730	1,840
Honduras	2,430	2,510	2,530	2,590	2,760	2,900
Jamaica	3,500	3,610	3,670	3,790	3,950	4,110
Mexico	8,690	8,760	8,830	8,980	9,640	10,030
Nicaragua	3,050	3,130	3,130	3,180	3,480	3,650
Panama	5,920	6,010	6,150	6,420	6,730	7,310
Paraguay	4,610	4,740	4,600	4,690	4,820	4,970
Peru	4,610	4,650	4,880	5,080	5,400	5,830
Puerto Rico	15,090	16,210	. . .	. . .	16,120	. . .
Saint Kitts and Nevis	10,150	10,310	10,550	10,740	10,910	12,500
Saint Vincent and the Grenadines	5,090	5,400	5,540	5,870	5,590	. . .
Saint Lucia	5,250	5,020	5,170	5,310	6,030	5,980
United States of America	34,690	35,320	36,260	37,750	39,820	41,950
Trinidad and Tobago	8,260	8,420	9,080	10,390	11,430	13,170
Uruguay	8,710	8,560	7,690	7,980	9,030	9,810
Venezuela	5,580	5,760	5,240	4,750	5,830	6,440

Source: World Bank. World Development Indicators, 2006.

The increase in social spending was not enough to repair the damage caused by the successive economic crises, however, nor did it alter existing differences between countries nor the distribution within them. While Argentina, Brazil, Costa Rica, Cuba, and Uruguay allocated more than 18% of GDP for social spending, Ecuador, El Salvador, the Dominican Republic, Guatemala, and Trinidad and Tobago assigned less than 7.5% to it. These variations mean that despite the efforts of poorer countries to boost social spending, the disparities in Latin America and the Caribbean continue in real terms (2).

Also in 2002–2003, it is estimated that Latin American and Caribbean countries directed most of their public spending into social security and social welfare (7.1%), followed by education (4.1%), with spending on health and housing amounting to just 2.9% and 0.9%, respectively (see Figure 6).

Spending on the health sector as a percentage of GDP in 2002–2003 is shown in Figure 7. Figure 6 shows changes in the patterns of public social spending, by sector, since 1990 in Latin America and the Caribbean; Figure 7 shows the large differences that persist in the percentage of GDP that the countries devote to social investments.

Investments in health, particularly targeting the most vulnerable groups, have an immediate impact on the population's productive prospects. Investments in the health of the most vulnerable persons are a necessary condition for facilitating their access to greater development benefits, such as the possibility of boosting their productivity, building their income, and transferring assets to their descendents. The pattern of social spending on education and health in Latin America shows a positive trend, exemplified by the increase in access to public services and the po-

33

FIGURE 3. Per capita gross national income (GNI) in US$ adjusted for purchasing power parity (ppp), by income quintile, countries of the Americas, 2005.

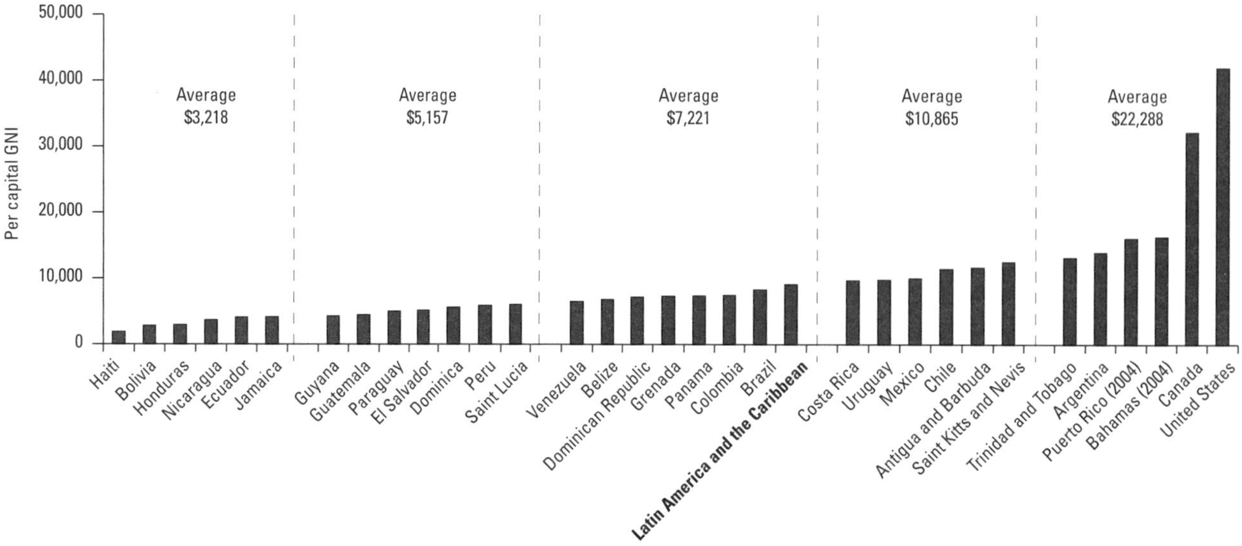

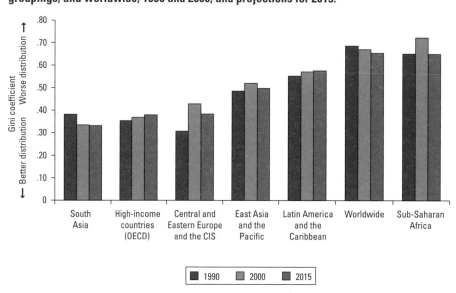

Source: World Bank. World Development Indicators, 2006.

FIGURE 4. Gini coefficient, Latin America and the Caribbean, various regions and country groupings, and worldwide, 1990 and 2000, and projections for 2015.

Sources: Dikhanov Y, Ward M. Evolution of the Global Distribution of Income 1970–1999. 2001. UNDP. Human Development Report 2005, p. 62.

litical will of governments during the 1990s to finance programs for the population's poorest segments, particularly at early life stages, as a way to break the intergenerational cycle of poverty. Social spending varies from country to country, however, and public spending on health shows wider differences than public spending on education. This pattern occurs both because of the structure of the countries' national health systems and of the fact that private sector spending contributes to provide health services. Finally, public spending on social security (pensions) is more regressive, in that it has a negative effect on the poorest sectors, favoring those

FIGURE 5. Inequity gap between the wealthiest quintile and the poorest quintile, selected countries of the Americas, 2000–2005.

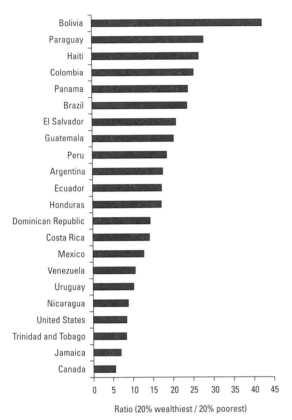

Ratio (20% wealthiest / 20% poorest)

Source: Human Development Report 2006, based on data on income or spending from World Bank (2006), World Development Indicators 2006.

who usually contribute to plans (medium- and high-income persons) and receive health care and pension benefits after they retire. The poor tend to work in the informal sector and do not receive a pension or protection from catastrophic events; rather, government resources to assist them are eaten away by the commitment to fund social security. This is a legacy from the recent past, given that social security plans do not provide universal access and only benefit employees in the formal economy.

In general, the low level of per capita public spending and of the amount of funding allocated to social spending by the poorest countries reflect their low tax revenues. Considered in a global context, Latin American and Caribbean countries' government revenues expressed as a percentage of GDP are also relatively low.

Along with the increase in public social spending, in the 1990s several Latin American and Caribbean countries received new financial resources from multilateral institutions, cooperation agencies, and privately funded global initiatives. The strongest economies and some mid-sized ones have been the main beneficiaries, followed by the poorest countries that are part of the Highly Indebted Poor Countries Initiative.

Subregional and Regional Integration

During the 1990s, opportunities arose for consolidating economic agreements in the Americas. In addition, various cooperation mechanisms were created to address political, economic, social, and cultural aspects important for Latin American and Caribbean countries.

These trade-oriented subregional integration processes were followed by social integration processes that have given rise to bodies and mechanisms designed to study various aspects of economic integration and its social repercussions. Chapter 5 analyzes in detail the Central American Integration System, the integration processes in the Caribbean, the Andean Community of Nations, the Southern Common Market, the Amazon Cooperation Treaty Organization, and the North American Free Trade Agreement.

Charting New Paths through Summits— Regional Political Cooperation

The First **Ibero-American Summit**, held in Mexico in 1991, was convened to establish a forum to advance along a common political, economic, and cultural process. These summits have been a favored forum for conducting political consultation and consensus-building so as to reflect on international challenges and promote cooperation and solidarity among the 22 member countries (Andorra, Argentina, Bolivia, Brazil, Chile, Colombia, Costa Rica, Cuba, Dominican Republic, Ecuador, El Salvador, Guatemala, Honduras, Mexico, Nicaragua, Panama, Peru, Paraguay, Portugal, Spain, Uruguay, and Venezuela). Since the first, 16 summits have been held. Early on, the issues under discussion did not reflect a central concern for health, but more recently, summits have given special attention to social development with emphasis on human development issues. This, in turn, has translated into commitments related to public health. The Declaration of the Thirteenth Ibero-American Summit, held in Santa Cruz de la Sierra, Bolivia, in November 2003, states that "health is a fundamental human right for sustainable development" and undertakes to "revisit primary health care, the goal of health for all, compliance with the Millennium Development Goals, and improvement of local management capacity in health." In the same declaration, the Heads of State and Government undertake to "target activities to excluded sectors, with the aim of reducing infant and maternal mortality rates and preventing the spread of infectious diseases such as AIDS" (3). The Fourteenth Ibero-American Summit, held in San José, Costa Rica, in November 2004, reaffirmed the commitment to the Millennium Development Goals, placing special emphasis on the need to reduce extreme poverty and hunger and to combat social injustice.

The Fifteenth Ibero-American Summit, held in 2005 in Salamanca, Spain, created the Ibero-American General Secretariat, a permanent body designed to support the institutionalization of the Ibero-American Conference and which is charged with promoting "cooperation programs in the field of health that help to combat pandemics and curable diseases" in relation to the MDGs.

TABLE 3. Public spending on social sectors, per capita (in 2000 US$) and as a percentage of GDP, selected countries of Latin America and the Caribbean, 2002–2003.

Country	Total social sector public spending		Public spending on education		Public spending on health		Public spending on social security[a]		Public spending on housing and others	
	Per capita	As a percentage of GDP	Per capita	As a percentage of GDP	Per capita	As a percentage of GDP	Per capita	As a percentage of GDP	Per capita	As a percentage of GDP
Argentina	1,284	19.4	279	4.2	291	4.4	642	9.7	72	1.1
Bolivia	136	13.7	66	6.7	16	1.6	51	5.1	3	0.3
Brazil[b]	678	19.2	128	3.6	102	2.9	444	12.6	4	0.1
Chile	764	14.8	209	4.0	155	3.0	390	7.6	10	0.2
Colombia[c]	268	13.5	86	4.3	87	4.4	76	3.8	19	1.0
Costa Rica	782	20.7	235	5.7	236	5.7	232	7.4	79	1.9
Cuba[d]	784	29.3	328	12.3	168	6.3	209	7.8	79	2.9
Dominican Republic	185	7.4	72	3.0	39	1.6	28	1.1	46	1.7
Ecuador	77	5.7	36	2.7	15	1.1	23	1.7	3	0.2
El Salvador	149	7.1	67	3.2	34	1.6	29	1.4	19	0.9
Guatemala	110	6.5	44	2.6	17	1.0	20	1.2	29	1.7
Honduras[e]	126	13.0	70	7.2	34	3.5	5	0.5	17	1.8
Jamaica	311	9.6	162	5.2	78	2.5	15	0.5	56	1.4
Mexico	603	10.5	233	4.1	136	2.4	144	2.5	90	1.5
Nicaragua	68	8.8	32	4.1	24	3.0	. . .	. . .	13	1.7
Panama	686	17.4	185	4.7	236	6.0	218	5.5	47	1.2
Paraguay	115	9.1	55	4.4	16	1.3	38	3.0	6	0.4
Peru[c]	158	7.8	50	2.5	36	1.8	67	3.3	5	0.2
Trinidad and Tobago	392	5.5	223	3.1	93	1.3	5	0.1	71	1.0
Uruguay	1,072	20.9	173	3.4	125	2.4	754	14.7	20	0.4
Venezuela[f]	489	11.7	213	5.1	67	1.6	170	4.1	39	0.9
Latin America and the Caribbean[g]	641	15.4	171	4.1	120	2.9	314	7.5	36	0.9

Source: ECLAC, based on information from the Commission's database on social spending.

[a]Includes spending on labor.

[b]The figure is an estimate for social spending at the three levels of government (federal, state, and municipal) based on information on social spending at the federal level.

[c]The figure corresponds to the average 2000-2001. This figure is not included in the averages.

[d]The figure in per capita dollars uses the official exchange rate (1 dollar = 1 peso).

[e]The figure corresponds to 2004 and is not included in the regional averages.

[f]The figures correspond to agreed social spending (budget and budget amendments at the end of each year).

[g]Weighted average for the countries, except El Salvador.

Also, the meeting agreed on the importance of "promoting concrete actions and initiatives to make the universal right to health a reality, placing this objective at the top of the political agenda in our countries and in Ibero-American cooperation" (*4*).

At the Sixteenth Ibero-American Summit, held in Montevideo, Uruguay, in November 2006, the leaders highlighted the importance of addressing the global migration issue from the standpoint of human rights and to acknowledge the cultural contribution that immigrants bring to the host countries.

To carry out the mandates issued from the Ibero-American summits, parallel meetings have been instituted of the Ibero-American Meetings of Ministers of Health, which have approved an Ibero-American space for health and the launching of the first four thematic networks for cooperation in health: the Ibero-American donation and transplant network; the drug policies network; the network to combat tobacco use; and the network for public health teaching and research. The Ibero-American forum has made it easier for the countries to reaffirm their shared values and principles, with a view to building consensus for improving living and health conditions in Member Countries.

At the urging of the United States, the **Summit of the Americas** met for the first time in 1994 in Miami (USA). From the outset, its objective was to lay the groundwork for a Free Trade Agreement of the Americas, but it was acknowledged that to achieve this goal, agreement would have to be reached and progress made in pending social issues. The Summit of the Americas meets every four years, and its decisions are summarized in a Declaration and an Action Plan signed by the participating presidents and heads of state. Two summits were held in the 1990s, the Miami summit in 1994 and the Santiago summit in 1998. The Third Summit was

FIGURE 6. Evolution of public social spending as a percentage of GDP, by sector, Latin America and the Caribbean, 1990–1991, 1996–1997, and 2002–2003.

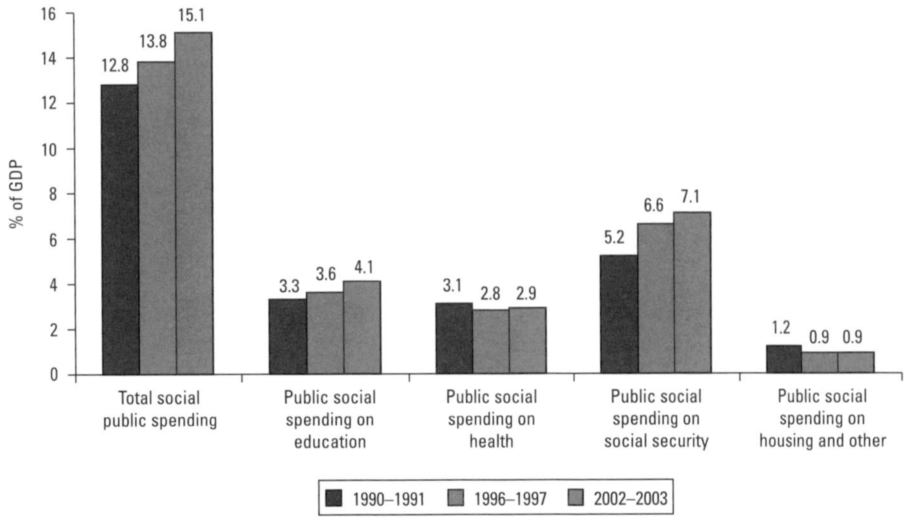

FIGURE 7. Distribution of public social spending as a percentage of GDP, by sector, Latin America and the Caribbean region and selected Latin American and Caribbean countries, 2002–2003.

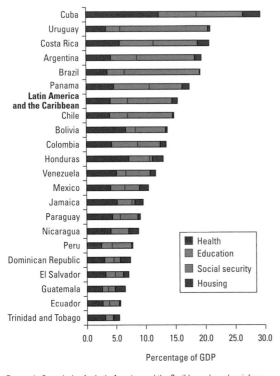

held in 2001 in Quebec City, Canada, and dealt with the commitment to strengthen democracy, create prosperity, and develop human potential. For the first time, the discussion about hemispheric security included the concept of new health threats, such as the HIV/AIDS pandemic and rising poverty levels (5). Discussions also stressed the need to work together on health sector reforms, emphasizing concern with the essential functions of public health, the quality of care, equality of access, and the preparation of standards to govern the performance of the public health profession. Commitments entered into at this summit included strengthening hemispheric programs for the prevention, control, and treatment of communicable and noncommunicable diseases, mental illnesses, violence, and accidents, as well as participating in negotiating a framework agreement to combat smoking (5).

In 2004, the Special Summit of the Americas was held in Monterrey, Mexico. Its declaration sets forth a commitment to reinforce the strategies for disease prevention and treatment, health promotion, and investments in health, emphasizing the social protection of health as a pillar of human development. Support was given to the World Health Organization's initiative to provide antiretroviral treatment for three million people worldwide by 2005, and participants committed themselves to provide treatment for at least 600,000 persons in the Americas by that year.

The Fourth Summit of the Americas was held in Mar del Plata, Argentina, in November 2005. The keynote theme was "Creating Jobs to Fight Poverty and Strengthen Democratic Governance." In addition to reaffirming the commitments made at the Millennium Summit of reducing poverty by 2015 (6), the summit

> *"The economic crisis of the 1980s aggravated the social debt, plunging more people into poverty while simultaneously limiting the resources available to the social sectors. The situation seems to be a vicious cycle: lingering economic problems lead to a lack of services that adversely affects the health of the population, but the countries need a healthy population in order to participate in economic and social development."*
>
> Carlyle Guerra de Macedo, 1992

supported the creation of a strategic intersectoral partnership among ministries of health, of education, of labor, and of the environment. Under this partnership, a commitment was made to promote public policies "to protect the health and safety of all workers and foster a culture of prevention and control of occupational hazards in the Hemisphere"(*6*). Lastly, the summit recognized the urgency of developing national preparedness plans to fight influenza and avian flu pandemics before June 2006 (*6*).

The purpose of the **Latin American, Caribbean, and European Union Summit**, first held in Rio de Janeiro in 1999, is to promote and develop a strategic association based on full respect for international law; on the United Nations Charter goals and principles; and on a spirit of equality, partnership, and cooperation. The Second Summit was held in Madrid, Spain, in 2002, and stressed the importance of gender equity in combating poverty, achieving sustainable and equitable development, and assuring the well-being of all boys and girls. To that end, it recognized the importance of strengthening assistance in health and social protection. In terms of HIV/AIDS, it recognized the importance of prevention and the need to facilitate access to antiretroviral treatment. The Third Summit, which was held in Guadalajara, Mexico, in 2004, reaffirmed the commitment to achieve the MDGs in 2015 and announced the launching of the EUROsociAL program, whose objective is to promote the exchange of experience, specialized knowledge, and good practices between Europe and Latin America, particularly in the education and health sectors. It also established a commitment to strengthen bi-regional cooperation mechanisms for indigenous peoples, women's empowerment, the rights of persons with disabilities, and children's rights. The Fourth Summit was held in Vienna, Austria, in 2006, and it reaffirmed the commitment to increase official development aid, bringing it up to 0.56% of GNI by 2010 and meeting the target of 0.7% by 2015, recognizing that additional resources are required to achieve the MDGs.

The summits have led to the establishment of commitments among heads of state and government, their respective ministries, and regional and international multilateral organizations to work jointly and determinedly to attain the MDGs in the Region. In this context, the fundamental role played by health in the

reduction of poverty and inequity has been strengthened. Consensuses also have been built that have had repercussions on social policy development and planning at the local level, and fundamental values have been disseminated throughout the Region. They include a recognition of the role of social determinants, the particular needs of the most vulnerable population groups, the importance of boosting the efficiency of social spending through a quest for synergies within government agencies, and the need to involve other social players, starting with their own beneficiaries, in social change actions.

THE SOCIAL CONTEXT

Individual health is not an isolated phenomenon. In fact, the greatest health determinants are social in nature, mainly poverty, undernutrition, and unemployment, but also gender, ethnic group, and race. The MDGs are commitments to reduce poverty, hunger, disease, illiteracy, environmental degradation, and gender inequity. They present a vision of development that goes far beyond economic growth, since it stresses health, education, and environmental conservation as the motors of development. Three of the eight objectives, eight of the 16 targets, and 18 of the 48 indicators are directly linked to health, and health also exerts an important influence on attaining other objectives (see the spread on the Millennium Development Goals in Latin America and the Caribbean on pp. 4–9).

The MDGs represent the first political consensus by heads of state and government, whereby they commit themselves, in an act of solidarity that transcends borders, to reduce poverty; at the same time, developed nations commit themselves to increasing official development assistance. Promoting and working towards the MDGs has led, once again, to the acknowledgment of the transcendental role played by social determinants in health, particularly in the health of the most vulnerable groups.

In 2005, the World Health Organization (WHO) established the Commission on the Social Determinants of Health to study the impact of socioeconomic and environmental conditions on health. The commission was set up to create a local and global agenda for the formulation, planning, and implementation of health policies, plans, and programs that would help to reduce health inequities and improve the quality of life and the health of individuals.

The commission stresses the role played by persistent inequalities, poverty, exploitation of certain population groups, violence, and injustice in the absence of health. Worldwide, socially disadvantaged persons have less access to basic health resources and to the health system as a whole. That is why persons belonging to more vulnerable groups become ill and die more frequently. Paradoxically, despite progress made in medical science and the fact that the planet has never had access to so much wealth, the inequity gap continues to widen. The commission underlines that health is not simply a biological and personal matter, but, by its very nature, it is the result of complex and changing relations and interactions between an individual's biology; the surroundings; and living conditions on the economic, environmental, cultural, and political fronts.

The MDGs and the social determinants of health are validated by the Universal Declaration of Human Rights adopted and proclaimed by the General Assembly of the United Nations on 10 December 1948 and, in turn, they reaffirm and strengthen it. In Article 25, the declaration clearly establishes the right to adequate standards of living for the health and well-being of persons and their families, when it affirms that: "Everyone has the right to a standard of living adequate for the health and well-being of himself and of his family, including food, clothing, housing and medical care and necessary social services, and the right to security in the event of unemployment, sickness, disability, widowhood, old age or other lack of livelihood in circumstances beyond his control." It adds that mothers and their small children have the right to special care and support.

The lack of access to health-related goods and services, as well as the absence of social protection plans, are key factors in explaining inequities in Latin American and Caribbean countries. In this context, it is clear that the efforts of society as a whole should focus on improving access to health systems for groups that are currently excluded, through the gradual expansion of health care service coverage and the elimination of barriers—economic, ethnic, cultural, gender-based, and labor-related—to access those services.

In order to attain the MDGs in Latin America and the Caribbean, the social and economic determinants that have a negative influence on equity must be addressed. In so doing, the probability of making headway in the reduction of existing inequality gaps and in building up the political, economic, and social rights of citizens will increase.

Poverty and Indigence

There is close correspondence between the MDGs and the major determinants of inequity. For example, the main determinant of health is poverty, and this is reflected in MDG 1, which proposes to eradicate extreme poverty and hunger.

Despite economic advances, poverty persists in all Latin American and Caribbean countries. The main elements that have caused existing high poverty rates include low growth rates, poor productivity, a limited pool of human capital, ineffective economic and social policies, and sometimes, the negative consequences of external factors.

Income often is used to measure poverty. MDG 1 proposes to reduce by half the percentage of persons earning under US$ 1 a day. For Latin America and the Caribbean, however, ECLAC establishes national indigence lines that consider the cost of purchasing a basic food basket. A broader definition, complementing the income definition, considers poverty as a human condition marked by the ongoing or chronic lack of resources, capabilities, options, security, and the power necessary to enjoy an adequate standard of living and other civil, cultural, economic, political, and social rights (7).

Indigence: A person is classified as "indigent" when the per capita income of the household in which he or she lives is below the "indigence line," or below the minimum income the members of a household must have in order to purchase the cost of a basic food basket, taking into consideration consumption habits, the effective availability of foodstuffs and their relative prices, as well as the differences between metropolitan areas, other urban areas, and rural areas.

Poverty: A person is classified as "poor" when the per capita income of the household in which he or she lives falls below the "poverty line"—or the minimum income the members of a household must have in order to meet their basic needs. To calculate the total value of the poverty line, the indigence line is multiplied by a constant factor of 2 for urban areas and 1.75 for rural areas. Poverty lines are expressed in each country's currency and are based on the calculation of the cost of a particular basket of goods and services, employing the "cost of basic needs" method.

According to the most recent calculations, the monthly equivalent in dollars of the poverty line varies between US$ 45 and US$ 157 in urban areas and between US$ 32 and US$ 98 in rural areas; the figure for indigence lines varies between US$ 23 and US$ 79 in urban areas and between US$ 18 and US$ 56 in rural areas (in all cases, the lowest values correspond to Bolivia and the highest to Mexico).

Source: Economic Commission for Latin America and the Caribbean (ECLAC), Social Panorama of Latin America 2006.

FIGURE 8. Indigence and poverty rates (A) and numbers of indigent and poor persons (B), Latin America and the Caribbean, 1980–2006.

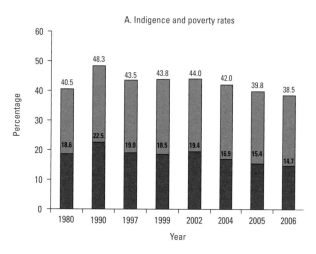

A. Indigence and poverty rates

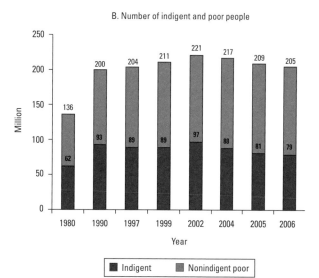

B. Number of indigent and poor people

Source: ECLAC. Social panorama of Latin America 2006.

FIGURE 9. Poverty and indigence rates, Latin America and the Caribbean, most recent available estimates.

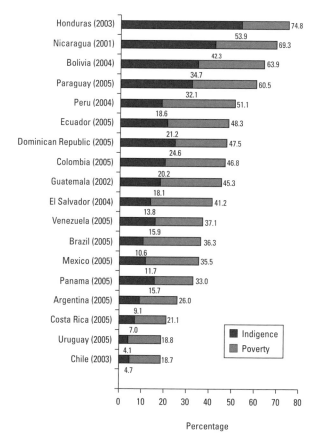

Source: Economic Commission for Latin America and the Caribbean. Social Panorama of Latin America 2006. Statistical Annex.

According to ECLAC estimates, there were significant reductions in poverty and indigence rates in Latin America and the Caribbean between 2002 and 2006. Over that period, the percentage of people living in poverty fell from 44% to 38.5% and the figures for indigence fell from 19.4% to 14.7%. In terms of numbers of poor and indigent, it is estimated that in 2006, 205 million people lived in poverty and 79 million in indigence (*8*) (Figure 8, A and B).

Moreover, the poverty rate is almost twice as high in rural areas as in urban ones and the indigence rate is almost triple.

With continuous migration to cities, however, the number of poor and indigent people continues to rise in urban areas.

ECLAC considers that the 2003–2006 period saw the best performance in social issues in the last 25 years. In 2006, the poverty rate fell below 1980 levels for the first time (*9*). In terms of progress toward MDG 1 and its goal of reducing indigence by half between 1990 and 2015, the estimated figures for 2006 indicate 68% progress for Latin America and the Caribbean (*9*).

In Latin American and Caribbean countries, however, poverty and indigence figures for 2002–2005 vary significantly. Despite progress made, several countries still have poverty levels above 60% (see Figure 9).

These results should be viewed with caution, given that they are national averages and can mask significant inequalities between different population groups or between geographic areas within the countries.

Poverty also expresses itself in terms of unsatisfied basic needs, including a lack of access to education (in terms of enrollment and number of completed years), housing (in quality and available per capita space), and certain public services (potable water, basic sanitation, and electricity).

Unlike changes in household income that come about as a result of changes in the economy, improvements in unmet basic needs come more slowly. According to ECLAC, in Latin America and the Caribbean the two most frequent unmet needs that affect more than 30% of the countries' population are the housing shortage, measured by the percentage of overcrowded houses (ranging from 5% in Uruguay to 70% in Nicaragua) and the lack of appropriate waste disposal systems in rural areas (ranging from 8% in Chile to 83% in Guatemala). At least 10% of the Latin American population is affected by one or the other of these needs (2).

Poverty is a determinant of health; moreover, poor health is both a cause and a consequence of poverty. Disease can reduce family finances, learning capacity, productivity, and quality of life, leading to the onset or perpetuation of poverty. In turn, poor people lack adequate nutrition and are more exposed to individual and environmental health risks and have fewer possibilities of gaining access to pertinent information and treatment. In short, the poor are at greater risk of disease and disability than other population groups.

Hunger and Undernutrition

One of the targets of MDG 1 is to reduce by half, between 1990 and 2015, the percentage of people who suffer from hunger. Two of the indicators for this target deal with nutrition. Indicator 4 measures "the prevalence of underweight children under 5 years of age" and indicator 5 evaluates the "proportion of population below the minimum level of dietary energy consumption." Undernutrition is as powerful a determinant of health as poverty, and, in most cases, poverty causes undernutrition. Large segments of the population experience social exclusion, having limited possibilities of living a healthy and productive life and, therefore, limited possibilities of escaping from poverty. Undernutrition is one of the leading ways that poverty and inequality get passed on from generation to generation. Undernourishment affects 10% of the Latin American and Caribbean population. Between 1990 and 2003, the number of undernourished persons in Latin America fell from 59

million to 52 million, which means that the region is moving apace toward MDG 1. Progress is uneven, however; most of the advances are concentrated in South America and the Caribbean, while increases in both numbers and in prevalence are observed in Central America (10).

According to ECLAC, between 1990 and 2003, the percentage of the Latin American and Caribbean population that suffered from undernutrition fell from 13% to 10%. Over the same period, out of 24 countries with available information, only 5 had been able to reach the goal of reducing hunger by half, achieving the target set for 2015. Nine other countries made significant progress, with about a 60% reduction in undernutrition compared to 1990. Another six, although they also made some progress, will not attain the 2015 goal (Figure 10). In the period in question, undernourishment increased in three countries (10).

Nutritional deficiencies have an impact throughout life, but their effects are more harmful during the early years. The development of human capacity requires adequate nutrition from early infancy. Undernutrition hampers the intellectual and physical development of children, placing them at multiple physical and cognitive disadvantages later on in life.

According to Food and Agriculture Organization (FAO) figures, in Latin American and Caribbean countries there are great differences in the percentage of persons who are unable to cover their minimum dietary energy requirements, with extremes ranging from 2% in Argentina, Barbados, and Cuba to 47% in Haiti (Figure 11). Overall, this situation also is reflected in the levels of underweight (low weight-for-age) among children under 5 years old, which ranges from 0.7% in Chile to 22.7% in Guatemala (Figure 12).

Undernutrition is the most direct consequence of hunger and has a series of negative effects on health, education and, over time, on a country's productivity and economic growth. Undernutrition makes individuals more vulnerable to various diseases and affects their survival. Undernourished children are more likely to become ill, which means that they often enroll late in the education system and are absent from school more often. Micronutrient deficiencies, particularly deficiencies in iron, zinc, iodine, and vitamin A, are linked to cognitive deterioration, which translates into decreased learning. These disadvantages, com-

---

Undernourishment: Food intake that is insufficient to meet dietary energy requirements continuously.

Undernutrition: The result of undernourishment, poor absorption and/or poor biological use of nutrients consumed.

Malnutrition: An abnormal physiological condition caused by deficiencies, excesses, or imbalances in energy, protein, and/or other nutrients.

Source: FAO glossary, available at http://www.fivims.net/glossary.

FIGURE 10. Trends in the rate of undernourishment, in terms of progress (%) towards MDG 1—which proposes to eradicate extreme poverty and hunger by 2015—Latin America and the Caribbean and selected countries, from 1990–1992 to 2000–2002.

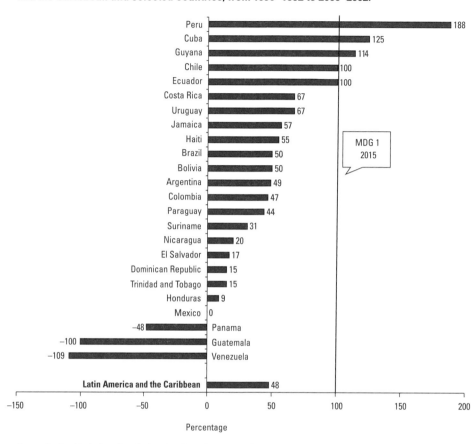

Source: Food and Agriculture Organization of the United Nations. The State of Food Insecurity in the World 2004.

pounded over the life cycle, can result in adults who cannot develop to their maximum intellectual or physical potential, nor reach their productive potential.

Unemployment

Employment is a basic health determinant that acts in various ways. Access to labor markets is a contextual determinant, income is a structural determinant, and labor conditions are intermediate determinants. Sustainable employment is crucial if Latin American and Caribbean countries are to reduce poverty and reach MDG 1.

Between 1995 and 2005, the unemployment rate[2] in Latin America and the Caribbean held steady at about 10%, while the employment rate tended to decline up to 2002, after which it began

to rise again (Figure 13). Employment in the informal sector represents a very high percentage of total employment, as does the informal economy's contribution to GDP (Figure 14).

The main disadvantages of working in the economy's informal sector include lack of access to social welfare and pension benefits, which leaves these workers vulnerable to unforeseen events such as serious illnesses, accidents, loss of income, or death. In 2005, 58.9% of the employed urban population in Latin America had health protection and/or pensions. However, informal workers continue to experience coverage rates that are significantly lower than those for the employed taken as a whole, since just 33.4% of them are covered by some kind of health protection and/or pension plan (11).

Juvenile unemployment is another expression of social exclusion in many Latin American and Caribbean countries. Youths' inability to find work leads to feelings of marginalization and uselessness and can contribute to their involvement in illegal activities. Furthermore, for many youths, not having a job means

---

[2]Number of persons who are not working, are available to work, or are seeking work, as a percentage of the total labor force.

FIGURE 11. Percentage of persons living below the minimum dietary energy level, Latin American and Caribbean countries, 2001–2003.

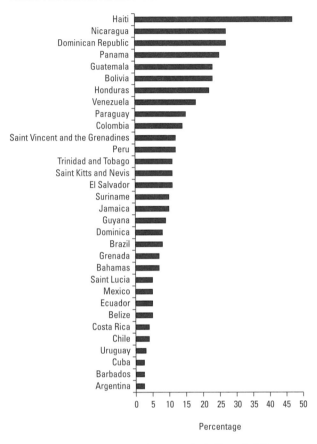

Percentage

Source: Economic Commission for Latin America and the Caribbean. Social Panorama of Latin America 2006.

FIGURE 12. Percentage of underweight (low weight-for-age) children under 5 years old, selected Latin American and Caribbean countries, most recent year available.

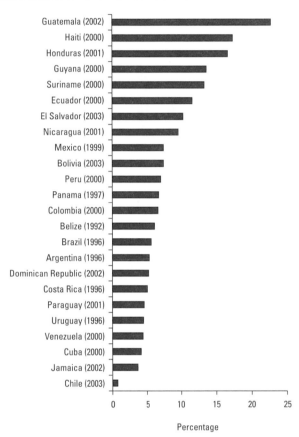

Percentage

Source: Economic Commission for Latin America and the Caribbean. Social Panorama of Latin America 2006. Statistical Annex.

not having the chance to escape from poverty, which helps to perpetuate the needs they have experienced practically since they were born. According to ECLAC, in 2003–2004, the unemployment rate among youths 15–24 years old in Latin America and the Caribbean averaged 19.6% for males and 26.2% for females. These figures were much higher than in 1990 (11.5% and 13.9%, respectively) (*12*).

Figure 15 shows the wide variations seen in youth unemployment in Latin American and Caribbean countries. In every case except for El Salvador, unemployment is higher among females than males. In Argentina, the unemployment rate is almost the same for both sexes, although the figures are high: one out of every three youths in Argentina is unemployed. Unemployment among males 15–24 years old ranges from a minimum of 5.6% in Mexico to a maximum of 34.1% in Uruguay, while the figures for females range from 7.6% in Mexico to just over 41% in Colombia and Uruguay. For the most recent year for which information is available, the average unemployment rate among females

15–24 years old is more than 8% higher than the rate for males in the same age group.

These figures often refer to urban or metropolitan areas, or only reflect open unemployment, failing to consider other aspects such as underemployment or employment in the informal sector, which is extremely high in some countries. Employment figures among youths do not take into account the quality of work or whether it pays sufficient wages or provides social protection mechanisms to enable young people to escape poverty.

Target 16 of MDG 8 refers to youth unemployment, extending the commitment to, "in cooperation with developing countries, develop and implement strategies for decent and productive work for youth." This commitment is consistent with the quest for labor conditions that will produce good health for future generations. And yet, according to data reported by the International Labor Organization (ILO), the percentage of underemployed youths is increasing, with some working for fewer hours than they would like and others working long hours without fair compensation (*13*).

43

FIGURE 13. Unemployment and employment rates (%), Latin America and the Caribbean, 1995–2005.

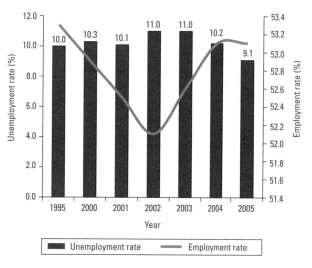

Source: Economic Commission on Latin America and the Caribbean. Economic Study of Latin America and the Caribbean, 2005–2006, p. 85. 2006.

Access to Education

The relationship between education and poverty is clear, particularly the relationship between years of schooling and extreme poverty. The poorest children have fewer opportunities for completing primary school, and by failing to do so they replicate the conditions of extreme poverty that halted their education in the first place. Given these circumstances, MDG 2 proposes the at-

tainment of universal primary education as a strategy for combating poverty.

The impact of education on the productive potential and income prospects of individuals has been widely documented (*14*). Many studies have also linked the amount of education to the health of individuals and that of their families. Figure 16 shows the relationship between the mother's years of schooling and infant mortality. The link between education and health problems and conditions such as maternal mortality, HIV/AIDS, obesity, and various lifestyle problems also has been proven (*15*).

Given the key role that education plays in the distribution of opportunities for well-being, particularly its impact on health, it is fundamental to pursue an approach to achieving the MDGs that is comprehensive, synergistic, and indivisible. Progress has clearly been made in attaining universal public education (*16*)— Latin American and Caribbean primary-school enrollment rates have increased, on average, from 86.2% in 1990 to 91.5% in 2004 (Figure 17). Yet, inequity in access by the most vulnerable groups and disparities within countries continue to be the greatest challenge in education.

An ECLAC analysis in 2002 found that at least one in four youths 15–19 years old from the poorest 20% of Latin American and Caribbean households failed to complete primary school. The same study indicated that the opportunities for completing primary school for children in rural areas are much lower than for children in urban areas, and that there also were significant differences in primary school completion rates between indigenous and nonindigenous populations, particularly in Bolivia, Brazil, Ecuador, Guatemala, Nicaragua, Panama, and Paraguay (*9*).

FIGURE 14. Urban employment in the informal sector and contribution of the informal economy to the GDP, selected Latin American countries, 2003–2005.

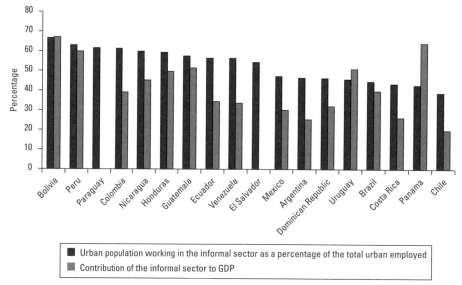

Sources: Economic Commission for Latin America and the Caribbean. ECLAC Review 88. 2006; World Bank, Doing Business Database.

FIGURE 15. Unemployment rate among 15–24-year-olds, by sex.

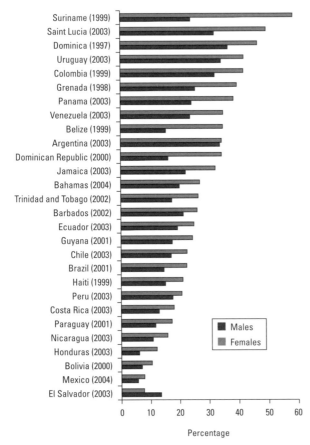

Percentage

Source: United Nations Statistics Division. Available from: http://mdgs.un.org/unsd/mdg/data.

One of the greatest challenges for reducing poverty, and one that has an impact on health determinants, is the educational lag in adults. Based on the 2000 round of censuses, in 2005 UNESCO estimated that 9.5% of the population older than 15 years old in 28 Latin American and Caribbean countries was illiterate, with figures of 8.8% for men and 10.3% for women (*17*). Although significant progress was made in attending to this priority group, wide gaps remain between countries, as shown in Figure 18. In Guatemala, Haiti, Honduras, and Nicaragua more than 20% of the adult population is illiterate and in Bolivia, Brazil, the Dominican Republic, El Salvador, and Jamaica more than 10% of the population is illiterate.

Inequities in Health Conditions

Inequities are inequalities that are described as and considered to be unfair and avoidable. Consequently, actions to reduce inequities in health seek to correct the injustice that poor health conditions of the most vulnerable groups represent. Inequality in health is a generic term used to designate differences, variations, and disparities in the population's health status. Most inequities in health between social groups (differences by class or race, for example) reflect an unfair distribution of social determinants of health (*16*).

The average health status in Latin America and the Caribbean is relatively good. However, an examination within subregions and within countries reveals inequities. Inequities in access to health services manifest themselves as wide gaps in subregional health indicators, some of which are exemplified in Table 4. In addition, inequities within countries are very pronounced. In a group of selected countries (Bolivia, Brazil, Colombia, Guatemala, Haiti, Nicaragua, Paraguay, and Peru) 34% of the poorest quintile

FIGURE 16. Trends in infant mortality rates, by level of schooling of the mother, selected Latin American and Caribbean countries, 1986–2003.

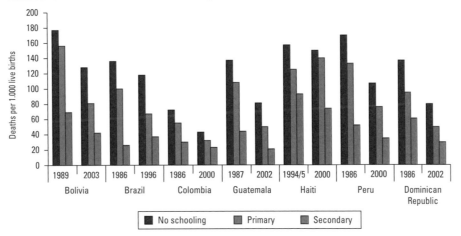

Source: Economic Commission for Latin America and the Caribbean. Millennium Development Goals: a Latin American and Caribbean Perspective. 2005.

FIGURE 17. Net primary-school enrollment rates, selected Latin American and Caribbean countries, 2004.

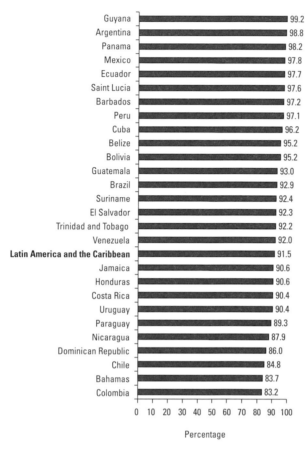

FIGURE 18. Trends in illiteracy rates, population older than 15 years of age, Latin America and the Caribbean and selected countries in the region, 2005.

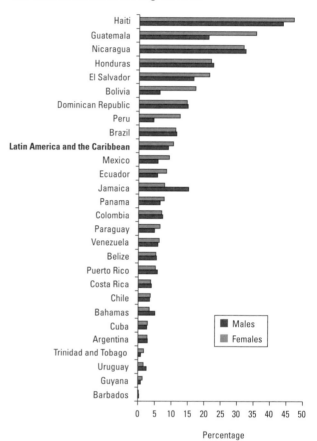

Source: Economic Commission for Latin America and the Caribbean. Social Panorama of Latin America, 2006. Statistical Annex.

Source: UNESCO-IEU. Online database.

and 94% of the wealthiest quintile have access to health care services (Table 5).

These levels of inequality in access translate into yawning gaps in health indicators, such as childhood malnutrition and maternal mortality. For the same group of eight countries, the simple average for undernutrition in children in the poorest quintile is 6.3 times higher than in the richest quintile. There are also large differences between countries, with the quotient ranging from 3.6 in the least unequal cases to 10.1% in countries with the greatest inequality. In Bolivia, for example, the percentage of births attended by health care professionals (an indicator for MDG 5) in 1998 was just 39% in the poorest quintile, compared to 95% in the richest. Moreover, the percentage of children 0–2 years old who were immunized against diphtheria, tetanus, and polio in the richest quintile is 9% higher than that in the poorest quintile (*18*).

The World Bank's concentration index (*1*) shows that in several Latin American countries, the greatest inequities in health

are concentrated in the poorest households.[3] For mortality in children under 5, the concentration index worldwide in 2002 was –0.12; it was –0.17 for Latin America, meaning that it was more concentrated in the poorest households there than in the rest of the world. The index was even higher in Brazil, Bolivia, and Peru, for –0.26, –0.25, and –0.22, respectively. In terms of underweight, Latin America again had a concentration index that was farther from zero than did the rest of the world (–0.28, while the global index was –0.17), with extremes such as the Dominican Republic and Peru with –0.44 and –0.40, respectively. Brazil, Paraguay, and Peru had values farthest away from zero in the prevalence rates for diarrheal diseases. In indicators such as the coverage of

---

[3] The concentration index is a measurement for determining the degree to which a variable is distributed unequally along the income profile of a population. Aspects such as infant mortality ("bad") produce a negative concentration index and aspects such as immunization ("good") produce a positive value. A concentration index of zero indicates absolute equity.

TABLE 4. Selected health indicators: worldwide; Latin America and the Caribbean; and Bolivia, Guatemala, Guyana, Haiti, Honduras, and Peru.

Indicator	World average	Latin America and Caribbean average	Countries with the greatest difference from Latin America and Caribbean average
Infant mortality rate[a]	54	27	Haiti 74 Bolivia 54 Guyana 48
Mortality rate among children under 5 years[b]	79	31	Haiti 117 Bolivia 69 Guyana 64
Percent childbirths attended by trained personnel	62	88	Haiti 24 Guatemala 41 Honduras 56
Maternal mortality rate[c]	410	194	Haiti 680 Bolivia 420 Peru 410

[a]Number of deaths among children under 12 months for every 1,000 live births.
[b]Number of deaths among children under 5 years for every 1,000 live births.
[c]Number of women per 100,000 who die from complications during pregnancy or delivery, according to the estimation model.
Sources: World Bank (2006) World Development Indicators Database 2004 and PAHO (2006) Regional Core Health Data Initiative.

TABLE 5. Access to health care services, by income quintile, selected countries in Latin America and the Caribbean, 1996.

Country	Average	1 (poorest)	2	3	4	5 (richest)
Bolivia	56.7	19.8	44.8	67.7	87.9	97.9
Brazil	87.7	71.6	88.7	95.7	97.7	98.6
Colombia	84.5	60.6	85.2	92.8	98.9	98.1
Guatemala	34.8	9.3	16.1	31.1	62.8	91.5
Haiti	46.3	24.0	37.3	47.4	60.7	78.2
Nicaragua	64.6	32.9	58.8	79.8	86.0	92.3
Paraguay	66.0	41.2	49.9	69.0	87.9	98.1
Peru	56.4	14.3	49.6	75.4	87.2	96.7

Source: Inter-American Development Bank (2004). Millennium Development Goals in Latin America and the Caribbean, p. 139.

basic universal vaccination plans, prenatal care, and assistance during childbirth by trained personnel, Latin America had concentration indexes that indicate that these "good" conditions are concentrated in the richest households more frequently than in the rest of the world.

For all the indicators analyzed, Latin America had concentration indexes farther away from zero than did the rest of the world, which is consistent with the findings of a study on socioeconomic inequality that indicated that Latin America appeared systematically as the most inequitable region on the planet (*19*).

Gender, Ethnic, and Racial Inequities

One of the most important social determinants in public health is inequity in access to goods and services. When examining these inequalities from the standpoint of gender, ethnic group, and race in Latin America and the Caribbean, it can be seen that poor women, indigenous people, and Afro-descendents are at a disadvantage in terms of access to health services.

Autonomy for women and gender equality are acknowledged to be key objectives in the Millennium Declaration. For Latin American and Caribbean countries, the pursuit of equity and the

TABLE 6. Estimates of the indigenous population as a percentage of the total population, selected countries of the Americas.

Percent of total population	Total indigenous population		
	<100,000	100,000 to 500,000	>500,000
More than 40%			Peru Guatemala Bolivia Ecuador
5%–40%	Guyana Belize Suriname	El Salvador Nicaragua Panama	Mexico Chile Honduras
Under 5%	Costa Rica Guyana Jamaica Dominica	Argentina Brazil Paraguay Venezuela	Canada Colombia United States

Sources: Reports on the Evaluation of the International Decade of the Indigenous Peoples of the World, PAHO, 2004. Hall G, Patrinos AH. Indigenous Peoples, Poverty and Human Development in Latin America: 1994–2004. Washington, DC: World Bank, 2005. Montenegro R, Stephens C. Indigenous Health in Latin America and the Caribbean [Indigenous Health 2]. Lancet 2006; 367:1859–69.

provision of culturally sensitive services for indigenous peoples and communities of African descent is a social debt that can no longer be postponed; an effective means to combat poverty, hunger, and disease; and a way to stimulate truly sustainable development (*10*). Because these are cross-cutting objectives, the adoption of policies that take into consideration gender, ethnic, and racial issues will contribute to attain all the MDGs, because the goals are related to the development of capabilities (education, health, nutrition); access to resources and opportunities (jobs, income, property rights, political participation); and security (protection from violence and abuse).

In Latin America and the Caribbean, cultural diversity is largely determined by the existence of some 40 million indigenous people, who represent more than 10% of the total population (see Table 6). There are about 400 different ethnic groups, each with a different language, view of the world, and social organization, as well as different forms of economic organization and modes of production responsive to their ecosystems (*20*). As shown in Table 7, different countries of the Americas face major challenges related to health care for indigenous populations. The Inter-American Development Bank (IDB) estimates that in countries where household surveys are broken down by ethnic group, up to one-fourth of the difference in income levels can be attributed simply to the fact of belonging to an indigenous or Afro-Latin ethnic group (*21*).

Causes of Inequity in Access to Essential Health Care Resources

Women, particularly indigenous women, suffer most from the consequences of poverty. In Bolivia, for example, illiteracy is highly concentrated among the indigenous women, affecting one out of four women over the age of 35. The same holds true in Peru, where indigenous women who are heads of households have 4.6 fewer years of schooling than nonindigenous women (*22*).

When society ascribes a domestic role to women, it limits women's opportunities to participate in the productive arena; the lack of recognition of the economic and social worth of women's work at work and at home is the root of gender inequity.

While indicators relating to women's education have shown progress, such is not the case for indicators of women's participation in the labor or political arenas. Women participate in the workforce less than men, and although the figure for urban women in Latin America rose from 37.9% to 49.7% between 1990 and 2002, the difference with men's participation averaged more than 30% for the period (*23*). Urban males' participation in the workforce ranged from 71% (Uruguay, 2004) to 83% (Venezuela, 2003 and Nicaragua, 2001), while the figures for women ranged from 45% (Costa Rica, 2004 and Chile, 2003) to 57% (Bolivia, 2002; Colombia, 2002; and Paraguay, 2000) (*2*).

Unemployment is higher among women in all Latin American countries, except for El Salvador, Mexico, Nicaragua, and Peru. In the Dominican Republic, open unemployment among urban males was 13% in 2003; for women, the figure was 31% (*2*). Women also earn less then men, and in Latin America they are paid 35% less, on average (*2*). In 2002, women earned 58% of what men earned in Guatemala and 77% in Colombia (*23*). Figure 19 shows the average income of women compared to men.

In Latin America and the Caribbean, the percentage of women working in the economy's informal sector and at part-time jobs is higher than for men. One of the reasons is that women seek to make their domestic and labor responsibilities compatible. But both informal and part-time jobs tend to receive less protection or to be left out of social security coverage and health insurance plans. In 2002, the average percentage of urban women working in low productivity sectors (informal sector) was 56%, while the figure for men was 48% (*2*). This difference is greater in Bolivia (76.7% and 58.5%, respectively) and in Peru (71.7% and 56.7%, respectively) (*24*).

During the 1990s, 40% of women and 20% of men worked part time in Argentina; 33% of women and 12% of men worked part time in Venezuela; and 41% of women and 17% of men worked part time in Bolivia (*25*).

Indigenous people and descendants of Africans tend to work at low-paying jobs, mainly in the informal economy, which means that they lack social protection and health insurance. Their work often entails health risks. In Bolivia, according to a 2000 study, indigenous people work at 67% of insecure jobs and 28% of semi-skilled jobs. Just 4% of indigenous workers have jobs that require

TABLE 7. Health care challenges for indigenous peoples.

Poverty

Ecuador. In rural zones in the sierra and the Amazon, which are areas with indigenous populations, it is estimated that 76% of children are poor (PAHO, 1998).

Illiteracy

Peru. In the Peruvian Amazon, 7.3% have no schooling whatsoever, compared with 32% in indigenous communities (INEI-UNICEF, 1997).

Unemployment

El Salvador. Unemployment among the indigenous population is 24% (PAHO, 2002).

Undernutrition

Guatemala. The chronic undernutrition rate is 67.8% among indigenous peoples and 36.7% among nonindigenous (PAHO, 2002).

HIV/AIDS

Honduras. Garífunas and English-speaking groups are most affected by HIV/AIDS (PAHO, 2002).

Basic services

El Salvador. Among the indigenous population, 33% has electricity, while 64% use candles; 91.6% drink river water or well water (PAHO, 2002).

Ethnic and cultural heterogeneity

Brazil. The indigenous population is estimated to be 350,000 persons belonging to nearly 210 different groups who speak 170 languages. Although they constitute 0.2% of the total population, indigenous people are present in 24 of the 26 states (PAHO, 2003).

Infant mortality

Mexico. The infant mortality rate among indigenous children was 59 per 1,000 live births in 1997, which is twice as high as the national rate (PAHO, 2002).

Maternal mortality

Honduras. The national average for maternal mortality is 147 deaths per 100,000 live births. In the departments of Colón, Copán, Intibucá, Lempira, and La Paz, which are areas with indigenous populations, the maternal mortality rate fluctuates between 255 and 190 deaths per 100,000 live births (PAHO, 1999).

Infectious diseases

Nicaragua: The municipalities affected by sickle-cell trait are located in the autonomous regions on the Atlantic coast, which is where indigenous people and Afro-descendents live (PAHO-NIC, 2003).

Diabetes, obesity, alcoholism

United States. The indigenous population has a far greater probability of dying from liver disease related to alcohol abuse that the general population (PAHO, 2003).

Suicide

Canada. The suicide rate is two to seven times higher among the indigenous population than the general population and is a cause of concern, particularly among young males in Inuit communities (PAHO, 2002).

Location

Indigenous populations are generally scattered, sometimes are on the move, and are difficult to reach; they mostly live in rural, marginal urban, and border areas. Several indigenous peoples are multinational, such as the Miskito of **Nicaragua** and **Honduras** and the Quechua of **Colombia, Ecuador, Peru, Bolivia, Argentina** (PAHO, 2002).

Culturally appropriate care

In the evaluation of essential public health functions, function 8 (human resources development and training in public health) ranks poorly in Latin America and the Caribbean (38%); the component for providing culturally sensitive care also rates poorly (17%) (PAHO, 2002).

Source: PAHO (2003) Health of indigenous peoples initiative. Strategic directions and plan of action 2003–2007.

higher skills. In 2000, one out of every five indigenous workers in Chile had a temporary job. In Guatemala, 81% of indigenous people worked in the informal economy (*26*)

Unemployment is also higher among indigenous people and Afro-descendents. In Brazil, unemployment is higher among Afro-descendents than among whites (13.8% for Afro-descendent women and 8.4% for men). In 2001, average wages earned by black women were 53% of white women's (*27*).

Women, indigenous people, and Afro-descendents have less access to social benefits and long-term health care plans. Also, given their roles in childbearing and in child rearing and because culturally they are the main caregivers for the elderly and the chronically ill, women experience more breaks in their work history, which diminishes their access to insurance. The gap in contributions between men and women is extremely large and widens with age in every Latin American country. On average, in 2002 among 15–64-year-olds, 19% of women and 32% of men, on average, made contributions to the social security system in 2002 (*23*). These factors translate into pensions for women at age 65 that are equivalent, on average, to 77% of the pensions received by men (*23*).

FIGURE 19. Average income of women compared to men, selected Latin American and Caribbean countries, most recent year for which information is available.

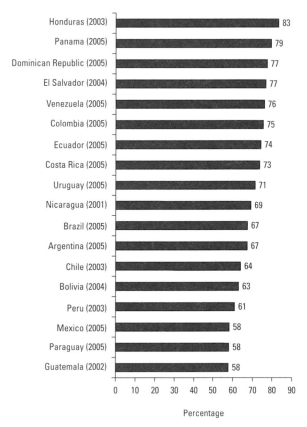

Percentage

Source: Economic Commission for Latin America and the Caribbean. Social Panorama of Latin America 2006. Statistical Annex.

Health and Equity in Gender, Ethnicity, and Race

Analyzing health status from the gender equity standpoint underlines conditions and problems that: (a) are exclusive to one sex or the other; (b) respond differently to risks by sex; (c) affect men and women differently; and (d) can be avoided. The categories that usually respond to these criteria are: sexual and reproductive health (fertility regulation, teenage pregnancy, maternal health, HIV/AIDS and other sexually transmitted infections); malignant neoplasms (breast and uterine cancer, prostate cancer, lung cancer); and several conditions that present clear differences by sex in prevalence and risks, such as accidents and violence (murder, suicide, violence against women), diseases of the circulatory system, nutritional problems, diabetes, and cirrhosis of the liver.

In all Latin American and Caribbean countries, women have longer life expectancy at birth and lower mortality than men in all age groups, except in the perinatal period and early infancy—in the Americas, women live an average of 5.9 years longer than men. The advantage ranges from 7 years longer in Argentina,

Brazil, and Uruguay and 1.3 years longer in Haiti. Women's greater longevity means that they are the majority of older adults. Women account for 56% of the population over 60 years old in Latin America and the Caribbean (*28*).

Women's greater longevity does not necessarily mean a better quality of life, however. Estimates of healthy life expectancy expressed in years of life free from disability indicate that differences by sex tend to be smaller when quality of life is included in the consideration. In the Americas, figures show that the gap in healthy life expectancy between men and women removes almost two years from the life expectancy at birth figure, and this difference is proportionally higher in the poorer countries (*29*). PAHO's SABE-2000 survey shows that in seven Latin American and Caribbean cities, the frequency of disability among persons 60 years old and older was 27% to 52% higher for women than for men (*30*). Although they live longer, women experience more illness and disability than men throughout their lives. This differential is more pronounced in cases of acute conditions and short-term disability during the reproductive years, and in chronic conditions and disabilities in the elderly. In contrast, men experience fewer illnesses and disabilities, but their health problems, when they occur, tend to be lethal (*31*).

There are also differences between the life expectancy figures of indigenous populations compared and those of nonindigenous persons, as well as between Afro-descendents and whites. A study conducted in Mexico comparing indigenous and non-indigenous municipalities found that in 1900–1996, indigenous Mexicans lived for 64 years and nonindigenous, for 68 (*32*). In Brazil, life expectancy in 2000 was 71 years for whites and 64 years for blacks (*27*).

The nature and size of the gender gaps related to length and quality of life vary substantially depending on the socioeconomic and the cultural contexts. WHO documented an example of the interaction between gender and socioeconomic inequality in 13 Latin American countries by estimating the risk of premature death (death between 15 and 59 years old) for poor and non-poor men and women (*33*). Calculation of the ratio for the risk of premature mortality between poor and non-poor persons showed the impact of poverty on the probability of survival of men and women. In 1990, in 10 Latin American and Caribbean countries, the risk of premature death among poor men was 2 to 5 times higher than that for non-poor men; for poor women, the same risk was 4 to 12 times higher than for non-poor women.

Women older than 60 years of age are the majority of the older adult population, and they also are one of the most vulnerable groups in society. These women are affected by loneliness, poverty, disease, and a lack of social and economic benefits. Women living longer means that that they experience higher rates of widowhood and years lived without a partner. In addition, the cumulative effect of their diminished participation in the workforce, lower wages and, consequently, lower contributions to retirement systems during their lives, means that women reach

FIGURE 20. Unmet contraception needs among women and adolescents with no schooling, selected Latin American countries, most recent year for which information is available.

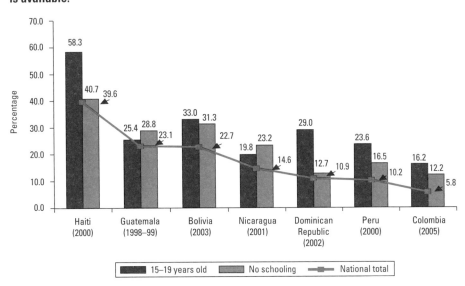

Source: Demographic and health surveys performed in each country.

old age at a disadvantage, not just in economic terms, but also in terms of their entitlements to health and social security benefits.

Gender and Access to Health Care

Inequities in access to health services vary by socioeconomic stratum and age and by type of service. In some poor countries and in low-income sectors, women's use of services for illness or injury deviates from the norm and is lower than men's. In terms of age, women in their childbearing years use services more than men; in some countries, the percentages of boys and girls who received treatment for illnesses revealed that when showing symptoms of fever, acute respiratory infection, or diarrhea, boys were brought to medical services more often than girls (*34*). Evidence shows that women tend to use preventive services more, while men resort to emergency services more often (*34*).

Information on the use of health services based on the specific needs of each sex has not been widely systematized and available data tend to relate to women's reproductive health services, for example:

Contraception. In 2000–2005, more than 60% of Latin American and Caribbean women regulated their fertility with modern contraceptive methods. Access to those methods is highly uneven, however, and disparities are tied to a given country's socioeconomic context, the national reproductive health policies, education, socioeconomic stratum, rural or urban residence, and a woman's ethnic origin. Another relevant inequality is related to distribution by sex of the respon-

sibility for obtaining and using modern contraceptive techniques, which women bear in 84% to 98% of cases (*35*).

Family planning. The unmet-needs index in family planning for a group of countries shows that the percentage of women with unmet contraceptive needs ranged from a minimum of 5.8% in Colombia (2005) to a maximum of 40.7% in Haiti (2000) (Figure 20). The highest levels of unmet demand were among adolescent women (17% to 58%), women with less education (13% to 41%), indigenous women (39%), and women living in rural areas (8% to 40%) (*36*).

Births delivered by qualified personnel. Although 91.4% of births in the Americas were delivered by qualified personnel, about 7 out of every 10 births in Guatemala (2004) and Haiti (2000) and 4 out of every 10 in Bolivia (1999–2003) received no qualified care (*37*). This indicator also reveals inequalities: in Ecuador, just 30% of deliveries among indigenous women were seen by qualified personnel, while 86% of white women and 80% of mixed-race women received such assistance (*38*).

Gender Equity and Health Care Financing

Gender inequity in access to health care services also is linked to how health care is financed. Systems that do not have solidarity-based financing place a disproportionate burden on women, since their more frequent need for care (particularly because of the reproductive function) means that women use more health services and spend more on them. Information from household surveys shows that in Chile, private insurance premiums for persons in childbearing age were 2.5 times higher for women than for men (39), and in Brazil, the Dominican Republic, Ecuador, Paraguay, and Peru, out-of-pocket spending on health care was between 16% and 60% higher for women (40). Given women's diminished economic capabilities, this absolute inequality in spending restricts their access to basic services or imposes a disproportionate financial burden on them.

Health care coverage for indigenous people is much lower than for non-indigenous groups. In Bolivia, where coverage rates are low, 10% of indigenous people are covered by the public system and 2% have private coverage. In Mexico, close to 45% of the population has health coverage, but just 18% of the indigenous population is covered. In Peru, access to health coverage is extremely low for the indigenous and the non-indigenous population alike, and 55% of Peruvians have no coverage at all. Close to 42% of Peruvians have public health coverage and just 1.1% of indigenous and 2.8% of non-indigenous have access to private plans (41).

THE ENVIRONMENTAL CONTEXT

Urban Growth

Latin America and the Caribbean have the highest rate of urbanization in the developing world: 77% of the population (433 million people) lives in cities, and projections suggest that the figure will rise to 81% by 2030.

Although urban settings have been recognized historically as a favorable health determinant, the unplanned urban growth currently occurring in the developing world can threaten health. The rapid growth of cities seriously affects the environment and the social context, and has detrimental consequences for the population's quality of life and health. Haphazard urban expansion, particularly in suburban areas, leaves the urban population's poorest sectors living in sites that are highly vulnerable to natural disasters and have limited access to basic services such as housing, electricity, drinking water, drainage, and solid waste removal. Violence and marginalization are growing at alarming rates.

Green spaces, recreational areas, and sports grounds that foster physical activity and entertainment and that strengthen the sense of community are increasingly scarce or nonexistent in large cities, particularly in marginal areas. Vast urban areas with scant natural spaces have produced so-called "hot zones," which can create conditions that favor infestations of disease-transmitting vectors. Finally, environmental pollution problems are aggravated by rapid economic development and industrialization in cities, and are associated with delays in adopting effective air pollution control measures.

The health repercussions from unplanned urban growth are manifested in an important group of infectious diseases (diarrhea, dengue, respiratory infections), chronic diseases (cancer, diabetes, obesity, cardiovascular problems), and accidents and injuries.

Access to Potable Water, Water Pollution, and Waste Disposal

Since ancient times, societies have acknowledged that water and sanitation are health determinants. Science has further demonstrated their causal relationship to health.

Although more than 90% of households in urban centers have access to water, there are large social and spatial inequities within cities. The cost of drinking water is rising, due to growing demand, to decreasing accessibility, and, particularly, to declining groundwater levels. Sewage treatment also is a major challenge in urban settings. In Latin America and the Caribbean, just 14% of sewage is adequately treated. Anecdotal evidence points to rising pollution of surface- and groundwater with nitrates and heavy metals, yet monitoring and systematic protection of water sources has only been introduced very recently, and it still is not a high priority on the research agenda. Water pollution has a significant impact on coastal areas, where 60 of the 77 major cities of Latin America and the Caribbean are located and 60% of the population lives (42).

Per capita solid waste production has doubled in the last 30 years and its composition has changed from waste that was fundamentally dense and organic to waste that is bulky and non-biodegradable. Almost 90% of the waste produced is collected, but more than 40% is not adequately disposed of and goes on to pollute land and water (43).

These services are extremely important for human health. In Latin America, mortality caused by infant diarrhea is a major consequence of the lack of water, poor quality water, and the lack of sanitation.

Air Pollution

Air quality is a basic determinant of health. Human beings take in oxygen from the atmosphere, and oxygen is one of the main elements that keep cells alive. Modern air pollution reduces the oxygen in the atmosphere, contaminating air and lungs.

Today, some mega cities, such as Mexico City and São Paulo, monitor and control air pollution from intensive use of fossil fuels in transportation and industry. Bogotá also has reduced air pollution from motor vehicles, but it still struggles to control emissions from several urban industries. Air pollution and its impact on health are rising in medium-sized and smaller cities, where resources and technologies for controlling it are less readily available. Indoor air pollution, which mainly affects poor urban dwellers who use biomass for cooking or heating, has an even lower profile on the urban agenda (42).

Although average per capita carbon dioxide emissions appear to have peaked in 1998 and have recently fallen, very few countries have improved their energy efficiency. Only one-third of Latin American countries have set air quality standards or emission limits. Urban sprawl has increased travel times and the demand for public transport, with an estimated combined cost of 6.5% of the region's GDP (43).

Air pollution contributes to infectious and chronic respiratory diseases, cancer, and cardiovascular disease. Air pollution seriously affects the health of 80 million people in Latin America and the Caribbean and is the primary cause of more than 2.3 million cases of respiratory insufficiency in children each year and more than 100,000 cases of chronic bronchitis in adults.

Shrinking Forests and Land Degradation

In the 1990s, 46.7 million hectares of forest were destroyed in Latin America and the Caribbean—half the global loss at twice the rate. Almost half of this loss occurred in Brazil. Unrestrained globalization, haphazard urbanization, and a lack of territorial planning are driving the conversion of forests into pastureland (to produce more livestock for export), an increase in monoculture plantations (including coca and soy), infrastructure growth (such as mega dam and road projects), and rising human settlements. Other pressures come from land speculation, wood harvesting (61.7% of the wood is used for fuel, mainly in Brazil and in Central America), and to meet demand for timber by Asian furniture industries that supply northern markets (44).

Deforestation depletes water sources and diminishes their quality; it increases soil erosion and the sedimentation of bodies of water, and is responsible for the severe decline or loss of biodiversity. Deforestation also is an important source of greenhouse gas emissions. Deforestation in Latin America and the Caribbean is responsible for 48.3% of total global carbon dioxide emissions.

Moreover, some 313 million hectares in Latin America and the Caribbean (15.7% of the territory) have been degraded (42). Degradation is more severe in Mesoamerica, affecting 26% of the territory; 14% is affected in South America (45). Erosion is the main culprit in degradation of the land, but the gradual intensification of agricultural production plays an important role in depleting nutrients from the soil and wind erosion also is significant in some areas. Desertification, which affects 25% of the territory, is largely determined by natural conditions, but also has been influenced by deforestation, overgrazing, and inadequate irrigation.

Shrinking forests and degraded land pose serious health risks, such as acute and chronic diseases caused by a lack of water, use of contaminated water, nutritional imbalances due to poor quality nutrients or their absence, and death and injury due to increased vulnerability to natural disasters.

Coastal Degradation and Ocean Pollution

Degraded coasts and polluted seas can harm health in various ways. More than half of the population in Latin America and the Caribbean lives within 100 km of the coast, compared to 38% globally (42). A 1996 estimate of global threats to coastal ecosystems indicates that 50% of South America's coast and 29% the coast in North and Central America was at moderate or high threat from cities, ports, and other sites with high population

> *The permanent denial of fundamental rights has led to the marginalization of the indigenous population, leading to alarming poverty rates, lack of land, low earnings, high unemployment, high rates of illiteracy especially among women, high rates of school dropouts, and an epidemiological profile with high rates of illnesses and premature death where preventable causes are predominant. The communities and municipalities with the highest percentage of indigenous population are those furthest from the goals set by the Millennium Declaration.*
>
> Mirta Roses, 2006

density (for example, tourism infrastructure), and oil or industrial pipelines (46). In the Caribbean, 61% of coral reefs are under moderate or high threat from sedimentation, marine- and land-based pollution sources, and overfishing. Coastal groundwater contamination (including salt-water intrusion) and depletion are occurring throughout the Region, taking an enormous economic toll (42).

Some 86% of sewage in Latin America and the Caribbean is dumped raw into rivers and oceans. In the Caribbean, the figure hits 90% (42). There is a high level of oil pollution from Greater Caribbean refineries, particularly in the Gulf of Mexico, and offshore drilling in the Gulf of Mexico and Brazil. Agrochemical runoff is also a source of pollution, and highly toxic concentrations have been found in Caribbean estuaries and in Colombia and Costa Rica. Shipping also contributes, with cargo volume doubling between 1970 and 2000. Hazardous waste, including radioactive materials from other regions of the world, is shipped around South America or through the Panama Canal. Many invasive species come in freight and ballast, such as crustaceans, mollusks, and insects that have inflicted great economic damage on infrastructure and crops.

Overfishing also is a matter of grave concern, particularly in the Caribbean. Estimates indicate that most central Caribbean local production systems are threatened by over-exploitation of commercially valuable species. The Caribbean deep-sea fishery peaked in 1994, accounting for nearly 28% of the global catch. Fish harvests in Peru and Chile, which represent most of the catch, doubled or tripled compared to the 1980s (47). Catch levels fell by 50% in 1998, however, although they climbed again by 2000, reaching 85% of the 1994 levels. These fluctuations are warnings of the dangers of overfishing.

The health effects of degraded coasts and polluted seas are seen in infectious diseases, injuries, and deaths caused by such factors as an increased vulnerability to natural disasters, malnutrition, and the violence associated with unemployment. Warm sea-surface temperatures promote algal growth that can play a part in cholera epidemics. Finally, rising sea levels also can increasingly threaten coastal communities (42).

Regional Variability and Climate Change

Climate change will damage health worldwide through direct effects, such as increased temperatures on the earth's surface, or through indirect effects, such as food shortages, water shortages in arid and semiarid regions in particular, a wider reach of vector-borne diseases (dengue, malaria), or an increase in vulnerability to natural disasters.

The Intergovernmental Panel on Climate Change has predicted that the impact of global warming and climate change in Latin America and the Caribbean will include rising sea levels, higher rainfall, increased drought risk, stronger winds and rain linked to hurricanes, and more pronounced floods associated with El Niño (47, 48).

Environmental, social, and productive pressures increase the vulnerability of Latin America and the Caribbean to this impact. Central America's tropical rainforests, the Amazon river basin, the Caribbean coral reefs and other tropical areas, the Andean mountain ecosystems, and wetlands are particularly vulnerable (49). Water cycle changes may affect arid and semiarid areas, with consequences to electric power generation and agriculture.

Rising temperatures, modification of land cover, changing precipitation patterns, and shrinking spending on health lie behind the re-emergence in Latin America and the Caribbean of epidemics that were once under control (42). Climate conditions linked to the El Niño Southern Oscillation (ENSO) or to global climate change cause temperature and precipitation extremes, contributing to the proliferation of vector-borne diseases such as malaria, dengue, yellow fever, and bubonic plague. The loss of plant cover and extreme weather events will help bring about water pollution and an increase in pests.

Glacier loss due to rising temperatures in the Andes and saltwater intrusion due to rising sea levels will put pressures on the availability of drinking water. Agricultural production, food security, and tourism will be affected.

The increase in extreme weather events since 1987, such as tropical storms and hurricanes, floods, landslides, and droughts is evidence of the impact of climate change. The number of episodes of this kind doubled in Central America between 1987 and 1997 and grew by nearly 60% in South America between 1998 and 2005. Loss of human life tripled in Central America and grew 4.3 times in the Caribbean islands and 6.5 times in South America, while economic damage doubled in Central America and grew by 80% in South America and by 50% in the Caribbean islands (42).

Where there is flooding or drought, respiratory diseases can increase due to overcrowding. Excess fungal growth also can cause respiratory diseases, and there often is a rise in psychiatric disorders such as anxiety and depression, probably related to damages to the domestic environment and financial losses. Higher suicide rates have been reported and the number of behavioral disorders in children can rise. Droughts can have an impact on health in developing countries owing to their adverse effects on food production and hygiene, given that water is mostly consumed, rather than used for cleaning. Finally, outbreaks of malaria also can occur during droughts as a result of geographic changes that affect the disease's vector (47).

INTERNATIONAL HUMAN RIGHTS LAW

Legal Sources for the Right to Health in Latin America and the Caribbean

The right to the highest attainable standard of health ("the right to health") is enshrined in different national and international legal sources. The right to health and/or the right to health protection is established in 19 of the 35 national constitutions of Latin American and Caribbean countries. The most important international sources of the right to health include the Constitution of the World Health Organization, international and regional human rights conventions, and international guidelines or standards on health and human rights. The United Nations System has a Special Rapporteur to cooperate with the States in promoting and protecting the right to health (50).

WHO's Member States have reached agreement on important principles related to public health that appear in the preamble to the Organization's Constitution. This document establishes a fundamental international principle to the effect that the enjoyment of the highest attainable standard of health is not just an individual concern but is "one of the fundamental rights of every human being without distinction of race, religion, political belief, economic or social condition."

With regard to international and regional conventions, Article 12 of the International Covenant on Economic, Social, and Cultural Rights sets forth "the right of everyone to the enjoyment of the highest attainable standard of physical and mental health" (51) and the measures that Member States should adopt to ensure that this right is effective, including the prevention and treatment of diseases and epidemics and the provision of medical treatment and services. Article 10 of the Protocol of San Salvador (Additional Protocol to the American Convention on Human Rights in the Area of Economic, Social and Cultural Rights) (52) also enshrines the right to health. International and regional human rights conventions have incorporated the principles established by the Universal Declaration of Human Rights, which is considered a fundamental legal source of civil, political, economic, social, and cultural rights, and fundamental freedoms.

At the international level, the most important conventions for the protection of human rights in the United Nations System include: the International Covenant on Civil and Political Rights (53); the Convention on the Rights of the Child (54); the Convention against Torture and Other Cruel, Inhuman, or Degrading Treatment or Punishment (55); and the Convention on the Elimination of All Forms of Discrimination against Women (56). The Inter-American system includes the American Convention on

Human Rights (57); the Inter-American Convention on the Elimination of All Forms of Discrimination against Persons with Disabilities (58); the Inter-American Convention on the Prevention, Punishment, and Eradication of Violence against Women; and Article 10 of the Protocol of San Salvador, mentioned earlier.

A series of declarations, recommendations, and reports promulgated by the General Assembly of the United Nations Organization; the General Assembly of the Organization of American States; the United Nations Commission for Human Rights; the United Nations Committee on Economic, Social, and Cultural Rights; the Inter-American Human Rights Commission; WHO; and PAHO also set forth important guidelines (although not binding) that can be incorporated into national plans, policies, legislation, and practices related to different areas of health.

Initiatives in Bioethics

In October 2005, UNESCO's General Conference approved by acclamation the Universal Declaration on Bioethics and Human Rights, whereby Member States undertake to respect and apply the fundamental principles of bioethics. The declaration represents a major step toward the recognition of rules that govern respect for the dignity of individuals, human rights, and fundamental freedoms in the field of bioethics.

As an applied discipline, bioethics deals with issues related to health; interventions involving life, death, and genetic heritage; and the social accountability of scientists, physicians, and other professionals. In Latin America and the Caribbean, equity in the access to health care services coupled with the provision of quality services remain as major challenges. The first of these issues is of concern to the authorities, opinion shapers, and service managers. The second has to do with financing, research, and human resource training, which entail bioethical responsibilities.

Bioethics demonstrates that improvements in health care and scientific and technological advances merit special attention. It is difficult to gauge the impact of work done on bioethics, since it is basically qualitative, but evaluations by health systems managers, health professionals, the public, and policymakers indicate that its inclusion in the policy-related and technical mandates of international organizations is fundamental.

References

1. De Ferranti D. Inequality in Latin America and the Caribbean: breaking with history? Washington, DC: World Bank; 2004.

2. Economic Commission for Latin America and the Caribbean. Social panorama of Latin America 2006. Santiago de Chile: ECLAC; 2006.

3. Declaration of Santa Cruz de la Sierra, XIII Ibero-American Summit in Santa Cruz, Bolivia, 2003.

4. Declaration of Salamanca, XV Ibero-American Summit in Salamanca, Spain, 2005.

5. Plan of Action of the III Summit of the Americas, Quebec, Canada, 20–22 April 2001.

6. Declaration of Mar del Plata, IV Summit of the Americas, Mar del Plata, Argentina, 2005.

7. United Nations, Committee on Economic, Social, and Cultural Rights. Cuestiones sustantivas que se plantean en la aplicación del Pacto Internacional de Derechos Económicos, Sociales y Culturales: la pobreza y el Pacto Internacional de Derechos Económicos, Sociales y Culturales. (E/C.12/2001/10). Geneva: UN; 2001.

8. Economic Commission for Latin America and the Caribbean. Briefing paper: Social panorama of Latin America 2006. Santiago de Chile: ECLAC; 2006.

9. Economic Commission for Latin America and the Caribbean. The Millennium Development Goals: a Latin American and Caribbean perspective. Santiago de Chile: ECLAC; 2005.

10. Food and Agriculture Organization of the United Nations. State of food insecurity in the world. Rome: FAO; 2006.

11. International Labor Organization. 2006 Labor overview. Latin America and the Caribbean. Lima: ILO; 2006.

12. Economic Commission for Latin America and the Caribbean. Social panorama of Latin America 2006. Statistical appendix. Santiago de Chile: ECLAC; 2006.

13. International Labor Organization. World and regional trends in youth employment. Prepared for the expert group meeting on the monitoring of the Millennium Declaration Goals (MDGs) of the Millennium Declaration. Geneva: ILO; 2004.

14. Psacharopoulos G, Patrinos HA. Returns to investment in education: a further update. Policy Research Working Paper Series 2881. World Bank; 2002.

15. Navarro J, Roses M. La salud y la educación para el cambio: más que un vínculo. Washington, DC: Organización Panamericana de la Salud; 2006. In press.

16. Kawachi I, Subramanian SV, Almeida-Filho N. A glossary for health inequalities. J Epidemiol Community Health 2002;56: 647–652.

17. United Nations Education, Scientific and Cultural Organization. Universal primary education in Latin America: Are we really that close? Regional report about the Millennium Development Goals related to education. Santiago de Chile: UNESCO; 2004. Available from: http://unesdoc.unesco.org/images/0013/001373/137330s.pdf.

18. Inter-American Development Bank. The Millennium Development Goals in Latin America and the Caribbean: challenges, actions and commitments. Washington, DC: IDB; 2004.

19. Wagstaff A, Watanabe N. Socioeconomic inequalities in child malnutrition in the developing world. World Bank Policy Research Working Paper 2434. Washington, DC: World Bank; 1999.

20. Deruyttere A. Pueblos indígenas, recursos naturales y desarrollo con identidad: riesgos y oportunidades en tiempos de globalización. Washington, DC: Inter-American Development Bank, 2001.

21. Dureya S. Measuring social exclusion. Washington, DC: Inter-American Development Bank; 2001.

22. Hall G, Patrinos H. Indigenous peoples, poverty and human development in Latin America: 1994–2004. Washington, DC: World Bank; 2005.

23. Economic Commission for Latin America and the Caribbean. Shaping the future of social protection: access, financing and solidarity. Santiago de Chile: ECLAC; 2006.

24. Pan American Health Organization. Gender, women, and health in the Americas. Basic indicators. Washington, DC: PAHO; 2005.

25. León F. Mujer y trabajo en las reformas estructurales latinoamericanas durante las décadas 1980 y 1990. Santiago de Chile: ECLAC; 2000. p.18.

26. Hopenhayn, M, Bello A, Miranda F. Serie Políticas Sociales N° 118. Los pueblos indígenas y afrodescendientes ante el nuevo milenio. Santiago de Chile: ECLAC; 2006.

27. Borges Martins R. Serie Políticas Sociales N° 82. Desigualdades raciales y políticas de la inclusión racial: resumen de la experiencia brasilera reciente. Santiago de Chile: ECLAC; 2004.

28. United Nations. Population by five-year age group and sex, medium variant 2005. In: World population prospects: the 2004 revision. New York: United Nations; 2005.

29. World Health Organization. The world health report 2004: changing history. Geneva: WHO; 2004. Available from: http://www.who.int/whr/2004/en/index.html.

30. Pan American Health Organization. Survey on Health, Welfare and Aging in Latin America and the Caribbean (SABE). Washington, DC: PAHO; 2001.

31. Verbrugge LM. Pathways of health and death. In: Apple R (ed). Women, health and medicine in America. New York: Garland Publishing; 1990. p. 62.

32. Bello A, Rangel M. Equity and exclusion in Latin America and the Caribbean: the case of indigenous and Afro-descendent peoples. CEPAL Review 76. April 2002.

33. World Health Organization. The world health report 1999: making a difference. Appendix table 7. Geneva: WHO; 1999.

34. Pan American Health Organization. Gender, equity and access to health services. Preliminary results. Washington, DC: PAHO; 2001.

35. United States Agency for International Development. Demographic and Health Surveys (DHS). [DHS by country, in 9 countries of the Region]. 2000–2005.

36. United States Agency for International Development. Measure DHS. STATcompiler. 2006. Available from: http://www.measuredhs.com.

37. Pan American Health Organization. Health situation in the Americas. Basic indicators. Washington, DC: PAHO; 2006.

38. Ecuador, Centro de Estudio de Población y Desarrollo Social. Encuesta Demográfica y de Salud Materna e Infantil (ENDEMAIN) 2004. Quito: CEPAR; 2005.

39. Vega J, Bedregal P, Jadue L, Delgado I. Equidad de género en el acceso de la atención de salud en Chile. Pan American Health Organization; 2001.

40. Gómez E. Género, equidad y acceso a los servicios de salud. Rev Panam Salud Publica 2002;(11):5–6.

41. Hall G, Patrinos H. Indigenous peoples, poverty and human development in Latin America: 1994–2004. Washington, DC: World Bank; 2005.

42. United Nations Environment Program. GEO Latin America and the Caribbean: environmental outlook 2003. UNEP; 2004.

43. Winchester L. Sustainable human settlements development in Latin America and the Caribbean. In: Serie Medio Ambiente y Desarrollo N° 99. Santiago de Chile: ECLAC; 2005.

44. United Nations Environment Program. GEO data portal. Available from: http://geodata.grid.unep.ch.

45. World Resources Institute; United Nations Environmental Program; United Nations Development Program; World Bank. World resources 1996–1997: a guide to the global environment: the urban environment. New York: Oxford University Press; 1996.

46. Heileman S. Technical notes on large marine ecosystems in Latin America and the Caribbean. Unpublished. 2006.

47. Intergovernamental Panel on Climate Change. Climate change 2001: impacts, adaptation, and vulnerability. Cambridge: Cambridge University Press; 2001.

48. Krug T. Vulnerabilidade, impactos e adaptação. O caso particular das florestas brasileiras. [Technical note]. Instituto Nacional de Pesquisas Espaciais; Instituto Interamericano para Pesquisa em Mudanças Globais. Unpublished.

49. Garea B, Gerhartz J. Technical Note for GEO-4. Unpublished.

50. Office of the United Nations High Commissioner for Human Rights. Special Rapporteur of the Commission on Human Rights on the right of everyone to the enjoyment of the highest attainable standard of physical and mental health. 2002. Available from: http://www.ohchr.org/english/issues/health/right/.

51. International Covenant on Economic, Social and Cultural Rights, G.A. res. 2200A (XXI), 21 UN GAOR Supp. (No. 16) p. 49, UN Doc. A/6316 (1966), 993 U.N.T.S. 3, entered into force January 3, 1976.

52. Additional Protocol to the American Convention on Human Rights in the Area of Economic, Social and Cultural Rights, "Protocol of San Salvador," O.A.S. Treaty Series No. 69 (1988), entered into force November 16, 1999, reprinted in Basic Documents Pertaining to Human Rights in the Inter-American System, OEA/Ser.L.V/II.82 doc.6 rev.1 at 67 (1992).

53. International Covenant on Civil and Political Rights, G.A. res. 2200A (XXI), 21 UN GAOR Supp. (No. 16) p. 52, U.N. Doc. A/6316 (1966), 999 U.N.T.S. 171, entered into force March 23, 1976.

54. Convention on the Rights of the Child, G.A. res. 44/25, annex, 44 U.N. GAOR Supp. (No. 49) at 167, U.N. Doc. A/44/49 (1989), entered into force September 2, 1990.

55. Convention against Torture and Other Cruel, Inhuman or Degrading Treatment or Punishment, G.A. res. 39/46, [annex, 39 U.N. GAOR Supp. (No. 51) at 197, U.N. Doc. A/39/51 (1984)], entered into force June 26, 1987.

56. Convention on the Elimination of All Forms of Discrimination against Women, G.A. res. 34/180, 34 U.N. GAOR Supp. (No. 46) at 193, U.N. Doc. A/34/46, entered into force September 3, 1981.

57. American Convention on Human Rights, O.A.S. Treaty Series No. 36, 1144 U.N.T.S. 123, entered into force July 18, 1978, reprinted in Basic Documents Pertaining to Human Rights in the Inter-American System, OEA/Ser.L.V/II.82 doc.6 rev.1 at 25 (1992).

58. Inter-American Convention on the Elimination of All Forms of Discrimination against Persons with Disabilities. G.A./ Res. 1608 (XXIX-0/99), entered into force September 14, 2001.

Chapter 2
HEALTH CONDITIONS AND TRENDS

In recent years, the demographic situation in the Americas continues to be characterized by a transition caused by low fertility and decreasing mortality rates. As a result, the population overall is aging and the "demographic dependence" of the young (0–14 years of age) and the old (64 years of age and older) on the potentially active (working) population (15–63 years of age) is decreasing. Regional, subregional, and national averages, however, mask persistent inequitable situations at various geographic and social levels and among certain population groups. Furthermore, migration within and between countries affects the distribution of the population and impacts the delivery of health services.

In the last quarter-century, life expectancy in the Americas has increased by 17 years, with the average age today over 70. The aging of the population varies greatly among countries of the Americas: aging is a significant phenomenon in Barbados, Cuba, Puerto Rico, and Uruguay; while in Bolivia, Haiti, Guatemala, Honduras, and Nicaragua the population is generally younger.

The mortality profile in the Americas has changed significantly over the past several decades. In almost every country, communicable diseases have been replaced as the principal causes of illness and death by chronic, degenerative diseases—circulatory system diseases, malignant neoplasms, chronic respiratory diseases, and diabetes—and by external causes such as traffic accidents and homicides. Among the factors contributing to this changed profile are the aging of the population, the control and reduction of a number of communicable diseases, and the appearance of new ones such as HIV/AIDS. Significant differences in mortality exist, however, among countries and subregions of the Americas.

Countries of the Americas have led the way in vaccine-preventable disease eradication (smallpox and poliomyelitis), elimination (endemic transmission of measles), and control (pertussis, diphtheria, tetanus, invasive diseases caused by *Haemophilus influenzae* type b, and hepatitis B). These achievements have been secured by attaining and maintaining high levels of immunization coverage, implementing effective surveillance, and conducting mass immunization campaigns. In 2003 the countries committed to eliminating rubella and congenital rubella syndrome by 2010. Using immunization to its full potential is critical to attaining mortality reduction and health development targets, which implies new challenges in immunization that extend to influenza, rotavirus, pneumococcus, and human papilloma virus.

Vector-borne diseases—especially malaria, dengue, and Chagas'—continue to compromise the health of a large proportion of the regional population. While the number of reported cases of malaria hit a peak in the late 1990s, the disease is still endemic in 21 countries and results in approximately one million cases reported annually—a significant economic impact, as two-thirds of those cases occur in working-age people. The incidence and epidemics of dengue have increased worldwide over the past 35 years; from 2001 to 2005, more than 30 countries in the Americas reported almost three million cases of dengue and dengue hemorrhagic fever. Chagas' disease, endemic in 21 countries of the Americas, is currently estimated to infect some 18 million people, primarily the poor in rural areas.

Zoonoses—diseases in animals that can be transmitted to humans—represent two-thirds of pathogenic species affecting humans and three-fourths of emerging pathogens. Given the serious threat they pose to public health and economic development, the countries of the Region vigorously pursue prevention and control programs to combat such zoonoses as plague, rabies, leishmaniasis, hydatidosis, brucellosis, and bovine tuberculosis.

At year-end 2005, an estimated 3.2 million people in the Americas were infected with HIV—60% of whom resided in Latin America and the Caribbean. Moreover, incidence of the disease is on the rise in the Region, with 220,000 new cases reported in 2005. Of the 10 regions with the highest HIV prevalence worldwide, the Caribbean ranks second, and, while the disease is concentrated in certain populations in the rest of the Region, in the Caribbean it is generalized throughout the population. The groups most affected by HIV are men who have sex with men, sex workers, and those who inject drugs. An estimated 50 million new cases of sexually transmitted infections (STIs) occur every year in the Americas.

Noncommunicable chronic diseases—cardiovascular diseases, cancer, diabetes, and chronic pulmonary obstructive diseases—cause two of every three deaths in the general population of Latin America and the Caribbean and almost half of all deaths in the under-70-year age group. In addition to leading to premature deaths, these diseases cause complications and disabilities, limit productivity, and require costly treatments. Together with genetic disposition and age, risk factors contributing to these diseases include poor diet, physical inactivity, smoking, and alcohol abuse; other factors range from hypertension, to high cholesterol, to overweight and obesity.

Mental health problems constitute one-fourth of the total disease burden in the Americas, as measured by disability-adjusted life years (DALYs) lost. Notwithstanding, in most countries a significant gap exists between the magnitude of mental health disorders and the health sector's response to them. Mental health care tends to concentrate on dealing with psychiatric problems—anxiety, depression, and substance abuse. Disasters are major a cause of mental disturbances.

Oral health continues to be a critical aspect of public health in the Americas, because of its contribution to overall morbidity, the high costs of treatment, and the increase in oral health inequities. While the prevalence of dental caries in the Region has dropped 35%–85% since 1995, oral disease continues to be high compared to other parts of the world. Poor oral health services and their limited coverage contributed to these high rates. Scientific evidence points to a causal relationship between oral health and health in general. Fluoridation programs, the promotion of simple technologies, and health systems that integrate oral health with general health care can lead to reduced oral disease.

In Latin America and the Caribbean, two-thirds of the incidence of eye disease—namely, blindness and visual impairment—can be attributed to treatable conditions such as cataracts, refractive errors, diabetic retinopathy, and glaucoma. According to national assessments, however, huge discrepancies exist in eye care service coverage—from close to 80% in well-developed urban areas to less than 10% in rural and remote areas—as well as in the quality of services provided. Prevention of eye disease has the potential to produce major savings for national economies; conversely, if large-scale preventive measures fail to be taken, the cost of eye disease is expected to more than double by 2020, to approximately US$ 10 billion.

Sexual and reproductive health involves mostly maternal and child health and the health of adolescents and adults. Some 16.2 million children are born every year in the Region, 11.7 of them in Latin America. The regional population is increasing, but birth and fertility rates are dropping, although rates differ greatly from country to country. The sexual and reproductive health situation in Latin America and the Caribbean represents 20% of the total burden of disease in women and 14% in men—a clear gap. The use of birth control methods exceeds 60%, but considerably less than that in some countries. Although reporting differs among sources, and huge disparities occur among countries of the Region, the World Health Organization (WHO) estimates that of the 16.2 million births registered in the Americas in 2003, 22,680 maternal deaths occurred—a rate of 140/100,000 live births—principally resulting from abortion, preeclampsia, and hemorrhage. WHO further estimated that 280,000 perinatal deaths had occurred in 2006. Again, disparities are wide: the risk of perinatal deaths in Latin America and the Caribbean is three times that in Canada and the United States. Sexual and reproductive health relates directly to the high rates of birth among adolescents in Latin America and the Caribbean, where one in three females under 19 years of age has had a child.

Malnutrition in children and noncommunicable chronic diseases in adults, which pose problems in all the countries of the Region, are in large measure the results of poor diet. The growing tendency for children to be over recommended weights places them at later risk for chronic diseases. Breast-feeding is the single most important practice to reduce infant morbidity and mortality and a significant and preventable mode of mother-to-child transmission of HIV, the main cause of pediatric HIV. Micronutrient deficiencies—of iron, vitamin A, zinc, vitamin B12, folate, and iodine—continue to be public health concerns that greatly impact human development and economic productivity. The coupling of nutritional problems with physical inactivity is a recipe for major increases in noncommunicable chronic diseases.

Disasters are a constant in the Americas and in large part correlate to geography: volcanoes in Central America and the Andean countries; storms and hurricanes in the Atlantic and Pacific oceans and in the Gulf of Mexico; flooding in the Southern Cone; and El Niño affecting almost the entire Region. These disasters have a huge impact as measured by numbers of persons affected, deaths, and economic damage.

Some 50 million indigenous people live in the Americas, and in some countries they represent the majority of the population. They tend to be poorer, less educated, more unemployed, and in worse health—with higher rates of maternal and infant mortality, malnutrition, and infectious diseases—than their compatriots. In some countries, alcoholism, suicide, drug abuse, and sexually transmitted infections are disproportionately higher among indigenous populations. Their poor health status is compounded by discrimination and inequity within the health system. To redress this situation, many countries have drafted national policies and established funding for indigenous-focused health programs.

The population of the Americas includes an estimated 250 million Afro-descendants. Most of the countries in the Region do not disaggregate data on this group, rendering an analysis of its health status difficult. Nevertheless, available information indicates that the situation with regard to Afro-descendants is extremely vulnerable in South America, where in a number of countries they are disproportionately poorer and less educated, suffer higher rates of infant and child mortality as well as of HIV and other poverty-related diseases, have less access to drinking water, and represent a smaller proportion of doctors and other health workers. While the situation is generally not as serious in Central America, in one country in the isthmus child mortality rates are higher and health professionals fewer among Afro-descendants.

The focus on family and community health integrates programs that enable individuals, as both family and community members, to manage their health throughout the life cycle and enables the greater coverage and efficiency of, as well as more direct participation in, health services. Health indicators improve significantly by emphasizing the role of the family in health promotion and protection, prevention of exposure to risks, and early diagnosis and rehabilitation.

Youth between the ages of 10 and 24 represent 28% of the population in Latin America and the Caribbean. Of the 161 million youth in the Region, the largest share lives in the poorest countries. Many indigenous youth live on the margins of the predominant culture, in their own communities. Approximately half of adolescents in the Region are sexually active, and about half of those use no birth control or protection of any kind. Dealing with the problem is hampered by cultural beliefs and practices. Another major problem afflicting the health of youths is violence, with homicide figuring as one of the principal causes of death among 10–19 year olds. Youths' health is further undermined by their lifestyle choices—the consumption of alcohol, tobacco, and drugs; poor nutrition and physical inactivity; and the growing prevalence of overweight and obesity.

Although the aging of the population varies considerably throughout the Americas, by the mid-21st century all but five of the countries of the Region will have as many inhabitants over 60 years of age as under 15 years, and a few countries will have twice as many elderly as young people. Reductions in infectious diseases and in infant and child mortality have translated into longer lives. More than three in four individuals born in Latin America and the Caribbean today will live to be older than 60, and two in five will celebrate their 80th birthday. The challenge for health policymakers and health systems will be to ensure that those living beyond 60 can celebrate not only their longevity but their good health and functionality.

Uniform epidemiological analysis regarding disabilities is lacking throughout the Americas, making it difficult to assess the dimensions of disability in the Region; reported prevalence rates range from over 14% in Brazil to less than 4% in Venezuela. The most common types of disability relate to mobility, communication, and social participation. The most frequent causes are age-related degeneration, chronic diseases, accidents, problems stemming from pregnancy and delivery, and occupational diseases.

Neglected diseases—infectious, parasitic diseases that afflict millions of poor people in Latin America and the Caribbean—are a patent expression of inequities in health. Included under the rubric of neglected diseases are intestinal helminthiasis, schistosomiasis, lymphatic filariasis, leptospirosis, leishmaniasis, cysticercosis, Chagas' disease, and onchocerciasis—all of which disproportionately affect indigenous populations, minority ethnic groups, slum and rural dwellers, and migrant workers. Together, the toll of these diseases on workers' productivity and, consequently, countries' economic development is huge. Yet inexpensive medications, health promotion, and environmental sanitation could effectively control and eliminate them.

Emerging and reemerging infectious diseases are becoming a growing threat to global health security, stemming from disease outbreaks in one country or region that can spread to others and from the intentional or accidental release of biological agents. Since 2001, the Region has experienced a series of significant disease outbreaks related to emerging and reemerging diseases that have required international public health interventions.

POPULATION CHARACTERISTICS AND TRENDS[1]

Consequences of the Demographic Transition

The concept of demographic transition[2] has been useful in describing the effect that the social, political, and economic changes have had on mortality and fertility trends in developed countries (the United States and Canada, in the case of the Americas). To some degree, this concept has also been theoretical food for thought, fueling speculations that the developing countries of the 20th century—accounting for practically all of the Americas—would undergo similar transitions and at more or less the same time frame. However, birth and mortality indicators in Latin American and Caribbean countries have evolved differently (due more to the spread of technological innovation in health than to sustained, equitable development) and in different time frames (because they evolved faster than in the more developed countries and have been less tied to economic, social, and political crises sweeping the Hemisphere in recent decades). This situation had led to consequences in terms of inequality, inasmuch as the so-called "population explosion"[3]—resulting from a slowdown in the decrease in the birth rate with respect to that of the mortality rate—has been sustained, for the most part, by the poorer segments of society.

What is certain nearly a century later is that the visible expressions of this process during the early years of the 21st century show certain characteristics that merit consideration and that define a continent with a very low population growth and low fertility and mortality rates, thus giving the appearance of stability and equilibrium. Indicators at the national level mask differences that need to be pointed out, given their impact on the population's characteristics and because these differences need to be considered in formulating social policy generally and health policy specifically. In terms of the Region as a whole, these characteristics can be summarized as follows:

- In little more than 30 years, median annual population growth rates in Latin American and Caribbean countries have decreased nearly 50%, dropping appreciably during the last two decades, from annual averages on the order of 2.7% during 1950–1955 to 1.5% at this writing. Consequently, the Region's population more than tripled between 1950 and 2000, skyrocketing from 161 million inhabitants in 1950 to 561 million in 2005. The population of the Region, expressed as a percentage of the world's total population, increased slightly over this same period (from less than 7% to nearly 9%).

- By 2005, most countries had either achieved low levels of fertility and stabilized mortality (in full demographic transition, characterized by low population growth) or were experiencing an advanced stage of demographic transition, with only slight or no population growth. Guatemala is the only country of the Region currently in a moderate stage of demographic transition, inasmuch as its fertility rate has remained higher than that of the other countries.[4]

- Annual population growth rates reveal the first important difference between the countries of the Region, ranging from 0.3% in Cuba to 2.5% in Honduras (Figure 1).

- Fertility rates in the Region, which were among the world's highest 40 years ago, are now at very low levels, and in many cases fall below the world average. Figure 2 illustrates the second significant difference among the Region's countries with respect to fertility: a difference of nearly three children per woman between the countries on either extreme.

- Mortality in the Region, which began a sustained decline during the first half of the 20th century, is reflected in a 20-year increase in life expectancy at birth for both sexes, increasing to 72 years over 2000–2005—or eight years higher than in all other developing regions of the world, although at levels experienced by developed countries 35 years ago. Figure 3 illustrates the third great difference among the countries of the Region: a nearly 30-year variation in life expectancy between the countries at either extreme.

The above-mentioned changes in fertility and mortality have altered the population structure, owing to differences in growth among age groups. Accordingly, this has brought about a shift in the distribution of the dependent population (ages 0–14 and age 60 and older) with respect to the economically active population (ages 15–59). This shift reveals two trends that merit closer examination: a declining population dependence (defined as the dependent population—or the sum of the 0–14 plus the 60 and older age groups—divided by the economically active popula-

---

[1]This section was prepared in conjunction with the United Nations Latin American and Caribbean Demographic Centre (CELADE, Population Division of the Economic Commission for Latin America and the Caribbean [ECLAC]), pursuant to an agreement between PAHO and ECLAC. The content is based on references 1–4; information cited in figures 1, 2, 3, and 5 was furnished by the PAHO Regional Core Health Data Initiative (RCHDI) (http://www.paho.org/Spanish/SHA/coredata/tabulator/newTabulator.htm).

[2]This concept makes it possible to describe the passage from high to low levels of mortality first and then of fertility, with consequences for population growth and population structure by sex and age.

[3]The transition from high to low birth and mortality rates has not occurred uniformly in the countries of the Americas and, with the exception of countries where this transition occurred earlier—Canada and the United States first, followed later by Argentina, Cuba, and Uruguay—most countries have experienced extremely high population growth rates due to persistent high fertility rates amid rapid drops in mortality. This process of rapid growth is known as the *population explosion.*

[4]Clear differences exist between countries in the process of demographic transition. Upon considering Canada and the United States within the group of developed countries in the original demographic transition model, said countries are actually in post-transition stages.

FIGURE 1. Annual population growth rate (%), Region of the Americas, 2005.

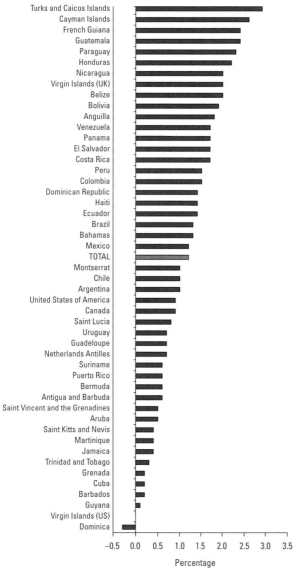

Source: PAHO Regional Core Health Data and Country Profile Initiative (RCHDI) (http://www.paho.org).

FIGURE 2. Total fertility rate, Region of the Americas, 2005.

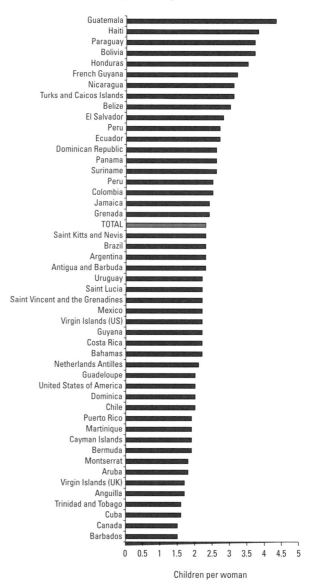

Source: PAHO Regional Core Health Data and Country Profile Initiative (RCHDI) (http://www.paho.org).

tion—or the 15–59 age group) and the aging of the population (understood as the portion of the population over age 60 years above a given percentage level).

The decline in the population dependency ratio is associated with the economic "burden" the economically-active population must assume to satisfy the demand of the dependent population. The lower the dependency ratio, the lower this burden, which is considered desirable for society as a whole. Projections indicate that for a certain period specific to each country (Figure 4), the dependency ratio will fall below 60, which is considered a "demo-

graphic dividend," meaning that the countries will experience a "dividend" in terms of less demand pressure from children. This dividend should be used to invest in productive sectors and to reallocate social spending, primarily as a means for improving the quality of education and health-sector reforms, with a view to changing the epidemiological profile. Once this window of opportunity closes (i.e., due to an increase in the proportion of older adults), the specific demand in the health sector will be much more costly than it was for children. Unfortunately, there is no evidence to suggest that countries are using this demographic

FIGURE 3. Life expectancy at birth (years), Region of the Americas, 2005.

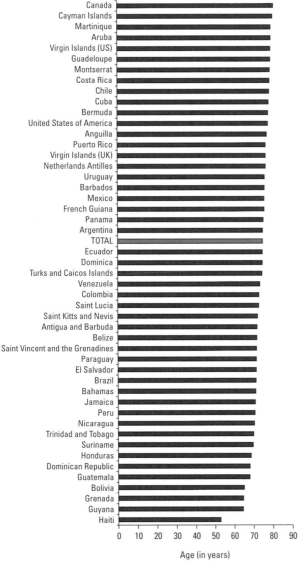

Age (in years)

Source: PAHO Regional Core Health Data and Country Profile Initiative (RCHDI) (http://www.paho.org).

FIGURE 4. Year the population dividend will "end," selected countries, Region of the Americas.

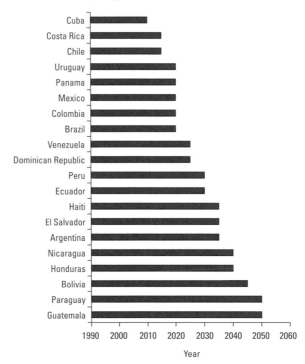

Year

Source: CELADE, Population Division of ECLAC, 2005.

Moreover, as the demographic transition progresses, the Latin American and Caribbean population is slowly and relentlessly aging, with annual rates of nearly 3.5%, much higher than the 1.5% average rate. In all countries of the Region, the proportion and absolute number of persons 60 years old and older will increase steadily over the next decades. The elderly population will grow between three and five times faster than the total population in 2000–2025 and 2025–2050, respectively. Consequently, the percentage of persons aged 60 and older will triple between 2000 and 2050. Social insurance and health systems could very well face definitive collapse without a redistribution of income and an equitable distribution of the opportunities derived from macroeconomic development.

In order to do this, men and women must be guaranteed equal employment and social protection opportunities, and health coverage must be ensured for the urban and rural poor, as well as for different ethnic groups in many countries of the Region. In terms of health, it will be necessary to redefine the role and characteristics of health care according to an approach based on the need to preserve the independence of older adults as long as possible, thus postponing disability; to initiate a reengineering of health systems with a view to training qualified human resources so they can provide comprehensive care of older adults; and to focus on disease prevention and health promotion actions targeted to

window of opportunity to their advantage, inasmuch as the job demand generated by the swelling ranks of the economically active population is being met instead with excessively flexible, precarious, and/or informal employment arrangements that are more beneficial to middle- and high-income households, which are precisely those that have experienced greater declines in fertility. If this "dividend" is to help poor sectors, income redistribution policies must be implemented to ensure that all of society can benefit from any resources freed up due to a lower dependency ratio.

each life-cycle stage, and not only to the elderly population. The longevity of women merits special attention, since its effects will need to be taken into account in health policies.

DIFFERENCES AND INEQUITIES IN FERTILITY AND MORTALITY

Despite the decline in fertility over the last 30 years and the limited impact of economic and social crises on these changing profiles, certain characteristics of the Region of the Americas should be pointed out, with a view to better understand the demands that health systems must cope with. The main challenges in this regard include:

- Fertility rates range from below the replacement level (fewer than two children per woman) in Canada, Cuba, the United States, and other Caribbean island nations to nearly four children per woman in Guatemala and Haiti (see Figure 2).
- Low total fertility stands in contrast with an increase in adolescent fertility, which has spiked in recent years in most countries, especially among young people under 18 years of age. This trend—which is much more frequent among poor segments of society—is linked to the school drop-out rate and has been steadily increasing among unmarried persons or those not in a stable union.
- Generally, there is a high negative correlation between fertility and certain economic and social development indicators, such as per capita gross domestic product, level of schooling, illiteracy, exposure to the mass media, and levels of poverty. If the use of contraceptives is factored into the analysis (i.e., prevalence use of modern methods among women in common law relationships), this variable in fact captures the main differences in fertility among countries, and most of the remaining variables lose statistical significance. Accordingly, this situation reinforces the need for effective, universally applied reproductive health policies.
- Disparities observed within countries are even greater than differences between countries, since fertility is highest among the poorest of the population—groups with lower levels of education and indigenous populations that have been historically marginalized. In some countries such as Bolivia, Guatemala, and Honduras, fertility among uneducated women is three times higher than among women who have completed secondary or higher education. This gap holds true in countries where vast segments of the population are still not using modern and safe birth control methods.
- In terms of differences in fertility among ethnic groups, census data (2000) show that indigenous populations continue to have high fertility rates.

Despite the significant reduction in mortality mentioned previously (especially among the young), which has brought about

FIGURE 5. Estimated infant mortality rate (per 1,000 live births), Region of the Americas, 2004.

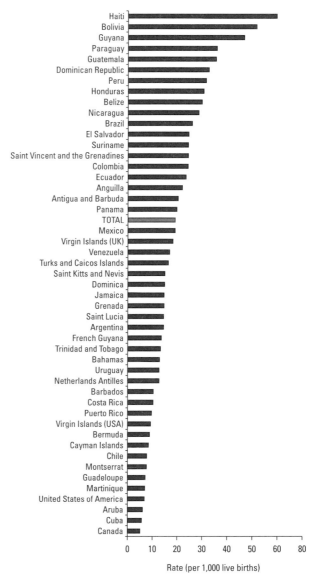

Rate (per 1,000 live births)

Source: PAHO Regional Core Health Data and Country Profile Initiative (RCHDI) (http://www.paho.org)

an increase in the life expectancy of the population of the Americas, and in light of important changes in the epidemiological profile of death and disease by cause (which points to an improvement in the health of the population), significant inequalities remain:

- Infant mortality in Latin America has dropped from an average of 128 deaths in children under 1 year old per 1,000 live births in 1950–1955 to only 28 deaths in 2000–2005. There are significant differences between countries, however (Figure 5). Moreover, this indicator continues to be higher among the most disadvantaged populations (indigenous groups, rural populations, and groups in which mothers have low levels of education), in which preventable causes constitute the leading causes of death. This points to the fact that the battle against premature mortality in the Region has yet to be won completely.

- Although the gap among countries with respect to life expectancy at birth is closing, significant inequalities remain that account for a difference of almost 30 years between countries on either extreme (see Figure 3).
- In all Latin American countries, female mortality is lower than male mortality. Consequently, life expectancy at birth for females is nearly seven years more than for males. Beyond biological differences between the sexes, there are some diseases that are unique to women, such as the complications of pregnancy and delivery, which have been battled with better success than diseases primarily affecting men, such as those associated with cardiovascular disease, external causes (violence), and certain types of malignant tumors. Moreover, men delay seeking timely health care compared to women.
- Maternal morbidity and mortality are considered among the most important public health problems of developing countries. Although their numbers are not terribly high, maternal morbidity and mortality are unacceptable because they can be easily avoided in most cases. According to available estimates, approximately half a million (515,000) women died worldwide due to this cause in 1995. In Latin America and the Caribbean, maternal deaths that year accounted for approximately 22,000 deaths, or approximately 4% of the total worldwide.
- Mortality has increased in some countries among certain age groups of the population, due to the persistence or re-emergence of epidemics of communicable diseases such as cholera, hantavirus, malaria, Chagas' disease, tuberculosis, and dengue—all of them diseases of poverty.
- The incidence of HIV/AIDS is lower in the Americas than in other regions of the world. Because it is lower, some countries have not made much effort to reduce mortality due to this cause, especially among specific population groups. In the Region, which accounts for approximately 8% of the world's population, some 1.5 million persons were infected with HIV by the end of 2002 (220,000 contracted the disease in 2005), representing 3.6% of the 42 million cases worldwide. The disease is most relevant in Haiti, Honduras, and other countries of the Caribbean.

International and Internal Migration

International and internal migrations are two aspects of the same process and are population components that underscore inequalities in terms of how people leave their countries and how they move around within their countries. This holds important

❝Acute respiratory infections—especially pneumonia in its various forms—and influenza continue to cause a major proportion of disease and suffering in the Americas.❞

Hugh Cumming, 1932

consequences for the well-being of significant contingents of people and can have negative health consequences for both migrants and for those who remain.

External migration is very much linked to earlier and current population changes in the Region. In recent years it has been characterized by a significant increase in migration to North America (especially to the United States and, to a lesser degree, to Canada) and to Europe (especially Spain). Migration within Latin America and the Caribbean has remained at the same levels as in the past, with migration flows largely targeting the traditional receiving countries, such as Argentina and Costa Rica. This phenomenon has not occurred uniformly among population groups, and the specific characteristics of this migration in terms of gender, age groups, and socioeconomic status have deeply affected the social and family structures of the Region's countries. The main characteristics of recent trends in this regard may be summarized as follows:

- It is estimated that 20 million Latin American and Caribbean persons currently reside outside their country of birth. This unprecedented figure is the result of a massive increase in migration that has been going on for more than a decade, mainly involving migrations to the United States (75% of migrants), as well as unprecedented new migratory flows to Europe, especially to Spain.
- Of this number, 15 million migrants were already in the United States by 2000, 54% of which were Mexican, followed by Cubans, Dominicans, and Salvadorans. Migrations to other destinations involved a total of five million people, three-quarters of whom went to Canada, some European countries (especially Spain and the United Kingdom), Japan, Israel, and Australia. The remaining two million migrated to other Latin American and Caribbean countries (Argentina, Costa Rica, and Venezuela continue to have the highest numbers). In the Caribbean, significant numbers of Haitians continue to migrate to the Dominican Republic.
- The flow of migrants—which is likely to continue and even to increase in the future, despite restrictions imposed by some countries—is fueled by difficulties in fulfilling the demand for new jobs and deteriorating standards of living in many of the Region's countries. Other factors that have fed the flow are technological innovations, better access to information regarding opportunities outside the homeland, improved transportation facilities, and migrant community networks.

- The lack of legal status that many immigrants must contend with and the absence of a social safety net for legal immigrant workers are important issues for consideration given their impact on migrant health, which is reflected in extremely weak and discriminatory integration mechanisms, which particularly affect women. Undocumented migrants with low levels of education and who work in unskilled jobs are more prone to risks and exclusion.

- Trends point to a significant "feminization" of migratory flows—a distinguishing characteristic of Latin American and Caribbean migration with respect to other regions of the world. The nature of migratory flows by sex is closely related to the complementary nature of the countries' labor markets, demand for service-based jobs, and the effects of family reunification. Female migration features specific characteristics that should be taken into account in health-sector planning and policies.

Internal migration, which has a long and deeply-rooted history in the Region, also results in inequities and disparities in terms of access to goods and services for a significant portion of the migrant population and for the receiving population. The main features of recent trends in this demographic component may be summarized as follows:

- Internal migration has resulted in the highest degree of urbanization in the developing world. Three of every four inhabitants of Latin America and the Caribbean live in urban areas. In most countries, migrants target large cities (one of every three persons of the Region resides in a city with more than one million inhabitants) and most settle in the largest city, accounting for more than one-quarter of a country's population and one-third of its urban population.

- Internal migration also occurs between cities and is selective, in that migrants tend to be women and young people. Generally, the likelihood of a person migrating increases with education level.

- In recent decades a trend toward migration to midsized cities has been observed, as well as migrations to areas specializing in producing raw material for export or that offer advantages in terms of trade (i.e., border areas).

- Recent years have witnessed: i) moderate internal migration within Latin America and the Caribbean at rates below that of the most developed countries, such as the United States and Canada; ii) a predominance of flows between urban areas; iii) persistent net outmigration from the countryside, which continues to greatly affect rural areas, inasmuch as it explains the intensified aging of their populations, which is beyond what would be expected as a result of these areas' stage in the demographic transition; iv) constant forced migrations as a result of internal conflicts in several of the Region's countries; v) ongoing migration from major metropolitan areas to more dynamic mid-sized cities that offer a better quality of life, some of which lie within metropolitan areas; vi) the persistent and significant allure for migrants of some small-country capitals, with highly advantageous urban systems; vii) the polarization of inter-metropolitan population transfers, with the poor tending to move to city outskirts and higher-income families moving to rural areas near cities, where they take advantage of urban services and infrastructure and from which they commute daily into the city to work or study; and vii) a revival of the downtown areas of some cities due to repopulation programs.

- Migrants show selectivity by age and above-average education, and persistence—although declining—of the traditional feminine bias of internal migration and the highest levels of unemployment among recent immigrants. Also observed, however, is the fact that migrants' income levels are equal to or higher than those of non-migrants (where key variables are controlled for, such as age, education, and family responsibility).

- With the exception of forced migration, migratory flows and the decision to migrate are fanned by expectations for better living conditions. Evidence suggests that migration has benefited many migrants, as evidenced in their higher median incomes, after controlling for other factors. However, significant numbers of migrants face difficulties integrating into the society where they settle, as is evidenced by higher rates of unemployment among recent immigrants, and difficult access to goods and services—to such a degree that some are unable to improve on their former living situation.

CONCLUSIONS

The analysis presented here summarizes the main demographic aspects that have a direct or indirect effect on the population's health. Aging and the future consequences of the rapid growth in the proportion of the elderly population are at the heart of an evaluation and prospects of current and future health care systems. The rise in adolescent fertility and the rising reports and confirmations of maternal deaths are yet additional examples of the intertwined nature of demographic and health trends. If infant mortality and life expectancy are to improve, health systems must act to control preventable childhood illnesses and other diseases affecting the adult population, such as HIV/AIDS. The absorption of massive numbers of immigrants and, conversely, the emigration of large groups of the population from one country to another, pose challenges for health systems, which may collapse in the receiving countries under the weight of the new demands for services or in the source countries where demand dries up. The growth of urban populations and consequent saturation of hospital supply in the most economically depressed urban areas with a significant poor population also pose challenges for public health.

Discussions point to the development of better mechanisms to close the current gaps, masked by national averages. Finally, access to demographic information at the national level, as well as the potential to access data for smaller areas where health events and disease occur, is an essential input for assessing the health situation, formulating health policies, and conducting follow-up and monitoring.

MORTALITY: EXTENT, DISTRIBUTION, AND TRENDS

OVERVIEW

The mortality profile for the Region of the Americas has undergone significant changes in recent decades. In almost all of the countries, chronic degenerative diseases have overtaken communicable diseases as the leading causes of disease and death. Diseases of the circulatory system, neoplasms, chronic respiratory diseases, and diabetes are among the leading causes of death, along with external causes such as traffic accidents and homicide.

Several factors have contributed to this evolving profile, including changes in the population structure (aging), improvements in disease control and a lowered risk of death due to several diseases (such as vaccine-preventable diseases and intestinal infectious diseases), and the emergence of other diseases (such as HIV/AIDS). Changes have not occurred uniformly or with the same intensity in every country. This section examines the leading causes of death by sex and broad age groups for each of eight countries or subregions: the Andean Area, Brazil, Central America, the Latin Caribbean, the non-Latin Caribbean, Mexico, North America, and the Southern Cone (see Box 1: Technical Notes).

With respect to the population as a whole, four causes of death are consistently present within the ten leading causes of death for all eight subregions: ischemic heart disease (ranking from the first to the third leading cause), cerebrovascular disease (first to the fourth), diabetes mellitus (first to the seventh), and pneumonia and influenza (first to the eighth). In fact, with the exception of Central America and the Latin Caribbean, these same causes figure among the ten leading causes of death and disease in men and women alike. Likewise, chronic respiratory diseases appear among the ten leading causes of death in five of the eight subregions, with the exception of Central America, the Latin Caribbean, and the non-Latin Caribbean.

BOX 1. Technical Notes

1. Subregions. For this mortality analysis, countries and territories were classified into the following subregions:
   —North America: Bermuda, Canada, and the United States
   —Mexico
   —Central America: Costa Rica, El Salvador, Guatemala, Honduras, and Nicaragua
   —Latin Caribbean: Cuba, French Guyana, Guadeloupe, Haiti, Martinique, Puerto Rico, and the Dominican Republic.
   —Non-Latin Caribbean: Anguilla, Antigua and Barbuda, Bahamas, Barbados, Belize, Cayman Islands, Dominica, Guyana, Montserrat, Saint Kitts and Nevis, Saint Lucia, Saint Vincent and the Grenadines, Suriname, Trinidad and Tobago, Turks and Caicos Islands, and the British and U.S. Virgin Islands.
   —Andean Area: Bolivia, Colombia, Ecuador, Peru, and Venezuela
   —Brazil
   —Southern Cone: Argentina, Chile, Paraguay, and Uruguay.

2. Data years. The source of data for each country or territory is the most recent available (past two to three years). On average, the data used for all subregions is circa 2002. Accordingly, the mortality rates appearing in the tables reflect the average of the corresponding period.

3. Rates. Specific mortality rates by cause and age have been calculated according to the methodology described in Health Statistics from the Americas, 2006 Edition (http://www.paho.org/english/dd/ais/hsa2006.htm).

4. Rank order. For this purpose, a specific list of the leading causes of death was prepared by PAHO and WHO in 2004 (A method for deriving leading causes of death, Bulletin of WHO, April 2006, 84(4) http://www.who.int/bulletin/volumes/84/4/297.pdf).

FIGURE 6. Mortality from ischemic heart disease, by sex, subregions of the Americas, circa 2002.

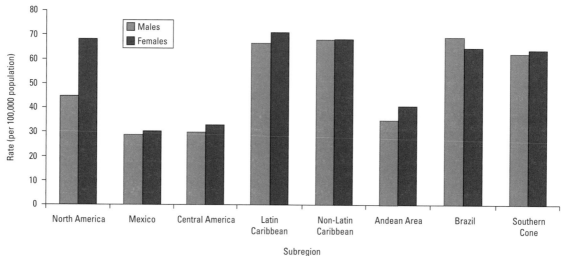

Source: Pan American Health Organization.

FIGURE 7. Mortality from cerebrovascular disease, by sex, subregions of the Americas, circa 2002.

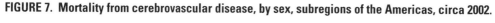

Source: Pan American Health Organization.

Figure 6 shows that men consistently have higher rates for **ischemic heart disease**. There are significant differences between subregions, with rates ranging between 35–50 per 100,000 population in Central America and Mexico, and up to more than 170 per 100,000 population in North America. Similarly, Central America and Mexico have lower mortality rates for **cerebrovascular disease** (Figure 7). In contrast to ischemic heart disease, mortality rates for cerebrovascular disease are highest among women in almost all subregions except for Brazil.

With regard to diabetes (Figure 8), although differences by sex have been decreasing in recent years, mortality rates continue to be higher among women than men. In the Southern Cone,

diabetes mortality rates are practically the same for men and women.

Mortality rates from **influenza and pneumonia** are highest among males in six of the eight subregions (Figure 9); North America and the Southern Cone being the exceptions.

Mortality rates from **chronic respiratory diseases** in Latin America range between 16 and 25 per 100,000 population for the population as a whole, and are consistently higher among men (Figure 10). In North America, these rates approach 42 per 100,000 population and are the same for both sexes. This group of diseases is not included among the leading causes of death for either sex in the non-Latin Caribbean.

FIGURE 8. Mortality from diabetes, by sex, subregions of the Americas, circa 2002.

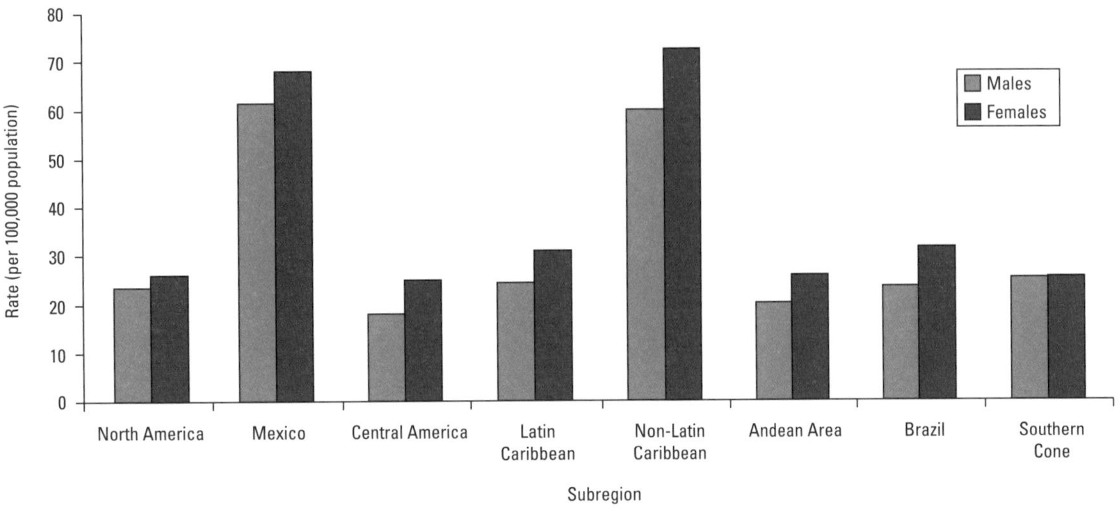

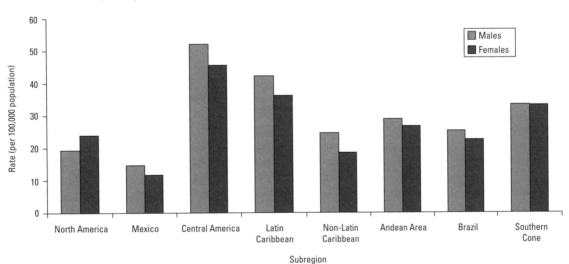

Source: Pan American Health Organization.

FIGURE 9. Mortality from pneumonia and influenza, by sex, subregions of the Americas, circa 2002.

Source: Pan American Health Organization.

Heart failure and complications and ill-defined descriptions of heart disease rank among the ten leading causes of death in all subregions except Mexico. On the one hand, this increases the relative weight of diseases of the circulatory system within overall mortality; on the other, it points to potential problems regarding imprecise medical certification of the causes of death, inasmuch as these conditions often are the terminal cause of death, but not necessarily the basic or underlying cause.

While the great majority of deaths from **conditions originating in the perinatal period** occur during the first months of life, they may also occur up to several years following birth. Although

infant mortality has decreased considerably in the subregions, there is still room to reduce it further. Moreover, because children continue to represent an important percentage of the overall population, these conditions continue to figure among the ten leading causes of death among the total population. Only in North America and in the Southern Cone countries, with their older populations and lower infant mortality rates, are these conditions not included among the ten leading causes of death for the total population. Nonetheless, they are the leading cause of death in children under 5 years old in all the subregions. In addition, **intestinal infectious diseases** continue to rank among the five

71

FIGURE 10. Mortality from chronic respiratory diseases, by sex, subregions of the Americas, circa 2002.

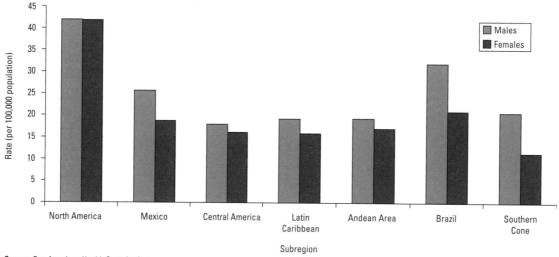

Source: Pan American Health Organization.

leading causes of death in children under 5 in all subregions except North America.

In Mexico, Central America, the Latin Caribbean, and the Andean Area the **maternal mortality** causes rank among the ten leading causes of death among females aged 10–59 years old, while in Brazil and the Southern Cone they are among the leading ten causes of death only in adolescent females aged 10–19 years old. In North America and the non-Latin Caribbean, the causes of maternal mortality do not rank among the ten leading causes of death for females in any age group. These findings, together with those discussed in the preceding paragraph suggest that much more progress will be needed to meet the Millennium Development Objectives (MDGs).

The impact of **external causes of death** on mortality also is important. Despite an observed decline in traffic accidents, they continue to rank among the leading causes of death in most of the subregions—only in the Southern Cone do traffic accidents not figure among the ten leading causes of death among males. Mortality due to homicide has been on the rise, particularly among young men and adolescent boys. Suicide constitutes an important component of mortality and is included among the leading causes of death in adolescents and young adults. In North America and the Southern Cone there are more suicides than homicides. Accidental drowning or submersion is also a significant cause of death.

ANALYSIS BY SUBREGION

North America

Ischemic heart disease accounts for 20.9% of all deaths in this subregion, for a mortality rate of 171.1 per 100,000 population

(the Region's highest), followed by cerebrovascular disease (6.9%) and malignant neoplasms of the trachea, bronchus, and lung (6.6%), the latter of which is the second leading cause of death among men (7.8% of deaths). Also important is the fact that dementia and Alzheimer's disease is the fourth cause of death among women and the fifth cause for the population as a whole; it does not figure among the ten leading causes of death in men (Table 1).

Other differences in mortality between the sexes can be seen with respect to malignant neoplasms. Neoplasm of the prostate is the sixth leading cause of death among men; breast cancer holds the corresponding rank for women. For men, malignant neoplasms of the hematopoietic and lymphatic systems account for the seventh leading cause of death, and malignant neoplasm of the colon for the ninth, although these diseases are not included among the ten leading causes of mortality in females.

Almost half of all deaths of children under 5 in both sexes are due to conditions originating in the perinatal period, with another more than 20% attributable to congenital malformations. External causes account for most of the remaining 30%, including traffic accidents, homicide, and accidental drowning or submersion.

Among the population aged 5–19, which is the group with the lowest risk of death overall, external causes contributed most to mortality in both sexes, with traffic accidents constituting the leading cause, followed by homicide. Suicide is the third leading cause of death among the population aged 10–19 years old, and affects both sexes equally. Mortality rates for all causes among 5–9-year-olds and 10–19-year-olds are the lowest in the Region, at 0.15 and 0.42 per 1,000 population, respectively.

Malignant neoplasms of the trachea, bronchus, and lung is the leading cause of death among women 20–59 years old in North

TABLE 1. Rates, percentage, and cumulative percentage (based on defined causes) of the ten leading causes of death, by sex, North America, circa 2002.

Deaths	Total				Males				Females			
	Rank	Rate (per 100,000 population)	%	Cumulative %	Rank	Rate (per 100,000 population)	%	Cumulative %	Rank	Rate (per 100,000 population)	%	Cumulative %
Total	—	830.7	100.0	—	—	830.4	100.0		—	831.0	100.0	
Ill-defined causes	—	—	1.3	—	—	—	1.3		—	—	1.3	
Defined causes	—	819.9	100.0	—	—	819.6	100.0		—	820.2	100.0	
Ischemic heart disease	1	171.1	20.9	20.9	1	177.6	21.7		1	164.9	20.1	
Cerebrovascular disease	2	56.6	6.9	27.8	3	44.6	5.4		2	68.1	8.3	
Malignant neoplasm of the trachea, bronchus, and lung	3	54.5	6.6	34.4	2	64.2	7.8		3	45.1	5.5	
Chronic diseases of the lower respiratory tract	4	41.8	5.1	39.5	4	41.9	5.1		5	41.8	5.1	
Dementia and Alzheimer's disease	5	32.0	3.9	43.4	—	—	—		4	44.6	5.4	
Diabetes mellitus	6	24.8	3.0	46.4	5	23.4	2.9		8	26.1	3.2	
Heart failure	7	22.4	2.7	49.2	—	—	—		7	26.5	3.2	
Pneumonia and influenza	8	21.7	2.6	51.8	10	19.4	2.4		9	23.9	2.9	
Malignant neoplasm of the colon, sigmoid, rectum, and anus	9	20.1	2.5	54.3	9	20.5	2.5		—	—	—	
Malignant neoplasm of the hematopoietic and lymphatic systems	10	19.6	2.4	56.7	7	21.3	2.6		6	28.8	3.5	
Malignant neoplasm of the breast	—	—	—	—	6	22.0	2.7		—	—	—	
Malignant neoplasm of the prostate	—	—	—	—	—	—	—		10	20.9	2.5	
Disease of the genitourinary system	—	—	—	—	8	21.3	2.6		—	—	—	
Traffic accidents (terrestrial)	—	—	—	—	—	—	—		—	—	—	

— Not among the ten leading causes.
Source: Mortality database, PAHO/HDM/HA.

America; nevertheless, despite representing only the fourth leading cause among men, the male mortality rate (20.4 per 100,000 population) for this cause is higher than that for the female population (16.9 per 100,000 population). Traffic accident rates are almost three times higher for males (24.7 per 100,000 population) than females (9 per 100,000 population), representing the second and fourth leading causes, respectively. Among men in this same age group (20–59), ischemic heart disease is the leading cause of death, and, as mentioned earlier, traffic accidents are the second, followed by suicide, lung cancer, cirrhosis, and homicide. Death from HIV/AIDS, which was among the highest ranking causes of death in the mid-1990s, began trending downward in the late 1990s. After lung cancer, ischemic heart disease is the second leading cause of death among women, followed by breast cancer, traffic accidents, cerebrovascular disease, and cirrhosis.

Beginning at age 60, for both sexes, the leading causes of death are diseases of the circulatory system (ischemic heart disease and cerebrovascular disease) and neoplasms (cancer of the lung for both sexes, of the breast in women, and of the prostate in men), in addition to dementia and Alzheimer's disease, chronic respiratory disease diseases, and diabetes, presenting similar profiles for both sexes and with slightly higher rates among men.

Mexico

The leading cause of death for Mexico's total population is diabetes mellitus, accounting for 12.8% of deaths; it is the leading cause among women, responsible for 15.7% of deaths, and the second leading cause among men, with 10.6% of deaths (Table 2). As does the non-Latin Caribbean, Mexico has one of the highest rates in the Americas for both sexes, with more than twice the rates of any other subregion.

Ischemic heart disease and cerebrovascular disease rank among the four leading causes of death in Mexico for both men and women, as in all other subregions. Cirrhosis is the country's third leading cause of death, for a rate of 32 per 100,000 population (49.5 among men and 15.4 among women). Moreover, Mexico is the only subregion in which cirrhosis is included among the ten leading causes of death in women (fifth leading cause). It is the leading cause of death among men aged 20–59 (15%) and the second leading cause among women (6.1%). For men, traffic accidents, chronic respiratory diseases, conditions originating in the perinatal period, and homicides continue to figure prominently. Among women, chronic respiratory diseases constitute the fourth leading cause, followed by cirrhosis, conditions originating in the perinatal period, hypertensive disease, diseases of the urinary system, pneumonia and influenza, and nutritional deficiencies and anemias (2.5% of all female deaths) rounding up the tenth cause—Mexico is the only subregion where this occurs.

Among children under 5 years old, conditions originating in the perinatal period and congenital malformations account for 60% of total deaths, followed, in order of importance, by pneu-

monia and influenza, intestinal infectious diseases, accidental obstruction of the respiratory tract, and malnutrition. The same holds true with respect to the leading causes of death among both boys and girls, although mortality rates are slightly higher among boys for all these diseases.

Among Mexico's female population aged 5–19 years old, the leading causes of death are traffic accidents, followed by malignant neoplasms of the hematopoietic and lymphatic systems, congenital malformations, diseases of the urinary system, suicide (third leading cause among the 10–19-year-olds), and homicide; complications of pregnancy, childbirth, and the puerperium is the seventh leading cause among the age group 10–19 years old. Traffic accidents are also the leading cause of death among males in the 5–19 age group, followed by homicide, malignant neoplasms of the hematopoietic and lymphatic systems, accidental drowning or submersion, and congenital malformations. Mortality rates for the age group 5–19 are consistently lower than those of other groups, although rates for males are always higher than for females, especially with regard to external causes. As is the case for the female population, suicide is the third leading cause of death among males.

Among the population 20–59 years old, diabetes is the leading cause of death for women and the second for men; cirrhosis is the first leading cause for men and the second for women. After these two causes, the causes of death for the male population, in rank order, are traffic accidents, homicides, ischemic heart disease, and HIV/AIDS. The third to sixth causes of death are ischemic heart disease, malignant neoplasms of the uterus, malignant neoplasms of the breast, and cerebrovascular disease.

After age 60 the leading causes of death for both sexes are diabetes, ischemic heart disease, cerebrovascular disease, and chronic respiratory diseases.

Central America

The leading cause of death for both sexes in this subregion are pneumonia and influenza (8.6% of total deaths), whose rate is more than double that seen in most of the other subregions. This may partly be due to shortcomings in the medical certification of death, inasmuch as pneumonias are often fatal but the basic or underlying cause is not stated on the death certificates. Among the male population, pneumonia and influenza are followed by homicide, ischemic heart disease, intestinal infectious diseases, and conditions originating in the perinatal period, whereas the corresponding order for the female population is ischemic heart disease, cerebrovascular disease, intestinal infectious diseases, and diabetes. It bears mentioning that Central America is the only subregion in which intestinal infectious diseases are included among the ten leading causes of death, accounting for the fourth leading cause in both sexes (Table 3).

Among children under 5, the leading causes of death for both sexes, in rank order, are conditions originating in the perinatal

TABLE 2. Rates, percentage, and cumulative percentage (based on defined causes) of the ten leading causes of death, by sex, Mexico, circa 2002.

Deaths	Total				Males				Females		
	Rank	Rate (per 100,000 population)	%	Cumulative %	Rank	Rate (per 100,000 population)	%	Cumulative %	Rank	Rate (per 100,000 population)	Cumulative %
Total	—	514.8	100.0	—	—	591.2	100.0	—	—	441.6	100.0
Ill-defined causes	—	—	2.0	—	—	—	1.8	—	—	—	2.3
Defined causes	—	504.5	100.0	—	—	580.6	100.0	—	—	431.4	100.0
Diabetes mellitus	1	64.7	12.8	12.8	2	61.3	10.6	10.6	1	67.9	15.7
Ischemic heart disease	2	55.1	10.9	23.7	1	63.1	10.9	10.9	2	47.4	11.0
Cirrhosis of the liver and other chronic liver diseases	3	32.3	6.4	30.1	3	49.8	8.6	8.6	5	15.5	3.6
Cerebrovascular disease	4	29.5	5.8	36.0	4	28.8	5.0	5.0	3	30.2	7.0
Chronic diseases of the lower respiratory tract	5	22.1	4.4	40.4	6	25.7	4.4	4.4	4	18.8	4.4
Conditions originating in the perinatal period	6	19.2	3.8	44.2	7	23.2	4.0	4.0	6	15.5	3.6
Traffic accidents (terrestrial)	7	16.5	3.3	47.5	5	26.5	4.6	4.6	9	11.8	2.7
Pneumonia and influenza	8	13.2	2.6	50.1	9	14.7	2.5	2.5	8	12.0	2.8
Disease of the genitourinary system	9	13.1	2.6	52.7	10	14.2	2.4	2.4	7	14.2	3.3
Hypertensive disease	10	12.5	2.5	55.1	—	—	—	—	7	14.2	3.3
Assault (homicides)	—	—	—	—	8	19.0	—	3.3	—	—	—
Malnutrition and nutritional anemias	—	—	—	—	—	—	—	—	10	11.0	2.5

— Not among the ten leading causes.
Source: Mortality database, HDM/HA/PAHO.

TABLE 3. Rates, percentage, and cumulative percentage (based on defined causes) of the ten leading causes of death, by sex, Central America, circa 2002.

Deaths	Total				Males			Females		
	Rank	Rate (per 100,000 population)	%	Cumulative %	Rank	Rate (per 100,000 population)	Cumulative %	Rank	Rate (per 100,000 population)	Cumulative %
Total	—	643.5	100.0	—	—	721.9	100.0	—	566.2	100.0
Ill-defined causes	—	—	11.9	—	—	—	10.8	—	—	13.3
Defined causes	—	566.9	100.0	—	—	643.9	100.0	—	490.9	100.0
Pneumonia and influenza	1	48.8	8.6	8.6	1	52.0	8.1	1	45.6	9.3
Ischemic heart disease	2	38.5	6.8	15.4	3	41.3	6.4	2	35.7	7.3
Cerebrovascular disease	3	31.4	5.5	20.9	6	29.9	4.6	3	32.8	6.7
Intestinal infectious diseases	4	28.5	5.0	26.0	4	31.3	4.9	4	25.8	5.3
Conditions originating in the perinatal period	5	26.4	4.7	30.6	5	30.6	4.8	6	22.1	4.5
Assault (homicides)	6	25.3	4.5	35.1	2	45.8	7.1	—	—	—
Diabetes mellitus	7	21.5	3.8	38.9	—	—	—	5	24.9	5.1
Heart failure	8	19.7	3.5	42.4	10	18.2	2.8	7	21.1	4.3
Cirrhosis of the liver and other chronic liver diseases	9	19.2	3.4	45.7	7	26.4	4.1	—	—	—
Diseases of the genitourinary system	10	16.6	2.9	48.7	9	21.0	3.3	—	—	—
Traffic accidents (terrestrial)	—	—	—	—	8	24.0	3.7	—	—	—
Chronic diseases of the lower respiratory tract	—	—	—	—	—	—	—	8	16.1	3.3
Cardiac arrest	—	—	—	—	—	—	—	9	14.4	2.9
Malignant neoplasms of the uterus	—	—	—	—	—	—	—	10	13.0	2.6

— Not among the ten leading causes.
Source: Mortality database, PAHO/HDM/HA.

period, intestinal infectious diseases, pneumonia and influenza, congenital malformations, and malnutrition. Central America and the Latin Caribbean are the only subregions of the Americas where vaccine-preventable diseases still rank among the ten leading causes of death for this age group (seventh leading cause in Central America and tenth in the Latin Caribbean).

Homicide is the leading cause of death among Central American males aged 5–19 years old, followed by traffic accidents, external causes of undetermined intent, pneumonia and influenza, and accidental drowning or submersion. Among females in this age group, the leading causes are pneumonia and influenza, intestinal infectious diseases, traffic accidents, and external causes of undetermined intent. Central America is the only subregion where vaccine-preventable diseases figure among the leading causes of death for this age group (eighth leading cause).

Among the Central American population 20–59 years old, homicide is the leading cause of death. The extent of male mortality from this cause is such that while only representing the tenth leading cause among females, it still ranks as the leading cause for the total population of this age group. Among males, the leading causes of death are homicide, cirrhosis, traffic accidents, adverse effects of psychoactive drugs (including alcohol), and external causes of undetermined intent. Among females, the leading causes of death are malignant neoplasms of the uterus, diabetes, cerebrovascular disease, pneumonia and influenza, and ischemic heart disease.

With regard to older adults (age 60 and over), the five leading causes of death for both sexes are ischemic heart disease, followed by cerebrovascular disease, pneumonia and influenza, diabetes (fourth among women, fifth among men) and heart failure (fifth among women, fourth among men).

Latin Caribbean

The three leading causes of death for both sexes are ischemic heart disease, cerebrovascular disease, and pneumonia and influenza (Table 4). Among women, these are followed by diabetes, hypertensive disease, and HIV/AIDS, and among men, by HIV/AIDS; malignant neoplasms of the trachea, bronchus, and lung; and intestinal infectious diseases. It is important to bear in mind that the presence of HIV/AIDS as a leading cause is heavily influenced by the number of deaths from this cause in Haiti, where the disease constitutes the leading cause of death. This is also the case in mortality from malnutrition and intestinal infectious diseases among the youngest age groups.

Among children 0–4 years old, the five leading causes of death are the same for both sexes: conditions originating in the perinatal period; malnutrition; intestinal infectious diseases; pneumonia and influenza; and congenital malformations.

Among the population aged 5–19, the four leading causes of death are the same for both sexes: traffic accidents; intestinal infectious diseases; HIV/AIDS; and external causes of undeter-

mined intent. In addition, the causes of maternal mortality constitute the second leading cause among the female population aged 10–19.

Among the population aged 20–59, the leading cause of death for both sexes is HIV/AIDS. Among men in this age group, HIV/AIDS is followed by ischemic heart disease, traffic accidents, homicide, and cerebrovascular disease; among women, it is followed by cerebrovascular disease, ischemic heart disease, and the causes of maternal mortality.

Mortality profiles have remained practically identical for both women and men after age 60, with only slightly higher rates among men. The three leading causes of death for both sexes are ischemic heart disease, cerebrovascular disease, and pneumonia and influenza. For females, these are followed by diabetes, hypertensive disease, and heart failure, and, for males, by malignant neoplasms of the prostate, malignant neoplasm of the lung, and heart failure.

Non-Latin Caribbean

The leading causes of death for both sexes in this subregion are ischemic heart disease, cerebrovascular disease, and diabetes (Table 5). As does Mexico, the non-Latin Caribbean subregion has one of the highest mortality rates from diabetes in the Americas (between 60 and 72 per 100,000 population); it also has the highest HIV/AIDS mortality rates in the Americas, at 37.7 per 100,000 population among the general population, 48.3 per 100,000 among males (fourth leading cause), and 27.3 among women (fifth leading cause).

With respect to children under 5, the six leading causes of death for both sexes are conditions originating in the perinatal period (53.9%), congenital malformations (11.1%), intestinal infectious diseases (5.5%), pneumonia and influenza (3.9%), HIV/AIDS (3.5%), and malnutrition (2%).

Traffic accidents are the leading cause of death for both sexes in the age group 5–19 years old, followed by HIV/AIDS, homicide, suicide (the leading cause among adolescent females), and accidental drowning and accidental submersion.

HIV/AIDS is the leading cause of death among men and women aged 20–59 years old, at 15.7% and 14.9% of deaths, respectively. Among males of this group HIV/AIDS is followed by ischemic heart disease (10.2%), homicide (6.2%), diabetes (6.2%), and suicide (5.9%); among females, by diabetes (10.9%), ischemic heart disease (7.9%), cerebrovascular disease (6.7%), and malignant neoplasm of the breast (5%).

After age 60, the three leading causes of death for both sexes—and in very similar proportion—are ischemic heart disease (17.2%), cerebrovascular disease (14.1%), and diabetes (12.5%). Mortality rates are higher for men in terms of the first two causes; among women, rates are higher for diabetes. Among men of this group, these causes are followed in importance by malignant neoplasms of the prostate and hypertensive disease, and among women, by hypertensive disease and heart failure.

TABLE 4. Rates, percentage, and cumulative percentage (based on defined causes) of the ten leading causes of death, by sex, Latin Caribbean, circa 2002.

Deaths	Total				Males			Females		
	Rank	Rate (per 100,000 population)	%	Cumulative %	Rank	Rate (per 100,000 population)	Cumulative %	Rank	Rate (per 100,000 population)	Cumulative %
Total	—	872.6	100.0	—	—	953.0	100.0	—	793.1	100.0
Ill-defined causes	—	—	15.3	—	—	—	15.7	—	—	14.8
Defined causes	—	739.1	100.0	—	—	803.4	100.0	—	675.7	100.0
Ischemic heart disease	1	83.5	11.3	11.3	1	90.2	11.2	1	76.9	11.4
Cerebrovascular disease	2	68.7	9.3	20.6	2	66.5	8.3	2	70.8	10.5
Pneumonia and influenza	3	39.2	5.3	25.9	3	42.2	5.3	3	36.2	5.4
HIV/AIDS	4	31.8	4.3	30.2	4	36.5	4.5	6	27.1	4.0
Diabetes mellitus	5	27.7	3.7	33.9	—	—	—	4	30.9	4.6
Hypertensive disease	6	26.8	3.6	37.6	10	24.7	3.1	5	28.8	4.3
Conditions originating in the perinatal period	7	26.4	3.6	41.1	7	26.7	3.3	8	26.0	3.8
Intestinal infectious diseases	8	25.8	3.5	44.6	6	27.8	3.5	9	23.8	3.5
Heart failure	9	25.3	3.4	48.1	—	—	—	7	26.2	3.9
Malignant neoplasm of the trachea, bronchus, and lung	10	19.0	2.6	50.6	5	29.1	3.6	—	—	—
Traffic accidents (terrestrial)	—	—	—	—	8	25.3	3.1	—	—	—
Malignant neoplasm of the prostate	—	—	—	—	9	25.2	3.1	—	—	—
Chronic diseases of the lower respiratory tract	—	—	—	—	—	—	—	10	15.9	2.4

— Not among the ten leading causes.
Source: Mortality database, HDM/HA/PAHO.

TABLE 5. Rates, percentage, and cumulative percentage (based on defined causes) of the ten leading causes of death, by sex, non–Latin Caribbean, circa 2002.

Deaths	Total				Males			Females		
	Rank	Rate (per 100,000 population)	%	Cumulative %	Rank	Rate (per 100,000 population)	Cumulative %	Rank	Rate (per 100,000 population)	Cumulative %
Total	—	683.4	100.0	—	—	766.5	100.0	—	602.6	100.0
Ill-defined causes	—	—	3.3	—	—	—	2.9	—	—	3.8
Defined causes	—	660.8	100.0	—	—	744.3	100.0	—	579.7	100.0
Ischemic heart disease	1	87.6	13.3	13.3	1	98.7	13.3	1	76.8	13.2
Cerebrovascular disease	2	68.0	10.3	23.5	2	67.9	9.1	3	68.1	11.7
Diabetes mellitus	3	66.3	10.0	33.6	3	60.0	8.1	2	72.4	12.5
HIV/AIDS	4	37.7	5.7	39.3	4	48.3	6.5	5	27.3	4.7
Hypertensive disease	5	33.5	5.1	44.4	6	31.2	4.2	4	35.7	6.2
Pneumonia and influenza	6	21.6	3.3	47.6	7	24.6	3.3	7	18.6	3.2
Heart failure	7	20.1	3.0	50.7	—	—	—	6	20.0	3.5
Conditions originating in the perinatal period	8	19.8	3.0	53.7	8	23.0	3.1	8	16.6	2.9
Malignant neoplasm of the prostate	9	16.4	2.5	56.1	5	31.9	4.3	—	—	—
Traffic accidents (terrestrial)	10	13.9	2.1	58.2	9	22.3	3.0	—	—	—
Assault (homicides)	—	—	—	—	10	21.3	2.9	—	—	—
Malignant neoplasm of the breast	—	—	—	—	—	—	—	9	16.3	2.8
Malignant neoplasm of the uterus	—	—	—	—	—	—	—	10	15.2	2.6

— Not among the ten leading causes.
Source: Mortality database, PAHO/HDM/HA.

Andean Area

Homicide is the leading cause of death among men (15.1% of all deaths) and constitutes the second leading cause among the total population in this subregion, despite its absence among the women's ten leading causes of death (Table 6). Male mortality from homicide, which is the highest of all the subregions, approaches 87.3 per 100,000 men. Within the subregion, rates are highest in Colombia, about three times that of the other countries in the subregion.

Among the general population and among women, ischemic heart disease is the leading cause of death. Ischemic heart disease is the second leading cause of death for men, followed by cerebrovascular disease, traffic accidents, pneumonia and influenza, and conditions originating in the perinatal period. With respect to women, ischemic heart disease is followed by cerebrovascular disease, pneumonia and influenza, diabetes, conditions originating in the perinatal period, and hypertensive disease.

Among the age group 0–4 years old, the five leading causes of death for both sexes, with very similar proportions and mortality rates, are conditions originating in the perinatal period (39.7% of deaths), congenital malformations (12.4%), pneumonia and influenza (11.5%), intestinal infectious diseases (6.1%), and malnutrition (4.6%).

Among males in the age group 5–19 years old, the five leading causes of death are external causes (more than 70% of total deaths); homicide is first among the external causes at 42%, followed by traffic accidents, external causes of undetermined intent, suicide (among adolescents), and accidental drowning or submersion. Among females of this group, the three leading causes of death are also external causes—traffic accidents, homicide, and suicide—followed in fourth place by malignant neoplasms of the hematopoietic and lymphatic systems, and in fifth, by external causes of undetermined intent. It is important to note that this last category includes homicides, suicides, and accidents of undetermined intent. This makes external causes even more important than the figures suggest.

Among the population aged 20–59, the mortality profile varies by sex. Among women, the leading causes of death are malignant neoplasms of the uterus (7.1% of total female deaths), cerebrovascular disease (7%), ischemic heart disease (6.6%), homicide (5.1%), and malignant neoplasms of the breast (5%). Among men, the leading cause is homicide, accounting for 28.8% of deaths, followed by ground transportation accidents (8.8%), ischemic heart disease (6.3%), external causes of undetermined intent (6%), and HIV/AIDS (3.5%).

Beginning at age 60, the six leading causes of death are the same for both sexes, albeit not in the same order. Ischemic heart disease is the leading cause of death for both sexes, accounting for 16% of total deaths, followed by cardiovascular disease (9.2%). Among women, these are followed by diabetes, hypertensive disease, pneumonia and influenza, and chronic respiratory diseases, accounting for 7.3%, 5.9%, 5.7%, and 5.3% of deaths in women,

respectively. Among men, chronic respiratory diseases (6%) are the third leading cause of death, followed by pneumonia and influenza (5.3%), diabetes (5%), and hypertensive disease (4.9%).

Brazil

As Table 7 illustrates, the two leading causes of death in Brazil are cerebrovascular diseases (10.6% of total deaths) and ischemic heart disease (9.8%), with similar percentages by sex. Among males, these causes are followed by homicide (7.8%, rate of 57.3 per 100,000 men), ground transportation accidents (4.4%), chronic respiratory diseases (4.3%), and conditions originating in the perinatal period (4.2%). Diabetes is the third leading cause of death among women, accounting for 6.1% of female deaths, followed by heart failure (4.7%), conditions originating in the perinatal period (4.4%), and pneumonia and influenza (4.3%).

Among children under 5, most deaths for both sexes are the result of conditions originating in the perinatal period (54.5%) and congenital malformations (12.1%), as is the case in all the subregions. These causes are followed by pneumonia and influenza (5.7%), intestinal infectious diseases (5%), and septicemia (3.1%). The mortality profile is roughly the same for children of both sexes in this age group, with rates slightly higher among boys.

Mortality due to external causes is the leading cause of death among the population aged 5–19, especially among males, for whom homicide ranks first (tenth leading cause among the 5–9-year-olds and first among 10–19-year-olds), accounting for nearly 40% of total deaths. Among the male population, these causes are followed by traffic accidents, accidental drowning or submersion, external causes of undetermined intent, and, in the case of adolescent boys, suicide. Among females, traffic accidents are the leading cause, followed by homicide and accidental drowning or submersion. Maternal mortality causes account for the fourth leading cause of death among adolescent girls, followed by suicide. Among girls aged 5–9, pneumonia and influenza, and malignant neoplasms of the hematopoietic and lymphatic systems are also significant causes of death.

Among the population aged 20–59 years old, the mortality profile by sex is quite different. The leading cause of death among women in this age group is cerebrovascular disease (11%), followed by ischemic heart disease (7.7%), malignant neoplasms of the breast (5.2%), diabetes (4.8%), and malignant neoplasms of the uterus (4.1%). Among men, homicide is the leading cause of death (15.9%), followed by traffic accidents (8.4%), ischemic heart disease (8.1%), cirrhosis (6.3%), and cerebrovascular disease (6.1%).

Beginning at age 60 the profile is practically the same for both sexes. Accordingly, cerebrovascular disease is the leading cause of death, accounting for 14.5% of deaths, followed by ischemic heart disease (12.9%). Chronic respiratory diseases are the third leading cause among men and fifth among women. Moreover, heart failure is the fourth leading cause for both sexes, while diabetes is fifth among men and third among women.

TABLE 6. Rates, percentage, and cumulative percentage (based on defined causes) of the ten leading causes of death, by sex, Andean Area, circa 2002.

Deaths	Total				Males				Females			
	Rank	Rate (per 100,000 population)	%	Cumulative %	Rank	Rate (per 100,000 population)	%	Cumulative %	Rank	Rate (per 100,000 population)	%	Cumulative %
Total	—	589.7	100.0	—	—	674.9	100.0	—	—	504.8	100.0	100.0
Ill-defined causes	—	—	5.8	—	—	—	5.2	—	—	—	—	6.5
Defined causes	—	555.5	100.0	—	—	639.8	100.0	—	—	472.0	—	100.0
Ischemic heart disease	1	56.6	10.2	10.2	2	62.8	9.8	9.8	1	50.4		10.7
Assault (homicides)	2	47.6	8.6	18.8	1	87.3	13.6	13.6	—	—		—
Cardiovascular disease	3	37.8	6.8	25.6	3	35.0	5.5	5.5	2	40.6		8.6
Pneumonia and influenza	4	27.8	5.0	30.6	5	28.9	4.5	4.5	3	26.7		5.7
Conditions originating in the perinatal period	5	23.9	4.3	34.9	6	27.1	4.2	4.2	5	20.7		4.4
Diabetes mellitus	6	23.0	4.1	39.0	8	20.1	3.1	3.1	4	25.9		5.5
Traffic accidents (terrestrial)	7	19.8	3.6	42.6	4	30.6	4.8	4.8	—	—		—
Hypertensive disease	8	18.4	3.3	45.9	10	17.4	2.7	2.7	6	19.5		4.1
Chronic diseases of the lower respiratory tract	9	18.3	3.3	49.2	9	19.4	3.0	3.0	7	17.1		3.6
Heart failure	10	15.4	2.8	52.0	—	—	—	—	8	15.9		3.4
Event of undetermined intent	—	—	—	—	7	20.2	3.2	3.2	—	—		—
Malignant neoplasm of the uterus	—	—	—	—	—	—	—	—	9	15.5		3.3
Diseases of the genitourinary system	—	—	—	—	—	—	—	—	10	12.6		2.7

— Not among the ten leading causes.
Source: Mortality database, PAHO/HDM/HA.

TABLE 7. Rates, percentage, and cumulative percentage (based on defined causes) of the ten leading causes of death, by sex, Brazil, circa 2002.

Deaths	Total				Males			Females		
	Rank	Rate (per 100,000 population)	%	Cumulative %	Rank	Rate (per 100,000 population)	Cumulative %	Rank	Rate (per 100,000 population)	Cumulative %
Total	—	729.1	100.0	—	—	851.7	100.0	—	609.4	100.0
Ill-defined causes	—	—	14.0	—	—	—	13.4	—	—	14.8
Defined causes	—	627.0	100.0	—	—	737.6	100.0	—	519.2	100.0
Cerebrovascular disease	1	66.7	10.6	10.6	2	69.0	9.4	1	64.5	12.4
Ischemic heart disease	2	61.7	9.8	20.5	1	72.3	9.8	2	51.4	9.9
Assault (homicides)	3	30.8	4.9	25.4	3	57.3	7.8	—	—	—
Diabetes mellitus	4	27.6	4.4	29.8	10	23.5	3.2	3	31.6	6.1
Conditions originating in the perinatal period	5	27.0	4.3	34.1	6	31.2	4.2	5	22.8	4.4
Chronic diseases of the lower respiratory tract	6	26.4	4.2	38.3	5	32.0	4.3	7	21.0	4.0
Heart failure	7	24.3	3.9	42.2	9	24.3	3.3	4	24.4	4.7
Pneumonia and influenza	8	23.9	3.8	46.0	8	25.3	3.4	6	22.5	4.3
Traffic accidents (terrestrial)	9	19.9	3.2	49.2	4	32.7	4.4	—	—	—
Hypertensive disease	10	19.0	3.0	52.2	—	—	—	8	20.0	3.9
Neoplasm of the breast	—	—	—	—	—	—	—	9	13.2	2.5
Malignant neoplasm of the uterus	—	—	—	—	—	—	—	10	10.4	2.0
Cirrhosis of the liver and other chronic liver diseases	—	—	—	—	7	25.8	3.5	—	—	—

— Not among the ten leading causes.
Source: Mortality database, PAHO/HDM/HA.

Southern Cone

This is the only subregion of the Americas in which external causes are absent from the ten leading causes of death for both males and females. The four leading causes are the same for both sexes, although in different order. Among males, ischemic heart disease (8.8%) is the leading cause, followed by cerebrovascular disease (8.1%) and heart failure (7.6%). Among women, heart failure (10.1%) is the leading cause, followed by cerebrovascular disease (10%) and ischemic heart disease (7.1%). Pneumonia and influenza are the fourth leading cause for both sexes, accounting for 5.2% of female deaths and 4.3% of male deaths (Table 8). The fifth leading cause among males is malignant neoplasms of the trachea, bronchus, and lung, followed by diabetes and cirrhosis. Among women, malignant neoplasm of the breast is fifth, followed by diabetes and respiratory failure.

The leading causes of death among children under 5 are the same for both sexes and similar in terms of rates and percentage: conditions originating in the perinatal period (44.5% of total deaths in this age group), congenital malformations (19.9%), pneumonia and influenza (6.4%), intestinal infectious diseases (3.6%), and septicemia (2.8%).

After North America, the age group 5–19 years old in the Southern Cone has the lowest mortality rates from all causes, both for the 5–9 (0.31 per 1,000 population) and the 10–19-year-old subgroups (0.51). The leading cause of death for both sexes of these subgroups is traffic accidents (12.9% among males and 10.6% females). Other relevant causes among children 5–9 years old include malignant neoplasms of the hematopoietic and lymphatic systems, congenital malformations, and accidental drowning or submersion. Other significant causes of mortality among adolescents aged 10–19 are homicide (leading cause among males, at 10.8%, and third leading cause among females, at 11.5%), suicide (second among females at 10.8% and third among males at 11.5%), and malignant neoplasms of the hematopoietic and lymphatic systems (third among females at 6.6% and sixth among males at 4.4%.

Among men in the 20–59-year-old age group, the leading causes of death are ischemic heart disease (7.7%), cerebrovascular disease (6.7%), traffic accidents (6.3%), cirrhosis (5.5%), homicide (5.3%), and suicide (5.3%). The leading causes of death among women in the same age group are malignant neoplasm of the breast (8.9%), cerebrovascular disease (8.7%), malignant neoplasm of the uterus (6.6%), ischemic heart disease (3.9), heart failure (3.6%), and diabetes (3.2%).

The mortality profile for the population aged 60 years old and older is similar for both sexes, with diseases of the circulatory system constituting the three leading causes—heart failure, ischemic heart disease, and cerebrovascular disease—and accounting for 30% of all deaths, followed by pneumonia and influenza with 5.5% of deaths. Among males in this age group, the next leading causes of death are malignant neoplasms of the tra-

chea, bronchus, and lung (4.4%), and diabetes (3.9%). Among females in this age group, diabetes is the fifth leading cause of death (4.4%), followed by respiratory failure (3.4%).

MORBIDITY

VACCINE-PREVENTABLE DISEASES

Immunization is one of the most cost-effective interventions available in public health. It plays a significant role in reaching the Millennium Development Goals of reducing child mortality and improving maternal health, and is a key tool for promoting socioeconomic development (5). The countries of the Americas have made immunization a top priority among the health interventions they pursue, and they have pioneered the effort to eradicate, eliminate, and control vaccine-preventable diseases (6)— the Region of the Americas was the first to eradicate smallpox and poliomyelitis, and the first to eliminate the endemic transmission of measles (5,6). These achievements have been possible through sustained high levels of immunization coverage in the regular program, implementation of high-quality surveillance, and mass vaccination campaigns designed to rapidly reduce large susceptible populations.

Responsible management of national immunization programs, the development and execution of annual and multi-year plans of action, municipal-level planning, the promotion of coordination among immunization partners through national interagency committees, the training of health workers, effective supervision, and regular and sustained program evaluation are some of the key tools that have been used to implement strategies for the eradication, elimination, and control of vaccine-preventable diseases. The close monitoring of coverage and surveillance data at the local level and the validation of data, such as rapid coverage monitoring and active case searches, also are important tools. Ongoing efforts to finance immunization programs with regular government funds by having a budget line for immunization in the national budget, and ensuring that immunization legislation is in place also been essential for successfully sustaining immunization programs in the Americas (6). Finally, PAHO's Revolving Fund for the Purchase of Vaccines has been instrumental in supporting national immunization programs in the countries of the Americas by ensuring an uninterrupted supply of quality vaccines at affordable prices; the Fund has earned increasing supplier confidence through prompt payment and better forecasting (7).

Yet, despite considerable gains, much remains to be done to address the unfinished immunization agenda, hold on to achievements, and confront the new challenges presented by an ever-changing and interdependent world. This section summarizes the main achievements in immunization in the Americas in 2001–2005 and highlights the challenges that loom ahead.

TABLE 8. Rates, percentage, and cumulative percentage (based on defined causes) of the ten leading causes of death, by sex, Southern Cone, circa 2002.

Deaths	Total				Males				Females		
	Rank	Rate (per 100,000 population)	%	Cumulative %	Rank	Rate (per 100,000 population)	%	Cumulative %	Rank	Rate (per 100,000 population)	Cumulative %
Total	—	757.5	100.0	—	—	826.0	100.0	—	—	691.3	100.0
Ill-defined causes	—	—	7.7	—	—	—	7.4	—	—	—	8.0
Defined causes	—	699.2	100.0	—	—	764.9	100.0	—	—	636.0	100.0
Cerebrovascular disease	1	63.0	9.0	9.0	2	62.2	8.1	8.1	2	63.7	10.0
Heart failure	2	61.2	8.8	17.8	3	58.2	7.6	7.6	1	64.0	10.1
Ischemic heart disease	3	56.0	8.0	25.8	1	67.3	8.8	8.8	3	45.1	7.1
Pneumonia and influenza	4	33.3	4.8	30.5	4	33.4	4.4	4.4	4	33.2	5.2
Diabetes mellitus	5	25.3	3.6	34.2	6	25.1	3.3	3.3	5	25.5	4.0
Malignant neoplasm of the trachea, bronchus, and lung	6	20.8	3.0	37.1	5	32.1	4.2	4.2	—	—	—
Diseases of the genitourinary	7	19.1	2.7	39.9	10	19.7	2.6	2.6	9	18.5	2.9
Respiratory failure	8	18.6	2.7	42.5	—	—	—	—	8	18.5	2.9
Septicemia	9	18.5	2.6	45.2	—	—	—	—	7	18.7	2.9
Chronic diseases of the lower respiratory tract	10	15.8	2.3	47.4	8	20.7	2.7	2.7	6	24.5	3.9
Neoplasm of the breast	—	—	—	—	—	—	—	—	6	24.5	3.9
Cirrhosis of the liver and other chronic liver diseases	—	—	—	—	7	22.3	2.9	2.9	—	—	—
Neoplasm of the prostate	—	—	—	—	9	20.5	2.7	2.7	—	—	—
Hypertensive disease	—	—	—	—	—	—	—	—	10	16.8	2.6

— Not among the ten leading causes.
Source: Mortality database, HDM/HA/PAHO.

FIGURE 11. Vaccination coverage of children under 1 year old, Latin America and the Caribbean, 2001–2005.

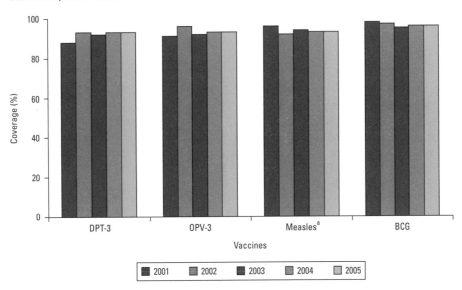

[a]Measles data reported for children aged 1 year, with the exception of Haiti.
Source: Country reports to PAHO, Family and Community Health, Immunizations.

Holding on to Achievements

Under the guiding principles of reducing inequities, strengthening public health infrastructure, fostering a prevention culture, and galvanizing political commitment, immunization programs in the Americas, have eradicated, eliminated, and significantly reduced the morbidity and mortality associated with vaccine-preventable diseases. Important by-products of this achievement have included strengthening the public health infrastructure, encouraging effective inter-sectoral coordination, promoting equity, and increasing the community's awareness about prevention (*8*).

An Umbrella of Protection

Immunization's umbrella of protection includes polio eradication; measles and neonatal tetanus elimination; and the control of pertussis, diphtheria, tetanus, invasive diseases caused by *Haemophilus influenzae* type b, and hepatitis B.

Regionwide, routine coverage for BCG,[5] DTP-3,[6] polio-3[7] and measles-containing vaccines[8] in children under 1 year old has been higher than 90% since 2002 (Figure 11). As a result of

this high coverage, the morbidity and mortality associated with vaccine-preventable diseases have been significantly reduced (Figure 12a, b, c, and d)

The countries of the Americas have expanded the umbrella of childhood protection by adding other vaccines to the six antigens of the original Expanded Program on Immunization (EPI). As of 2006, all countries in the Region, except Haiti, include measles-mumps-rubella (MMR), *Haemophilus influenzae* type b (Hib), and hepatitis B vaccines; 31 countries are using the pentavalent vaccine, which combines DTP, Hib, and hepatitis B antigens.

Poliomyelitis

More than 20 years have passed since PAHO Member States unanimously approved a resolution to eradicate the transmission of wild poliovirus from the Western Hemisphere (*9*). After the last case of poliomyelitis caused by a wild poliovirus that occurred in Peru in 1991, the countries of the Americas have remained free of the circulation of the indigenous wild poliovirus (*10*).

At the global level, significant progress has been made towards the goal of polio eradication: only 2,033 wild-polio cases were reported in 2005,[9] and the number of polio-endemic countries is at the lowest in history (*11*). Recent episodes of the spread of wild poliovirus to countries that had interrupted transmission in Africa and Asia, however, highlight the constant risk for polio importation to the Americas (*12*). In addition to the risk of wild

---

[5]BCG: bacille Calmette-Guérin, a vaccine against severe forms of tuberculosis.

[6]DTP: vaccine against diphtheria-pertussis-tetanus; DTP-3: third-dose of DTP, as DTP or a combination vaccine.

[7]Polio-3: third dose of polio vaccine (oral polio vaccine (OPV) or inactivated polio vaccine).

[8]Measles-containing vaccines refer to measles vaccines as a single antigen or in combination, most commonly as measles-mumps-rubella vaccine (MMR).

[9] Data as of 22 June 2007, WHO Global Polio Eradication Initiative. http://www.who.int/immunization_monitoring/diseases/poliomyelitis/en/

FIGURE 12a. Umbrella of protection: measles elimination, Region of the Americas, 1980–2005.

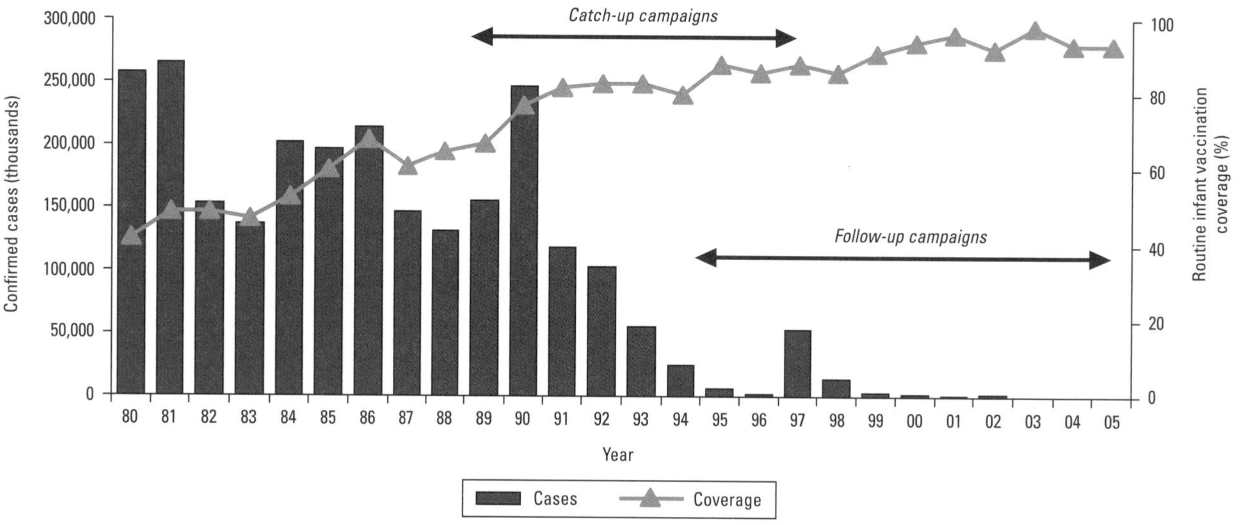

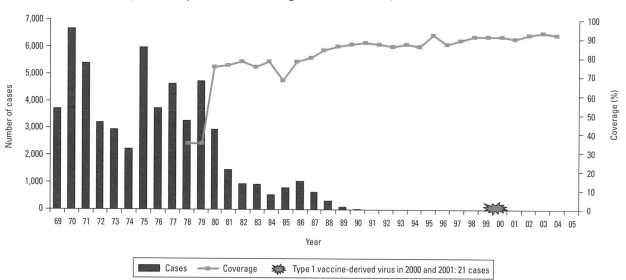

Note: 81 confirmed cases in 2005.
Source: Country reports to PAHO, Family and Community Health, Immunizations.

FIGURE 12b. Umbrella of protection, polio eradication, Region of the Americas, 1969–2005.

Source: Country reports to PAHO, Family and Community Health, Immunizations.

poliovirus importations, the outbreak of vaccine-derived poliovirus in the Dominican Republic and Haiti in 2000–2001 that resulted in 21 cases (*13*), a similar occurrence in the Philippines (*14*), and the 2005 circulation of vaccine-derived polio in the United States in a religious community that generally refuses vaccination (*15*), emphasize the risk of low oral polio vaccine (OPV) coverage in countries, municipalities, and communities,

as well as the risk of failing to timely detect poliovirus circulation. That said, the lack of spread of vaccine-derived poliovirus from isolated cases, such as a case of paralysis in an immunocompromised child in Peru in December 2003 (*16*), shows that high coverage will halt the circulation of the poliovirus.

As of 2006, all Latin American and Caribbean countries had continued to vaccinate against polio and maintained acute flaccid

FIGURE 12c. Umbrella of protection: neonatal tetanus elimination, Region of the Americas, 1985–2005.

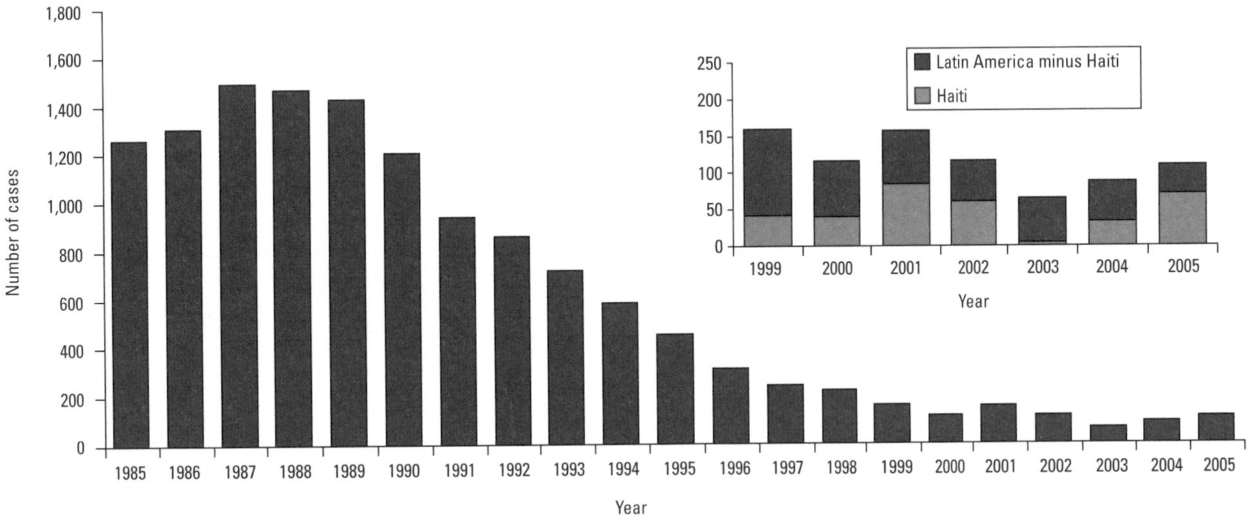

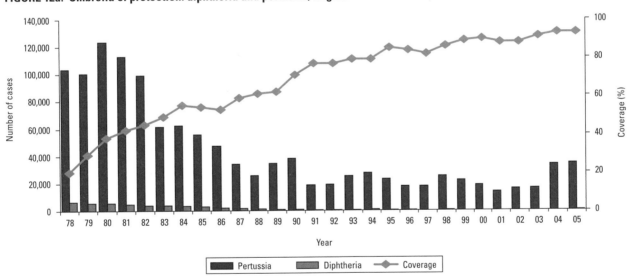

Source: Country reports to PAHO, Family and Community Health, Immunizations.

FIGURE 12d. Umbrella of protection: diphtheria and pertussis, Region of the Americas, 1978–2005.

Source: Country reports to PAHO, Family and Community Health, Immunizations.

paralysis surveillance according to international standards. As stated earlier, polio-3 vaccination coverage is over 90% Region-wide, and most countries continue to administer OPV during supplementary immunization activities, such as the Vaccination Week in the Americas. The Regional acute flaccid paralysis rate remains at more than 1 per 100,000 children under 15 years old, and the proportion of cases with adequate specimens remains

close to 80%. It should be said, however, that these achievements are not uniform, and most countries have at-risk areas within their borders.

To minimize the risk for reintroduction of wild poliovirus from laboratories, the Region's countries carry out a containment plan for all poliovirus strains in laboratories. Phase I of the containment plan, inventorying all laboratories that have poliovirus or potentially infected material, is expected to be ready by the end of 2006 (*17*).

Measles

In 1994, the countries of the Americas became the first in the world to commit themselves to interrupting the indigenous transmission of measles (*18*). In the 1990s, the annual number of measles cases diminished dramatically, from approximately 250,000 in 1990 to 2,109 in 1996 (Figure 12a). However, a large outbreak that began in São Paulo, Brazil, in 1997, resulted in 52,284 confirmed cases and 61 deaths in Brazil, spreading to neighboring countries (*19*). The outbreak underscored the need for aggressively implementing the elimination strategy developed by PAHO in order to eliminate measles (*20*).

To achieve and maintain high levels of measles immunity, the elimination strategy adopted by the Latin American and Caribbean countries includes a three-tiered vaccination approach: a one-time-only "catch-up" campaign to interrupt virus circulation; "keep-up" vaccination or routine immunization to maintain the interruption of measles virus circulation; and "follow-up" vaccination campaigns among preschoolers to counter the inevitable buildup of measles-susceptible children. In addition, special intensive efforts, known as "mop-up" vaccination, may be required to provide measles vaccine to children living in high-risk areas who have missed vaccination (*21*). When the PAHO vaccination strategy is fully implemented, virtually all children will receive one dose of measles vaccine, and most will receive more than one dose.

Caribbean and Latin American countries conducted catch-up campaigns between 1989 and 1995, and have been conducting follow-up campaigns since 1994 (*6, 19*). Additionally, several countries have vaccinated adolescents and adults with measles-rubella (MR) vaccines since 2001, as part of rubella elimination campaigns. Routine coverage has increased from 80% in 1994 to more than 90% since 1999. In 2005, the lowest coverage levels for routine vaccination were reported in Haiti (59%), Venezuela (76%), Bolivia (89%), and Colombia (89%).

A large measles epidemic that affected Venezuela between September 2001 and November 2002 can be viewed as the last instance of widespread endemic transmission of the measles virus in the Americas. This outbreak originated from an importation from Europe. It resulted in 2,501 cases (109 in 2001 and 2,392 in 2002) reported from 17 of the country's 27 states (Figure 13); only 18% of the confirmed cases had received a measles-containing vaccine (*22*). The outbreak spread to Colombia, leading to 140 confirmed cases between January and September 2002 (*23*). The outbreak in Venezuela was controlled thanks to mass vaccination efforts that had solid political commitment.

Since 2003, only about 100 cases have been reported in the Americas annually (119 in 2003, 108 in 2004, and 85 in 2005) and most of them can be positively linked to importations from other regions of the world. As of 2006, no other region in the world had interrupted the endemic circulation of the measles virus.

Between 2003 and 2006, the following outbreaks were reported in the Americas (*24*):

- In 2003–2004, Mexico reported outbreaks totaling 108 cases related to an H1 virus genotype indigenous to the Far East.
- In 2005, Brazil reported an outbreak of six cases linked to an imported case infected in South Asia related to a D5 virus genotype.
- From November 2005 to February 2006, Canada, Mexico, and the United States have reported cases related to a B3 virus genotype, a strain indigenous to Central and West Africa;
- From February to June 2006, Venezuela reported 81 cases, the primary case-patient having a travel history to Spain. The virus isolated from this outbreak was B3, the same genotype circulating in Spain.
- In May 2006, the United States reported an outbreak of 18 cases in Boston related to an imported case likely infected in Southeast Asia.
- In November 2006, Venezuela reported another outbreak that resulted in 12 cases, all residents of the Camaguan municipality, Guarico State. The genotype of the virus isolated was B3.
- Finally, between October and November 2006, the state of Bahia, Brazil, confirmed 57 measles cases. The measles genotype in this outbreak was D4, genetically related to measles that had been imported to Canada this year. The D4 genotype circulates widely in Europe and Africa. The source of this outbreak could not be identified.

Molecular epidemiology of circulating measles viruses has provided a better understanding of measles virus transmission around the world. Transmission of the D6 measles virus genotype—which caused large outbreaks in Argentina, Bolivia, Brazil, the Dominican Republic, and Haiti, starting in 1995—was interrupted in September 2001. Subsequent transmission of the D9 measles virus genotype in Venezuela was interrupted in November 2002 (*25*). All genotypes identified from outbreaks occurring since 2003 have been nonindigenous to the Americas (*26*).

Epidemiological surveillance remains critical to maintaining measles elimination in the Americas. The PAHO-recommended measles surveillance strategy, which now is fully integrated with rubella surveillance, encompasses weekly reporting of suspected cases, including zero-case reporting; laboratory confirmation of suspected cases using serology or viral isolation; active case-searches in areas reporting cases and in silent municipalities; measles virus genotyping; and classification of confirmed cases by source of infection as imported, imported-related, or unknown. Periodic active-case finding in institutions also is recommended to monitor the quality of the surveillance system. For the early detection of imported cases, private-sector health facilities that care for tourists and intercontinental travelers should be in-

FIGURE 13. Distribution of confirmed measles cases, by age group and week, Venezuela, 2001–2002.

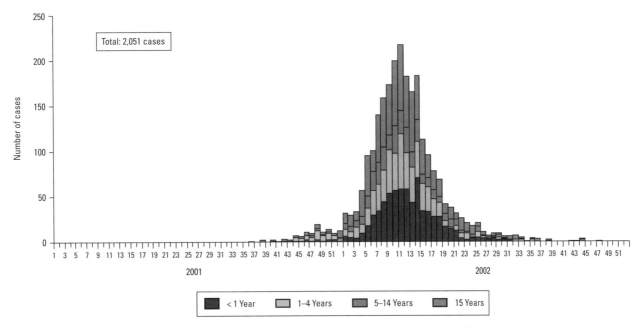

Source: Graph presented at XVI Meeting of the Technical Advisory Group on Vaccine-preventable Diseases, Mexico City, November 2004.

cluded in the surveillance system, as illustrated by recent outbreaks following importations.

PAHO recommends using standardized measles/rubella surveillance indicators to allow a transparent and uniform monitoring of surveillance data across countries (*26*). The percentage of cases discarded by negative laboratory results has consistently been over 95% since 2001. The percentage of sites reporting weekly and the percentage of cases with adequate samples have exceeded 80% at the Regional level since 2002, and the percentage of laboratory results released within four days reached 80% in 2004. Nevertheless, the timely submission of samples to the laboratory and the timely reception of results (Regional average <80%) are indicators that have not been consistently met.

Neonatal Tetanus

Ten years after the World Health Assembly called for the global elimination of maternal and neonatal tetanus by 1995, global efforts have been successful in eliminating neonatal tetanus (NNT) in 104 out of 161 developing countries (*27*). In the Americas, the elimination of neonatal tetanus (NNT) as a public health problem—defined as fewer than 1 case per 1,000 live births in each district or municipality—has been achieved, except in Haiti (*17*).

PAHO-recommended strategies to eliminate NNT include a high-risk district approach and a strategy to investigate each NNT case in detail and vaccinate all women of childbearing age with at least two doses of tetanus vaccine. It should be noted that PAHO recommends the administration of tetanus and diphtheria toxoid (Td), rather than tetanus toxoid (TT) alone, because Td

provides maintains immunity to both diphtheria and tetanus in adults (*28, 29*). In the Americas, a single case of NNT is considered a failure of the health services. In order to prevent new cases, therefore, each case should be subject to a thorough evaluation to determine how it could have been averted (*26*).

Following the implementation of Regional strategies in the 1980s, the number of reported NNT cases in the Americas fell more than 50% in the first four years and has continued to decline in the 1990s and 2000s, registering a 94% decline from 1986 to 2005. Nevertheless, as of 2006, Haiti continued to report close to 50% of the Region's total cases and the country's national average NNT incidence is twice the threshold of 1 per 1,000 live births. NNT incidence in Haiti exceeds that threshold in 10 out of 12 departments, and in one-third of the districts. Furthermore, districts where the incidence is under the threshold in some cases may represent "silent" districts. In Haiti, NNT is ranked sixth among neonatal death causes, accounting for 4% of all neonatal deaths.

Non-neonatal Tetanus

Tetanus cases have declined following the widespread administration of tetanus toxoid to children and to women of childbearing age as part of the effort to prevention neonatal tetanus. Nevertheless, the disease continues to occur in unvaccinated populations that are at risk of wounds and in places where there are *Clostridium tetani* spores; in other words, in rural, poor, livestock-raising areas with populations that do not have adequate health services. More than 7,000 cases of tetanus were reported in 1980, and fewer than 1,000 non-neonatal tetanus cases have been reported in the Region annually since 2001 (479 in 2001; 387 in 2002; 881 in 2003; 825 in 2004; and 972 in 2005). The vast majority occurred in persons 15 years of age or older, and the male:female ratio is approximately 4–5:1. As vaccinated cohorts reach adulthood and countries provide tetanus booster doses, the incidence of tetanus should continue to decrease.

Pertussis

The number of pertussis cases reported in the Americas has dropped dramatically with the widespread use of pertussis vaccines, decreasing from more than 120,000 cases reported in 1980 to fewer than 35,000 reported in 2005.

In Latin America, pertussis has continued to decline in recent years, dropping from 9,421 cases in 1999, to a low of 4,921 cases in 2003. However, 4,928 cases were reported in 2004 and 6,807 in 2005, and outbreaks continue to occur, some of them drawing significant media attention (30).

In recent years, more than 70% of all pertussis cases reported in the Americas came from the United States. There, pertussis incidence has been gradually increasing since the early 1980s. In 2004, a total of 25,827 cases were reported, the largest number since 1959. In the United States, adolescents (11–18 years old) and adults (20 years old and older) have accounted for an increasing proportion of cases. During 2001–2003, the annual incidence of pertussis among 10–19-year-olds increased from 5.5 per 100,000 in 2001, to 6.7 in 2002, and 10.9 in 2003. In 2004, approximately 60% of cases were among persons 11 years old and older. Increased recognition and diagnosis of pertussis in older age groups have probably contributed to this increase of reported cases among adolescents and adults (31). This shift in the ages of those presenting with the disease led the United States to recommend a booster of pertussis vaccine in adolescents, using a recently licensed vaccine that contains smaller doses of acellular pertussis (32).

There is no information by age group for the Region as a whole. However, a review of the number of pertussis cases reported in selected Latin American countries for which information is available (Chile, El Salvador, Guatemala, Honduras, Panama, Paraguay, and Peru) indicated a downward trend in disease incidence between 2000 and 2004 in children under 1 and in adolescents.

In Latin America and the Caribbean, the main challenges in pertussis control are the standardization of surveillance definitions and improvements in laboratory diagnosis.

Diphtheria

In 1978, before the Expanded Program on Immunization (EPI) was fully implemented, 6,857 diphtheria cases were reported in the Americas. Between 1999 and 2003, approximately 100 cases were reported annually for the entire Region. However, 181 cases were reported in 2004 and 272 in 2005, following a diphtheria out-

break in the Dominican Republic and Haiti. The cases in these two countries accounted for 88% and 92% of the total number of cases in the Americas in 2004 and 2005, respectively (Figure 14).

Since 2000, outbreaks have occurred in Colombia (2000), following a sustained decrease in DTP coverage in the late 1990s after a major reorganization of the health care system (33); in Paraguay (2002), related to low vaccination coverage and delays in case notification and implementation of control measures (34); and in the Dominican Republic and Haiti (2004–2005), affecting mostly low-coverage areas. The case-fatality rate of this last outbreak was as high as 47% in Haiti in 2005 (35).

Vaccination is the main strategy to prevent diphtheria. To control outbreaks, the priority is to intensify vaccination through a combination of mass vaccination efforts targeting affected areas and areas with low coverage levels, and the strengthening of routine services for the provision of DTP in infants and booster doses, as DT/Td vaccines, in older children and adults. Strengthening case management, including the early use of diphtheria antitoxin, also should be a priority in high-risk countries (34).

Haemophilus Influenzae Type B

Haemophilus influenzae type b (Hib) is an important cause of bacterial meningitis, pneumonia, and other forms of invasive disease in children aged under 5 years old. Before the introduction of the vaccine, 20,000 cases of Hib disease were estimated to occur in the United States (36) and another 20,000 cases of Hib meningitis were estimated to occur in the Latin America and the Caribbean every year (37). Reported annual incidence rates of Hib meningitis in children under 5 years old ranged from 12.8 per 100,000 in the Dominican Republic to 68.6 in Alaska (U.S.), not including studies in special-risk groups (38–40). Most cases of Hib meningitis in the Americas occurred in children aged under 23 months old, with 60% or more of the cases occurring in children 0–11 months old (38). The annual mortality rate for Hib meningitis in children aged under 5 years old was estimated to be around 2 per 100,000 for the Region (38). However, case-fatality rates and sequelae vary significantly by country, with the lowest rates occurring in industrialized countries.

Since 1997, PAHO has recommended the introduction of Hib vaccine in all countries of the Americas (41). However, Hib vaccine is considerably more expensive than vaccines traditionally included in EPI. Given this, PAHO's Technical Advisory Group on Vaccine-preventable Diseases has emphasized the need to consider sustainability when introducing Hib vaccine into national routine schedules and has recommended purchasing Hib vaccine in combination with DTP or DTP/HepB (as a pentavalent vaccine) through the PAHO Revolving Fund for the Purchase of Vaccines (41).

As of 2006, all of the Region's countries and territories (except Haiti) include Hib vaccine in their childhood immunization schedule: 36 use combination vaccines (32 as pentavalent). Hib-3 coverage Regionwide exceeded 90% in 2004 and 2005. A dramatic

FIGURE 14. Reported diphtheria cases, Region of the Americas, 1999–2005.

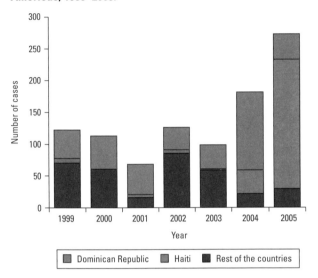

Source: Country reports to PAHO, Family and Community Health, Immunizations.

reduction in Hib disease has been demonstrated in those countries of the Region where well-performing Hib surveillance exists. An estimated 85% decrease in Hib meningitis cases has occurred in Latin America and the Caribbean, based on coverage levels achieved, 95% vaccine effectiveness, and the 20,000 cases estimated in the pre-vaccine era (*42*).

Hepatitis B

Routine universal infant vaccination against hepatitis B is the main strategy for the control of hepatitis B and its severe consequences. In addition to infant vaccination, PAHO recommends routinely vaccinating health care workers (*43*). The decision to add a dose at birth is based on the prevalence of carriers in the general population—recommended when the hepatitis B virus seroprevalence exceeds 8%—and on the country's resources (*44*). The endemicity of hepatitis B virus infection in the Americas varies from low to intermediate; the highest prevalence rates are in the Amazon basin, at 8%, and the lowest in the southern portion of South America (*45–49*).

The introduction of hepatitis B vaccine into childhood immunization schedules in the Americas has been progressive, with most countries having introduced the vaccine between 1997 and 2000 (*44*). As of 2006, all countries of the Americas, except Haiti, included hepatitis B in their infant immunization schedule, and 13 countries/territories included a hepatitis B dose at birth. Coverage levels for the third dose of hepatitis B vaccine have been higher than 90% at the Regional level since 2004, and are generally higher than 80% in the countries. However, hepatitis B vaccine coverage overall is lower than that for the third dose of DTP in countries that were not using them in combination. At this

writing, information is insufficient to assess the use of hepatitis B vaccine in health care workers in the Americas.

Moving from Child to Family Immunization

Immunization programs in the Americas are rapidly shifting from targeting children exclusively to including the entire family. The rubella elimination strategy (discussed below) has led to the vaccination of more than 76 million adolescent and adult men and women against rubella and measles. In recent years, countries have accelerated the introduction of seasonal influenza vaccine into routine schedules for adult populations at risk. Finally, the recent licensure of safe and effective vaccines against human papillomavirus has made the determination of the burden of cervical cancer an urgent matter. The many lessons learned from vaccinating adults in the Americas will serve as a model for other Regions of the world, and will also serve as the basis for developing HIV immunization strategies, once a vaccine against that virus becomes available (*50*).

The Unfinished Immunization Agenda

Elimination of Rubella and Congenital Rubella Syndrome

In 2003, the Region of the Americas embarked on an effort to eliminate rubella and congenital rubella syndrome (CRS) by 2010. The elimination of rubella and CRS in the Americas has been defined as the successful interruption of the endemic transmission of rubella in all the countries, without the occurrence of CRS cases associated with endemic transmission.

The rubella elimination initiative came when surveillance carried out as part of measles elimination clearly highlighted how significant a public health problem rubella and CRS were for the Western Hemisphere (Figure 15). Moreover, most rubella outbreaks and CRS cases in the United States in the late 1990s occurred in persons of Hispanic background (*51*). Based on available epidemiological data, it was estimated that in non-epidemic years, approximately 20,000 children were born with CRS in the Region each year (*52*). Furthermore, economic analyses in the Caribbean determined that the cost to care for a child with CRS throughout the child's life was between US$ 50,000 and US$ 63,900 (not accounting for indirect and social costs), and that mass campaigns were highly cost-beneficial and cost-effective (*53*). In light of these data, and of the significant experience in the reduction of rubella in Cuba and the English-speaking Caribbean through enhanced childhood rubella vaccination and mass vaccination campaigns targeting adults, PAHO's Technical Advisory Group on Vaccine-preventable Diseases recommended the accelerated control of rubella in 1997 (*41*). The Caribbean Community (CARICOM), comprising the English-speaking Caribbean countries and Suriname, went one step further by setting a goal to eliminate rubella and prevent the occurrence of CRS cases in its Member States by 2000 (*54*).

FIGURE 15. Impact of rubella and measles elimination strategies, Region of the Americas, 1980–2005.

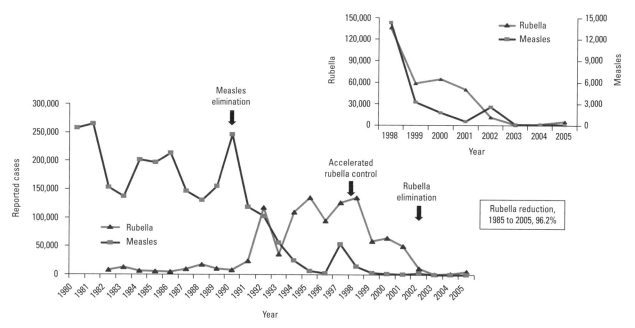

Source: Country reports to PAHO, Family and Community Health, Immunizations.

The main strategies recommended for rubella and CRS elimination in the Americas, based on knowledge about the disease, the vaccine, and rubella control experiences, are as follows (*55*):

- Introducing the rubella vaccine in routine immunization schedules and reaching vaccination coverage of more than 95% in the target population in each municipality.
- Implementing a one-time mass vaccination campaign of men and women in all countries with endemic transmission, in order to significantly reduce the time to interrupt rubella virus circulation and rapidly prevent the occurrence of CRS.
- Continuing to use the measles-rubella vaccine in "follow-up" campaigns for measles elimination.
- Integrating rubella surveillance into the epidemiological surveillance system used for measles elimination.
- Implementing CRS surveillance.
- Strengthening the laboratory diagnosis of rubella and CRS, as well as viral isolation.

As of 2005, approximately 99% of new birth cohorts in the Americas have access to the combination measles, mumps, and rubella (MMR) vaccine. Only Haiti has yet to include the vaccine in its vaccination schedule. In 2002, all the Region's countries had conducted "follow-up" campaigns for children under 5 years old using the measles-rubella (MR) vaccine, and had achieved over 90% coverage. Before the Regional elimination resolution, Chile

in 1999 and Brazil in 2001–2002 conducted mass rubella campaigns targeting only women, aiming to prevent CRS. Additionally, from 1998 to December 2005, the English-speaking Caribbean, Colombia, Costa Rica, Ecuador, El Salvador, Honduras, Nicaragua, and Paraguay conducted adult vaccination campaigns targeting men and women, in most cases reaching coverage levels higher than 95%. Venezuela conducted the first stage of its campaign in June 2005, vaccinating persons younger than 17 years old. Countries such as Canada, Cuba, Panama, the United States, and Uruguay have included the rubella vaccine in their childhood immunization schedules and have reached high coverage levels for several years. In the United States endemic rubella virus transmission has been declared eliminated (*56*). To reach the Regional elimination goal, the remaining countries plan to conduct vaccination campaigns between 2006 and 2008.

All countries have integrated rubella and measles surveillance, although it still needs strengthening. As of 2005, some countries continued to report rubella cases that were not included in the measles/ rubella surveillance system, and, therefore, were not properly investigated.

Since the rubella vaccine was introduced and vaccination campaigns were carried out, rubella incidence declined 96%, from 135,000 reported cases in 1998 to 5,296 cases in 2005 (*57*). In 2005, 88% of all rubella cases reported in the Region came from countries that had not yet launched campaigns. No cases were reported from countries after they conducted mass vaccination campaigns targeting adult men and women. Rubella outbreaks in Canada and Chile (among institutionalized men) in 2005, and continued transmission of rubella and occurrence of CRS cases in Brazil highlight the need to include men in vaccination strategies in order to interrupt rubella virus transmission in the Americas.

The number of countries and territories in the Americas that conduct CRS surveillance has increased from 13% (18 countries) in 1998 to 100% since 2003. In 2005, countries started reporting suspected CRS cases on a weekly basis. Between 2001 and 2003, 79 CRS cases were reported, 27 in 2004 and 20 in 2005. Nevertheless, CRS surveillance is still not complete. Of the 1,952 suspected cases reported in 2005, 99% came from only six countries (Brazil, Chile, Colombia, El Salvador, Honduras, and Peru). Argentina, Brazil, Costa Rica, the Dominican Republic, El Salvador, and Peru also have conducted retrospective studies in children's and obstetric hospitals, schools for the deaf and blind, and the community to identify children with CRS; these studies allowed for the identification of many more probable or confirmed CRS cases among infants. The lessons learned in CRS surveillance in the Americas will certainly help define good public health practices for establishing CRS surveillance and detecting suspected cases at the primary care level with the involvement of specialists (58).

An area that needs more attention is the detection and isolation of rubella virus from cases of rubella and CRS reported from countries of the Americas. Viral isolation and molecular typing is critical to help determine the source of infection and rubella virus variations. Phylogenetic studies of rubella viruses have shown two virus clades and seven genotypes. In the Americas, the 1C rubella virus has been identified as endemic. Clade 2 viruses have not been found circulating in the Region (59).

Implementing the rubella elimination strategy helps to consolidate the elimination of measles in the Region, greatly contributes to the reduction of inequities in maternal health outcomes, strengthens the political commitment for immunization services, and promotes a culture of prevention (50, 60). CRS surveillance can reinforce the health services' diagnostic capacity to promptly detect and treat infant disabilities. In addition to CRS prevention, women's health care can be further improved by the strengthening of adult health services, staff education, improvements in epidemiological surveillance, decentralization of decision-making, better program management, enhanced health awareness, and community participation that result from the implementation of the strategy (17, 50, 60).

Reaching the Underserved

Immunization's umbrella of protection does not yet extend to all children and at-risk women in the Region. Even though national coverage levels are high, much disparity exists among municipalities within countries, reflecting vast inequities. In Latin America and the Caribbean in 2005, 39% of the more than 15,000 municipalities or districts had not reached the Regional goal of 95% coverage with DTP-3 (61, 62). Furthermore, approximately

"The population in some countries still suffers such epidemic diseases as typhoid, smallpox, plague, malaria, and dysentery; child mortality is excessive, nutrition inadequate, modern hospitals practically nonexistent and average life expectancy low."

Fred Lowe Soper, 1951

one child in three in Latin America and the Caribbean lives in a district where coverage with DTP-3 does not reach 80% (63). Completing the unfinished agenda for immunization requires that these unreached children and their families have equitable access to the benefits of immunization. Identifying municipalities at risk and targeting them for focused interventions remains critical.

Vaccination Week in the Americas

Vaccination Week in the Americas is a Regionwide effort that aims to reach the unreached, strengthen the regular immunization program, and foster political commitment to immunization. This initiative, originally proposed by the Ministers of Health of the Andean Region and then endorsed by the Directing Council of the Pan American Health Organization (64), is based on the principles of equity, access, and Pan-Americanism. This annual hemispheric event, held every April, allows countries to target high-risk population groups and underserved areas, gather political support for disease elimination and control, and promote Regional and cross-border coordination.

In 2003, 19 countries and territories participated in the Vaccination Week in the Americas and over 16 million persons were vaccinated. The number of countries and territories participating increased to 35 and 36 in 2004 and 2005, respectively. The number of persons vaccinated during the Week reached 43.7 million in 2004. In 2005, five countries reported having vaccinated over 48,000 children aged 1 to 4 years who had never received a dose of DTP or pentavalent before. Colombia, Guatemala, Honduras, Mexico, and Panama reported vaccinating more than 539,000 women of childbearing age who had not received a previous dose of Td (17).

Besides vaccinating vulnerable populations, countries have used the Vaccination Week in the Americas to introduce new vaccines; conduct rubella-measles campaigns; launch immunization awareness campaigns among health workers and in the community; and provide other health interventions such as vitamin A supplementation, distribute antiparasitic drugs and instructions on preparing oral rehydration solution, conduct eye examinations, and provide health education. The political commitment from national authorities and public health stakeholders with immunization during the event has been illustrated by 30 cross-border launchings and the participation of five presidents; four first ladies;

and ministers of health, local authorities, representatives from international organizations, and other immunization partners.

Following the example from countries of the Americas, and using the lessons learned there, WHO's European Region launched its First Annual European Vaccination Week in October 2005.

Yellow Fever

Yellow fever remains a serious public health problem in several tropical areas in the Americas. Although yellow fever vaccine 17D, considered to be a safe and effective vaccine, has been available since the 1930s, the disease is yet to be adequately controlled. Occasional cases of jungle yellow fever, the occurrence of outbreaks, and the proliferation of *Aedes aegypti* across the Region are evidence of the continued risk of the reurbanization of the disease.

Cases of jungle yellow fever are confined to areas of South America, including Bolivia, Brazil's east-central region, Colombia, Ecuador, French Guiana, Guyana, Peru, Suriname, and Venezuela, and to Trinidad and Tobago in the Caribbean. Panama has enzootic areas, but has not reported cases in several decades. No urban cases of yellow fever have been reported since 1942.

The epidemiology of yellow fever infection has cyclical characteristics—there have been three major epidemic spikes since 1994. The highest number of cases was recorded in 1995, resulting from a major outbreak in the western Andean region of Peru. Between 2001 and 2005, 662 cases and 315 deaths were reported, which is a reduction of almost half compared to the figures for 1995–2000. In 2003, there was an increase in yellow fever incidence due to outbreaks in Colombia (112 cases), Brazil (64 cases), Venezuela (34 cases), and Peru (26 cases). Limited outbreaks and isolated cases were reported between 2004 and 2005. Cases continue to occur mostly among young adults 15–40 years old, predominantly in males. Migrants to enzootic areas also are a vulnerable group.

National plans of action have included vaccinating all residents of enzootic areas and travelers to those areas; strengthening syndromic jaundice-fever surveillance and epizootic surveillance (appearance of the disease or death in monkeys in jungle areas); and promptly responding to outbreaks. Additionally, Bolivia, Colombia, French Guiana, Guyana, Peru, Trinidad and Tobago, and Venezuela, seven of the eleven countries or territories with enzootic areas, have introduced yellow fever vaccine for all children 1 year old at the national level. In six of those seven, coverage rates are comparable to those achieved for MMR vaccine.

New Challenges in Immunization

Using immunization to its full potential is critical to attain global targets of mortality reduction and development. The Global Immunization Vision and Strategy (GIVS) developed by WHO and the United Nations Children's Fund (UNICEF), calls for a two-thirds reduction in mortality from vaccine-preventable diseases by 2015 as compared with 2000 levels. GIVS is a major global policy aimed at "protecting more people against more diseases by expanding the reach of immunization to every eligible person, including those in age groups beyond infancy" (65). In addition to improving vaccination coverage levels, particularly in low-coverage districts, other proven public health interventions need to be integrated with immunization strategies and new and under-utilized vaccines targeting priority diseases need to be introduced into routine immunization programs. Examples of integration of immunization with other public health interventions are delivery of antihelminthics during Vaccine Week in the Americas; vitamin A supplementation; integration of CRS surveillance with perinatal and infant programs; implementation of rotavirus surveillance in the context of childhood diarrhea surveillance and the integrated management of childhood illness (IMCI) strategies; pneumococcus surveillance in the context of other bacterial invasive diseases in children and IMCI; and human papillomavirus vaccination initiatives integrated to secondary screening, adolescent health programs, and cancer monitoring.

New and Under-utilized Vaccines

Several new vaccines against killer diseases are either available or in the pipeline; the decision whether to introduce them or not, more than ever needs to be supported by local evidence. Because these new-generation vaccines are much more expensive than traditional ones, they create new sustainability challenges for immunization programs.

Previous experiences with the introduction of vaccines such as MMR, Hib, and pentavalent in countries of the Americas has made it clear that before a vaccine is introduced, the following factors must be considered: disease burden, the definition of at-risk groups, cost-effectiveness studies, vaccine availability, possible adverse events attributable to the new vaccine, the vaccine's impact on the national budget and on the cold chain infrastructure, effects on the country's immunization schedule, adequacy of surveillance, political commitment, competing health priorities, opportunity costs, and financial sustainability (7, 26). Strengthening national regulatory authorities to evaluate new vaccines that may not be licensed in their country of origin and improving the monitoring of adverse events after the vaccine has gone on the market are also important areas of work in Latin America and the Caribbean.

In consideration of the above-mentioned factors regarding vaccine introduction, an analysis of new and under-utilized vaccines available in the pipeline shows that vaccines against influenza, rotavirus, pneumoccocus, and human papillomavirus should be considered as priorities in the Region of the Americas.

Influenza

Influenza is a viral disease that strikes millions of people worldwide and causes fatal complications in approximately one million people every year (*66*). Even though the burden of influenza in Latin America and the Caribbean has not been well-documented, studies from selected countries suggest that seasonal influenza is a major cause of morbidity and mortality associated with respiratory infections, mainly in older adults and young children (*67, 68*). Many of these cases and deaths can be avoided through the use of safe, highly effective vaccines. Influenza vaccine administered seasonally has been considered as perhaps the most under-utilized vaccine in the Region (*17*).

Since 2000, the Region's countries have made significant progress in increasing influenza vaccination coverage in the population 60 years old and older, chronically ill individuals, immunocompromised persons, health professionals, and pregnant women. Of the 39 Latin-American and Caribbean countries and territories that responded to a survey of national immunization program managers aimed to determine the status of influenza vaccination in the Region by the end of 2005, 19 reported having public policies for influenza vaccination (Anguilla, Argentina, Bahamas, Bermuda, Brazil, British Virgin Islands, Cayman Islands, Chile, Colombia, Costa Rica, Cuba, El Salvador, French Guiana, Honduras, Mexico, Netherlands Antilles, Panama, Paraguay, and Uruguay). Of these, 84% vaccinate health workers and 16% immunize persons who come in contact with birds. In many of the other countries, influenza vaccine is only available through the private sector. The routine immunization of children younger than 23 months old has been introduced in Bahamas, Bermuda, Cayman Islands, Colombia, El Salvador, Mexico, Panama, and Uruguay; Chile, Costa Rica, and Honduras vaccinate children under 5 years old who suffer from high-risk conditions. The United States has been using influenza vaccine since the 1970s; in 2006, the country expanded its recommendation to include all children up to 5 years of age (*69*). This represents marked progress compared to 2001, when only nine Latin American and Caribbean countries reported including influenza in their routine schedule.

Countries need to implement or strengthen their epidemiological surveillance for influenza. Although 84% of the respondent countries report having a routine surveillance system for influenza, the countries or territories surveyed do not have consistent or complete information on viral circulation patterns. Surveillance data are key in determining the burden of influenza, the cost-effectiveness ratio of introducing influenza immunization, and in deciding the best vaccination strategy, particularly in tropical areas. It also is necessary to generate vaccination coverage data in all target groups in order to evaluate program effectiveness and impact.

There is a limited global production capacity for influenza vaccine, and countries have faced vaccine shortages, mainly vaccine formulated in the Northern Hemisphere. Strategic partnerships with manufacturers and technology transfer to Latin American countries such as Argentina, Brazil, and Mexico will be critical for ensuring adequate vaccine supply. Also, the demand created by administering influenza vaccine seasonally may increase the likelihood that a supply of pandemic vaccine will be available for the Region's countries.

Rotavirus

Rotavirus is one of the most common causes of severe diarrhea worldwide. It accounts for approximately 40% of diarrhea hospitalization in children aged under 5 years old and for more than 600,000 estimated deaths per year. Even though rotavirus affects children in both developed and developing countries, 82% of all rotavirus deaths occur in developing countries (*70*). Disease burden estimates indicate that rotavirus diarrhea constitutes an important public health problem in most of the Region's countries, causing more than 15,000 deaths and an estimated 75,000 hospitalizations each year (*70*).

In 2006, two rotavirus vaccines entered the market. Results from clinical trials indicate that both are safe and effective in preventing severe rotavirus diarrhea (*71*). None of these vaccines have been associated with an increased risk of intussusception, the adverse event that led to the withdrawal of an early rhesus-based tetravalent rotavirus vaccine from the market in 1999 (*71–73*).

In July 2004, representatives of ministries of health of countries of the Americas called upon PAHO and the PAHO Revolving Fund for the Purchase of Vaccines to facilitate the introduction of vaccines against rotavirus at prices accessible to all the Region's countries as soon as a vaccine becomes available (*74*). In preparation for vaccine introduction, significant progress has been made in implementing hospital-based surveillance in the Region. As of July 2006, Bolivia, El Salvador, Guatemala, Guyana, Honduras, Paraguay, Saint Vincent and the Grenadines, Suriname, Trinidad and Tobago, and Venezuela had implemented surveillance using standardized case definitions and protocols, and routinely reporting to PAHO. Of the suspected cases, almost 40% were positive for rotavirus in 2005 and almost 52% were positive in 2006 (preliminary data as of May 2006) (Table 9). The seasonality of rotavirus infection has become evident in most countries, with incidence peaks during winter months. The predominant genotype in the Region is P[8]. The G9 serotype seems to be emerging, and the similar frequency of the G3 and G9 serotypes may indicate that G9 is replacing G3 (*75–78*). These findings again emphasize the importance of continued strain surveillance in the Region, since it can provide important insights for adjusting the next-generation vaccine composition.

In the first half of 2006, Brazil, Panama, Venezuela, and priority areas in Mexico began using rotavirus vaccine for infants 2–4 months old. That year, the United States also reintroduced its recommendation for the routine use of rotavirus vaccine in its childhood immunization schedule in 2006 (*62*).

Pneumoccocus

Worldwide, pneumonia is the leading cause of death in children, ranking higher than HIV, tuberculosis, or malaria (*79, 80*).

TABLE 9. Data and indicators of rotavirus hospital-based sentinel surveillance, reporting countries, Region of the Americas, 2005.

INDICATORS	Bolivia Nov–Dec	CAREC[a] Jan–Dec	El Salvador Jan–Dec	Guatemala Jan–Dec	Honduras Jan–Dec	Paraguay Jan–Dec	Venezuela[b] Jan–Nov	TOTAL
Number of hospitalizations in children under 5 years old	1,826.0	388	15,275	18,568	37,127	2,281	1,279	76,744
Number of hospitalizations due to diarrhea in children under 5 years old	326.0	214	3,105	2,502	2,420	326	200	9,093
% of hospitalizations due to diarrhea in children under 5 years old	17.9	55.2	20.3	13.5	6.5	14.3	15.6	11.9
Number of children under 5 years old that meet the case definition	180.0	150	1,109	1,391	1,133	223	598	4,784
% of suspect rotavirus cases	55.2	70.1	35.7	55.6	46.8	68.4	...	52.6
Number of children with complete form and stool sample collected	173.0	46	388	1,035	587	196	598	3,023
% of suspect cases with form and stool sample collected	96.1	30.7	35.0	74.4	51.8	87.9	100.0	63.2
Number of cases with positive results for rotavirus	31.0	14	106	616	78	106	254	1,205
% of confirmed rotavirus cases	17.9	30.4	27.3	59.5	13.3	54.1	42.5	39.9

[a]The four countries reporting rotavirus data to the Caribbean Epidemiology Center (CAREC) are Guyana, Saint Vincent and the Grenadines, Suriname, and Trinidad and Tobago.
[b]Does not include data for number of total hospitalizations for diarrhea from three hospitals.
Source: Country reports to the rotavirus database, PAHO, Family and Community Health, Immunizations.

Streptococcus pneumoniae, or pneumococcus, causes an estimated 1.6 million deaths, 800,000 of which occur in children (*81*). The rates of invasive disease are highest in children aged younger than 2 years old, but disease continues to occur in other age groups, particularly among the elderly. In industrialized countries, the disease has the highest mortality rate among the elderly.

Data obtained from the Regional Vaccine System (SIREVA), a network for the surveillance of pneumococcus established in 1993, indicate that the circulating serotypes in the Americas have not changed significantly in the six participating countries between 1993–1999 and 2000–2003. Serotype 14 was the leading serotype isolated in most countries (*80*).

Since 2000, a conjugated 7-valent vaccine has been available to prevent invasive pneumococcal disease in infants. In 2005, this vaccine was only routinely being used in Bermuda, Canada, and the United States. Chile and Panama have introduced it for children with immune disorders and other chronic pathologies. In addition, 9-valent and 11-valent vaccines are being evaluated, and it is expected that they will become available in the near future. Based on serotype data from SIREVA, the 7-valent vaccine would cover 59%, 9-valent would cover 71%, and 11-valent would cover 77% of the serotypes circulating in Latin America (*80*).

In preparation for pneumococcus vaccine introduction, PAHO is working with the countries to expand surveillance of invasive bacterial diseases and conduct population-based epidemiological studies in the Region (*80*). In addition to conducting epidemiological studies, countries are preparing to evaluate the economic implications of introducing pneumococcus vaccine. The vaccine's cost, at US$ 53 per dose purchased through the Revolving Fund in 2006, has been the main limitation preventing the vaccine's introduction.

Human Papillomavirus

Cervical cancer persists as a significant public health problem in Latin America and the Caribbean, despite the long-standing availability and application of secondary prevention through Papanicolaou (PAP) smear cytology. Every year, 86,532 new cases of cervical cancer and 38,435 deaths occur among women in the Americas, with Latin America accounting for 71,862 deaths and the Caribbean, for 32,639 deaths annually (*82*). In addition to these cases of invasive cervical cancer, women with low- and high-grade precancerous cervical lesions (dysplasias and carcinoma *in-situ*) also contribute to the disease burden and to the high costs associated with screening, diagnosis, and treatment of this disease.

Two prophylactic recombinant human papillomavirus (HPV) vaccines, one bivalent (16 and 18 virus-like types) and the other tetravalent (16, 18, 6, and 11 virus-like types) have been developed. Both vaccines have shown excellent results in terms of their immunogenecity, safety, and efficacy in preventing incident and persistent HPV infections, as well as cervical cancer precursor le-

sions (cervical intraepithelial neoplasia) (*83–85*). The tetravalent vaccine has also been shown to be efficacious against genital warts (*condyloma acuminata*) and vulvar and vaginal intraepithelial neoplasias (*86*). The tetravalent vaccine was licensed in its country of origin in 2006, for use in women 9–26 years old.

HPV vaccination complements secondary cervical cancer prevention efforts. PAHO is advocating and supporting the conduct of economic impact and cost-effectiveness studies related to cervical cancer and HPV vaccines in Member States, so that countries will have good data and information for rational public health decision-making regarding the feasible and sustainable introduction of this vaccine (*17*).

Ensuring Program Sustainability in the Context of New Vaccine Introduction

To hold on to achievements, address the unfinished immunization agenda, and introduce new vaccines, countries of the Americas will require substantial additional financing for their national immunization programs.

In 2005, only three Latin American countries reported financing less than 95% of their routine vaccines using government funds. In most countries (21 of 24 with data available) at least 90% of the national immunization program recurring costs were financed using government funds. All Latin American and Caribbean countries (except Haiti) reported having a budget line for purchase of vaccines (in two Caribbean countries vaccines are included in the budget line for purchase of all medications) (*62*). It should be said, however, that the existence of a budget line does not always secure the necessary funds for vaccines or the immunization program.

As several new vaccines are rapidly becoming available, it is critical that decision-making on new vaccine introduction be based on the best evidence, in order to be able to prioritize interventions. If these new vaccines are to contribute to overall prevention effectiveness in a sustainable way, economic evidence must be considered along with the usual epidemiologic, demographic, and management data. National committees on immunization practices should participate fully in this assessment process. In order to strengthen immunization program capabilities to gather evidence and set priorities for these new technologies, PAHO has launched the Pro-Vac Initiative. This initiative encompasses multiple country-level training, data collection, and development of economic analysis steps in the context of new vaccine introduction. It is anticipated that this will generate greater demand for, and promote the informed use of, relevant economic studies to support policy-making at country and regional levels (*17*).

New approaches to sustainable financing are currently being explored, focusing on securing longer-term and reliable funding flows for immunization programs, mainly through the creation of fiscal opportunities. A fiscal opportunity is the flexibility in a national budget that allows for the provision of resources without jeopardizing overall financial sustainability or economic stability.

Specific strategies to create fiscal space include re-prioritizing expenditures for immunization, increasing efficiency and transparency, improving the efficiency of tax collection, and increasing indirect taxes on products that cause significant public health problems, such as tobacco, alcohol, and firearms. Additional strategies include developing new sources of revenue, such as proceeds of national lotteries, and increasing external support (87).

Strengthening vaccine legislation can reduce a country's costs associated with the procurement of vaccines and immunization supplies. Legislation also contributes to reliable and effective program financing and the creation of fiscal opportunities for immunization. Legislation can also contribute to secure the necessary funds for the functioning of strong and sustainable immunization programs (88).

Finally, with new-generation vaccines already available, Pan-American cooperation through the Revolving Fund will enable the Region to continue its spectacular immunization achievements and maximize the Fund's benefits to the countries. As of 2006, 37 countries were making regular use of the Revolving Fund to procure up to 45 different vaccine products. The Fund is streamlining its integrated services to countries by further reducing costs of vaccine procurement, holding, distribution, and use along the supply chain. At the close of 2005, the Revolving Fund was capitalized at just over US$ 34 million and total expenditures exceeded US$ 154 million that year. The Revolving Fund, as a highly efficient procurement agency, is positioned to continue its strategic role in strengthening the sustainability of national immunization programs throughout the Region.

VECTOR-BORNE DISEASES

Malaria

The highest number of malaria cases reported in the Region since records have been kept was 1.3 million, recorded in 1995 and 1998 (Table 10) (89). Since that last year, the total number of cases has continued to decline, with 882,361 cases reported in 2004. This figure represents a 23% decrease from the 1.15 million cases reported in 2000, when countries of the Region officially adopted the Roll Back Malaria Initiative (90, 91).

Despite the reduction in morbidity, very little change has been seen in the age distribution of cases. Annual reports from 2002 to 2004 indicate that 63%–64% of cases occur in persons older than 15 years old; 20%–24% occur in persons 5–15 years old; and 11%–12% occur in children under age 5. Fewer than 5% occur in undetermined age groups or among persons older than 59 years old. During the same period, the proportion of males among persons suffering from malaria rose from 54% to 62% (92). These figures continue to highlight the economic impact of the disease, as it afflicts people in the most productive years of their lives.

Brazil consistently accounts for the majority of the cases, with 52.6% of total cases in the Region in 2004. Other countries that account for considerable proportions of the total number of cases in the Americas include Colombia (13.3%), Peru (10.6%), Venezuela (5.3%), Guatemala (3.3%), Guyana (3.3%), Ecuador (3.3%), and Honduras (1.8%). Collectively, countries that share the Amazon rainforest (Bolivia, Brazil, Colombia, Ecuador, French Guiana, Guyana, Peru, Suriname, and Venezuela) reported 91% of all cases in 2004. Meso-America, which here refers to Mexico, Central America (Belize, Costa Rica, El Salvador, Guatemala, Honduras, Nicaragua, and Panama), the Dominican Republic, and Haiti, accounts for almost 9%. In 2004, 1,263 cases were reported in a number of countries in the Region that had previously been declared as transmission-free for malaria. All these cases were imported from endemic countries within and outside the Americas (92).

While less than one million cases are currently reported in the Americas, 264 million people, or 30% of the Region's population, live in areas where the disease is transmitted, 41.5 million of whom are in areas of high (more than 10 cases per 1,000 population) and moderate (1 to 10 cases per 1,000 population) transmission risk. It is estimated that 94% of cases occur in these areas (90, 91).

At present, malaria is endemic in 21 countries (93), but Argentina, El Salvador, Mexico, and Paraguay are likely to eliminate malaria in the next few years. Belize, Costa Rica, Nicaragua, and Panama also are considered malaria-endemic.

The annual parasitic index in all risk areas is 3.35 per 1,000. For populations living in moderate- and high-risk areas, the index more than triples, at 10.8 per 1,000 (93). Countries with the highest indices in the reporting period were Colombia, French Guiana, Guyana, Suriname, and Venezuela. Most cases in the Americas are caused by *Plasmodium vivax* (74%); 25.6% of cases are caused by *P. falciparum*, and there are very few reported cases caused by *P. malariae* (<0.4%), most of which occur in Suriname (89, 92).

Trends in the distribution of cases by parasite species in the countries varied very little from 2000 to 2004. In Brazil, 76.2% of the cases were caused by *P. vivax*, while 22.7% were due to *P. falciparum*. Bolivia, Colombia, Ecuador, Peru, and Venezuela in the Andean Area follow a similar trend, with 75% of cases caused by *P. vivax* and 25% by *P. falciparum*. Cases in Argentina and Paraguay in the Southern Cone are almost always due to *P. vivax*, with very few exceptions. From 2000 to 2004, French Guiana, Guyana, and Suriname—the countries that make up the Guyana Shield—had a decrease in the proportion of *P. falciparum* cases (65% to 54%) and an increase in *P. vivax* cases (35% to 43%). Mexico and the Central American countries reported that 94% of the cases were due to *P. vivax* and 6%, to *P. falciparum*. In Haiti and the Dominican Republic, the only Caribbean countries where the disease is transmitted, *P. falciparum* is essentially responsible for all cases (89, 92).

Mortality from malaria in the Region is associated with the pathogenesis of *P. falciparum*. Mortality decreased by 55% be-

TABLE 10. Malaria morbidity, Region of the Americas, 1994–2004.

Year	Population (in thousands)		Blood slides			Case detection (per 100,000 inhabitants)	
	Total for the countries	Risk areas[a]	Examined	Positive	Slide positivity rate	Total for the Americas	Malarious areas
1994	763,305	231,323	8,261,090	1,114,147	13.49	145.96	481.64
1995	774,712	248,978	9,022,226	1,302,791	14.44	168.16	523.26
1996	786,055	298,128	8,601,272	1,139,776	13.25	145.00	382.31
1997	793,582	306,521	9,037,999	1,075,445	11.90	135.52	350.86
1998	803,546	308,323	9,148,633	1,289,741	14.10	160.51	418.31
1999	818,273	298,453	10,174,427	1,207,479	11.87	147.56	404.58
2000	832,863	293,196	10,210,730	1,140,329	11.17	136.92	388.93
2001	835,814	293,560	9,456,093	960,792	10.16	114.95	327.29
2002	849,361	262,382	7,785,398	884,744	11.36	104.17	337.20
2003	858,563	302,981	6,980,597	909,788	13.03	105.97	300.28
2004	867,142	264,139	6,980,789	882,361	12.64	101.76	334.05

[a]Population in areas of the Americas ecologically favorable for transmission; includes areas without active transmission.
Source: Pan American Health Organization. Epi-Data: Status of Malaria Tables, 1994–2004. [Online]. 2006 [cited 2006 July 20]. Available from: http://www.paho.org/english/ad/dpc/cd/mal-status-2004.pdf.

tween 2000 and 2004, from 348 deaths to 56 (*90, 91*). Annual reports from the countries for the last three years of the above-mentioned period reflect a consistently increasing proportion of cases among the population older than 15 years old, from 74.3% in 2002 to 85.1% in 2004. Deaths among children under 5 years old, on the other hand, decreased from 8.8% in 2002 to 4.6% in 2004. More deaths were recorded among males (67% and 74%) than females (33% and 26%) (*92*).

Passive case detection (diagnostic examination performed in general health services and hospitals or by volunteer collaborators only on patients with clinical symptoms) is used more widely in the Region, except in Argentina, Costa Rica, the Dominican Republic, Panama, and Paraguay, which rely more on active case detection (diagnostic examinations performed for screening, epidemiologic investigations, and follow-up purposes). The proportion of passive case detection use in the Region between 1998 and 2004 ranged from 68% to 81%. To date, official data on access and availability of case detection modalities is limited, but microscopy is known to still be most widely used (*89–91*).

Aminoquinolines remain the most widely used anti-malarial medication in the Region. *P. falciparum*, the most pathogenic of the malaria parasites, is now known worldwide to be capable of developing resistance to anti-malarials. The phenomenon, which was first reported in Colombia in 1958, continues to be one of the greatest challenges in the global battle against the disease. In the Americas, resistance has only been suspected or confirmed in countries that share the Amazon rainforest (*89–91*).

At least eight different species of *Anopheles* mosquitoes are considered significant vectors for malaria in the Region. *Anopheles albimanus* is found in Belize, Colombia, Costa Rica, the Dominican

Republic, Ecuador, El Salvador, Guatemala, Haiti, Honduras, Mexico, Nicaragua, Panama, and Peru; *A. albitarsis* is found in Brazil; *A. aquasalis*, in Venezuela; *A. benarrochi*, in Peru; *A. darlingi*, in Belize, Bolivia, Brazil, Colombia, French Guiana, Guatemala, Guayana, Honduras, Paraguay, Peru, Suriname, and Venezuela; *A. marajoara*, in Venezuela; *A. pseudopunctipennis*, in Argentina, Bolivia, Guatemala, Mexico, and Peru; and *A. vestitipennis*, in Belize, Guatemala, and Mexico. As of 2004, most of the 21 endemic countries include a malaria vector control component in their national programs, but reports or information on these components' effectiveness and efficiency are few (*89–91*).

The most commonly used insecticides in the Americas are organophosphates and pyrethroids. No country reports the use of the organochlorine DDT, which is among the insecticides recommended by the WHO Pesticide Evaluation Scheme (WHOPES) for indoor residual spraying against malaria vectors (*94*). Several countries also rely on fogging, principally to reduce *Aedes aegypti*, but also to decrease anopheline densities. Mexico and the Central American countries also engage in environmental management activities, use biologic control options, and enlist the community's participation in reducing vector breeding sites through the Regional Action Program and Demonstration of Sustainable Alternatives for Malaria Vector Control without Using DDT (Global Environment Facility – DDT Project) (*89–91*).

Current Strategies and Program Impact

Since the Global Malaria Control Strategy was adopted in 1992, the 21 countries of the Americas with active malaria transmission applied, in varying degrees, the four technical elements of the strategy in their national programs: early diagnosis and prompt treatment; planning and implementation of selective and sustainable preventive measures, including vector control; early detection, containment, and prevention of epidemics; and strengthening of local capacities in basic and applied research to permit and promote the regular assessment of a country's malaria situation, particularly the disease's ecological, social, and economic determinants (95–98). Efforts fostered the expansion of the health sector's national and local-level operating capacity for early diagnosis and treatment. The number of blood tests for malaria screening and diagnosis performed peaked at 10.2 million in 2000 (89, 92). The notable decline in the number of blood slides examined from 2001 to 2004 is due to unavailability of data from Peru, which examines approximately 1.5 million blood slides annually.

In 1998, the World Health Organization, along with partner institutions from the United Nations system, the World Bank, national governments of malaria-endemic countries, bilateral cooperation organizations, non-governmental organizations, and civil society, launched the Roll Back Malaria Initiative, with the goal of halving the global burden of malaria by 2010. During the 42nd Directing Council of the Pan American Health Organization in September 2000, the nations of the Americas committed themselves to the goals and ideals of the initiative (99).

Activities pursued through the Roll Back Malaria Initiative in the Region focused on supporting the health ministries' efforts related to malaria prevention and control; promoting synergies with related health programs, especially those dealing with environmental health, pharmaceuticals, maternal and child health, HIV/AIDS, and tuberculosis; promoting the participation of communities and civil society; engaging the private sector in the delivery of prevention and treatment; identifying best practices, partnerships, and finance mechanisms for extending interventions; preparing managerial tools and support measures; building capacity; and promoting collaboration among countries (90, 91, 95–98).

Along with the financial support extended through the Initiative, Member States harness national resources, contributions from other sources, loans, and PAHO technical and programmatic support to carry out malaria activities. The strategic framework has resulted in several successful collaborations and attempts to more efficiently mobilize resources. Highlights among these include the Amazon Network for the Surveillance of Anti-malarial Drug Resistance/Amazon Malaria Initiative, in which eight Amazon region countries participate and that receives financial support of the United States Agency for International Development (USAID); the approval of and successful use of funds allocated for the joint Andean proposal (Colombia, Ecuador, Peru, and Venezuela) and individual country proposals for Bolivia, Guatemala, Guyana, Haiti, Honduras, Nicaragua, and Suriname to the Global Fund to Fight AIDS, Tuberculosis, and Malaria; the Regional Action Program and Demonstration of Sustainable Alternatives for Malaria Vector Control without Using DDT (Global Environment Facility – DDT Project) in Mexico and Central America; and the research collaboration with the World Bank, United Nations Development Program, and WHO's Program for Research and Training in Tropical Diseases (90, 91).

As of 2004, 15 out of the 21 malaria-endemic countries reported decreases in the total number of cases. Eight of them have so far reached the Roll Back Malaria Initiative target of at least 50% case reduction by 2010 (Argentina, Bolivia, Ecuador, El Salvador, Honduras, Mexico, Nicaragua, and Paraguay); another seven registered decreases in case numbers but still have not reached the goal (Belize, Brazil, Costa Rica, French Guiana, Guatemala, Haiti, and Suriname); and six continue to report increases (Colombia, the Dominican Republic, Guyana, Panama, Peru, and Venezuela) (90, 91).

In 2001, Peru and Bolivia became the earliest adopters of artemisinin-based combination therapy against malaria. With an increased focus on research on drug resistance and the use of evidence-based treatment regimens, Bolivia, Ecuador, Guyana, Peru, Suriname, and Venezuela are now using various artemisinin-based treatment combinations as first-line therapy against *P. falciparum* malaria. Brazil and Colombia are expected to implement this policy in 2006. These eight countries account for 92% of all *P. falciparum* cases reported in the Region. Malaria cases in Haiti and the Dominican Republic, almost all of which are caused by *P. falciparum*, are still reported to be sensitive and non-resistant to chloroquine (90, 91).

The Regional Strategic Plan for Malaria, 2006–2010

The malaria situation in the Americas is permeated with strong sociopolitical, economic, behavioral, environmental, educational, administrative, and policy overtones. Sociopolitical and economic factors remain important aspects of the problem of malaria in the Region, including poor housing conditions, particularly among itinerant groups and isolated populations; various sociopolitical problems that impede access to programs; lack of political commitment to implement the Global Malaria Control Strategy in the local health services; illegal activities in some areas that prevent the identification of cases; an increase in demand and a reduction in resources in marginalized settlements; and lack of basic sanitation in marginalized settlements. The high level of migration among populations where prevention and control is most difficult—miners, loggers, banana and sugarcane plantation workers, indigenous groups, and populations living in areas of armed-conflict—is also linked directly to sociopolitical and economic conditions (90, 91).

Migration makes almost every aspect of malaria prevention and control extremely difficult to implement and monitor. Other behaviors reported to be an ongoing cause of malaria transmission include the tendency among the population to remain outside the home or protective shelter during the known period of increased hematophagous activity of vectors; limited community participation; limited social commitment and social mobilization; high rate of noncompliance to treatment regimens; improper self-medication; and use of expired or low-quality medications (90, 91).

Environmental factors such as the presence of natural breeding sites, favorable ecological conditions for the reproduction of vectors, the existence of virtually inaccessible or outrightly isolated communities, and the presence of multiple vectors, are likewise considered as important causes or aggravating factors (*90, 91*).

Many countries do not have enough health professionals trained in malaria (90, 91). Moreover, there is a need to conduct education on malaria prevention and control among the most affected groups.

The malaria problem's policy and administrative dimensions are the aspects that have the greatest potential for the most concrete interventions. At least 11 countries cited various administrative and policy issues that contribute to the persistence of malaria transmission in the Region, including a lack of budgetary allocations; limited health service coverage in malaria-endemic areas; a lack of intersectoral cooperation; a lack of stratification in control strategies; problems regarding the sustainability of measures; drug-supply problems; a lack of transportation; a lack of insecticide supplies; a delay in the release of funds; a delay in the approval and execution of projects; administrative and management problems in municipalities related to the decentralization process; disruption of country programs due to outbreaks of other infectious diseases such as dengue; inadequate vector control; and a lack of human and financial resources (*90, 91*).

The total expenditure (national and external contributions) for malaria reported by endemic countries increased from US$ 107,798,405 in 2000 to US$ 172,524,015 in 2004. The per capita expenditure of the reported population at risk of malaria in the Americas grew by 76%; from US$ 0.37 in 2000 to $0.65 in 2004 (Table 11) (*90, 91, 100*).

Notwithstanding the reduction in mortality related to *P. falciparum*, malaria remains an important public health problem in the Region, particularly the persistent transmission rate of *P. vivax*, which is more difficult to control because of its characteristic life cycle in humans. It is imperative that entomological research and surveillance be strengthened alongside health surveillance and disease management. Current investments aimed at combating the disease should at least be sustained, if not increased, and must be aimed at both immediate and long-term health reforms so that the desired results may be attained. Operational research must be enhanced, and adequate attention must be given to specific target populations that include pregnant women, children, persons living with HIV/AIDS, travelers, miners, loggers, banana and sugarcane plantation workers, indigenous groups, populations in areas of armed or social conflict, and persons living in areas of common epidemiologic interest or in border areas. National capabilities to address and manage special situations such as epidemics; complex emergencies; malaria in urban areas; and malaria in remote border and low-incidence areas where elimination may be possible, must likewise be built and reinforced. Investment on human resource development also is paramount.

The 2006–2010 Regional Strategic Plan for Malaria comprehensively addresses the current malaria challenge in the Region and discusses PAHO's priority areas for technical cooperation as it fulfills its commitment to the Roll Back Malaria target. Achieving this goal fulfills the UN Millennium Development Goal of halting and beginning to reverse the incidence of malaria (and other major diseases) by 2015. In September 2005, PAHO's Directing Council proposed an additional 25% reduction (*101*).

Dengue

Dengue is caused by a virus of the genus *Flavivirus* (family Flaviviridae), which in the Americas is transmitted by the *Aedes aegypti* mosquito. There are four related but antigenetically distinct dengue serotypes (DEN-1, DEN-2, DEN-3, and DEN-4) that produce classic dengue fever or dengue hemorrhagic fever and dengue shock syndrome, the last two being the most serious clinical forms of the disease. The incidence of dengue and the numbers of outbreaks of the disease have risen in the last 35 years everywhere in the world. Prior to the 1950s, only nine countries had reported any cases of dengue. By the 1980s, 26 countries were reporting dengue cases and, since 1990, more than 100 countries around the globe have reported cases of the disease (*102*). The year with the largest number of reported cases of dengue was 2002, in which the disease struck 69 countries. Today, dengue is the leading viral disease transmitted by arthropods and represents a growing public health problem (*102*). On average, the burden of disease attributable to dengue is 658 disability-adjusted life years per 1,000,000 population (*103*).

Dengue and Dengue Hemorrhagic Fever in the Americas, 2001–2005

In 2001–2005 more than 30 countries of the Americas reported 2,879,926 cases of dengue and dengue hemorrhagic fever. The number of reported cases reached alarming proportions in 2002, with 1,015,420 cases (Table 12). There were 65,235 cases of dengue hemorrhagic fever during this same period, with the largest number of cases (15,500) reported in 2001 (Table 13). The number of deaths from dengue fever in the Region totaled 789 for the period as a whole, with the largest number of deaths (255) reported in 2002 (Table 12). All four dengue virus serotypes circulated in the Region (Table 14); in given years in the period, they were present simultaneously in Barbados, Colombia, El Salvador, French Guiana, Guatemala, Mexico, Peru, Puerto Rico, and Venezuela (*104*).

The following section analyzes the situation of dengue and dengue hemorrhagic fever in 2001–2005 by subregion.

Southern Cone

This subregion reported 64.6% of all cases of dengue and dengue hemorrhagic fever in the Americas in 2001–2005, with 1,859,259 and 4,509 cases reported, respectively, and 258 deaths. Brazil reported the most cases of dengue and dengue hemorrhagic fever (99.6%) and the most deaths from dengue in each year in the period (Table 12). In contrast, Chile and Uruguay were the only

TABLE 11. National budget for and nonbudgetary contributions to malaria control programs, Region of the Americas, 2000–2004.

Countries	2000 National malaria budget	2000 Contributed funds, loans, and other sources	2001 National malaria budget	2001 Contributed funds, loans, and other sources	2002 National malaria budget	2002 Contributed funds, loans, and other sources	2003 National malaria budget	2003 Contributed funds, loans, and other sources	2004 National malaria budget	2004 Contributed funds, loans, and other sources
Argentina	2,580,000	...	2,580,000	...	2,580,000	...	2,580,000	...	2,580,180	...
Bolivia	845,764	944,187	935,101	601,656	918,145	550,887	750,327	476,743	750,327	189,000
Brazil	44,766,876	2,477,870	21,517,299	805,197	21,411,765	1,137,503	40,695,955	523,926	40,695,955	523,926
Colombia	9,950,000	—	11,363,636	—	11,363,636	225,000	13,049,962	—	13,702,460	—
Costa Rica	3,380,000	—	2,500,000	—	2,880,000	—	3,840,000	—	2,980,000	—
Dominican Republic	1,410,013	157,238	1,443,223	29,722	1,220,721	5,000	25,860,927	1,200,675	448,254	15,676
Ecuador	...	...	3,155,525	180,000	3,815,603	180,000	5,235,182	92,954	5,396,634	...
El Salvador	...	...	4,555,000	...	...	...	2,142,205	...	1,698,141	3,675
Guatemala	702,703	—	...	—	...	...	...	...	...	—
Haiti	...	...	...	...	...	—	...	—	...	...
Honduras	2,597,868	3,605,010	2,352,572	1,450,000	81,250	54,039	388,888	7,289,800	4,850,000	7,285,000
Mexico	17,652,182	—	17,157,485	—	19,576,235	—	19,576,235	—	28,060,594	—
Nicaragua	333,333	—	333,333	175,500	333,333	175,500	333,333	175,500	...	...
Panama	5,066,318	—	4,680,289	—	3,986,849	—	2,751,541	...	5,024,766	88,417
Paraguay	1,932,103	—	1,061,490	—	1,064,936	1,164,935	175,000	1,147,905	202,404	...
Peru	1,900,915	58,572	4,109,728	130,000	3,900,000	200,000	3,500,000	200,000	3,600,000	200,000
Venezuela	5,411,675	960,000	...	...	2,065,933	200,000	20,834,228	...	48,263,202	...
Subtotal	**98,529,750**	**8,202,877**	**77,744,681**	**3,372,075**	**75,198,406**	**2,727,929**	**142,703,718**	**10,134,598**	**159,198,418**	**8,508,098**
Guyana	1,000,000	—	800,000	10,000	800,000	100,000	800,000	...	600,000	3,112,871
Belize	...	...	...	...	...	...	...	...	100,000	238,000
French Guiana	...	...	...	...	...	...	...	...	...	...
Suriname	65,778	—	178,363	636,000	160,628	536,000	160,628	606,000	160,628	606,000
Subtotal	**1,065,778**	**8,202,877**	**978,363**	**646,000**	**960,628**	**636,000**	**960,628**	**606,000**	**860,628**	**3,956,871**
Total	**99,595,528**	**8,202,877**	**78,723,044**	**4,018,075**	**76,159,034**	**3,363,929**	**143,664,346**	**10,740,598**	**160,059,046**	**12,464,969**
Grand Total		**107,798,405**		**82,741,119**		**79,522,963**		**154,404,944**		**172,524,015**
$US funds per person in malarious areas		**$0.37**		**$0.28**		**$0.30**		**$0.51**		**$0.65**

Note: Funds per person derived only from countries reporting national malaria budget data (information incomplete).
— Not applicable
... Information not available.
Source: Pan American Health Organization. Epi-Data: Status of Malaria Tables, 1994–2004. [Online, cited 2006, July 20.]. Available at: http://www.paho.org/english/ad/dpc/cd/mal-status-2004.pdf.

TABLE 12. Cases of dengue and dengue hemorrhagic fever (DHF), incidence and number of deaths from dengue, Region of the Americas, 2001–2005.

COUNTRY	2001			2002			2003			2004			2005		
	Cases of dengue & DHF	Incidence[a]	Deaths	Cases of dengue & DHF	Incidence[a]	Deaths	Cases of dengue & DHF	Incidence[a]	Deaths	Cases of dengue & DHF	Incidence[a]	Deaths	Cases of dengue & DHF	Incidence[b]	Deaths
Anguilla	25	208.33	0	5	41.67	—	2	16.67	0	0	0	—	0	0	—
Antigua and Barbuda[b]	20	30.77	0	5	7.69	—	0	0	—						
Argentina	11	0.03	0	214	0.57	0	135	0.36	0	3.284	8.77	—	34	0.09	0
Aruba	0	...	—	25	...	—	—	0	—	173	166.35	—	—	0	—
Bahamas	0	...	—	0	0	—	180	58.44	0	1	0.32	—			
Barbados	1,043	389.18	0	740	276.12	—	557	207.84	0	349	130.22	0	320	119.4	—
Belize[b]	3	1.3	—	41	16.4	—	0	0	—	2	0.87	—	380	164.5	0
Bermuda	0	0	—	0	0	—	0	0	0	0	0	0	2	3.17	0
Bolivia	176	14.67	0	892	74.33	1	6,548	327.4	6	7.39	369.5	0	4.443	222.15	0
Brazil	413,067	239.38	29	780,644	452.39	145	341,902	198.14	38	112.928	65.44	3	203,789	118.1	43
British Virgin Islands[b]	23	95.83	—	0	0	—	0	0	0	0	0	—	0	0	0
Cayman Islands	0	0	0	1	2.5	—	1	2.5	0	0	0	0	1	2.5	0
Chile[c]	—	—	—	636	—	—	0	0	0	0	0	0	0	0	0
Colombia	55,437	272.71	54	76,996	210.3	27	52,588	258.7	7	27,523	135.39	20	30,475	149.92	47
Costa Rica	9,237	818.16	0	12,251	314.53	0	19,669	606.32	0	9,408	290.01	0	37,798	1.165.17	2
Cuba	11,32	101.58	2	3,011	26.75	1	0	0	0	—	0	0	75	0.67	—
Curaçao	0	0	—	—	—	—	0	0	—	4	5.63	—	265	122.12	—
Dominica[b]	5	7.04	0	0	0	—	0	0	0				11	15.49	—
Dominican Republic	3,592	42.28	0	3,194	37.6	14	6,163	72.55	75	2,476	27.66	13	2.86	33.67	18
Ecuador	10,919	84.77	0	5,833	45.29	0	10,319	80.12	5	6,165	47.86	2	12,131	94.18	14
El Salvador	1,093	17.09	4	18,307	286.05	11	7,436	116.24	8	13,344	201.02	1	15,290	226.28	0
French Guiana	2,830	1664.71	0	280	164.71	—	2,178	1281.18	0	3,147	1851.18	—	4,365	2.567.65	0
Grenada[b]	12	12.77	0	84	89.36	—	17	18.09	0	7	7.45	—	0	0	0
Guadeloupe	0	0	—	93	21.58	—	495	114.85	0	0	0	—	3,364	780.51	—
Guatemala	4,516	38.64	2	7,599	65.02	6	6.75	57.76	3	6,352	54.35	4	6,341	54.26	1
Guyana	60	60	—	202	26.47	—	33	4.33	—	47	6.16	—	178	23.33	0

TABLE 12. (Continued).

COUNTRY	2001			2002			2003			2004			2005		
	Cases of dengue & DHF	Incidence[a]	Deaths	Cases of dengue & DHF	Incidence[a]	Deaths	Cases of dengue & DHF	Incidence[a]	Deaths	Cases of dengue & DHF	Incidence[a]	Deaths	Cases of dengue & DHF	Incidence[b]	Deaths
Haiti													—	0	
Honduras	9,077	138.05	0	32,269	490.78	17	16,559	251.85	11	19,971	303.74	2	18,843	286.59	6
Jamaica	39	39	0	90	3.46	—	52	2	0	9	0.35	—	46	1.77	—
Martinique	4,471	4471	4	392	101.55	—	791	204.92	0	0	0	—	6,083	1.575.91	4
Mexico[d]	6,210	6.19	0	9,844	9.81	6	5,018	5	—	8,202	8.17	13	16,862	16.8	0
Montserrat	1	1	0	1	12.5	—	1	12.5	—	0	0	—	0	0	0
Nicaragua[d]	2,104	40.4	21	2,157	41.42	12	2,799	53.74	4	1,035	19.87	2	1,735	31.64	12
Panama	1,545	53.29	1	711	24.53	0	293	10.11	0	373	12.87	2	5,489	137.98	1
Paraguay	38	0.67	0	1,871	33.2	0	137	2.43	0	164	2.91	0	405	7.19	0
Peru	23,329	89.41	4	8,875	34.01	1	3,637	13.94	0	9,774	37.46	1	6,358	24.36	0
Puerto Rico	5,233	132.41	4	2,906	73.53	1	3,735	94.51	0	3,288	83.2	3	5,701	144.26	7
Saint Kitts and Nevis[b]	89	89	0	20	52.63	—	2	5.26	—	4	10.53	—	0	0	—
Saint Lucia[b]	292	195.97	0	51	34.23	—	5	3.36	—	11	7.38	—	1	0.67	0
Saint Vincent and the Grenadines[b]	3	2.63	0	125	109.65	—	3	2.63	—	4	3.51	—	8	7.02	0
Suriname	760	181.38	0	1,104	263.48	—	285	68.02	—	375	89.5	—	2,853	680.91	—
Trinidad and Tobago	2,244	172.62	0	6,246	480.46	12	2,289	176.08	12	546	42	—	411	31.62	0
Turks and Caicos Islands	0	0	0	0	0	0	2	11.76	0	1	5.88	—			
United States[e]	96	8	0	29	2.42	0	40	3.33	0	0	0	0	1	5.88	—
Uruguay	—	—	—	—	—	—	0	0	0	0	0	0	0	0	0
Venezuela	83,180	337.69	15	37,676	152.96	1	26,996	109.6	7	30,693	124.61	5	4,198	171.31	4
TOTAL	652,212		140	1,015,420		255	517,617		164	267,050		71	427,627		159

[a] Incidence per 100,000 population.
[b] Data provided by the Caribbean Epidemiology Center (CAREC).
[c] Cases from Easter Island.
[d] Only confirmed cases.
[e] Imported cases.
Source: Pan American Health Organization, dengue web page: http://www.paho.org/english/ad/dpc/cd/dengue.htm, accessed on November 2006.

TABLE 13. Cases of dengue hemorrhagic fever, Region of the Americas, 2001–2005.

	2001	2002	2003	2004	2005
Anguilla	0	0	0	—	—
Antigua and Barbuda[a]	0	0		—	—
Argentina	0	0	0	—	0
Aruba		—		—	—
Bahamas	0	0	0	—	—
Barbados	14	0	0	—	—
Belize[a]		0		0	0
Bermuda	0	0	0	0	0
Bolivia	0	1	47	25	10
Brazil	679	2,607	713	77	433
British Virgin Islands		0	0	0	0
Cayman Islands	0	0	0	0	0
Chile[b]		0	0	0	—
Colombia	6,563	5,269	4,878	2,815	4,306
Costa Rica	37	27	69	11	52
Cuba	0 69	12	0	0	—
Curaçao		—		—	—
Dominica[a]	0	0	0	—	4
Dominican Republic	4	76	252	136	84
Ecuador	55	158	416	64	334
El Salvador	54	405	138	154	207
French Guiana	0	0	0	0	0
Grenada[a]	0	3	0	0	0
Guadeloupe		0	0	—	6
Guatemala	4	47	22	39	32
Guyana		2		0	0
Haiti					—
Honduras	431	863	458	2.345	1.795
Jamaica	0	0	0	—	—
Martinique	3	0	0	—	3
Mexico[d]	191	1,429	1,419	1,959	4,255
Montserrat	0	0	0	0	0
Nicaragua[d]	458	157	235	93	177
Panama	7	5	0	4	2
Paraguay	0	0	0	0	0
Peru	251	13	15	35	16
Puerto Rico	36	23	5	11	19
Saint Kitts and Nevis[a]	4	0		—	—
Saint Lucia[a]	0	0	0	0	0
Saint Vincent and the Grenadines[a]	0	2	0	0	0
Suriname	12	23	1	7	141
Trinidad and Tobago	86	273	80	49	0
Turks and Caicos Islands	0	0	0	—	—
United States of America[c]	0	0	0	0	0
Uruguay			0	0	0
Venezuela	6,541	2,979	2,246	1,986	2,681
TOTAL	15,500	14,374	10,994	9,810	14,557

[a]Data for the non-Latin Caribbean furnished by the Caribbean Epidemiology Center (CAREC).
[b]Cases from Easter Island.
[c]Imported cases.
[d]Only confirmed cases.
Source: Pan American Health Organization. Available at: http://www.paho.org/english/ad/dpc/cd/dengue.htm, accessed November 2006.

TABLE 14. Circulating dengue virus serotypes, Region of the Americas, 2001–2005.

	2001	2002	2003	2004	2005
Anguilla	DEN 3	DEN 2 , 3	DEN 3	DEN	DEN
Antigua and Barbuda[a]	DEN 3	DEN 3	DEN	DEN	DEN
Argentina	All imported	DEN 1, 3	DEN 1, 2, 3	DEN 3	DEN 2
Aruba		—	DEN	DEN 3	DEN
Bahamas		—	DEN 2, 3	DEN	DEN
Barbados	DEN 1, 2, 3, 4	DEN 3	DEN 1, 3	DEN 3	DEN 1, 3
Belize[a]		DEN 2	DEN	DEN 3, 4	DEN 1, 2, 3
Bermuda		—	DEN	DEN	DEN
Bolivia	DEN 1	DEN 1, 2	DEN 1, 2, 3	DEN 1, 2, 3	DEN 2, 3
Brazil	DEN 1, 2, 3	DEN 1, 2, 3	DEN 1, 2, 3	DEN 1, 2, 3	DEN 1, 2, 3
British Virgin Islands	DEN 2, 3	—	DEN	DEN	DEN
Cayman Islands		—	DEN	DEN	DEN
Chile[b]		DEN 1	DEN	DEN	DEN
Colombia	DEN 1, 2, 4	DEN 1, 3, 4	DEN 1, 2, 3	DEN 1, 2, 3, 4	DEN 1, 2, 3
Costa Rica	DEN 2	DEN 1, 2	DEN 1, 2	DEN 1, 2	DEN 1
Cuba	DEN 3	—	DEN	DEN	DEN
Curaçao		—	DEN	DEN	DEN
Dominica[a]	DEN 3	—	DEN	DEN	DEN
Dominican Republic		DEN 2	DEN 2	DEN 2, 4	DEN
Ecuador	DEN 2, 3	DEN 2, 3	DEN 3	DEN 3, 1, 4	DEN 1, 3
El Salvador	DEN 2	DEN 1, 2, 3, 4	DEN 2, 4	DEN 1, 2, 4	DEN 2, 4
French Guiana	DEN 1, 2, 3	DEN 3	DEN 1, 3	DEN 1, 3, 4	DEN 1, 2, 3, 4
Grenada[a]	DEN 2, 3	DEN 3	DEN	DEN	DEN
Guadeloupe		—	DEN 3	DEN	DEN 2, 3, 4
Guatemala	DEN 2, 4	DEN 2, 3, 4	DEN 1, 2, 3, 4	DEN 1, 2, 3, 4	DEN 1, 2, 3, 4
Guyana	DEN 2	DEN 3	DEN	DEN	DEN
Haiti					DEN
Honduras		DEN 2, 3, 4	DEN 2, 4	DEN 1, 2, 4	DEN 1, 2, 4
Jamaica		—	DEN	DEN	DEN
Martinique	DEN 2, 3	DEN 3	DEN	DEN	DEN 2, 3, 4
Mexico[d]		DEN 1, 2 , 3	DEN	DEN 1, 2, 3, 4	DEN 1, 2, 3
Montserrat		DEN 2, 3	DEN	DEN	DEN
Nicaragua[d]	DEN 2, 3	DEN 1, 2, 4	DEN 1	DEN 1, 2, 4	DEN 1, 2, 4
Panama	DEN 2	DEN 2	DEN 2	DEN 1, 2, 3	DEN 1, 2
Paraguay	DEN 1, 2	DEN 1, 2, 3	DEN 3	DEN 3	DEN 2
Peru	DEN 1, 2	DEN 1, 2, 3	DEN 1, 2, 3	DEN 1, 2, 3	DEN 1, 2, 3, 4
Puerto Rico	DEN 1, 2, 3, 4	DEN 1, 3	DEN 1, 2, 3	DEN 2, 3, 4	DEN 2, 3, 4
Saint Kitts and Nevis[a]	DEN 2	DEN 2	DEN	DEN	DEN
Saint Lucia[a]	DEN 3	DEN 3	DEN	DEN	DEN 4
Saint Vincent and the Grenadines[a]	DEN 3	DEN 3	DEN 3	DEN	DEN 3
Suriname	DEN 3	DEN 3	DEN 2	DEN 3	DEN 1, 2, 3
Trinidad and Tobago	DEN 2, 3	DEN 2 (15%), 3 (85%)	DEN 3	DEN	DEN 3
Turks and Caicos Islands		—	DEN	DEN	DEN
United States of America[c]	DEN 1	—	DEN	DEN	DEN
Uruguay	DEN 2, 3	DEN 2, 3	DEN	DEN	DEN
Venezuela	DEN 1, 2, 3, 4	DEN 2, 3, 4	DEN 1, 2, 3	DEN 1, 2, 3, 4	DEN 1, 2, 3, 4

[a]Data for the non-Latin Caribbean furnished by the Caribbean Epidemiology Center (CAREC).
[b]Cases from Easter Island.
[c]Imported cases.
[d]Only confirmed cases.
Source: Pan American Health Organization. Available at: http://www.paho.org/english/ad/dpc/cd/dengue.htm, accessed November 2006.

South American countries that retained their transmission-free status. DEN-1, DEN-2, and DEN-3 circulated in Argentina, Brazil, and Paraguay during the period, with DEN-1 reported circulating on Easter Island, Chile, in 2002 (Table 14) (*104*).

Andean Area

Bolivia, Colombia, Ecuador, Peru, and Venezuela, reported only 21.1% of all cases of dengue and dengue hemorrhagic fever (580,589 cases), but accounted for the largest share of cases of dengue hemorrhagic fever (63.9%, or 41,704 cases) in 2001–2005. The subregion also reported 221 deaths from dengue. Bolivia had the subregion's highest rates per 100,000 population in 2003 (327.4), 2004 (369.5), and 2005 (222.15) (Table 12), while Colombia reported 70% of all deaths (155). All four serotypes circulated in Venezuela in 2001, 2004, and 2005 and in Peru in 2005; the number of serotypes circulating in Bolivia went from a single serotype in 2001 (DEN-1) to three serotypes in 2003 and 2004 (DEN-1, DEN-2, and DEN-3). Different combinations of the four serotypes circulated in Colombia and Ecuador.

Central America and Mexico

Central America reported 289,929 cases of dengue and dengue hemorrhagic fever, accounting for 10.6% of all cases in the Americas, including 8,519 cases of dengue hemorrhagic fever and 133 deaths. The countries reporting the largest number of cases in 2005 were Costa Rica and Honduras, followed by Mexico, El Salvador, Guatemala, Panama, and Nicaragua (Table 12). The number of reported cases in El Salvador rose sharply between 2001 and 2005, from 1,093 to 15,290. Costa Rica had the subregion's highest rate in 2005 (1,165 per 100,000 population). It was Nicaragua, however, which reported most deaths in the subregion, 51 for the period as a whole (Table 12) Though all four serotypes circulating in the subregion, the most prevalent ones are DEN-1 and DEN-2 (*104*).

The Caribbean

This subregion reported 76,222 cases of dengue and dengue hemorrhagic fever between 2001 and 2005 (2.6% of all cases in the Americas), including 1,271 cases of dengue hemorrhagic fever. The highest numbers of cases of dengue were reported in 2001 (19,023) and 2005 (19,103).

Latin Caribbean. Cuba had the most cases of dengue and dengue hemorrhagic fever in this subregion (11,432) in 2001 in the wake of an epidemic outbreak, followed by Puerto Rico (5,233), and the Dominican Republic (3,592). The Dominican Republic reported the most cases of dengue hemorrhagic fever (552 cases) in 2001–2005 (Table 13), along with 120 deaths, for a case fatality rate of 21.7%, one of the highest in the Region. All four dengue virus serotypes circulated in Puerto Rico, while the Dominican Republic reported the presence of serotypes DEN-2 and DEN-4 (*104*).

Non-Latin Caribbean. Of the countries and territories in this subregion, French Guiana, Martinique, and Trinidad and Tobago reported the largest numbers of cases of dengue and dengue hemorrhagic fever in the reporting period. Martinique reported 6,083 cases in 2005, followed by French Guiana (4,365), Guadeloupe (3,364), and Suriname (2,853). All four serotypes circulated simultaneously in Barbados in 2001 and in Guyana in 2005, though the most prevalent serotypes in this group of countries in 2001–2005 were DEN-2 and DEN-3 (*104*). In 2001, Halstead and colleagues documented the hyperendemic transmission of the hemorrhagic dengue virus in Haiti, despite the absence of the disease itself (*105*). There are no official reports on the number of cases of dengue in that country, however.

Dengue Prevention and Control Strategies

Thanks to highly effective campaigns for the eradication of the *Aedes aegypti* mosquito throughout the 1950s and 1960s, by 1972, the vector had been successfully eliminated in 21 countries of the Americas. However, programs became unsustainable or were abandoned altogether, and eventually the countries were re-infested (*106*). This, and a combination of ecological, economic, political, and social macrofactors, contributed to the vector's re-emergence, prompting the design of a new generation of dengue prevention and control programs currently serving as the cornerstone of the Regional prevention and control strategy (*107*).

PAHO's Regional Program on Dengue is designed to focus public health policies on promoting multisectoral, interdisciplinary integration for the framing, implementation, and strengthening of an Integrated Management Strategy (IMS) at the subregional and country level. The goal is to foster the functional integration of the activities in six key program components, namely mass communication, entomology, epidemiology, laboratory techniques, patient care, and the environment. To date, Central America has established a subregional Integrated Management Strategy, and there are efforts under way to promote the development of such a strategy in the MERCOSUR countries. There are 11 functioning Integrated Management Strategies at the country level (Brazil, Colombia, Costa Rica, the Dominican Republic, El Salvador, Guatemala, Honduras, Nicaragua, Panama, Paraguay, and Venezuela), with ongoing field operations designed to promote their development in other countries around the Region. These strategies apply the COMBI (Communication for Behavioral Impact) method specifically to dengue, replacing the information dissemination strategy used by programs for the past 15 years (*108–110*). This new approach offers an effective way to change the practices and behavior of individuals and communities with a view to promoting their "ownership" of prevention and control measures. Training activities in the COMBI method have been conducted in more than 22 countries in the Region.

The laboratory techniques component is essential to enable countries to diagnose cases of dengue. To this end, technical capabilities of existing laboratories have been strengthened and efforts are under way to establish proficiency programs for laboratories in the Americas and, where applicable, bolster existing programs with direct support and assistance from PAHO/WHO collaborating centers for dengue. There is a proposal for a Region-wide interprogrammatic integrated vector management plan for the implementation of cost-effective strategies for controlling the vector for dengue and other diseases in the Americas (111, 112).

The Regional Program's epidemiological surveillance component has helped to improve the reporting of statistical data on dengue fever through its network known as DENGUE-NET (113). The International Network of Eco-Clubs is yet another strategic alliance for the prevention of dengue, as it pursues community-based dengue prevention and control activities (114).

Dengue Research and Development: Remaining Challenges

The complexity of dengue transmission dynamics has prompted studies of different factors that contribute to the circulation and persistence of this virus (115). Various international initiatives and organizations, such as the Special Program for Research and Training on Tropical Diseases, the Pediatric Dengue Vaccine Initiative (116), WHO and its regional offices, the Canadian International Development Research Center, and the European Union Research Program are all promoting research work in this area (117–119). As of this writing, most funding is being channeled into research for the discovery of second-generation vaccines and the development of new or improved approaches to vector control (118, 119).

Chagas' Disease

Chagas' disease is a zoonosis unique to the Americas and is endemic in 21 countries. It is a vector-borne disease caused by the protozoan parasite *Trypanosoma cruzi*, following a chronic course. The disease is a byproduct of adverse socioeconomic conditions that affect vast portions of Latin America's population, particularly in rural areas (120). Chagas' disease is a chronic, systemic, parasitic infection with an important autoimmune component, whereby 20% to 30% of infected individuals develop serious forms of cardiopathy or digestive megaformations (megacolon or megaesophagus) (121).

WHO estimates the current number of cases of human infection in the Americas at 18 million, of which approximately 5.4 million will develop into serious heart conditions and 900,000 into abnormal enlargements of digestive organs. There are an estimated 200,000 cases of the disease each year, with 21,000 yearly deaths directly related to this parasitic infection. Some 40 million people in Latin America are at risk of contracting the infection (122).

In 1993, the World Bank calculated the annual burden of Chagas' disease at 2.74 million disability-adjusted life years (DALYs),

representing an economic cost of more than US$ 6.5 billion a year for endemic Latin American countries (123).

According to a 2000 cost-effectiveness study conducted as part of Brazil's Control Program for Chagas' Disease (124), US$ 516.68 million had been spent on prevention and control measures between 1975 and 1995, during which period there were 387,000 deaths from this disease, or 17,000 deaths per year. In those same years, 50% of potential vector-borne transmissions were averted, representing 277,000 new cases of infection and 85,000 deaths. Moreover, 1.62 million DALYs were gained by averting 45% of potential deaths and 59% of potential disabilities. Control measures against transfusion-transmission of the disease prevented 5,470 new cases of infection and 200 deaths, gaining 17,900 DALYs by averting 8% of potential deaths and 92% of potential disabilities.

The estimated annual cost of treating patients suffering from Chagas' disease is somewhere around US$ 19.78 million in Chile and US$ 6.10 million in Uruguay. However, Chagas' disease control programs in both countries—with annual operating costs of US$ 2.02 million and US$ 133,000, respectively—successfully interrupted the disease's transmission nationwide in Chile in 1999 and in Uruguay in 1997 (125).

Disease prevention and control measures include: a) integrated vector control of triatomine species in households as a way to eliminate imported vectors and control indigenous species; b) screening of potential blood donors by blood banks as part of a safe-blood strategy; c) blood testing of pregnant women to detect maternal infections liable to be transmitted to the fetus via the placenta; and d) diagnosis, management, and treatment of infected individuals.

There are many ongoing national Chagas' disease control programs throughout the Region carrying out prevention and control efforts with different track records and varying levels of success. These programs all operate within the framework of international or subregional initiatives and horizontal technical cooperation programs. These initiatives are complemented by joint efforts such as the partnership between PAHO and WHO under the Control Program for Neglected Tropical Diseases, which help to globalize technical cooperation activities.

Argentina, Bolivia, Brazil, Chile, Paraguay, and Uruguay are participating countries in the **Southern Cone Initiative for the Elimination of Chagas' Disease**. The following are highlights of the Initiative's achievements:

- 1997—Vector-borne and transfusion transmission of *T. cruzi* was interrupted in Uruguay.
- 1999—Vector-borne transmission of *T. cruzi* was interrupted in Chile.
- 2000—Vector-borne transmission of *T. cruzi* by *Triatoma infestans* was interrupted in most endemic areas of Brazil.
- 2001—Vector-borne transmission of *T. cruzi* was interrupted in the endemic provinces of Jujuy, Neuquén, Río Negro, and La Pampa in Argentina.

- 2002—Transmission of *T. cruzi* was interrupted in Amambay Department in Paraguay and control programs continued to cover most endemic areas.
- 2002—A control program for Chagas' disease was established in Bolivia with assistance from the Inter-American Development Bank, PAHO, and the United Nations Development Program.
- 2004—After situation assessments were conducted in Río Grande do Sul (Brazil) and Entre Ríos (Argentina), the interruption of *T. cruzi* transmission was confirmed.
- 2006—Interruption of vector-borne transmission was confirmed in 711 municipalities in 13 states in Brazil, including all dispersal areas for *T. infestans*, thereby interrupting its transmission nationwide.

Belize, Costa Rica, El Salvador, Guatemala, Honduras, Nicaragua, and Panama participate in the **Initiative of Central American Countries for the Control of Chagas' Disease**, whose objectives are to interrupt vector transmission and eliminate transmission of *T. cruzi* by transfusion. Accomplishments in the subregion include expansions in coverage and improvements in the quality of vector control measures and blood-bank screening; transmission also has been interrupted in some areas. In addition, the number of sites infested with *Rhodnius prolixus* have been reduced, and it has been almost completely eliminated in El Salvador, Guatemala, Honduras, and Nicaragua; household infestations with *Triatoma dimidiata* have dropped 60% throughout the subregion. Strategic alliances with the Japanese International Cooperation Agency and the Canadian International Development Agency (CIDA) have played a pivotal role.

Participants in the **Andean Initiative to Control Vector Transmission and Transmission by Transfusion of Chagas' Disease** include Colombia, Ecuador, Peru and Venezuela. Given the differences in ecological and epidemiological conditions, and in the vector-borne transmission of the disease in this subregion, the participating countries decided to rely on a risk-approach for establishing control measures. To this end, and with a view to establishing a basic control strategy, a special workshop on this topic was conducted in Guayaquil in June 2004. Peru, for its part, has entered into a technical cooperation partnership with CIDA. The countries' national control programs have expanded their coverage.

Bolivia, Brazil, Colombia, Ecuador, French Guiana, Guyana, Peru, Suriname, and Venezuela are part of the **Intergovernmental Initiative for Surveillance and Prevention of Chagas' Disease in the Amazon Region**. The Initiative's goal is to integrate existing health programs and to develop a surveillance system for Chagas' disease that is linked to existing systems that operate within the framework of subregional integration projects or agencies. The Initiative grew out of an International Meeting on Surveillance and Prevention of Chagas' Disease in the Amazon

Region held in Manaus, Brazil, in September 2004, at which the nine participating countries acknowledged that American trypanosomiasis is a disease with an emerging epidemiology in that subregion and recommended the creation of an efficient and effective, adequate, sustainable, and responsive surveillance system with diagnostic capacity for coping with new situations (*126*). Brazil and Ecuador are setting up a surveillance system in their Amazon regions that is tied into the malaria surveillance system. All countries in the subregion have organized health care activities for Chagas' disease.

Given its scope and unique epidemiology, **Mexico** is dealing with Chagas' disease control through a national initiative. In 2002, nonetheless, the country set up a shared discussion space with the Initiative of Central American Countries for the Control of Chagas' Disease on control and elimination of *R. prolixus*, which has strengthened the formulation of control measures. Mexico declared the control of this disease to be a priority at a National Workshop for the Control of Chagas' Disease conducted in Huatulco, Oaxaca, in September 2003. The country has strengthened its vector-control strategies, its blood-bank screening, and the provision of care for persons who have contracted Chagas' disease.

It should be said that coverage has increased and the quality of blood screening for *T. cruzi* has improved in every endemic country. Moreover, efforts to coordinate and standardize the treatment of Chagas' disease have increase in all the subregions.

As of this writing, in the wake of improvements in socioeconomic conditions in the Region of the Americas, its various subregions, and its countries and given existing control and surveillance measures, the current epidemiological pattern of Chagas' disease underscores a number of interesting facts and challenges, namely (*127*):

- Overall, thanks to a new approach, Chagas' disease is under better control in the Region of the Americas.
- Control measures have been able to successfully interrupt the vector-borne transmission of Chagas' disease in large areas, but they lie alongside areas of active transmission with high morbidity and mortality rates.
- Rural-to-urban migration has affected the disease's vector-borne, transfusional, and congenital transmission and has led to a growing trend towards the urbanization of Chagas' disease.
- The incidence and prevalence of the disease are higher among socially disadvantaged groups and ethnic groups.
- New ecological and epidemiological niches for endemic areas of Chagas' disease have emerged or been identified, such as the Amazon subregion.
- New or newly recognized transmission modes are materializing or are on the rise, such as transmission via the digestive tract and through transplants.

- The coverage and quality of health care services must be improved, particularly in regard to the treatment of ill and infected individuals (*128*).
- Migration to non-endemic countries within or outside the Region is creating diagnostic, health care, and treatment needs at destination points.
- Prevention, surveillance, control, and care activities for Chagas' disease need to be reorganized in line with new epidemiological realities.

ZOONOSES

The link between animal and human health is highly important from a public health standpoint—61% of all species of organisms known to be pathogenic to humans and 75% of pathogens associated with emerging diseases are zoonotic (*129*).

In the countries of the Americas, technical cooperation activities that target zoonotic diseases are channeled along three broad directions: achieving the objectives of the unfinished agenda, as in the case of plague; sustaining existing achievements against diseases such as human rabies transmitted by dogs; and meeting new challenges such as that presented by leishmaniasis. The health ministries in the countries of the Region of the Americas have prevention and control programs for various zoonotic diseases, and they receive regular support and assistance from PAHO. However, there are several zoonoses that pose serious public health risks that have been neglected for many years and for which there are no existing control policies.

PAHO/WHO is the coordinating body for regional reporting systems to which the health ministries regularly report on information regarding human and animal rabies cases (*130*) and

human cases of plague. (*131*) The ministries of health and the World Organization for Animal Health (OIE) also furnish data on human and animal cases of other zoonotic diseases (*132*).

Rabies

The downturn in the number of cases of human rabies transmitted by dogs and canine rabies continued throughout 2001–2005. The decline in human rabies cases is attributable to the countries' efforts to strengthen epidemiological surveillance, conduct mass canine vaccination campaigns, and treat infected persons. A review of trends in rabies cases in the Americas in 1982–2005 shows an 81% drop in the number of human cases, from 332 to 64, and also a decrease in the number of canine rabies cases, which dropped by 89%, or from 12,524 to 1,427, during the same period (Figure 16). There were 11 cases of human rabies transmitted by dogs reported in the Americas in 2005. (*130*)

According to a PAHO study (*133*), most human rabies cases reported in 2001–2003 occurred in low-income groups residing in the outskirts of large cities such as Port-au-Prince (Haiti) and San Salvador (El Salvador), and in some Brazilian municipalities. These areas generally have higher densities of stray dogs bypassed by vaccination campaigns. Moreover, living and working conditions for residents of these areas curtail their access to treatment for dog bites. There was a sharp deterioration in the epidemiological situation of canine rabies in Bolivia in 2004, with outbreaks in La Paz, Cochabamba, and Santa Cruz de la Sierra. That same year, there were also concerns over the situation in Venezuela's State of Zulia.

Given the current status of rabies in the Americas, epidemiological surveillance is crucial. A study of the frequency of canine

FIGURE 16. Cases of human and canine rabies, Region of the Americas, 1982–2005.

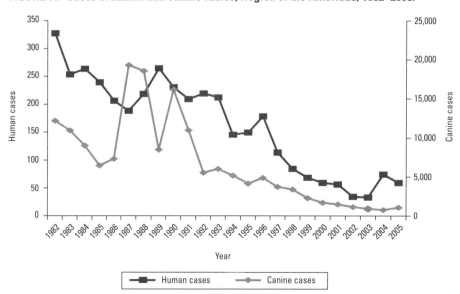

Source: Regional Information System of Epidemiological Surveillance of Rabies (SIRVERA), PAHO, 2006.

rabies cases in relation to epidemiological surveillance activities by subnational geopolitical units (states, departments, and provinces) in 2001–2003 classified the Region into five different epidemiological areas, namely: 1) areas free of canine rabies for more than 10 years; 2) areas free of canine rabies for the last three years that had adequate epidemiological surveillance (annual sampling of a minimum of 0.1% of the estimated canine population); 3) areas free of canine rabies for the last three years and that have passable epidemiological surveillance (annual sampling of 0.09%–0.01% of the estimated canine population); 4) areas free of canine rabies for the last three years that have no epidemiological surveillance (silent areas with sampling rates of under 0.01%); and 5) areas with active circulation of rabies virus variants 1 and 2 in the canine population (134). The same study (134) classified the following countries and areas as free of canine rabies for more than 10 years: Costa Rica and Panama in Central America; Argentina (except for its border area with Bolivia); all of southern Brazil (including the states of São Paulo and Rio de Janeiro); Chile; certain departments of Peru; and Uruguay in the Southern Cone. At the other end of the spectrum is a zone of active circulation of the rabies virus in the canine population confined to limited geographic areas, including large portions of Bolivia, northern and northeastern Brazil, parts of El Salvador and Guatemala, the State of Zulia in Venezuela, and the Argentine/ Bolivian, Bolivian/Peruvian and Guatemalan/Mexican borders.

Progress in the control of canine rabies is basically attributable to a strategy centered on mass canine rabies vaccination campaigns and timely prophylactic treatment for humans exposed to the disease (135). Some 44 million dogs are vaccinated every year in Latin America and one million or so humans at risk of contracting the disease are treated, 25% of whom receive post-exposure treatment. There is one health post administering rabies treatments for each 34 persons in Latin America (133). For detection and surveillance purposes, there is a rabies diagnosis network with over 100 national and regional laboratories processing close to 74,000 canine samples a year (133).

Prior to 2003, dogs were the main transmitters of rabies in the Americas. In 2004, the number of cases of human rabies caused by blood-feeding (vampire) bats for the first time outstripped the number of cases caused by dog bites (136). There were 51 reported cases of human rabies caused by blood-feeding bats in 2005 in the Amazon areas of Brazil, Colombia, and Peru, where many persons living in remote areas were bitten, with no readily accessible health facilities. A review of previous similar but smaller scale situations, showed that most outbreaks were associated with ecological changes or occurred in areas characterized by specific economic activities, such as gold mining and clearing of vegetation (137).

Plague

Plague, which has been around for more than a thousand years, has been responsible for millions of deaths in previous centuries, mainly in three major pandemics beginning in the years 542, 1346, and 1894 (138). While the number of reported cases is currently relatively low, this disease is a reflection of wide health gaps in many countries around the globe. According to WHO, there are 2,000 reported cases of plague each year worldwide. Only Bolivia, Brazil, Ecuador, Peru, and the United States have reported cases of plague in the Americas; all other countries in the Region are considered disease-free. Countries in which the disease remains have ongoing control programs coordinated by their respective governments. The last reported outbreak in the Andean area in 1994, with reports of 1,128 suspected cases of the disease, was followed by a sharp plunge in the number of cases. On average, 12 cases a year were reported to PAHO by countries with endemic areas in 2001–2005 (131). Peru reported the largest number of cases in 2005; that year, there were 16 reported cases of plague in humans. In Latin America, the disease generally strikes impoverished communities in remote rural areas. Persons living there have limited access to health facilities and no basic infrastructure; moreover, their dwellings expose them to the elements and to epidemiological risk factors. The causative agent of plague (*Yersinia pestis*) is still found in wild rodent populations in these countries, whose fleas (*Xenopsylla cheopis*) can transmit the disease to household rats (*Rattus norvegicus* and *Rattus rattus*) that feed on crops stored by peasant farmers inside their homes. Domestic guinea pigs (*Cavia porcellus*) are part of the disease's causal chain in Andean countries due to the custom of breeding these animals inside the home. The circulation of *Y. pestis* in wild animal populations is the main obstacle to the elimination of this disease.

All countries have active surveillance programs for wild and domesticated animals (dogs) and ongoing control programs for household rodents and fleas in endemic areas. It should be said, however, that there is general consensus that any attempt to address this health problem and develop a comprehensive solution to it should include poverty-reduction policies established within the framework of commitments in furtherance of the Millennium Development Goals (MDGs), as well as active participation by local governments; collaboration among the health, agriculture, and housing sectors; and active community organization and participation.

Visceral Leishmaniasis

Visceral leishmaniasis is endemic in Latin America, with risk factors for the disease detected in areas of Argentina, Bolivia, Brazil, Colombia, Costa Rica, El Salvador, Guatemala, Honduras, Mexico, Nicaragua, and Venezuela. Most cases of the disease in the Region were reported by Brazil, with an average of 3,000 cases a year (139). Brazil has had an epidemiological surveillance program and system for this disease since the 1980s, but not all countries have such a system in place.

Although the disease is typically found in rural areas, recent reports indicate the emergence of cases in urban areas of large

> "*Latin America is in a period of transition; it has not yet taken on the characteristics of the technologically advanced societies; and the dominant diseases are of the acute or chronic type and are governed by environmental factors that are susceptible to preventive measures.*"
>
> Abraham Horwitz, 1964

cities around the Region. This shift may have something to do with socioeconomic problems that have led to an increase in rural-to-urban migration and ecological changes that have bolstered the proliferation of the disease's causative agent and vector.

Animals, mainly dogs, are the main reservoirs of visceral leishmaniasis. Humans are not reservoirs of the disease unless it is associated with other health problems; consequently it is basically a zoonotic disease (transmitted from animals to humans). Humans simultaneously infected by causative agents of leishmaniasis and AIDS may have high *Leishmania* loads in their blood, transforming them into reservoirs of the disease. This presents specific problems for the diagnosis and treatment of coinfected patients and poses a risk of outbreaks of anthroponotic forms of the disease.

The identification and mitigation of the risk factors for leishmaniasis are essential to minimize its impact on public health. This requires efficient multidisciplinary coordination for successful vector control, reduction of rates of infection in animal populations operating as reservoirs of the disease, and the timely and effective diagnosis and treatment of infected individuals.

Echinococcosis/Hydatidosis

Cystic echinococcosis is a serious economic and public health problem in parts of the world whose economy is based mainly on livestock-raising. South America is one of the areas hardest hit by this disease, although there is no aggregate data on disease incidence due to differences in data collection methods (*140*). There are three species of the genus *Echinococcosis* present in the Region of the Americas—*E. granulosus, E. oligarthus,* and *E. vogeli*—the first of which is especially important because it is the only species prevalent in both humans and animals. Moreover, the extent of the disease's socioeconomic impact and its significant effect on livestock production makes it a public health problem. It is perpetuated mainly through dog-sheep cycles in endemic areas, although it can also involve other ruminants and pigs (*138*). The species *E. vogeli* and *E. oligarthus,* causative agents of polycystic hydatid disease found mainly in Central America and the northern reaches of South America (Brazil, Colombia, Ecuador, and Venezuela), are perpetuated mainly through cycles involving wild hosts. The species *E. multilocularis,* causative agent of alveolar echinococcosis, is found primarily in arctic zones of North America. The hardest hit areas of South America are Argentina (Río

Negro, Chubut, Tierra del Fuego, Corriente, and Buenos Aires provinces), Brazil (the state of Río Grande do Sul), Chile (primarily Regions VII, X, XI and XII), Uruguay, and mountainous areas of Peru and Bolivia (*140*).

There is an ongoing cooperation-among-countries initiative for the control and surveillance of this infection, with PAHO and the FAO serving as its technical secretariat. Since 2004, the Southern Cone Subregional Program for the Control and Surveillance of Hydatid Disease (Argentina, Brazil, Chile, and Uruguay) has coordinated many operations carried out by the national control programs in each member country (*140*).

Brucellosis

Bovine brucellosis caused by *Brucella abortus* was eliminated from Canada in 1989 and from Jamaica in 1994 (*4*); it has had a limited presence in the United States since 2003 (*141*), and is present in most Latin American countries. Human brucellosis transmitted by small stock animals is also a serious public health problem in several countries. According to OIE reports, there have been no problems with caprine and ovine brucellosis in Brazil since 2001, in Chile since 1975, in Panama since 2001, or in the United States since 1999. There were, however, reports of cases of the disease in sheep and goats in limited areas of Argentina, Mexico, and Peru prior to 2004 (*132*). Up to 2004, there had been no cases of porcine brucellosis, presumably caused by *B. suis,* in Barbados, Belize, the British Virgin Islands, Canada, Costa Rica, the Falkland Islands, Guatemala, Haiti, Jamaica, Saint Vincent and the Grenadines, and Trinidad and Tobago. The last reported case in Brazil was in 2003, Chile in 1987, and Panama in 2001. The disease is still found in Argentina, Cuba, Mexico (where its presence is limited to certain regions), Nicaragua, Uruguay, and Venezuela (also limited to certain regions) (*132*).

There are inconsistencies in the reporting of cases of human brucellosis. Estimates show that most countries are likely to have sizeable numbers of undiagnosed or unreported cases of the disease (*142*).

Bovine tuberculosis

Bovine tuberculosis is being eliminated from Canada and the United States, where only limited areas have yet to be certified as disease-free. According to country reports to the OIE, as of 2004, there had been no reported cases of the disease in Barbados since 1978, in Belize since 1991, in Jamaica since 1989, and in Trinidad and Tobago since 2001. Argentina, Bolivia, Chile, Colombia, Costa Rica, Cuba, the Dominican Republic, Guatemala, Uruguay, and Venezuela all have reported cases of bovine tuberculosis. It has a limited presence in certain areas of Bolivia, Mexico, Nicaragua, Panama, Paraguay and Peru. (*132*) Plans for controlling bovine tuberculosis in Latin America are based on the segregation of animals with positive tuberculin tests. As in the case of bovine brucellosis, the involvement of private veterinarians accredited by animal health agencies and supported by the private sector has had clear benefits, mainly in the dairy industry. The establishment of effective systems for segregating animals with positive tuberculin tests is imperative.

The inspection of slaughterhouses is the main surveillance activity for bovine tuberculosis conducted by animal health services in Latin America (*143*). Enteric transmission of the *Mycobacterium bovis* to humans is basically a result of the consumption of raw milk from tubercular cows. Since the 1950s, the main preventive measure has been the mandatory pasteurization of milk. There is still a risk of contracting tuberculosis from *M. bovis,* even in industrialized countries, however, due to the consumption of raw milk in certain rural areas. The elimination of bovine tuberculosis is considered a necessary prerequisite for the sustainable elimination of human tuberculosis from *M. bovis* (*143*).

HIV/AIDS AND OTHER SEXUALLY TRANSMITTED INFECTIONS

In 2001–2005, there were several positive forces at work at the global and Regional levels[10] that could have a direct effect on people's lives, provided they are sustained and expanded. Substantial year-by-year increases in funding to support Regional and national efforts, coupled with a greater commitment from government, civil society, the private sector, and the international development community, could change the course of the epidemics of HIV/AIDS and sexually transmitted infections (STIs) in the Americas. The period saw a renewal of the health sector's response to these diseases worldwide with the launching of WHO's and UNAIDS' "3 by 5" initiative; at the Regional level, with the launching of PAHO/WHO's Regional HIV/STI Plan for the Health Sector, 2006–2015; and at the country level with the build-up of health services, particularly treatment. The challenges ahead for the health sector include strengthening its capacity for implementing public health interventions that combine prevention, care, and treatment to more effectively reduce the number of new HIV infections and to provide care and support to those living with HIV. The quest for universal access to prevention, care, and treatment will be the focus of the health sector's interventions in the coming decade.

Epidemiologic Overview for HIV/AIDS and STIs

WHO and UNAIDS estimate that at the end of 2005 there were approximately 3.23 million people living with HIV in the Americas (*144*). Of these, 60% (1.94 million) lived in Latin America and the Caribbean. The epidemic is currently on the rise; at least

220,000 people were newly infected with the virus during 2005. Up to December 2005, a cumulative number of 1,540,414 AIDS cases had been reported to PAHO/WHO, of which 30,690 (2%) were in persons under 15 years old. It is estimated that these numbers are far from accurate due to under-registration and reporting delays. In Latin America and the Caribbean the epidemic is diverse, and all modes of transmission coexist. The most affected subregion is the Caribbean, which ranks second among the world's ten regions for HIV prevalence, with rates among adults of 2%–3%. The epidemic in the Caribbean is generalized, but is concentrated in most parts of Latin America and North America.[11]

PAHO/WHO and UNAIDS have reported (*145*) that the four groups that most commonly have prevalence rates of more than 5% in a concentrated epidemic are men who have sex with men, male commercial sex workers, injection drug users, and female commercial sex workers (Table 15). Recent surveys have shown HIV prevalence rates among men who have sex with men as high as 17.7% in El Salvador and 15% in Mexico. Rates in this group are also high in the Andean Area (for example, in Lima, Peru, the prevalence was as high as 21% in 2002). In Puerto Rico in 2003, 50% of all infections were associated with injectable drug use. In Argentina in 2003, the HIV prevalence rate among injecting drug users was 7.8%, compared to 0.3% among pregnant women. A recent multi-centric study conducted in Central America showed that HIV prevalence among female sex workers ranged from under than 1% in Nicaragua to more than 10% in Honduras. In 2000 in the Dominican Republic, the prevalence rates in female sex workers varied between 4.5% and 12.4% in the study sites. In Jamaica, HIV prevalence among female sex workers in Kingston was 10% and in Montego Bay, 20% in 2001. In Suriname, 21% of female sex workers were infected by HIV in 2003, while in neighboring Guyana the prevalence rate among the same group was 31% in 2000.

Other groups with high HIV prevalence rates are prisoners, migrant workers, members of the armed forces, truckers and other transport workers, and workers in mines and other isolated settings (*145*). HIV prevalence among prisoners is extremely high throughout the Region. In the Caribbean, a series of surveys conducted in 2004–2005 showed that prevalence rates among prisoners varied between 2% and 4%, while in the Dominican Republic and Argentina, the rate was 19% and 18.4%, respectively. Similarly, the rate of HIV infection in Mexican migrant workers who travel to the United States is 10 times higher than Mexico's national rate. The HIV seroprevalence among migrant workers in Guyana was 6% in 2001 (*146*).

---

[10]MDGs, UNGASS Declaration of Commitment on HIV/AIDS June 2001, WHO/UNAIDS "3 by 5" Initiative; December 2003, Summit of the Americas, PAHO/WHO Regional HIV/STI Plan for the Health Sector 2006–2015, UNGASS Declaration of Commitment on Universal Access; June 2001.

[11]UNAIDS and WHO have recently classified HIV epidemics into three broad categories: low-level, concentrated, and generalized epidemics. In a low-level epidemic, HIV prevalence has not exceeded 5% in any subpopulation, although it may have existed for many years. In a concentrated epidemic, HIV has spread substantially, and the prevalence is consistently 5% in at least one subpopulation, is below 1% in pregnant women in urban areas, and has not been well established in the general population. In a generalized epidemic, HIV is firmly established in the general population and the prevalence is consistently 1% among pregnant women.

TABLE 15. HIV prevalence in men who have sex with men and in female commercial sex workers, Central American and Andean countries, various surveys, 1999–2002.

	Number Surveyed	Percent with HIV
Men who have sex with men		
El Salvador (2002)	356	17.70%
Guatemala (2002	165	11.50%
Honduras (2001)	349	13%
Political capital, Tegucigalpa	171	8.20%
Economic capital, San Pedro Sula	178	16.00%
Nicaragua (2002)	199	9.30%
Panama (2002)	432	10.60%
Bolivia, La Paz (1999–2001)	48	14.60%
Santa Cruz (2001–2002)	186	23.70%
Three other cities (2002)	52	15.40%
Colombia, Bogotá (2002)	660	19.70%
Ecuador, Quito (1999–2001)	263	14.40%
Guayaquil (1999–2001)	227	27.80%
Four other port cities (2001–2002)	142	2.80%
Peru, Lima (1999–2000)	7,041	13.70%
Provinces, rural (1999–2000)	3,898	6.10%
Female commercial sex workers		
El Salvador (2002)	491	3.60%
Guatemala (2002)	536	4.50%
Honduras (2001)	535	n/a
Economic and political capitals (2001)	369	10.90%
Ports, Puerto Cortés and San Lorenzo (2001)	163	8.20%
Nicaragua (2002)	463	n/a
Capital, Managua (2002)	324	0.00%
Ports, Corinto and Bluefields (2002)	139	1.40%
Panama (2002)	432	n/a
Capital, Panama (2002)	291	1.90%
Colón (2002)	141	2.10%
Bolivia, Santa Cruz (2001)	195	0.50%
Three cities on the Argentine border (2002)	77	0%
Colombia, Bogotá (2001–2002)	514	0.80%
Ecuador, Quito (2001–2002)	200	0.50%
Guayaquil (2001–2002)	1,047	2.10%
Peru, Lima (1999–2000)	3,347	1.60%
Provinces, rural (1999–2000)	4,930	0.60%
Venezuela, Isla Margarita (2002)	652	0.00%

Sources: Montano, SM et al (2005). Prevalences, Genotypes, and Risk Factors for HIV Transmission in South America. Journal of Acquired Deficiency Syndrome. Vol. 1. September 2005.

Central American Multi-site HIV/STI Prevalence and Behaviour Study (results published in 2003 and available, by country, at: http://pasca.org/english/estudio_informes_eng.htm.

Even though an important proportion of countries still exhibit concentrated epidemics, there is a trend towards generalized epidemics in most of the Region's countries, with few exceptions (*144*). In 2005, 30% of adults living with HIV/AIDS in the Americas were women, ranging from 25% in North America to 31% and 51% in Latin America and the Caribbean, respectively (*144*). The male:female sex ratio in reported AIDS cases is declining rapidly in the Region. Regionwide, the proportion of all reported adult cases (for which sex is reported) among women has increased over time, from 6.1% before 1994, to 15.8% in 1999, and to 16.5% in 2002. In Brazil, the male:female ratio declined from 24:1 in 1985 to 1.5:1 in 2004; in Argentina, it declined from 15:1 in 1985 to 2.5:1 in 2004. In Trinidad and Tobago, the ratio declined from 6.25:1 in 1985 to 1.5:1 in 2002 (*146*). More and more young people are being affected by the epidemic. UNAIDS estimates that in Latin America and the Caribbean, the number of children under 15 years old who are infected with HIV increased from 130,000 in 2003 to 140,000 in 2005. Limited recent data exist regarding HIV infection in indigenous people, Canada, however, reports indigenous peoples in that country are being disproportionately affected by the HIV virus (*146*).

To date, most infections are due to unprotected sexual intercourse, although in several Southern Cone countries, injectable drug use is the major driving factor behind transmission. (*144*)

Despite the introduction of antiretrovirals, deaths due to AIDS continue to increase in the Region (*144*). The estimated number of deaths due to AIDS in adults and children increased from 97,000 in 2003 to 104,000 in 2005. However, a decline in reported mortality was observed in some countries that had introduced antiretrovirals early on (Bahamas, Brazil, Canada, and the United States) (*146*).

HIV/Tuberculosis Coinfection

In 2005, almost all the Region's countries reported some prevalence rates of HIV infection among tuberculosis (TB) patients. The reported prevalence rate of HIV infection in TB patients ranges from under 1% in some countries with low levels of or concentrated epidemics to more than 30% in some countries of the English-speaking Caribbean that offer HIV testing on a routine basis to TB patients.

Sexually Transmitted Infections

While responding to the threat posed by the HIV/AIDS epidemic, the Region continues to be challenged by the spread of STIs. It is estimated that 50 million new cases of STIs occur in the Americas each year. Surveys conducted in some Caribbean countries found that STI patients are seriously affected by the HIV epidemic. In several instances, HIV prevalence rates are two to six times higher among STI patients than in the general population. The magnitude of the STI epidemic in the Region is difficult to measure, given limited data, underreporting, and weaknesses of the surveillance systems. Examples of data from different countries obtained by various methods illustrate the problem. In a sentinel site in Chile, of 10,525 STI consultations between 1999 and 2003, 22% of patients were diagnosed with condyloma, 10.4% with latent syphilis, and 10.1% with gonorrhea. A similar situation was observed regarding cases of gonor-

TABLE 16. Prevalence of syphilis and congenital syphilis, reporting countries, Latin America and the Caribbean.

Country	Year	Prevalence of syphilis in pregnant women (%)	Congenital syphilis (per 1,000 live births)	Method
Bahamas	2004	2.4	1.3	Routine
Belize	2004	1.5	0.13	Routine
Bolivia	2004	4.9	12	Survey
Brazil	2004	1.6	4	Routine
Costa Rica	2004	NA	1.3	Routine
Cuba	2003	1.8	0	Routine
Ecuador	2002	NA	1.11	Routine
El Salvador	2003	6.2	0.9	Routine
Haiti	2004	4.2	NA	Survey
Honduras	2003	3.5	2.5	Routine
Jamaica	2003	NA	0.7	Routine
Mexico	2004	0.62	0.06	Routine
Nicaragua	2004	NA	0.06	Routine
Panama	2004	0.4	0.1	Routine
Paraguay	2003	6.3	1.9	Routine
Peru	2004	1	1.7	Routine

Sources: Ministries of Health of the reporting countries; Bolivia's Population Council.

rhea and syphilis among STI patients in Nicaragua during 2000–2002. A population-based survey (*147*) conducted in 2004 among adults in Barbados found that 14.3% of that population was infected by gonorrhea or chlamydia. In the United States, cases of primary and secondary syphilis declined between 1990 and 2000. However, the number of annual cases of syphilis increased during 2000–2002 and continued to increase from 2002 (6,862 cases) until the end of 2003 (7,177 cases). Surveys conducted to determine the prevalence of syphilis among different at-risk populations have demonstrated that vulnerable groups in Latin America are heavily affected by STIs. For example, in 2003, the prevalence of syphilis in Paraguay was 4.3% among blood donors and 6% among pregnant women, compared with a high prevalence rate of 37.4% among female sex workers. In 2004, a survey conducted by the Ministry of Health of Guyana found that 27% of female sex workers were infected with syphilis. In 2003, 15,570 cases of congenital syphilis were reported from 11 Latin American and Caribbean countries; during the same year, PAHO estimated that 110,000 cases had occurred, indicating serious underreporting of cases of congenital syphilis. The prevalence of syphilis among pregnant women and the incidence of congenital syphilis are summarized in Table 16. In countries where cases of congenital syphilis are reported annually, an increasing trend is observed (*148*). In Venezuela, cases increased from 50 in 2000 to 135 in 2002, and in Brazil, the rate of congenital syphilis per 1,000 live births increased from 1 in 2001 to 1.5 in 2003. Coverage and access to syphilis screening and treatment services continues to

be a public health issue in the Region, even in countries that have expanded their services to prevent mother-to-child transmission of HIV (for example, in 2003 only 17.3% of pregnant women diagnosed with syphilis were treated, even though Brazil's coverage for syphilis screening is 56.5%).

Socioeconomic Determinants and Compounding Factors in HIV Transmission

Socioeconomic marginalization increases the vulnerability to HIV transmission. This vulnerability, combined with gender inequities and a tendency towards risky behavior, including engaging in unprotected sex and alcohol and drug use, render persons younger than 25 years old (30% of the Region's population) particularly susceptible to HIV and other STIs (*146*). In a PAHO/WHO survey in the Caribbean in 2003, around one-third of young people (ages 10–18) reported that they were sexually active. Of these, nearly one-half said that their first sexual experience had been forced, and almost two-thirds stated that they had had intercourse before age 13. Of sexually active young people, only one-quarter always used a birth control method. Many of the sexually active youth reported being worried about getting AIDS, but only slightly more than half had used a condom during their last intercourse (*149*). In Latin America and the Caribbean, between one-quarter and two-thirds of young women marry during adolescence (*150*). Marriage of girls prior to age 18 places them at greater risk of HIV infection than sexually active unmarried girls (*151*). Many international and national AIDS prevention messages encourage abstinence until marriage, implying that marriage provides complete protection against HIV (*150*), when, in fact, for many adolescent girls, marriage results in a transition from virginity to frequent unprotected sex. Moreover, a recent review of adolescents worldwide found that "there is reason to believe that marriages of young women and older men are less equitable" than other marriages (*152*).

Children orphaned by HIV are particularly disadvantaged. Even HIV-negative orphaned children still lack the support and nurturing offered by a stable family environment, which can increase their vulnerability and likelihood to engage in high-risk behaviors.

For those infected, pediatric formulations of antiretroviral medicines remain highly inadequate. Only a handful of the antiretrovirals in the current WHO guidelines are available in formulations that are affordable, feasible, or acceptable for use in infants and young children. The global market for pediatric AIDS drug formulations is not attractive for originator or generic companies; in wealthy countries very few children are being born with HIV, and in developing countries, where most of the infected children are, pediatric formulations are not considered a priority or a lucrative market (*153*).

Gender inequity continues to be a central issue to HIV in the Region. In 2005, more than one-third of new HIV infections worldwide were among women with long-term partners (*144*). In Latin America and the Caribbean, a large number of women with HIV have been infected by their husbands or regular partners. For example, in Colombia in 2005, 72% of women testing HIV-positive at projects aimed at preventing the transmission of HIV from mother to child were in stable relationships, and 90% described themselves as "housewives"(*144*). The major interventions known to have an impact on HIV transmission—abstaining from sex, having sex with only one uninfected partner, or using male condoms—are often not under women's control due to a variety of societal norms and social conditions. In most countries in the Region, men have the most power in sexual relationships, with women at a disadvantage in protecting themselves from HIV (*154*). Using a female condom is difficult without the knowledge and consent of a woman's sexual partner, and transactional sex and sex work may be necessary for many women for economic survival. "For many women, current prevention methods are inadequate—women often do not have the social and economic power to refuse sex or negotiate condom use" (*155*).

A high prevalence of violence and sexual coercion also puts women at risk. There is a link between HIV and gender-based violence (*156, 157*). Women and adolescent girls threatened by violence and rape, including married women, cannot negotiate condom use. A study in Haiti among married women aged 15–19 years old found that 25% had experienced violence at the hands of their husbands (often sexual violence), within the 12 months prior to the Survey (*158*). Gender norms that validate coercive sex, acceptability of gender-based violence against sex workers, and males' gender-based violence need to be changed (*159*). Violence is also perpetrated against gay, lesbian, transgender, and bisexual populations in the Region. Homophobia places men at risk by ignoring the health needs of men who have sex with men. Also damaging is the definition of "being a man" as having sexual relations with multiple female sexual partners (*160*). Discrimination forces men who wish to engage in sexual activities with other men to go underground and deny the existence of the risk behavior. This deters prevention programs from reaching them and puts their unknowing female sexual partners at risk. In the Region, prevailing gender norms dictate that men have multiple sexual partners as a way to validate their masculinity, but the practice ends up validating ignorance about sexuality and submissiveness for young girls and women, which can lead to increased rates of HIV (*161*). A study of 148 HIV-positive women in São Paulo, Brazil, found that more than half (53%) did not perceive themselves to be at risk of HIV before learning they were HIV-positive, and 29% only went for testing after their partners became ill (*162*). Demographic Health Surveys in the Region found that men were four to five times more likely to report a greater number of casual sexual partners in the last year than women.

The mobility of populations plays an important role in the spread of HIV. Populations on the move, including migrant workers, are at risk because of complications derived from their poverty, lack of access to services, and lack of information, as well as their transient nature and the fact that they spend long periods away from their families, leading them to engage in transactional sex. Migrant workers who lack the necessary documentation to remain legally in their host country may face difficulties in receiving health care services or may hesitate to seek services out of fear of being deported (*146*).

Injecting drug use plays an important role in the spread of the epidemic, particularly in North America, Brazil, and the Southern Cone. In some cities in Brazil, the HIV prevalence rate among injecting drug users in 2004 was 60 times higher than the rate in the general population. Although injecting drug use has become a significant factor in the epidemic Regionwide, with infection rates reaching 60% in some cities, there is limited political support for developing programs to address this issue.

The Health Sector's Response: Key Achievements

The Region of the Americas has, since the epidemic began, swiftly responded to the challenges of HIV infection. The health sector established and maintained national AIDS programs. Most countries also have set up national AIDS committees or councils to function as intersectoral collaboration mechanisms. In Latin America and the Caribbean at least 15 countries have national networks, social organizations, and community-based organizations dealing with HIV/AIDS, covering a myriad of focus areas that include advocacy, promoting adherence to treatment, the conduct of operational research, and the pursuit of more integrated perspectives. Several countries in the Region are using a comprehensive approach to tackle HIV that seeks to give equal weight to prevention and treatment efforts. Most countries have successfully launched prevention interventions, which have had a positive effect. In Haiti, for example, the percentage of HIV-infected pregnant women declined by half from 1993 to 2003–2004 (*144*), despite the fact that Haiti is one of the Region's poorest countries. Programs to promote testing and counseling in various modalities—such as voluntary counseling and testing (VCT) or provider initiated testing and counseling (PITC)— have expanded and been effective in changing behaviors to reduce HIV transmission. A randomized control trial in Kenya, Tanzania, and Trinidad and Tobago found that persons who received VCT significantly changed their risk behaviors compared to those who only received health education. For instance, the percentage of persons who reported having unprotected intercourse with non-primary partners declined by 35% among men and 49% among women who received VCT, as compared to 13% of men and women who only received health education (163). Health programs that increased access to condoms and media campaigns that promote condom use have resulted in increased condom use. In Brazil in 2004, 51.6% of adults 15–54 years old, 58.4% of young adults 15–24 years old, and 66.9% of men who have sex with men reported regular condom use with casual partners. In the same age groups and the same year, 76%, 74.1%, and 80.7%, respectively, reported that they had used a condom in their last intercourse with a casual partner (*164*). Sex education has been shown to delay initiation of sexual intercourse and reduce risky sexual behavior. Providing skills has been more effective than merely providing information. In 2005, a review was conducted of 83 evaluations of curriculum-based efforts to reduce adolescent sexual risk behaviors that promoted abstinence but also discussed or promoted condom use and/or contraception (including 18 studies in Brazil, Chile, Jamaica and Mexico). Results found that many programs had positive effects on knowledge, awareness of risks, values, attitudes, self-efficacy, and intentions (*165*). The evaluations found significantly increased condom use and none found decreased condom use; half of the evaluations found significantly decreased sexual risk-taking behavior and none found increased sexual risk-taking (*165*). However, abstinence-only education has not been shown to delay the onset of intercourse (*167, 168*). A review of the impact of abstinence-based programs on risk behaviors in developing countries "found little evidence of the effectiveness of these types of programs in changing individual behavior in developing countries (*168*)." Interventions for specific vulnerable groups, however, have proven to be effective. Brazil has successfully kept the prevalence of HIV at a low and stable rate of 6% among sex workers, with 74% of sex workers in 2004 reporting consistent use of condoms with clients (*164*). Prevention of mother-to-child transmission services have resulted in a significant reduction in the number of HIV-infected children in some of the Region's countries (*146*).

PAHO/WHO's "3 by 5" Report indicated that all countries in the Region have achieved an unprecedented acceleration in the provision of antiretroviral treatment, especially during 2004 and 2005. The goal of treating at least 600,000 people in the Region who require treatment has been met and exceeded. Since January 2004, more than 100,000 new treatments have been initiated in Latin America and the Caribbean alone. However, there are important gaps in the Region (Figure 17). For the first time, the Region has access to the necessary resources to begin to match the need for care and treatment. The Global Fund has disbursed US$ 480 million to 28 countries in the Region and to subregional venues such as the Pan-Caribbean Partnership Against HIV/AIDS (PANCAP). Moreover, lower prices obtained through negotiations between the countries and pharmaceutical companies have resulted in greatly reduced prices for first-line antiretrovirals. In several countries in the Region where ART has been provided through the health system for several years, dramatic declines in death rates have been observed. Bahamas, Brazil, Canada, Costa Rica, Haiti, and the United States, for example, have experienced impressive declines. These countries recognized early on that treatment is key for prevention and control, as well as for direct, positive impact on the lives of people with HIV. By 2003, the Bahamas had experienced a 56% reduction in AIDS deaths overall and a reduction of 89% of deaths among children since the introduction of ART.

FIGURE 17. Estimated percentage of people under anti-retroviral treatment (ART) and treatment gap, by subregion,ᵃ 2004–2005.

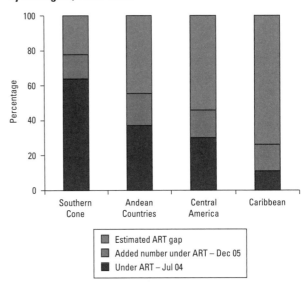

ᵃExcludes Brazil, Mexico, Canada, and the United States.
Source: PAHO/WHO. Toward Universal Access to HIV Prevention, Care and Treatment: 3 by 5 Report for the Americas.

Completing the Unfinished Agenda: 2006 and Beyond

The negative impact of the HIV epidemic on demographic trends in the Region has been well documented. If current trends continue, AIDS will be responsible for reducing life expectancy by at least 10 years by the end of 2010 in hard-hit countries such as the Bahamas, Guyana, and Haiti. According to PAHO/WHO projections (*146*), in order to halt and reverse the spread of HIV by 2015 (MDG 6), new infections will have to be reduced by 50% by 2010, with an additional 50% reduction by 2015. This will only be possible by strengthening the health sector response so as to be able to scale up HIV/AIDS activities in the Region. In most countries, services are still centralized in specialized clinics located in large cities, and the integration of services at the primary level of care is still very limited. The provision of vertical services in specialized HIV and STI clinics is a known barrier for access to care because it further isolates people suffering from these illnesses and may even perpetuate stigmatization and discrimination.

The spontaneous demand for counseling and testing, essential for the early detection of HIV-positive individuals, is also compromised due to the limited availability of community-level quality services that are backed up by adequate referral systems. While prevention is key to the success of the fight against HIV, primary health care services are not equipped to provide comprehensive prevention services for vulnerable groups, such as youth, injecting drug users, men who have sex with men, and commercial sex workers. Similarly, the prevention and treatment of STIs, diseases that are an important risk factor for HIV, have not received adequate attention in the health sector in recent years. Rapid scale-up of comprehensive care and treatment requires an array of essential support services that, until now, are largely inadequate in most countries of the Region. Drug procurement and management systems have not expanded rapidly enough to effectively support the provision of direct patient care. The supply of antiretroviral drugs and laboratory diagnostics has been hampered by inconsistent pricing policies by the Region's manufacturers. Obtaining further reductions in prices, particularly in second-line medicines and diagnostics, is a priority for the Region.

The extension and expansion of services for people with HIV is occurring within a context of limited qualified human resources. Health providers may not be equipped or motivated to provide comprehensive care and treatment; they often lack the necessary training and specialization and they may not be deployed to the areas where services are most needed. There is a lack of human resource strategic planning and management processes to inform the ministries of health on critical issues related to policies, staffing, cost, and accreditation needs. Moreover, some fiscal policies implemented by countries impose limitations on the ministries of health regarding the hiring and retention of staff. The benefits package offered by the public health sector generally cannot compete with that offered by the private sector or even that offered by externally funded projects within the public sector.

The proliferation of services in the for-profit and nonprofit sectors has contributed to the rapid expansion of HIV services and has improved access to care for specific population groups or people living in specific areas. Nonetheless, these services can present a challenge for improving public health systems because public services may lack the authority to regulate private services, resulting in a lack of consistency in guidelines and treatment protocols, as well as poorly defined referral systems. Scaling up services also presents challenges in the areas of management, monitoring, and evaluation. The majority of countries do not have adequate health information systems, and challenges exist in regard to collection of HIV data, assurance of confidentiality, and integration into existing systems. The lack or limited availability of good and timely data has been recognized as a major obstacle to inform country and Regional efforts.

While the increased investment in HIV/AIDS in Latin America and the Caribbean by a variety of development initiatives has clearly benefited the countries, it also leads to the fragmentation of local responses and puts considerable pressure on the countries' limited human and financial resources. Despite wide acknowledgement of the importance of the "Three Ones" principles for the coordination of national AIDS responses, development partners continue to stress their own agendas, including separate monitoring and evaluation mechanisms. In order to cope with these pressures, national programs are forced to make strategic choices in order to make the most of the increased support. They face the challenge of streamlining efforts to avoid parallel processes and to ensure a balanced investment in multiple sectors of society.

To support the strengthening of the health sector's response in the Region of the Americas, PAHO/WHO launched the "Regional HIV/STI Plan for the Health Sector, 2006–2015" in November 2005 (Box 2). The Plan is a "further step to promote effective prevention and care." The Regional Plan will guide PAHO's work in the years to come.

CHRONIC COMMUNICABLE DISEASES

Tuberculosis

Tuberculosis is one of the oldest diseases; its effective treatment was discovered in the middle of the 20th century. It is still very far from being eliminated as a public health problem in the Region of the Americas, however. Despite progress made toward tuberculosis control in the 1990s, this preventable, treatable, and curable disease still has a prevalence rate of more than 466,000 cases in the Region, and is responsible for more than 50,000 deaths per year (168). Although tuberculosis can affect any segment of the population, regardless of socioeconomic status, it is the poorest and most vulnerable population groups—migrants, persons living in urban marginalized areas, prisoners, people with HIV/AIDS, and indigenous populations—who carry the greater burden of disease.

BOX 2. Critical Lines of Action for the Regional HIV/STI Plan for the Health Sector

1. Strengthen health sector leadership and stewardship and foster the engagement of civil society.
2. Design and implement effective, sustainable HIV/AIDS/STI programs and build human resource capacity.
3. Strengthen, expand, and reorient the health services.
4. Improve access to medicines, diagnostics, and other commodities.
5. Improve information and knowledge management, including surveillance, monitoring and evaluation, and dissemination.

In the Americas, marked differences exist among countries in terms of the burden of tuberculosis. In countries that have established market economies, such as the United States, Canada, and some English-speaking Caribbean countries, the incidence of tuberculosis is estimated at five cases per 100,000 population. In countries with fewer resources, the incidence rate is much higher; for example, it is estimated that it is 61 times higher in Haiti, 43 times higher in Bolivia, and 35 times higher in Peru (Table 17). There also are differences in incidence rates within countries. The countries that have assigned priority for tuberculosis control include Bolivia, Brazil, Colombia, the Dominican Republic, Ecuador, Haiti, Honduras, Guatemala, Guyana, Mexico, Nicaragua, and Peru, which together account for 80% of the cases reported in the Region.

In 1994–2004, there was a slight downward trend in the reported incidence rate for all forms of tuberculosis (Figure 18), from 32 cases per 100,000 at the beginning of the period to 27 per 100,000 in 2004, the most pronounced decline since 1998. When the analysis is conducted exclusively on Latin America and the Caribbean, a similar downward trend is observed, but with higher incidence rates: from 46 to 38 cases per 100,000 population at the beginning and end of the period.

Tuberculosis can present at any time in life, but children and older adults are at a greater risk. However, nearly 40% of cases with positive bacilloscopy correspond to men 15–44 years old. High morbidity from tuberculosis in children is particularly relevant in public health, because it indicates the high degree of *Mycobacterium tuberculosis* transmission in the community.

The Directly Observed Treatment Short-course (DOTS)[12] in the Region has helped improve tuberculosis control since it was consistently implemented beginning in 1996. In 2004, 35 countries were applying the strategy, and at the end of that year, its coverage reached 82% of the general population of those countries. DOTS programs reported a total of 175,100 new cases and relapses in 2004, more than 95,000 of which were bacilliferous cases. These represent 59% of the estimated incidence in the Region, still far from the goal of 70% established by WHO in 2005 for this indicator. The average treatment success rate in patients following DOTS in 2003 was 82%, quite close to the goal of 85% proposed for that indicator in 2005 (Table 17 and Figure 19).

The emergence of new obstacles for tuberculosis control—such as the HIV/AIDS epidemic, multidrug-resistant tuberculosis,[13] health sector reforms, the weakening of the health system,

and the human-resource crisis in health—facilitated WHO's launching of the Stop TB strategy (*169*). The strategy, which was drafted based on experiences in the countries with the implementation of DOTS, adds a comprehensive approach to tuberculosis control. It has provided the bases for the Stop TB Partnership's Global Plan to Stop Tuberculosis, 2006–2015 (*170*), which lays down in detail the steps to reach the MDG pertaining to tuberculosis[14] and constitutes an appeal for mobilizing resources that will allow tuberculosis elimination as a public health problem in the long-term.

The Regional Plan for Tuberculosis Control, 2006–2015, is consistent with the Global Plan; its vision is a tuberculosis-free Region and its mission is to guarantee each patient with tuberculosis full access to quality diagnosis and treatment in order to reduce the social and economic burden as well as the inequity caused by this disease (*171*). The six strategic lines of work of the Plan are presented in Box 3.

The Region's Response within the Framework of the New Stop TB Strategy

HIV/TB Coinfection

The HIV infection epidemic has had a negative impact on the tuberculosis epidemic. First, it generates an increase in the number of tuberculosis cases, largely due to latent tuberculosis infection progressing to disease; second, case-fatality from tuberculosis is higher in patients with HIV infection or AIDS. Both situations threaten the achievements of the programs for tuberculosis control.

WHO has estimated that 10% of the Region's tuberculosis patients are also HIV-infected. This situation complicates not only the clinical treatment of patients, given the increasing access to antiretrovirals and the possible interactions between these and the tuberculostatics, but also the application of effective measures for the prevention of tuberculosis among people with HIV.

Many countries are responding to the HIV/TB coinfection problem by progressively implementing activities established by WHO to address both diseases (*172*). For example, with respect to epidemiological coinfection surveillance, in 2005 almost all the countries in the Region had estimates of the prevalence of HIV infection among people with tuberculosis; this prevalence goes from less than 1% in countries with early or concentrated HIV epidemics, to more than 30% in some English-speaking Caribbean countries that routinely test tuberculosis patients for HIV.

Resistance to Anti-tuberculosis Drugs

Multidrug-resistant tuberculosis also jeopardizes the success of many tuberculosis control programs, given its complex and ex-

---

[12] Directly Observed Treatment Short-course (DOTS) is the internationally recognized strategy for tuberculosis control. It typically has five components: 1) political commitment with sustainable and increasing financing; 2) case detection by sputum smear microscopy with quality control; 3) standardized treatment regimen, with patient supervision and support; 4) an effective pharmacological management system, and 5) a system of surveillance and evaluation, including assessment of treatment results.

[13] Multidrug resistant tuberculosis is defined as the appearance of resistance to isoniazid and rifampicin, which may be accompanied by resistance to other tuberculostatics.

[14] Target eight of MDG 6 states: "Halt and begin to reverse the incidence of malaria and other major diseases by 2015." In terms of tuberculosis, objective six defines the indicators of impact and implementation.

TABLE 17. Leading epidemiological and operational indicators for tuberculosis control, Region of the Americas, 2004.

	Estimated incidence, all forms[a]		New cases and relapses notified, all forms[b]		New cases of positive bacilloscopy (BK+)[c]		DOTS coverage[d] %	BK+ cases detected under DOTS[e] %	Treatment success, DOTS[f] %
	Number of cases	Rate	Number of cases	Rate	Number of cases	Rate			
Anguilla	3	25	0	0	0	0	0	ND	ND
Antigua and Barbuda	5	7	ND	ND	ND	ND	ND	ND	ND
Argentina	16,537	43	10,619	28	4,760	12	100	64	66
Bahamas	124	39	53	17	37	12	100	68	62
Barbados	31	11	19	7	19	7	100	139	100
Belize	128	49	83	31	34	13	100	60	89
Bermuda	3	4	6	9	0	0	0	ND	ND
Bolivia	19,568	217	9,801	109	6,213	69	60	71	81
Brazil	109,672	60	86,881	47	42,881	23	52	46	83
Canada	1,662	5	1,517	5	428	1	100	58	35
Cayman Islands	2	4	1	2	1	2	100	115	ND
Chile	2,567	16	2,664	17	1,297	8	95	114	85
Colombia	22,357	50	11,242	25	7,640	17	25	17	83
Costa Rica	612	14	712	17	419	10	100	153	94
Cuba	1,119	10	782	7	454	4	100	90	93
Dominica	12	15	ND	ND	ND	ND	ND	ND	ND
Dominican Republic	7,946	91	4,549	52	2,720	31	79	71	81
Ecuador	17,101	131	6,122	47	4,340	33	64	42	84
El Salvador	3,624	54	1,406	21	926	14	100	57	88
Grenada	5	5	2	2	2	2	0	ND	ND
Guatemala	9,469	77	3,313	27	2,339	19	100	55	91
Guyana	1,050	140	603	80	164	22	42	27	57
Haiti	25,707	306	14,533	173	7,044	84	55	49	78
Honduras	5,451	77	3,282	47	2,012	29	ND	83	87

	Incidence[a]	Total cases[b]	Rate[b]	Positive bacilloscopy[c]	Rate[c]	% population under DOTS[d]	% cases detected[e]	% treatment success[f]
Jamaica	197	7	116	4	69	3	100	79	53
Mexico	33,529	32	15,101	14	11,214	11	92	71	83
Montserrat	0.4	9	0	0	0	0	100	0	ND
Netherlands Antilles	16		11	6	8	4	0	ND	ND
Nicaragua	3,390	63	2,220	41	1,327	25	100	87	84
Panama	1,443	45	1,691	53	882	28	92	133	74
Paraguay	4,269	71	2,300	38	1,201	20	27	21	85
Peru	49,174	178	33,082	120	18,289	66	100	83	89
Puerto Rico	191	5	123	3	65	2	100	76	66
Saint Kitts and Nevis	5	11	2	5	0	0	100	0	ND
Saint Lucia	26	16	15	9	11	7	100	93	89
Saint Vincent and the Grenadines	34	28	8	7	5	4	100	33	ND
Suriname	290	65	94	21	38	9	0	ND	ND
Trinidad and Tobago	116	9	177	14	81	6	ND	0	ND
Turks and Caicos Islands	5	20	ND	ND	ND	ND	ND	ND	ND
United States of America	13,877	5	14,517	5	5,219	2	100	85	70
Uruguay	967	28	727	21	373	11	100	86	ND
Venezuela	10,946	42	6,808	26	3,776	14	98	77	82
Virgin Islands (UK)	3	15	2	9	2	9	100	0	ND
Virgin Islands (US)	12	11	ND	ND	ND	ND	ND	ND	ND
Region	363,245	41	235,184	27	126,290	14	82	59	82

ND: No data available.

[a] Incidence estimated by WHO, all forms of tuberculosis. For estimation methods, consult sources cited.

[b] Total number of cases reported to WHO, which include new cases and relapses. A new case is one that has never received treatment for tuberculosis. Relapse is defined as a case that has been declared cured of tuberculosis with negative microscopic examination and presents the disease again with positive bacilloscopy. Rate per 100,000 population.

[c] Total number of cases with positive bacilloscopy in sputum. Rate per 100,000 population.

[d] Percentage of population that live in a geographical location whose health facilities apply the DOTS strategy.

[e] Percentage of cases detected by BK+ under the DOTS programs. Estimation methods are described in the sources cited.

[f] Percentage of treatment success of BK+ cases under DOTS. Estimation methods are described in the sources cited.

Source: Tuberculosis Control: surveillance, planning, financing. WHO report 2005. Geneva; 2006. (WHO/HTM/TB/2006.362).

FIGURE 18. Trend in reported tuberculosis incidence, all forms, Region of the Americas, 1994–2004.

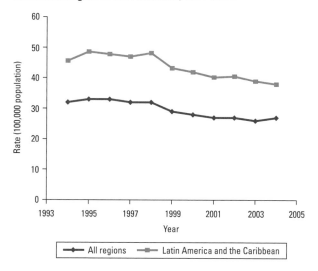

Source: World Health Organization. Global Tuberculosis Control: surveillance, planning, financing. WHO report 2005. Geneva; 2006. (WHO/HTM/TB/2006.362).

FIGURE 19. Leading indicators of tuberculosis control, Region of the Americas, 1996–2004.

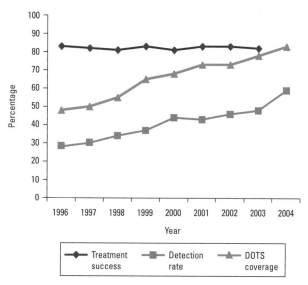

Source: World Health Organization. Global Tuberculosis Control: surveillance, planning, financing. WHO report 2005. Geneva; 2006. (WHO/HTM/TB/2006.362).

pensive diagnosis and treatment. The estimated prevalence of this type of tuberculosis is higher in those populations that lack access to the DOTS strategy and among the vulnerable population groups. It is estimated that there are more than 11,000 cases of multidrug-resistant tuberculosis in the Americas, although the case burden varies from country to country. The average prevalence of primary resistance to any tuberculosis drug is 11%

(ranging between 3.2% and 41%) and that of multidrug-resistant tuberculosis is 1.2% (between 0.3% and 6.6%). The average prevalence of secondary multidrug-resistant TB is 26% (ranging from 3% to 31%) (Table 18).

All of the Region's countries are working to confront drug resistance. Belize, Bolivia, Costa Rica, the Dominican Republic, Ecuador, El Salvador, Haiti, Honduras, Mexico, Nicaragua, Paraguay, and Peru have put in place projects to address multidrug resistance that have been approved by the Light Green Committee. This committee controls access to second-line quality drugs at a lower cost and controls for their rational use; provides technical assistance; and facilitates the adoption of internationally accepted policies for the medical care of multiple-drug resistance in low- and middle-income countries. Preliminary data indicate that a cure rate of 61% to 82% is achieved worldwide for multidrug-resistant tuberculosis cases, with proven cost-effectiveness measured in DALYs, in Estonia, Peru, the Philippines, and Russia (*173*).

The improper use of second-line drugs generates resistance to them; in tuberculosis this problem is called extreme drug-resistance (TB-XDR), for which a world alert is currently in place.

Strengthening the Health Systems

The Practical Approach to Lung Health initiative aims to improve the quality of care of patients with respiratory symptoms, strengthen primary health care services, and, indirectly, contribute to the sustainability of tuberculosis control programs in countries with low prevalence (*174*). Currently, 20 countries in the world, four of them in the Americas (Bolivia, Chile, El Salvador, and Peru), are carrying out activities related to this initiative. The initiative's feasibility study in Bolivia (2005) showed that 23% of patients that go to the health services do so due to respiratory symptoms; 90% of them have acute respiratory infections, and 0.4% have tuberculosis. Thanks to the approach proposed in this initiative, hospital referrals decreased 35% and the use of antibiotics, 16%. There was a 32% reduction in the total cost of prescribed medication and 37% in that of antibiotics. These results are similar to those in other countries (*175*).

Leprosy

The Strategic Plan for the Elimination of Leprosy, 2000–2005, whose goal is to achieve a prevalence rate lower than one case per 10,000 population by the end of 2005, has succeeded in increasing the coverage of the control activities in every country of the Region. In fact, with the exception of Brazil, every country achieved the goal of elimination of leprosy before 2002. The Plan evolved into the Global Strategy, 2006–2010, to Reduce the Burden of Leprosy and Sustain Leprosy Control Activities (*176*), which is endorsed by the partners that support leprosy control programs worldwide. In addition, the strategy aims to further reduce the disease burden due to leprosy by providing comprehensive care with equity and justice for every case.

BOX 3. Regional Plan for Tuberculosis Control, 2006–2015: Strategic Lines of Work

Strategic Line 1. Expand and strengthen the DOTS strategy, ensuring its quality.

Strategic Line 2. Implement and/or strengthen:
- TB and HIV/AIDS interprogram collaborative activities.
- Prevention and control activities for multidrug-resistant tuberculosis.
- Community strategies for neglected populations (for example, indigenous people, prisoners, peri-urban overlooked populations).

Strategic Line 3. Strengthen the health system, emphasizing primary care, a comprehensive approach to respiratory diseases, the laboratory network, and the development of human resource policies for tuberculosis control.

Strategic Line 4. Improve the population's access to tuberculosis diagnosis and treatment by including all public and private health care providers.

Strategic Line 5. Empower the affected persons and the community by implementing advocacy, communication, and social mobilization strategies in TB control activities.

Strategic Line 6. Include operational, clinical, and epidemiological research in national TB control program plans.

TABLE 18. Prevalence of primary and secondary resistance to antituberculosis drugs, selected countries, Region of the Americas, 1994–2005.

Country	Year	Global[a]	Primary multidrug resistance[b]	Secondary multidrug resistance[b]	Combined multidrug resistance[b]
Argentina	1999	10.2	1.8	9.4	3.1
Bolivia	1996	23.9	1.2	4.7	2.1
Brazil	1995	8.6	0.9	5.4	1.3
Canada	2000	8.5	0.7	3.4	0.9
Chile	2001	11.7	0.7	4.8	1.4
Colombia	2005	11.78	2.38	31.4	8.8
Cuba	2000	5	0.3	2.6	0.5
Dominican Republic	1994	40.6	6.6	19.7	8.6
Ecuador	2002	20	4.9	24.3	7.2
El Salvador	2001	5.7	0.3	7	0.8
Guatemala	2002	34.9	3	26.5	7.4
Honduras	2002	17.2	1.8	6.9	2.0
Mexico[c]	1997	14.1	2.4	22.4	7.3
Nicaragua	1997	15.6	1.2	—	—
Paraguay	2002	11.1	2.1	4	—
Peru	1999	18	3	12.3	4.3
Puerto Rico	2001	12	2	—	—
United States of America	2001	12.7	1.1	5.2	1.4
Uruguay	1999	3.2	0.3	—	—
Venezuela	1998	7.5	0.5	13.5	1.7

[a]Global resistance: percentage of tuberculosis strains resistant to any tuberculostatic.

[b]MDR: multidrug resistance, defined as the appearance of resistance to isoniazid and rifampicin, which may be accompanied by resistance to other tuberculostatics.

[c]Study conducted in three states.

Source: Results of MDR national surveys, published in: Antituberculosis Drug Resistance in the World. First Global Report, WHO/TB/97.229; Antituberculosis Drug Resistance in the World. Second Global Report, WHO/CDS/TB/2000. 279; Antituberculosis Drug Resistance in the World. First Third Global Report, WHO/HTM/TB/2004.343.

TABLE 19. Profile of newly recorded cases of leprosy, countries that reported more than 100 cases, Region of the Americas, 2005.

Country[a]	Number of cases reported	Multibacillary cases (%)	Cases in women (%)	Cases in children (%)	Grade II disability cases (%)
Argentina	484	79.1	40.9	1.3	1.6
Brazil	38,410	50	46.3	8.4	4.9
Bolivia	114	35.9	41.2	9.6	1.7
Colombia	585	68.7	—	3.2	9.7
Cuba	208	83.1	44.7	3.8	3.3
Dominican Republic	155	63.8	50.3	16.1	3.2
Ecuador	116	62.9	35.3	0	0
Mexico	289	75.4	37.3	2.7	11.7
Paraguay	480	77.7	38.5	3.9	7.9
Venezuela	768	64.5	33.9	7.2	6.1

[a]Countries that reported more than 100 cases in 2005.
Source: Annual leprosy reports from the countries, 2005.

In 2005, the Region registered a prevalence rate of 0.39 per 10,000 population and a detection rate of 4.98 per 100,000 population. Upon analyzing the profile of new cases recorded in 2005 in countries reporting more than 100 cases (Table 19), a great variety in the proportion of multibacillary cases is observed, ranging from 36% in Bolivia to 83% in Cuba. The variation in the proportion of children under 15 affected by the disease ranges from 1% in Argentina to 16% in the Dominican Republic. This indicator deserves special attention, since the proportion of grade II disability is an indicator of timely detection. There is currently great variation in this percentage, ranging from the lowest (1.6%) registered in Argentina to the highest (11.7%) in Mexico. The proportion of new cases with grade II disability and that of younger children are two indicators that allow for the characterization of the endemic disease.

In the Region of the Americas, significant achievements have been observed in leprosy control. In addition to having reached the goal of eliminating the disease before 2002 in almost every country, the Strategic Plan for the Elimination of Leprosy in the Americas has attained:

- The political commitment of countries with a high burden of disease.
- The diagnosis of more than 200,000 cases, which have already completed their treatment in 2000–2005.
- A policy of integrating leprosy control measures into the general health services, which is being implemented in 75% of the Region's countries.
- The reduction of registered cases in children under 15 from 10% in 2000 to 8% in 2005.
- A 30% reduction of new cases with grade II disability between 2000 and 2005.
- Greater participation of governmental and nongovernmental organizations (NGOs) in control activities.

The ongoing efforts to control leprosy will be strengthened by the implementation of the Global Strategy to Reduce the Burden of Leprosy and Sustain Leprosy Control Activities (Box 4). In the Region, the health authorities of some endemic countries (Costa Rica, the Dominican Republic, Ecuador, El Salvador, Paraguay, Peru, and Uruguay) began to develop an implementation strategy tailored to the epidemiological situation in each country.

CHRONIC NONCOMMUNICABLE DISEASES

Cardiovascular diseases, chronic obstructive respiratory diseases, cancer, and diabetes mellitus are the chronic noncommunicable diseases of greatest interest for public health in Latin America and the Caribbean (*177, 178*). In both subregions, noncommunicable chronic diseases are responsible for two out of three deaths in the general population (*177*) and nearly one-half of deaths among those under 70 years old (*179*). This group of disorders is the leading cause of mortality in men and women, and continues to increase at an extremely fast pace worldwide and in Latin America and the Caribbean (*177*). Of the 3,537,000 deaths registered in Latin America and the Caribbean in 2000, 67% were caused by these chronic diseases. Ischemic heart disease and cancer accounted for the majority of deaths in those 20–50 years old. Noncommunicable diseases contributed 76% of the DALYs to the overall disease burden.

In addition to early mortality, chronic noncommunicable diseases lead to complications, sequelae, and disability that limit functionality and productivity. Furthermore, these diseases require onerous treatments at enormous financial and social costs that undermine resources in both the health systems and social security. For example, the cost of diabetes in Latin America and the Caribbean in 2000 was estimated at US$ 65.2 billion, of which US$ 10.7 billion were direct costs and US$ 54.5 billion, indirect costs (*180*). Direct and indirect diabetes costs in the United States

---

> ## BOX 4. Main Objectives of the Global Strategy to Reduce the Leprosy Burden and Sustain Leprosy Control Activities
>
> * Provide high-quality services to all persons affected by leprosy.
> * Improve cost-effectiveness by decentralizing leprosy control activities and integrating them into primary care services.
> * Sustain political commitment and increase control activities in collaboration with all partners at the global, regional, and national levels.
> * Strengthen surveillance, monitoring, and supervision components.
> * Build capacity among health workers in integrated setting.
> * Enhance advocacy efforts in order to reduce the stigmatization and discrimination against persons affected by leprosy and their families.

were estimated at US$ 132 billion in 2002, and the medical care for chronic diseases represents 75% of the total health care cost in the country (*181*). In Mexico in 2006, it was estimated that the cost of hospitalization services for hypertension and diabetes mellitus exclusively, was higher than the cost of hospital and outpatient services for most infectious diseases (*182*). A 2002 study in Jamaica estimated the costs associated with diabetes and hypertension at US$ 33.1 million and US$ 25.6 million, respectively (*183*).

Primary prevention of chronic diseases could reverse their cost to the health care systems and to individuals. It is estimated that if only 10% of adults in the United States increased their physical activity by walking regularly, for example, US$ 5.6 billion could be saved in heart disease related costs (*184*).

Cardiovascular Diseases

These diseases (which include ischemic heart disease, cerebrovascular disease, hypertensive disease, and heart failure) represented 31% of the mortality burden and 10% of the total disease burden in the world in 2000 (*177*). The age-and sex-adjusted mortality rate for cardiovascular diseases (Figure 20) was highest in Nicaragua, the Dominican Republic, and Trinidad and Tobago, exceeding 200 per 100,000 population. The rate in Barbados, Canada, Chile, Costa Rica, Ecuador, El Salvador, Mexico, Peru, and Puerto Rico was below 150 per 100,000 population.

The latest available data (2000–2004) show that mortality from diseases of the circulatory system was higher in men (223.9 per 100,000 population) than in women (179.3 per 100,000). There also are vast differences among the subregions, from 35 to 50 per 100,000 population in Mexico and Central America, respectively, to 170 per 100,000 in North America (*185*).

A study that compared mortality trends for cardiovascular diseases in 10 Latin American countries between 1970 and 2000 found a strong and steady decline in mortality from coronary and cerebrovascular diseases in Canada and the United States. In Latin American countries in the same period, however, a decline in mortality from ischemic heart disease was reported only in Argentina, and a decline in mortality from cerebrovascular diseases only in Argentina, Chile, Colombia, Costa Rica, and Puerto Rico. The same study found less pronounced drops in mortality from ischemic heart disease in Brazil, Chile, Cuba, and Puerto Rico, and mortality from that cause increased in Costa Rica, Ecuador, Mexico, and Venezuela. That increase could be the consequence of unfavorable changes occurring in most Latin American countries with respect to the risk factors for this disease, such as improper diet, obesity, lack of physical activity, and smoking, in addition to a somewhat ineffective hypertension control and disease management (*186*).

A study on the risk for acute myocardial infarction conducted in four Latin American countries, found that high serum cholesterol, smoking, hypertension, high body mass index, and a family history of coronary heart disease were, as a whole, responsible for 81% of all cases of acute myocardial infarction in Cuba, 79% in Argentina, 76% in Venezuela, and 70% in Mexico (*187*).

Stroke claimed 271,865 lives in 27 countries in the Region in 2002 (*187*). The burden of stroke ranged between 5 and 14 potential years of life lost due to disability per 1,000 population. This figure was higher in the countries of the Americas than in most countries of the developed world. Stroke was the leading cause of death in Brazil in 2003; Mexico and Central America had the lowest mortality rates from that disease. In nearly all the subregions of the Americas, mortality from cerebrovascular disease was higher in women than in men. Mortality due to stroke dropped 10%–49% between 1970 and 2000 in most Latin American and Caribbean countries, with the exception of Mexico and Venezuela, whose mortality from stroke remained unchanged. In Canada and the United States, on the other hand, there was a more pronounced drop, around 60%, between the same years. Mortality from cerebrovascular diseases in 2000 was between twice and

FIGURE 20. Mortality from cardiovascular diseases,[a] adjusted by age and sex, selected countries, Region of the Americas, latest available year.

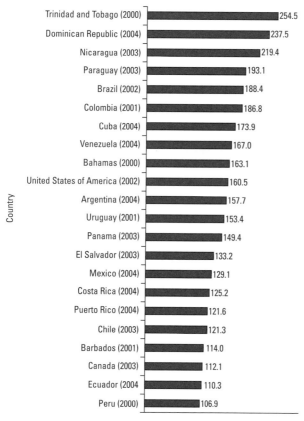

Country

Age- and sex-adjusted rate (per 100,000 population)

[a]Includes ICD-10 codes I20 to I25, I60 to I69, I10 to I15, and I50.
Source: PAHO, Health Analysis and Information Systems, Regional Mortality Database, 2006.

four times greater in Latin America and the Caribbean than in the United States (*186*). The reasons for these differences are not well known, although it is suspected that there are significant differences in the incidence of cerebrovascular events, access to services, quality of medical care for stroke, and risk-factor control.

Malignant Neoplasms

In 2005, there were 7.6 million estimated deaths due to cancer worldwide; in other words, 13% of all deaths and 21.6% of deaths from chronic diseases. Cancer is responsible for 5% of the total burden of disease worldwide. Mortality from malignant neoplasms of lung and breast in women increased in most Latin American countries between 1970 and 2000. For example, between 1970 and 1994, mortality from breast cancer in Costa Rica rose from 6.97 per 100,000 women to 13.42; in Cuba, from 12.33

per 100,000 to 15.82; in Mexico, from 4.99 to 9.04; and in Argentina, from 18.64 to 20.99. In contrast, mortality from breast cancer in North America declined between 1985 and 2000.

In 2002, Uruguay had the highest mortality from all malignant neoplasms in men, with an age-adjusted rate of 193.3 per 100,000. This rate was higher than that of Canada and the United States, which had rates of 156.6 and 152.6 per 100,000, respectively, similar to those of Argentina. Peru and Colombia had the highest age-adjusted cancer mortality rates in women, with 146.4 and 122.5 per 100,000, respectively. The lowest total mortality rates from cancer in men were found in El Salvador, Mexico, and Nicaragua; the lowest in women were found in Brazil and Mexico (Figures 21 and 22). In Argentina and Chile, mortality from cancer in men showed a downward trend between 1970 and 2000, while it increased in Colombia and Cuba (*188*).

Malignant Neoplasms of Bronchus and Lung

In 2002, Uruguay and Cuba had the highest age-adjusted mortality rates of malignant neoplasms of bronchus and lung in Latin America, 48.1 and 38 per 100,000 population, respectively. The lowest rates were registered in El Salvador and Guyana (5.7 and 7.2 per 100,000, respectively). Mortality from lung cancer in women increased between 1970 and 2000. These trends correlate with smoking patterns in Latin American men and women (*188–189*). On the other hand, mortality from lung cancer in women in Latin America and the Caribbean (10, per 100,000) was significantly lower than that in North America (26.7 per 100,000). In Argentina, mortality from lung cancer in women rose from 5.8 per 100,000 women in 1970 to 6.43 in 1994; in Chile during the same period, mortality from lung cancer rose from 5.48 to 6.37 per 100,000 and in Mexico, from 3.93 to 5.92 per 100,000.

Malignant Neoplasm of Stomach

Mortality from stomach cancer was very high among men in most Latin American countries in 2002, with rates above 11 per 100,000 in the Caribbean and Central America, and higher than 18 per 100,000 population in South America.

Among the countries with highest mortality are several in the Andean Area—Colombia (15.7 per 100,000 in women, 27.8 per 100,000 in men), Ecuador (22.1 per 100,000 in women and 31 per 100,000 in men), and Peru (24.1 per 100,000 in women, 29.5 per 100,000 in men). Chile's high rates (32.5 per 100,000 in men and 13.2 in women) are similar to those of Costa Rica (30.1 per 100,000 in men, 17.0 per 100,000 in women). Although the rates of countries such as Cuba and Mexico were below 10 per 100,000 population, they were higher than those observed in the United States (4.2 per 100,000 in men and 2.2 per 100,000 in women). Mortality from stomach cancer in the most Latin American countries declined steadily between 1970 and 2000, probably due to changes in diet, improvements in food preservation and refrigeration, and a reduction in the prevalence of *Helicobacter py-*

FIGURE 21. Cancer mortality rates (per 100,000 population), by sex, Region of the Americas, 2002.

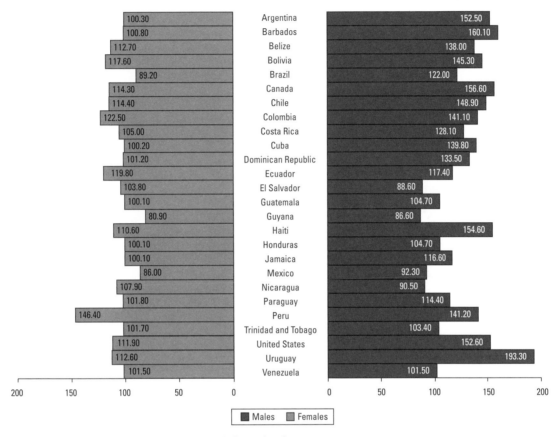

	Females	Country	Males	
	100.30	Argentina	152.50	
	100.80	Barbados	160.10	
	112.70	Belize	138.00	
	117.60	Bolivia	145.30	
	89.20	Brazil	122.00	
	114.30	Canada	156.60	
	114.40	Chile	148.90	
	122.50	Colombia	141.10	
	105.00	Costa Rica	128.10	
	100.20	Cuba	139.80	
	101.20	Dominican Republic	133.50	
	119.80	Ecuador	117.40	
	103.80	El Salvador	88.60	
	100.10	Guatemala	104.70	
	80.90	Guyana	86.60	
	110.60	Haiti	154.60	
	100.10	Honduras	104.70	
	100.10	Jamaica	116.60	
	86.00	Mexico	92.30	
	107.90	Nicaragua	90.50	
	101.80	Paraguay	114.40	
	146.40	Peru	141.20	
	101.70	Trinidad and Tobago	103.40	
	111.90	United States	152.60	
	112.60	Uruguay	193.30	
	101.50	Venezuela	101.50	

■ Males □ Females

Source: GLOBOCAN 2002 database, International Agency for Research on Cancer.

lori infection, as well as a possible reduction in smoking among men (*188, 190*).

Malignant Neoplasms of the Cervix and of the Breast

Cervical cancer remains as one of the leading causes of death for women in many parts of the world, despite the introduction of early detection programs more than 30 years ago. Latin America and the Caribbean recorded 71,862 new cases and 32,639 deaths from this cause in 2002 (*189*), some of the highest figures in the world. The age-adjusted mortality rates for the Region in 2002 were close to 15 per 100,000 women in the Caribbean and Central America, nearly 13 per 100,000 in South America, and much higher than the rate of 2.3 per 100,000 in North America. It is alarming that this detectable disease can have such a high mortality as Bolivia's (30.4 per 100,000 women), Haiti's (48.1), Nicaragua's (22.3), and Paraguay's (24.6).

Breast cancer has high mortality rates among women in the Caribbean and South American countries. In 2002, the highest age-adjusted mortality from breast cancer was found in Barba-

dos (25.5 per 100,000 women), Uruguay (24.1), and Argentina (21.8). In North America, rates hovered around 19.2 per 100,000. In recent years, mortality from breast cancer in women increased in most of the Latin American and Caribbean countries, especially in those that had the lowest rates, such as Colombia (5.2 in 1969 to 9.1 in 1994), Costa Rica (7.0 in 1970 to 12.7 in 1995), and Mexico (4.9 in 1970 to 9.5 in 1994). Trends were stable in Chile and Cuba. In North America, mortality from breast cancer declined from 23.8 per 100,000 in 1970 to 22.0 per 100,000 in 1994 in Canada, and from 22.5 in 1970 to 20.7 in 1994 in the United States (*189, 190*). Between 1963 and 1982, nine studies in Europe and Canada have shown that mammography, as a method to screen for breast cancer in women 50–69 years old, has been effective in reducing mortality by 23% (*191*). In the United States, Australia, and some European countries, it is recommended that physicians conduct case-by-case evaluations in order to determine the desirability recommending mammographies for women 40–49 years old (*189*). The relatively high ratios between mortality and incidence in many Latin American and Caribbean

FIGURE 22. Cancer mortality rates, by cancer site and sex, Region of the Americas, 2002.

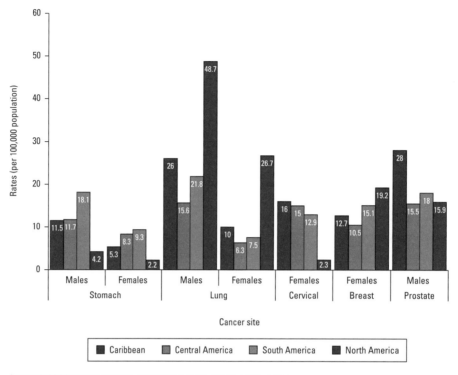

Source: GLOBOCAN 2002 database, International Agency for Research on Cancer.

countries show that breast cancer cases are not being adequately treated, indicating the need to provide ample access to appropriate diagnostic and therapeutic services (*191*).

Malignant Neoplasm of Prostate

The Caribbean and South America present extremely high age-adjusted mortality rates from prostate cancer, 28.0 and 18.0 per 100,000, respectively; the rate in Canada was 16.6 per 100,000, and in the United States, 15.8 per 100,000. In 2002, the highest mortality from prostate cancer occurred in Barbados (55.3 per 100,000), Belize (35.2), and the Dominican Republic (42.2), followed by Costa Rica, Guyana, Peru, and Uruguay, with rates close to 20 per 100,000. The lowest mortality was found in El Salvador and Mexico, comparable to that in North America at around 15 per 100,000. Between the 1970s and 2000, there was an increase in mortality from this cause in all Latin American countries, especially in Costa Rica and Mexico.

Diabetes

Diabetes mellitus was the fourth cause of death in Latin America and the Caribbean in 2001, accounting for 5% of total deaths (*185*). In Mexico it was the leading cause of death in the total population in 2002, with 12.8% of deaths (it was the leading cause among women, with 15.7%, and the second in men, with

10.5%). The highest diabetes mortality rates in the Americas (circa 2002) were in Mexico and in the non-Latin Caribbean (60 and 75 per 100,000, respectively) (*179*).

The estimated number of people with diabetes in Latin America was 13.3 million in 2000, a figure that is expected to reach 32.9 million by 2030 (more than doubling the number of cases) as a consequence of the aging of the population and urbanization (*192*). Given the increase in the prevalence of obesity in many of the world's countries, and obesity's importance as a risk factor for diabetes, the number of cases in 2030 could, in fact, be much higher (*192*). Even if the prevalence of obesity were to remain unchanged until 2030, it is estimated that the diabetes epidemic would continue. In the United States, the increase in the prevalence of diabetes has been explained by a similar increase in the proportion of obese persons, rather than by an increase in the absolute risk for presenting diabetes (*193*). According to the American Diabetes Association, people whose fasting blood sugar is between 100 mg/dl and 126 mg/dl are classified as having altered blood glucose values, or prediabetes, a term that indicates a greater risk of presenting the disease clinically. Prediabetes is also related to the metabolic syndrome, which also includes obesity or accumulation of abdominal fat, lipid disorders, and hypertension (*194*).

In the 1990s, there was an increase in the prevalence of diabetes and prediabetes in children and adolescents in the United States. This rise has been attributed to an increase in obesity due

FIGURE 23. Mortality from diabetes mellitus,ᵃ adjusted by age and sex, selected countries, Region of the Americas, latest year available.

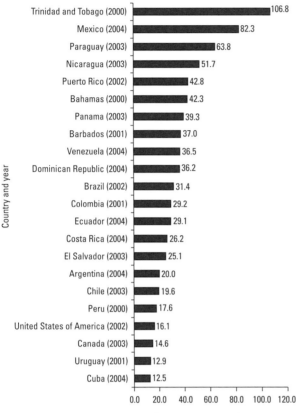

Country and year

Country and year	Age- and sex-adjusted rate (per 100,000 population)
Trinidad and Tobago (2000)	106.8
Mexico (2004)	82.3
Paraguay (2003)	63.8
Nicaragua (2003)	51.7
Puerto Rico (2002)	42.8
Bahamas (2000)	42.3
Panama (2003)	39.3
Barbados (2001)	37.0
Venezuela (2004)	36.5
Dominican Republic (2004)	36.2
Brazil (2002)	31.4
Colombia (2001)	29.2
Ecuador (2004)	29.1
Costa Rica (2004)	26.2
El Salvador (2003)	25.1
Argentina (2004)	20.0
Chile (2003)	19.6
Peru (2000)	17.6
United States of America (2002)	16.1
Canada (2003)	14.6
Uruguay (2001)	12.9
Cuba (2004)	12.5

Age- and sex-adjusted rate (per 100,000 population)

ᵃIncludes ICD-10 codes E10–E14.
Source: PAHO, Health Analysis and Information Systems, Regional Mortality Database, 2006.

to dietary changes and to a considerable reduction in physical activity among youth (*195*). Similar changes are taking place in Latin American and Caribbean countries, although the prevalence of obesity in children and adolescents has not yet reached the magnitude reported in the United States. In some localities in the north of Mexico, however, obesity rates are close to those observed in the United States (*196*).

The underreporting of mortality from diabetes is well known (*180, 197*). This is due to the fact that when people with diabetes die, the direct cause of death registered is often one of its chronic complications, such as cardiovascular disease or nephropathy. The latest available data indicate that the highest age-adjusted mortality rates from diabetes mellitus were observed in Mexico and Trinidad and Tobago; the lowest were found in Cuba, Canada, the United States, and Uruguay (Figure 23).

A study carried out in people aged 60 and older in seven Latin American and Caribbean cities found a self-reported prevalence of diabetes of 15.7%; the highest corresponded to women in

Bridgetown, Barbados (21.3%) and the lowest to men in Buenos Aires, Argentina (12.0%). In addition, a strong association was found between the prevalence of diabetes, and the body mass index (BMI) and lower educational levels (*198*).

Table 20 shows the crude and standardized prevalence of diabetes, hypertension, and overweight in adult populations, according to studies conducted in Barbados (*199*), Belize (*200*), Canada (*201*), Chile (*202*), Costa Rica (*203*), El Salvador (*204*), the United States (*205–207*), Guatemala (*208*), Haiti (*209*), Honduras (*210*), Mexico (*211–213*), and Nicaragua (*214*). According to studies carried out in persons 20 years old and older (Table 20), the adjusted diabetes prevalence was higher in Belize (15.3%), Nicaragua (11.9%), and Costa Rica (10.7%); the United States (9.3%), El Salvador (9.8%), and Honduras (8.0%) had prevalence rates higher than 7% but lower than 10%, whereas Chile and Haiti had prevalence rates of 7%. The Barbados study carried out in persons 40 years old and older (*199*), using glycosylated hemoglobin (A1c) as a diagnostic test, found a 19.4% crude prevalence of diabetes (18.6% standardized). The prevalence increased with age for both women and men, and was higher in women. Further, a study conducted in the United States-Mexico border region found that 15.7% of the respondents suffered from diabetes (*215*).

Chronic Respiratory Diseases

In Latin America and the Caribbean these diseases caused 3% of all deaths. The latest available data in the Region (circa 2000) indicate that mortality from chronic respiratory diseases ranges between 16 and 25 per 100,000 population; in most of the countries, mortality from this cause was higher among men. In the United States, the crude mortality rate in 2002 was 42.9 per 100,000 for both sexes. This group of diseases caused 2.5% of the global burden of disease in 2001, 3.5% of the burden in high-income countries, and 2.4% in low- and medium-income countries (*177*).

The highest age-adjusted mortality rates for chronic respiratory diseases (asthma, chronic obstructive pulmonary disease, emphysema, and chronic bronchitis) were found in Brazil, Colombia, Costa Rica, Cuba, Mexico, Nicaragua, Panama, the United States, and Uruguay, with rates between 30 and 20 per 100,000 population, according to the latest available data (circa 2000). Argentina, Belize, Canada, Chile, the Dominican Republic, El Salvador, Puerto Rico, Suriname, Trinidad and Tobago, and Venezuela had intermediate rates, between 20 and 10 per 100,000. The lowest rates were in the Bahamas, Barbados, Ecuador, Paraguay, and Peru, with fewer than 10 cases per 100,000 population.

Hypertensive Diseases

Hypertension is a major risk factor for heart disease and cerebrovascular disease. An analysis of age-adjusted mortality from hypertensive diseases (Figure 24) in selected countries of the Region shows Bahamas with the highest rate (44.8 per 100,000 pop-

TABLE 20. Prevalence of diabetes mellitus, hypertension, and overweight in adults, by sex, selected countries of the Americas, most recent available year.

Country	Year	Age (years)	Crude			Standardized[a]		
			Males	Females	Total	Males	Females	Total
Diabetes mellitus								
Barbados	2002[b]	40 and older	16.5	21.5	19.40	16.21	20.93	18.57
Belize	2006	20 and older	8.56	16.29	12.41	10.57	20.24	15.34
Chile	2003	20 and older	6.10	6.50	6.30	7.30	6.70	7.00
Costa Rica	2005	20 and older	8.30	7.60	7.90	11.52	9.97	10.67
El Salvador	2004	20 and older	7.68	7.09	7.37	10.79	9.05	9.85
Guatemala	2003	20 and older	8.84	7.72	8.23	11.30	10.05	10.65
Haiti	2002	20 and older	4.72	8.83	7.30			7.00
Honduras	2004	20 and older	6.41	5.88	6.12	8.79	7.35	8.00
Mexico	2000	20–69			10.70			14.50
Nicaragua	2004	20 and older	8.93	9.02	8.98	11.63	12.03	11.91
United States of America	2001–2002	20 and older	10.20	8.50	9.30	10.60	8.20	9.30
Hypertension								
Barbados	2002[b]	40 and older	49.8	59.6	55.4	50.55	58.74	54.64
Belize	2006	20 and older	27.11	30.73	28.91	31.76	38.33	33.54
Chile	2003	20 and older	36.70	30.80	33.70	41.50	36.60	38.30
Costa Rica	2005	20 and older	26.13	25.04	25.57	28.57	28.05	28.30
El Salvador	2004	20 and older	21.20	21.17	21.18	24.61	24.44	24.52
Guatemala	2003	20 and older	11.97	13.92	12.96	17.99	21.86	19.96
Haiti	2003	20 and older	48.52	45.68	46.74			41.30
Honduras	2004	20 and older	23.62	21.56	22.48	25.29	24.23	24.70
Mexico	2000	20–69	34.2	26.3	30.05	30.90	36.90	33.90
Nicaragua	2004	20 and older	24.02	25.09	24.59	30.62	33.51	32.18
United States of America	1999–2002	20 and older	25.10	25.70	25.50	25.20	25.80	25.50
Overweight (BMI ≥25)								
Belize	2006	20 and older	58.64	74.56	66.57	59.93	76.15	67.99
Canada[c]	2000	12 and older	51.80	37.80	44.80	56.62	40.49	48.56
Chile	2003	20 and older	43.20	32.70	37.80	62.95	66.09	64.52
Costa Rica	2005	20 and older	62.00	55.80	58.80	67.16	58.69	62.66
El Salvador	2004	20 and older	69.56	63.09	66.17	70.93	65.12	67.89
Guatemala	2003	20 and older	54.77	63.94	59.73	55.07	66.49	61.21
Honduras	2004	20 and older	51.94	59.95	56.36	52.69	61.48	57.57
Mexico	2000	20–69	60.7	65.3	62.0			
Nicaragua	2004	20 and older	59.04	71.40	65.61	63.08	74.40	69.19
United States of America	2000–01	20 and older	70.80	61.80	66.30	69.90	60.60	65.30

Notes:

Costa Rica, El Salvador, Guatemala, Haiti, Honduras, and Nicaragua conducted studies in urban populations in their capitals. Belize's data comes from a national-level study.

Diagnostic criteria for diabetes: Barbados HbA1c > 10%, or previous diabetes diagnosis; Chile, El Salvador, Mexico, and the United States—fasting glucose level ≥ 126 mm/l or previous diabetes diagnosis; Belize, Costa Rica, Guatemala, Haiti, and Nicaragua—two-hour glucose tolerance test ≥ 200 mm/l of fasting glucose ≥ 126 mm/l, or previous diabetes diagnosis.

Diagnostic criteria for hypertension: systolic arterial pressure ≥ 140 mm Hg, or dyastolic arterial pressure ≥ 90 mm Hg, or previous hypertension diagnosis.

[a]By age and sex, using Segi's population as a standard (Segi, M. Kurihara. Trends in Cancer Mortality for selected sites in 24 countries, 1950–1959, Department of Public Health. Tohoku University School of Medicine, Senday, Japan, 1963.)

[b]Year published.

[c]Age-standardized rates for persons 40 years old and older.

Source: Barbados (*199*), Belize (*200*), Canada (*201*), Chile (*202*), Costa Rica (*203*), El Salvador (*204*), United States (*205–207*), Guatemala (*208*), Haiti (*209*), Honduras (*210*), Mexico (*211–213*), and Nicaragua (*214*).

FIGURE 24. Mortality rates from hypertensive diseases,[a] adjusted by age and sex, selected countries of the Americas, latest available year.

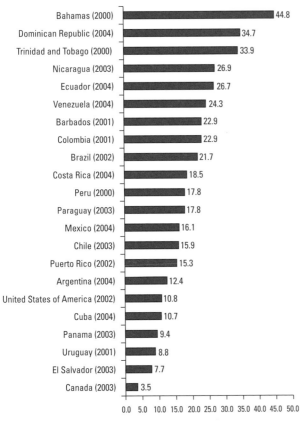

Country	Rate
Bahamas (2000)	44.8
Dominican Republic (2004)	34.7
Trinidad and Tobago (2000)	33.9
Nicaragua (2003)	26.9
Ecuador (2004)	26.7
Venezuela (2004)	24.3
Barbados (2001)	22.9
Colombia (2001)	22.9
Brazil (2002)	21.7
Costa Rica (2004)	18.5
Peru (2000)	17.8
Paraguay (2003)	17.8
Mexico (2004)	16.1
Chile (2003)	15.9
Puerto Rico (2002)	15.3
Argentina (2004)	12.4
United States of America (2002)	10.8
Cuba (2004)	10.7
Panama (2003)	9.4
Uruguay (2001)	8.8
El Salvador (2003)	7.7
Canada (2003)	3.5

Age- and sex-adjusted rate (per 100,000 population)

[a]Includes ICD-10 codes I10 to I15.
Source: PAHO, Health Analysis and Information Systems, Regional Mortality Database, 2006.

ulation) and Canada, El Salvador, Panama, and Uruguay with the lowest.

Data from several population studies in the Region (Table 20) reveal that the highest prevalence of age- and sex-adjusted hypertension among the population 20 years old and older was found in Haiti (41.3%) and Chile (38.3%); Belize, Costa Rica, the United States, Mexico, and Nicaragua presented prevalence rates between 25% and 34%, while El Salvador, Guatemala, and Honduras had prevalence rates lower than 25%. A survey and follow-up study carried out in Barbados in persons 40 years old and older, found a prevalence of hypertension of 54%; hypertension was more frequent among women and it increased markedly with age (*216*). In Mexico, the National Survey of Chronic Diseases and the National Health Survey showed that hypertension rose from 26% to 30% between 1998 and 2000 (*217, 218*). In Cienfuegos, Cuba, a prevalence of hypertension of 19.9% was reported in adults, and it was more frequent among men (*219*).

Inadequate blood pressure control can increase a hypertensive's risk of premature mortality. A study in Barbados (*216*) and another in Mexico (*220*) showed a high percentage of persons that were unaware that they had hypertension, as well as people with elevated blood pressure values, despite ongoing treatment. These studies also found greater general mortality from all causes among people with hypertension than among the general comparable population.

Risk Factors for Chronic Noncommunicable Diseases

Several risk factors common to many noncommunicable diseases (such as diabetes, cardiovascular diseases, and several forms of cancer) can be modified; the most important ones are an unhealthy diet, lack of physical activity, smoking, and alcohol abuse (*221*). In turn, those factors are manifested through others of intermediate risk, such as hypertension, hyperglycemia (diabetes and pre-diabetes), hypercholesterolemia (especially low-density lipoproteins), overweight, and obesity. The risk factors subject to modification, together with those that cannot be modified, such as age and heredity, explain the majority of the chronic diseases. All these factors are determined by demographic, social, cultural, political, and economic conditions, such as poverty, urbanization, globalization, and the population's structure and dynamics (*222*). The likelihood of success of preventive actions increases considerably when these factors are targeted (*180, 201, 223–225*).

Tobacco Use

Smoking is linked to several diseases, including lung and other types of cancer, heart disease and cerebrovascular diseases, emphysema, and peripheral vascular disease, (*226, 227*). Smoking is also harmful to pregnancy.

WHO has estimated that half of the current smokers (650 million people) will die between the ages of 35 and 69. It is estimated that tobacco caused 100 million deaths in the 20th century, and it is expected to cause one billion deaths in the 21st century (*226*). In the United States, cigarettes are responsible for more than 440,000 deaths per year, or one of every five deaths. Of these, nearly 10% occur as a result of exposure to second-hand smoke. All cancer cases caused by smoking could be prevented. At least 30% of all cancer deaths in the United States are due to smoking; furthermore, it is estimated that the habit is responsible for eight out of ten lung cancer cases. Some 8.6 million people have at least one serious disease caused by cigarette smoking. In the United States, the direct and indirect costs of the diseases associated with cigarette smoking total more than US$ 157 billion annually (*227*). Smoke also poses a serious threat to the health of non-smoking adults and children exposed to cigarette smoke—in the United States alone, cigarette smoke is responsible for the death from lung cancer of approximately 3,000 non-smokers each year (*226*). Among adult men, the countries with greater proportion of

131

smokers in the Americas are Cuba (48%), Ecuador (45.5%), Trinidad and Tobago (42.1%), and Peru (41.5%). Among adult women, tobacco use is more prevalent in Venezuela (39.2%), Argentina (34%), Brazil (29.3%), and Cuba (26.3%). Among adolescents 13–15 years old, smoking is more prevalent among males in Chile (34%), Bolivia (31%), and Peru (22%); it is more prevalent among females in Chile (43%), Argentina (30%), and Uruguay (24%). For all the countries, prevalence is higher in males than in females, both for adults and adolescents (228).

According to the United States risk factor surveillance system, in 2002, 23% of adults in that country (25% of men and 20% of women) claimed to be current smokers (defined as having smoked at least 100 cigarettes during their lifetime and currently smoking every day or some days). In 2001, 28.5% of high school students who participated in a survey reported having smoked cigarettes one or more days during the 30 days prior to the survey; the survey also reported that the average age at which they started smoking was 15.4 years (227). In 2000, 21.5% of Canadians 12 years old and older were daily smokers (201).

Diet and a Lack of Physical Activity

More than half the population of the Americas is sedentary, defined as not engaging in the recommended minimum of 30 minutes of moderate physical activity per day at least five days a week. In several countries, the proportion of the population whose health is at risk due to the lack of physical activity is close to 60%.

It is estimated that in Brazil, Chile, Mexico, and Peru, more than two-thirds of the population does not engage in physical activity based on levels recommended for deriving health benefits. The level of participation in physical activities is lower in women than in men; it is greater in people with higher income and it decreases with age, in both sexes (229).

In the United States in 2002, 25% of adults (28% of women and 22% of men) reported that they did not engage in physical activity during their spare time. The percentage was 37% for Hispanics, 33% for African Americans, and 22% for whites. More than three-fourths of adults (80% of men and 71% of women) reported that they did not consume the recommended daily amounts of fruits and vegetables (227). Among high school students, 48% indicated that did not participate in physical education classes (44% of males and 52% of females) (227) and 79% (77% of males and 80% of females) consumed less than five servings of fruit and vegetables per day. In the United States, it is estimated that at least 300,000 deaths each year are related to improper diet and lack of physical activity (227). In Canada, according to the Canadian Community Health Survey, 53.5% of persons 12 years old and older were sedentary; a lack of physical activity was more prevalent in women (57%) than in the men (49.6%) (201). A lack of physical activity is not a problem only in developed countries. According to an adult population survey. in Guatemala City's *municipio* of Villanueva (208), it was observed

that only 25% of respondents were physically active (150 minutes or more per week of moderate physical activity).

These risk factors unfold within a social, cultural, political, and economic context that can erode the population's health, unless measures are put in place to build a health promotion environment. In many developing countries, however, food policies continue to focus only on malnutrition and do not yet target chronic disease prevention (230).

Overweight and Obesity

People who are obese, defined as a body mass index (BMI) of $\geq 30 \text{ kg/m}^2$, are at greater risk of suffering from heart disease, hypertension, diabetes mellitus, breast cancer, colon cancer, vesicular lithiasis, and arthritis (227). In 2005, more than one billion people in the world were overweight, 805 million of which were women; more than 300 million were obese. If current trends persist, it is estimated that more than 1.5 billion persons will be overweight in 2015 and the BMI will increase in almost all the countries of the world. Every year, at least 2.6 million people die because of overweight or obesity (231).

In 2005, it was estimated that the prevalence of overweight in women 30 years old and older exceeded 50% in all the countries of the Region; in some countries, such as Jamaica and other Caribbean countries, Mexico, Nicaragua, and the United States, the prevalence was higher than 75% (231). In the United States, obesity has reached epidemic proportions, doubling its prevalence in the last two decades. In 2000, the direct and indirect costs attributed to obesity in the United States were US$ 117 billion. In that country in 2001, 11% of high school students were overweight (14% of males and 7% of females); furthermore, 14% were at risk of becoming overweight (227). In 2000, 44.8% of Canadians aged 12 years old and older were overweight (51.8% of males and 37.8% of females), which makes overweight a problem that cuts across all ages, but which mainly affects persons 35–64 years old. In addition, 19% were overweight and led a sedentary lifestyle simultaneously, and the percentage of those who simultaneously were overweight, led a sedentary lifestyle, and used tobacco was 5.3% (201).

The age- and sex-adjusted prevalence of overweight (BMI ≥ 25) for people aged 20 and older was highest in Nicaragua, El Salvador, and the United States (65% to 70%), while Chile, Costa Rica, and Guatemala presented an adjusted prevalence that ranged from 60% to less than 65%. In Honduras, the prevalence was 57.6%, and Canada presented the lowest adjusted prevalence (48.5%), although the data include people 12 years old and older (Table 20).

Hypercholesterolemia

Hypercholesterolemia is one of the major independent risk factors for heart disease and cerebrovascular disease. Total blood cholesterol levels are considered a risk factor when they reach $\geq 200 \text{ mg/dl}$. A 10% reduction in the total cholesterol levels can reduce the incidence of coronary disease by 30%. It has been estimated that in 2001, 105 million citizens of the United States (30.9% of the total population; 32.2% of men and 29.8% of women) had total cholesterol levels above the standard values, and that 80% of these people were not under treatment (*227*). In Mexico, the 2001 and 2002 National Health Survey found a global prevalence of hypercholesterolemia of 43.3% (*232*).

In Argentina's 2005 National Survey of Risk Factors, 27.8% of respondents that had had their cholesterol measured reported having high levels (*233*). In Chile, the 2003 Health Survey found a prevalence of elevated total cholesterol of 25% (*234*). In 2003–2004, the Central American Diabetes Initiative carried out a multinational survey on diabetes mellitus, hypertension, and their risk factors, which showed that the general prevalence of hypercholesterolemia was 19.7% in Managua, Nicaragua (*214*), 45.7% in San José, Costa Rica (*203*), and 35.5% in Villa Nueva *municipio*, Guatemala (*208*).

Alcohol Abuse

Alcohol abuse is considered a risk factor for cardiovascular diseases such as hypertension, stroke, and diabetes. A national study conducted in Canada (2000) found a prevalence of this risk factor of 7.8% for men and 4.3% for women (*201*). In Argentina (2005), 9.6% of regular alcohol consumption (defined as an average of more than one glass per day among women or two drinks per day among men) and 10.1% of excessive episodic alcohol consumption (defined as the consumption of five or more drinks on a single occasion on at least one day in the 30 days prior to the interview) (*233*). In a population study carried out in 2004 in Managua, Nicaragua, it was found that 18% (36% of men and 7.9% of women) reported having consumed five or more alcoholic beverages at least once in the four weeks that preceded the interview (*214*).

Educational Level and Economic Status

Having a low educational level has been used as an indicator of inequity in the Region of the Americas. Several studies have shown that people with little formal education are at a greater risk for noncommunicable diseases (*198, 233–235*). Diabetes has been related to low educational levels in many population studies of adults (*234, 235*) and older adults (*198*). Chile's 2003 National Health Survey also showed that the prevalence of hypertension, obesity, sedentary lifestyle, and chronic respiratory tract diseases was significantly higher among people with low educational levels.

People with lower incomes are more vulnerable to noncommunicable diseases and their consequences. In Argentina, according to the National Survey of Risk Factors, the proportion of people with hypertension or with poorly controlled blood pressure (blood pressure >140/90, with treatment) was greater in low-income groups and among those without social security coverage (*233*). Likewise, studies carried out in adults in several cities of Peru showed that a higher level of education and access to health information offers protection against overweight in women; it also found that as the socioeconomic status decreases, the prevalence of several risk factors (such as high cholesterol, diabetes, overweight, and obesity) for chronic diseases increases. The relative risk of presenting cardiovascular disease in the lowest socioeconomic strata was four times higher than that in the highest strata (*236, 237*). Other studies conducted in Brazil, Chile, and Peru showed that people in lower-income groups were the least likely to engage in physical activity (*229*).

The incidence of and mortality from cervical cancer was also related to poverty, limited access to services, rural residence, and low educational levels, as well as to cultural and psychosocial aspects. For example, an analysis carried out in 2004 found that in Ecuador, incidence rates and mortality from cervical cancer were higher among women of the poorest sectors, especially those in rural areas. In Bolivia, wide variations in the incidence and mortality from cervical cancer within the country were related to the access to services, the educational level, and poverty (*238*).

The Health System's Response

Available information, although limited, indicates that chronic diseases constitute an enormous and growing health problem for Latin America and the Caribbean. The cost-effective strategies for the prevention and control of noncommunicable diseases are well known and well documented. The integrated responses to noncommunicable diseases include a combination of a population strategy (healthy public policies, media campaigns, social marketing, and reorientation of the health services) and an individual strategy (management of both risk factors and chronic noncommunicable diseases), as well as an epidemiological surveillance system.

Although there has been some progress in the prevention and control of chronic diseases in Latin America, results have yet to be reflected in health conditions. Multisectoral strategies and the reorientation of the models of care toward prevention, risk control, and timely chronic disease treatment are still absent in all the countries of the Region. In 2001 and 2005, WHO conducted surveys to evaluate national capabilities to respond to noncommunicable diseases (*239*); the results indicate that some progress has been made in noncommunicable disease prevention and control in Latin America and the Caribbean. Of the 25 Latin American and Caribbean countries that responded to the 2005 survey, 81% had a department of chronic diseases in the ministry of health, compared to 59% in the 2001 survey. The proportion of countries that reported a specific budget item for chronic diseases rose from 23% in 2000 to 59% in 2005. Similarly, the proportion of countries that included noncommunicable diseases in the annual health report rose from 72% in 2000 to 96% in 2005, and those with noncommunicable disease surveillance systems in place rose from 50% in 2000 to 63% in 2005. Although a considerable number of Latin American countries seem to have surveillance systems for chronic diseases, there is little published data to evaluate the current noncommunicable disease situation

133

in them. Only publications from Argentina, Barbados, Brazil, Chile, and Mexico showed national data that show noncommunicable disease prevalence rates or related risk factors.

More than 80% of the countries reported having protocols for diabetes, hypertension, and cancer; 68% of the countries reported having policies for chronic diseases, mostly related to the health system or the information system. The Framework Convention on Tobacco Control and the Strategy on Diet, Physical Activity, and Health consider intersectoral population-based and noncommunicable disease risk prevention health policies. WHO's survey on national capabilities shows that only 16% of the countries had formulated plans to implement the aforementioned strategy. In Latin America, 27 countries (up to August 2006) had signed the Framework Convention on Tobacco Control. Although more than 80% of the countries signed the Convention, it is still too early to see its impact on mortality.

PROMOTING HEALTH

MENTAL HEALTH

Mental health is an area of public health that encompasses several spheres. In terms of health, it includes outreach and primary prevention; in terms of illness, it includes the recovery of mental health and the reduction of disabilities caused by mental health disorders. This section concentrates on the treatment of psychiatric disorders, as this is the target of most countries' efforts.

The Burden and Magnitude of Mental Health Disorders

Epidemiological studies conducted in the 1990s decade clearly establish a need for action in mental health. In 1990, psychiatric and neurological conditions accounted for an estimated 8.8% of DALYs in Latin America and the Caribbean; by 2002, the figure had more than doubled to 22.2% (240, 241).

Despite the extent of the burden of mental disorders, the countries' responses have been limited or inadequate. This paradoxical situation in which the burden is great and the response insufficient translates into treatment lags for mental health disorders and shortcomings in the mental health service models (241).

A review of the Region's most important epidemiological studies of health mental disorders reveals that the estimated average prevalence rate was 1% for nonaffective psychosis (including schizophrenia), 4.9% for major depression, and 5.7% for alcohol abuse or dependency. Yet, more than one-third of persons suffering from nonaffective psychosis, more than half of persons suffering from anxiety disorders, and approximately three-quarters of persons dependent on or abusing alcohol did not receive any type of psychiatric treatment at a specialized or general service (241).

Studies in several countries reveal these gaps by providing the percentage of individuals in need of treatment who did not receive it. Table 21 shows the treatment gap for various disorders in São Paulo, Brazil; Chile; and the Federal District, Mexico (242–244).

In short, only a minority of persons needing mental health services receives them, notwithstanding the extent of suffering and disability caused by mental disorders and the emotional and economic impact on families and communities. And the toll exacted by mental disorders is greater among those in the lowest socioeconomic strata, who have even less access to services.

Disasters and Mental Health

Many countries in the Region are exposed to natural disasters and internal armed conflicts, which leave psychosocial wounds and scars and raise the rates of psychiatric morbidity and other emotional problems. A study conducted in Honduras after Hurricane Mitch found elevated rates of symptoms consistent with post-traumatic stress disorder, major depression, and alcohol abuse. Among the low-income population, the prevalence rates

TABLE 21. Mental illness treatment gap,[a] Brazil, Chile, and Mexico.

Disorder	São Paulo, Brazil (month preceding the survey)	Chile (six months preceding the survey)	Mexico City, Federal District (entire life)
Nonaffective psychosis	58.0	44.4	—
Major depression	49.4	46.2	43.4
Dysthymia	43.8	32.4	78.5
Bipolar disorder	46.0	50.2	74.1
Generalized anxiety	41.1	44.2	72.2
Panic disorders	47.8	22.7	70.0
Obsessive-compulsive disorder	—	27.6	92.1
Alcohol abuse or dependence	53.3	84.8	—

[a]Gap expressed in terms of the percentage of people in need of treatment who did not receive it.
Source: Kohn R, Levav I, Caldas de Almeida JM, Vicente B, Andrade L, Caraveo-Anduaga JJ, Saxena S, Saraceno B. Los trastornos mentales en América latina y el Caribe: Asunto prioritario para la salud pública. Rev Panam Salud Pública 2005; 18 (4/5): 229–240.

for these conditions were 15.7%, 25.9%, and 8%, respectively, in the three months following the disaster (245).

The Response

There are several indicators that measure the countries' responses to mental health needs. Roughly 73% of the Region's countries have national policies and plans that deal specifically with mental health, but the biggest challenge at present is implementing them. In addition, 75% have laws specific to mental health in place, although they have not been updated in all the countries. Finally, 78.1% of the countries allocate budgetary resources to mental health, but in several of them this budget accounts for only approximately 1% of the total health budget. For example, according to an exhaustive study of mental health systems in Central American countries, El Salvador, Guatemala, and Nicaragua spend 1% or less of their total health budgets on mental health, and approximately 90% of this amount goes to psychiatric hospitals (246). This pattern of spending deters the establishment of alternative, community-based mental health models.

The control of psychiatric disorders requires, among other therapeutic modalities, pharmacological and psychosocial interventions that can be offered through primary health care. However, according to the aforementioned Central American study, many health clinics do not have essential psychopharmaceuticals.

Another way of measuring country response is by gauging the number of available specialized professionals. There are two psychiatrists per 100,000 population in the Americas, which is a fraction of the number in Europe (9.8 per 100,000 population). The comparison between Europe and the Americas is more favorable in terms of psychology professionals, of whom there are 3.1 and 2.8 per 100,000 population, respectively (247).

Prospects for Change

Since 1990, with the adoption of the Declaration of Caracas, Latin American and Caribbean countries have made the restructuring of psychiatric care a key component of their strategies, with the goal of transferring the care provided in mental institutions to the community.

This transformation strategy was ratified by nearly every country in the Region in Brasilia in November 2005, at the Regional Conference on Mental Health Services Reform: "15 Years after the Caracas Declaration," which evaluated the change process. However, in four of five countries, most psychiatric beds are still in psychiatric hospitals instead of in general hospitals, and one in four countries have yet to develop community-based psychiatric care. Nevertheless, important changes have been made that suggest that reforms will continue (248).

The final declaration of the Brasilia conference states that mental health services must address the new technical and cultural challenges that have emerged over the past 15 years, such as

Although the true magnitude of the sexually transmitted disease problem remains essentially unknown throughout the Americas, significant progress has been achieved in stimulating a new awareness of their seriousness.

Héctor R. Acuña, 1982

psychosocial vulnerability, which includes the problems faced by indigenous communities and the adverse effects of unplanned development in the Region's large cities; the increase in morbidity and psychosocial problems among children; higher societal demand for services that allow for the adoption of effective measures for the prevention and early treatment of suicidal behavior and alcohol abuse; and growing levels of violence in its different forms, which requires the active participation of mental health services, particularly victim services.

Mental health issues have unmistakably been rising in importance on citizens' and national agendas, as demonstrated by the 2001 Resolution of the Governing Bodies of the Pan-American Health Organization on mental health issues, successful local and national experiences, the emergence of new associations of mental-health-service users and families, and increased efforts to advance the cause. There are increasingly greater opportunities for cost-efficient interventions (249), which suggests that the response, while still limited, will strengthen over time.

ORAL HEALTH

Oral health is still a critical aspect of the overall health conditions in the Americas, given its important contribution to total morbidity, high treatment costs, and inequality in oral health care. These factors are exacerbated by poor quality oral health services, limited coverage, an increase in treatment costs, and low investment in public oral health programs. Since 1995, 40 national oral health surveys have been conducted in the Americas, and their results show a decrease of between 35% and 85% in the prevalence of dental caries (250). And yet, morbidity due to oral problems in the Region remains high in comparison with other regions of the world (251). In response, strategies have been developed to reduce morbidity due to oral problems and promote more equitable access to odontological services. These strategies are based on successful fluoridation programs carried out in recent decades; the promotion of simple, cost-effective technologies; and the establishment of comprehensive health care systems that combine oral and general health services (252).

Dental Caries

In 1999, the Pan American Health Organization proposed a goal of reducing dental caries by 50% throughout the Region (253). To this end, the Organization, in cooperation with each

135

country, is pursuing the conduct of epidemiological surveillance of dental caries through clinical cross-sectional studies targeting specific groups (cohorts), in accordance with protocols established by WHO (*254*).

In 2000, WHO set the oral-health target of achieving a decayed, missing, or filled teeth (DMFT) index of under 3 among 12-year-old children, known as DMFT-12. Anguilla, Antigua and Barbuda, Aruba, Bahamas, Barbados, Belize, Bermuda, the Cayman Islands, Canada, Colombia, Costa Rica, Cuba, Curaçao, Dominica, Ecuador, El Salvador, Grenada, Guyana, Haiti, Jamaica, Mexico, Nicaragua, Peru, Saint Kitts and Nevis, Suriname, Trinidad and Tobago, Turks and Caicos Islands, the United States of America, Uruguay, Venezuela, and several states in Brazil achieved an average DMFT of 3. Bolivia, the Dominican Republic, and several regions of Chile, still have an average DMFT higher than 4 (*255*). Two geographical patterns emerge when countries in the Region are classified by the percentage of children without caries. In Belize, the Cayman Islands, Guyana, Jamaica, and the United States, for example, 40% or more of 12-year-old children have no caries. In Bolivia, the Dominican Republic, Ecuador, Honduras, Nicaragua, Panama, and Paraguay, on the other hand, the figure is between 10% and 25% (*255*).

Although percentage reductions of dental caries since the 1980s vary greatly (from 2.5% in the Bahamas to 89.5% in Belize), as Table 22 shows, the average DMFT-12 index has fallen in every country (*255*). In Guatemala, Suriname, and Trinidad and Tobago—countries that carried out surveys of oral health between 2002 and 2004—the percentage reductions in dental caries were 35.8%, 71.2%, and 87.8%, respectively, as measured against data from surveys conducted in the 1980s (Figure 25). If the trend continues, most of the Region's countries are expected to reduce the prevalence of dental caries to an average DMFT-12 below 1.5 by 2015. Gradual declines are expected in the Andean, Caribbean, and Southern Cone subregions, and a more pronounced reduction is expected in Central America (Figure 26). These projections are estimates of the percentage reduction of dental caries, calculated using data from countries that have conducted epidemiological studies at least every 10 years.

Despite the decrease in the DMFT, and particularly the caries component, major disparities between countries remain when the contribution of missing and filled teeth to the DMFT is analyzed. There is a stark contrast between countries such as the Cayman Islands, Costa Rica, and the United States, which have high percentages (49% to 71%) of filled teeth, and countries such as Bolivia, the Dominican Republic, Ecuador, Honduras, Panama, and Paraguay, where untreated teeth account for more than 80% of the DMFT (*255*).

PAHO has developed a typology for identifying a country's oral health profile based on the DMFT-12 and to be able to make comparisons between countries (*250*). This typology identifies three stages of dental caries severity: 1) *Emerging*, defined by a DMFT-12 higher than 5 and the absence of a national fluoridation program; 2) *Growth*, defined by a DMFT-12 of 3–5 and the absence of a national fluoridation program; and 3) *Consolidation*, defined by a DMFT-12 of under 3 and the existence of a national fluoridation program. Progress in reducing dental caries is reflected in the major epidemiological changes that have occurred throughout the Region. Between 1996 and 2005 (Table 23), the number of the Region's countries that moved into the consolidation stage increased by 51.3%, and some 22% moved from the *emerging* stage to the *growth* stage, or directly to the *consolidation* stage, as was the case with Belize, El Salvador, Haiti, Nicaragua, and Peru.

Fluoridation in the Americas

The incorporation of systemic fluorides into water and salt for human consumption has been proven to be beneficial for the prevention of dental caries in several countries in the Americas and Europe (*256–258*). Fluoridation of drinking water has contributed significantly to the reduction in the prevalence of dental caries in North America (*259*); beneficial effects have also been reported from the ingestion of fluoridated salt (*260–262*).

In 1994, PAHO launched a multi-year Regional Plan for the Prevention of Dental Caries through Salt and Water Fluoridation. The plan was shaped by three operating principles: 1) prevention of dental caries; 2) creation of technical capability; and 3) sustainability of programs. Fluoridation programs in the Region vary by type of system used (water or salt), coverage, and status. As of this writing, Argentina, Bolivia, Brazil, Canada, Chile, Colombia, Costa Rica, Cuba, the Dominican Republic, Ecuador, Jamaica, Mexico, Peru, the United States, Uruguay, and Venezuela have water or salt fluoridation systems, or both; Belize, El Salvador, Guatemala, Nicaragua, Panama, Paraguay have initiated the development of some type of system; and Grenada, Guyana, and Suriname have plans to import fluoridated salt. Only Argentina, Brazil, Canada, Chile, Panama, and the United States have national water fluoridation systems; coverage is 65% in São Paulo, Brazil, and 67% in the United States (*255*).

The most successful experiences with salt fluoridation have been in Costa Rica, Jamaica, and Mexico. The first two began fluoridation programs in 1987, and Mexico followed suit in 1991. Epidemiological data from the second half of the 1980s and the first half of the 1990s show annualized percentage reductions in dental caries in the permanent teeth of 12-year-old children of between 6.6% (Mexico) and 15.2% (Jamaica) (*255*). Similar trends are expected in other countries in the Region, including Ecuador, Peru, and Uruguay, which launched salt fluoridation programs in the mid-1990s. Other vehicles for administering fluoride have been used successfully in the Region, as demonstrated by the

TABLE 22. Decayed, missing, or filled teeth (DMFT) index and percentage reduction among 12-year-old children, selected countries, Region of the Americas, 1980–2004.

Country	Year/period	DMFT	Year/period	DMFT	Reduction (%)	Annualized reduction (%)
North America						
Canada	1982	3.2	1990	1.8	43.8	6.9
United States	1986–1987	1.8	1988–91	1.4	21.8	7.9
Mexico	1988	4.4	1997–98	3.1	29.6	3.5
	1987	4.6	2001	2.0	45.7	6.5
Central America and Panama						
Guatemala	1987	8.1	2002	5.2		
Belize	1989	6.0	1999	0.6	89.5	20.2
El Salvador	1989	5.1	2000	1.4	74.5	11.7
Honduras	1987	7.7	1997	4.0	48.4	6.4
Nicaragua	1983	6.9	1997	2.8	60.0 (1983–97)	6.3
	1988	5.9				
Costa Rica	1988	8.4	1992	4.9	42.2 (1988–92)	12.8
			1999	2.5	72.5 (1988–99)	10.6
Panama	1989	4.2	1997	3.6	13.3	1.8
Andean Area						
Venezuela	1987	3.7	1997	2.1	42.2	4.1
Colombia	1977					
	1980	4.8	1998	2.3	52.1	3.7
Ecuador	1988	5.0	1996	2.9	40.5	5.9
Peru	1988	4.8	1990	3.1	N/D	
Bolivia	1981	7.6	1995	4.6	39.3	3.5
Chile	1987	6.0	1992	4.7	47.8 (1987–99)	7.0
			1996	4.1		
			1996	3.4	12.8 (1992–96)	3.4
Southern Cone and South America's northeastern area						
Argentina	1987	3.4				
Uruguay	1983–1987	8.5	1992	4.2		
		6.0	1999	2.5	40.6 (1992–99)	7.2
Paraguay	1983	5.9	1999	3.8	35.1	2.7
Brazil	1986	6.6	1996	3.1	54.0 (1986–96)	7.5
Suriname			1992	2.7		
			2002	1.9		
Guyana	1983	2.7	1995	1.3	51.9	5.9
Caribbean						
Anguilla	1986	7.5	1991	2.5	66.7	19.7
Bahamas	1981	1.6	2000	1.3	2.5	0.1
Cayman Islands	1989–		1995	1.1		
	1990	4.6	1999	0.9	63.0	16.6
Jamaica	1984	6.7	1995	1.1	83.9	15.2
Dominican Republic	1986	6.0	1997	4.4	26.0	2.0
Saint Kitts and Nevis	1979–1980	5.5	1998	2.6	53.4	3.8

Source: Estupiñán-Day, S. Promoting Oral Health: The Use of Salt Fluoridation to Prevent Dental Caries, Pan American Health Organization, Scientific and Technical Publication No. 615, Washington, D.C., PAHO, 2005.

FIGURE 25. Reduction in the number of decayed, missing, or filled teeth (DMFT) in children 12 years old, Guatemala, Suriname, and Trinidad and Tobago, 1980s and 2002–2004.

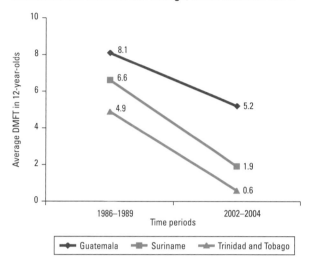

Source: Estupiñán-Day, S. (2005). "Promoting Oral Health: The Use of Salt Fluoridation to Prevent Dental Caries." Pan American Health Organization, (PAHO/WHO), Washington, D.C. Scientific and Technical Publication No. 615, Reviewed by John J. Warren, DDS, MS. Journal of Public Health Dentistry, 2006.

FIGURE 26. Average number of decayed, missing, and filled teeth (DMFT) at age 12, by subregion, Region of the Americas, 1980–2015.

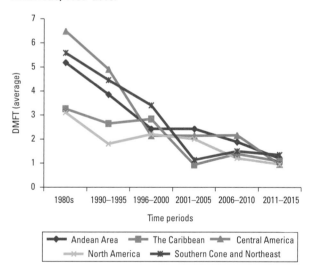

Source: Tellez, M. Progress Report No. 1 (Development Stage of Chapter Oral Health). Pan American Health Organization, July 2006.

fluoridation of milk in Codigua, Chile, between 1994 and 1999 (*263*). Roughly 400 million Latin American and Caribbean people are expected to have access to salt or water systemic fluoridation by 2010 (*255*).

Dental Fluorosis

Dental fluorosis is not considered to be a disease, as is dental caries, but rather a change in the mineralization of the dental enamel resulting from high exposure to fluoride during the formation and maturation of teeth. For all prevention programs in which systemic fluoride is administered to children under the age of 8, a 10% to 15% increase in the prevalence of the milder forms of fluorosis can be expected. Accordingly, it has been recommended that fluorosis be included in the Region's oral epidemiological surveillance programs.

Epidemiological studies conducted in the second half of the 1990s found that the prevalence of fluorosis ranged from 2.3% (Honduras) to 25.6% (Chile). A high prevalence of fluorosis is due not only to the consumption of fluoridated water or salt, but also to the use of fluoridated toothpaste; prevention programs that deliver fluoride supplements, as is the case in the Bahamas (where the prevalence rate of fluorosis is 24%); and high concentrations of fluoride occurring naturally in the water (greater than 1.5 mg/L) in Belize, Bolivia, Costa Rica, the Dominican Republic, and Paraguay. More recent cross-sectional studies in Colombia (*264*), the United States (*265*), and Mexico (*266, 267*), have found an increase in the prevalence of dental fluorosis, particularly among schoolchildren and young adults.

A literature review found that the prevalence of fluorosis (mild to severe) in Mexico ranges from 30% to 100% in areas with natural fluoride in the water, and from 52% to 82% in areas where fluoridated salt is used (*266, 267*). In Colombia, 1,061 children in primary school in the central region of Caldas were examined, and 63% were found to have some degree of fluorosis (56% had mild or very mild fluorosis, 7% had moderate or severe fluorosis) (*264*).

Practice of Atraumatic Restoration

In Latin America, the traditional restorative treatment for dental caries is the amalgam treatment, which is expensive and not very accessible, particularly among low-income groups. Atraumatic restorative treatment (ART), widely used elsewhere in the world (*268–270*), is a successful treatment that holds much promise in the Region. The technique involves removing carious tooth tissue with manual instruments only and filling the prepared cavity with an adhesive material, such as glass-ionomer, which supports the minimum intervention restorative concept (*271*). The purpose of the technique is to remove external, demineralized dental tissue; the technique does not require anesthesia, significantly reducing pain and fear in patients (*268, 269*). However, the lack of information on the cost-effectiveness of this technique, compared with conventional amalgam treatments, and its success when nontraditional personnel (dental assistants) perform the restorations prompted WHO and the IDB to conduct a prospective clinical study (*272*).

The study, which was carried out in Ecuador, Panama, and Uruguay, considered the countries' geographical, epidemiologi-

TABLE 23. Changes in the stages of the oral health typology,[a] Region of the Americas, circa 1996 and 2005.

	1996			2005		
	Emerging	Growth	Consolidation	Emerging	Growth	Consolidation
Anguilla						✓
Argentina		✓			✓	
Aruba						✓
Bahamas			✓			✓
Barbados						✓
Belize	✓					✓
Bermuda			✓			✓
Bolivia		✓			✓	
Brazil		✓				✓
Canada			✓			✓
Cayman Islands						✓
Chile		✓			✓	
Colombia		✓				✓
Costa Rica		✓				✓
Cuba			✓			✓
Curaçao						✓
Dominica			✓			✓
Dominican Republic	✓				✓	
Ecuador		✓				✓
El Salvador	✓					✓
Granada						✓
Guatemala	✓			✓		
Guyana			✓			✓
Haiti	✓					✓
Honduras	✓				✓	
Jamaica			✓			✓
Mexico		✓				✓
Nicaragua	✓					✓
Panama		✓			✓	
Paraguay	✓				✓	
Peru	✓					✓
Puerto Rico		✓				
Saint Lucia				✓		
Suriname		✓				
Trinidad and Tobago		✓				✓
Turks and Caicos						✓
United States			✓			✓
Uruguay		✓				✓
Venezuela		✓				✓

[a]Emerging stage, DMFT >5; growth stage, DMFT 3–5; consolidation stage, <3.
Source: Estupiñán-Day, S. *Promoting Oral Health: The Use of Salt Fluoridation to Prevent Dental Caries*, Pan American Health Organization, Scientific and Technical Publication # 615, Washington, D.C., PAHO, 2005.

cal, and economic differences. Approximately 1,630 children between the ages of 6 and 9 years who presented carious lesions in the enamel or tissue, or both, of their first permanent molars participated in the study. The children were randomly assigned to a treatment group (ART or amalgam) and reexamined 12 and 24 months later (and scheduled for reexamination at 36 months) to evaluate the restorations (in accordance with criteria set for ART restorations and by the United States Public Health Service) and

identify new lesions. In order to compare possible differences between restoration failure rates and service provider costs, both dentists and dental assistants were enlisted to perform the ART technique. During each procedure, information was recorded on the materials used and the time required for application; an estimate of the cost-effectiveness also was noted (*272*).

The study's preliminary findings clearly show the superiority of the ART technique over the amalgam treatment in terms of

FIGURE 27. Cost-effectiveness[a] of atraumatic restorative treatment (ART) and of amalgam treatment, by service provider, Ecuador, Panama, and Uruguay, 2006.

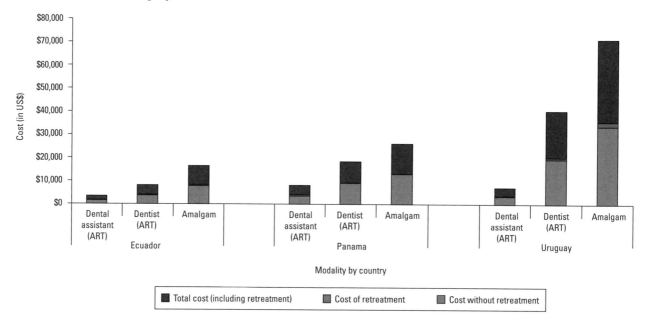

[a] At one year considering mainly planned treatments (figures in US$)

Note: Total costs including retreatment were calculated based on the following number of failed restorations in a one-year period: Ecuador—dental assistant/ART, 159; dentist/ART, 105; dentist/amalgam, 57. Panama—dental assistant/ART, 157; dentist/ART, 19; dentist/amalgam, 9. Uruguay—dental assistant/ART, 58; dentist/ART, 40; dentist/Amalgam, 58.

Source: Estupiñán-Day S., Milner T., Tellez M. (2006). "Oral Health of Low Income Children: Procedures for Atraumatic Restorative Treatment (PRAT). Final Report. Pan American Health Organization and Inter-American Development Bank. Washington, D.C. ATN/JF-7025-RG-Project No. 091024.

cost-effectiveness. Despite the fact that restorations were more likely to fail in Ecuador and Panama when dental assistants, as opposed to dentists, performed the ART technique, the cost savings could be significant. Taking into consideration the equipment and materials, personnel per procedure, and replacements of failed restorations, the annual total cost associated with the treatment and replacement of restorations by dental assistants is half the cost of ART procedures performed by dentists, and less than one-third of the cost of amalgam procedures performed by dentists (Figure 27) (*272*). Relying on the ART technique as a new model for the large-scale delivery of oral health services integrated into primary health care systems, and one in which professionals with different levels of academic training (dentists, dental assistants) participate, could reduce disparities in access to health services (*272*).

Periodontal Disease and Its Association with Systemic Disease

Periodontal disease is one of two major oral conditions that affect the world's population with high prevalence rates and severity (*273*). At this writing, the most valid clinical indicators of the disease are loss of clinical attachment and loss of bone mass. However, very few representative studies in the Region have used these indicators (*274*). The most commonly used indicator is the community periodontal index (CPI), recommended by WHO to

generate population profiles of periodontal disease in the Region's countries and to carry out comparisons internationally (*254*). Although it is a practical indicator for epidemiological studies, its validity has been questioned on several occasions on grounds that it is insufficiently sensitive to evaluate the extent and severity of the disease (*274*).

Gingivitis is widespread in the Region, although it is more prevalent among low-income groups and affects men at higher rates than women (*274*). The overall prevalence of severe periodontal disease ranges between 4% and 19% (*274*). These variations in the Region are due, in part, more to methodological differences than geographical variations. The risk factors for periodontal disease are consistent with nontransmissible disorders or conditions, such as tobacco use, malnutrition, excessive alcohol consumption, stress, diabetes mellitus, and other systemic disorders (*273*). A focus on behavioral and environmental risk factors is critically important for the development of effective disease prevention strategies.

Dental caries harbor opportunistic microorganisms and infections that can affect other organs of the body. A number of risk factors for systemic diseases are correlated with oral diseases, and these have been associated with cardiovascular disease, diabetes, and infarctions (*275*). Infections that affect pregnant women can cause changes in the hormonal system that regulates gestation, which can lead to preterm birth, early rupture of membranes, and low birthweight (*276, 277*). Controlled clinical studies in the Region have documented the association between periodontal disease and preterm birth or low birthweight. Periodontal disease may have similar pathogenic mechanisms to other maternal infections, as documented in controlled clinical studies of the Chilean population (*278, 279*).

Ocular Health

Blindness and Loss of Vision

The International Classification of Diseases, 10th Revision, categorizes visual impairment as a visual acuity under 20/70 (6/18), and blindness as a visual acuity under 20/400 (3/60) in the best eye. The burden of visual impairment is not distributed uniformly; in many Latin American and Caribbean countries it is estimated that for every million persons, 5,000 are blind and 20,000 are visually impaired. At least two-thirds are attributable to treatable conditions such as cataracts, refractive errors, diabetic retinopathy, and glaucoma (Figure 28). About 85% of blindness occurs in adults 50 years old and older (*280–282*).

Between 1999 and 2005, PAHO and the Christoffel–Blindenmission (CBM) promoted and supported the conduct of national-level rapid assessments of avoidable blindness and cataract surgical services in Cuba, Paraguay, and Venezuela. Similar urban studies were done in Buenos Aires, Argentina; Guadalajara, Mexico; and Campinas, Brazil. Rural rapid assessments were developed in Piura and Tumbes in Peru, and in Chimaltenango, Guatemala (*283*).

According to national surveys, the prevalence of blindness in people 50 years old and older varied from 2.3% to 3% (*283*); the prevalence in urban areas of Campinas, Brazil, and Buenos Aires, Argentina is 1.4% (*284*), and in rural areas of Guatemala and Peru, the prevalence nears 4% (*285*).

The proportion of blindness due to cataract in people aged 50 years old and older varied from 39% in the urban areas of Brazil and Argentina (*284*) to about 65% in the rural areas of Guatemala and Peru (*285*). National assessments revealed that close to 60% of blindness is due to cataracts (*283*). In Latin America, eye care services coverage for visual acuities under 20/200 is close to 80% in well developed, urban areas and under 10% in rural and remote areas (*283*).

The quality of surgery is highly variable. In rural areas, up to 30% of eyes operated with intraocular lenses may have a visual acuity under 20/200, compared to about 8% of eyes operated with intraocular lenses in urban, well-developed areas (*283*).

The Barbados eye studies found a prevalence of 42% with lens opacities, 7% with open angle glaucoma, and less than 1% with age-related macular degeneration among 40–84-year-olds (*286*). Prevalence of open-angle glaucoma varied among different ethnic groups, from 0.8% in whites, to 3.3% in mixed-race persons and 7% in blacks (*286*).

Diabetic retinopathy in Latin America is one of the main causes of blindness, after cataracts and glaucoma (*282*). A dia-

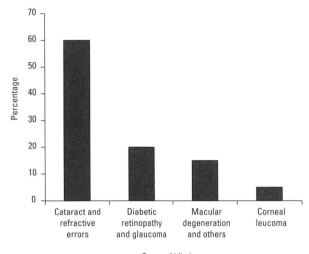

FIGURE 28. Causes of blindness, Latin America and the Caribbean, 2007.

Source: PAHO/WHO estimates.

betes and blindness survey in the Dominican Republic found that 5% of blindness was due to diabetic retinopathy (*287*). The Barbados eye studies found that among people of African origin, 1 in 17 had diabetic retinopathy; among diabetics, 29% had retinopathy (*288*).

Uncorrected refractive errors is the most common cause of bilateral visual impairment across all decades of life (*289*). In the Caribbean population 40–84 years old, myopia occurs in 22% and hyperopia in 47% (*290*). A study conducted in Santiago, Chile, among 6,998 schoolchildren found that more than 7% could benefit from proper spectacles, but 70% of that group had not had their vision corrected at the time of the eye exam (*291*).

In Latin America, onchocercosis is regionally clustered in 13 foci in Brazil, Colombia, Ecuador, Guatemala, Mexico, and Venezuela. The disease affects about one-half million persons, but it is not a major cause of blindness or visual impairment; currently, the Onchocerciasis Elimination Program for the Americas (OEPA) provides technical and financial support. Treatment with Mectizan® is given twice a year in endemic communities; 12 out of 13 foci are close to reaching the expected 85% coverage (*292*).

Vitamin A deficiency in Latin America and the Caribbean is usually subclinical. In the 1980s, it was reported as a public health problem in Bolivia, Haiti, Honduras, and Nicaragua (*293, 294*). Interventions to eliminate vitamin A deficiency are linked to nutrition, immunization, and primary health care systems.

Trachoma is caused by *Chlamydia trachomatis* infection and it is not a major cause of blindness in Latin America. Some foci have been identified in Brazil, Guatemala, and Mexico (*295*). Brazil has a trachoma control program at the federal level that is conducting a national trachoma school survey in 11 states. A prevalence of active disease was found in 5.2% children 1–9 years old. The program provides antibiotic treatment, and there is no data on trichiasis surgery (*296*). In Guatemala, trachoma is present in 92 communities; an NGO screens people 1–40 years old and provides antibiotics and trichiasis treatment. The State of Chiapas in Mexico put in place the Trachoma Prevention and Control Program implementing the surgery, antibiotics, facial hygiene, and environmental change (SAFE) strategy (*296*). The program is close to eliminating the disease in the state (no other state in Mexico reported active cases of trachoma).

The estimated prevalence of childhood blindness in Latin America is 4 to 6 per 10,000 children (*297*); between 34% and 44% of cases of childhood blindness are preventable or treatable. The most common preventable causes are rubella, toxoplasmosis, and ophthalmia neonatorum, while the most common treatable diseases are congenital cataracts, congenital glaucoma, and retinopathy of prematurity (ROP) (*297*). Various studies revealed that ROP is the most common etiology in the Region, especially in countries that have introduced neonatal intensive care services for low birthweight infants (*297, 298*).

Cost of Blindness

The annual gross domestic product (GDP) loss from blindness is being calculated by direct and indirect costs related to visual impairment, including direct medical costs; loss of earnings; cost to caregivers, including their loss of earnings; aids; equipment; home modifications; and suffering. In 2000, the annual GDP loss from blindness and low vision in Latin America and the Caribbean was calculated at US$ 3.2 billion. Prevention of blindness programs generate enormous savings for national economies. For 2020, the annual GDP loss in Latin America and the Caribbean from blindness and low vision has been estimated at US$ 10 billion, compared to US$ 3.7 billion if prevention of blindness programs were implemented in every country of the Region (*299, 300*).

Successes in Disease Control

In Latin America and the Caribbean, the annual cataract surgical rate per 1,000,000 varies according to a country's social and economic development. The rate has being increasing over time in most countries: in 1999, just 17% of countries had annual cataract surgical rates above 1,500 (*301*); in 2006, about half of the countries had such a rate. In 1995, just 25% of countries had a specialized low-vision service providing visual aids to persons who could not improve their vision by regular eyeglasses or medical or surgical treatment. At this writing, most countries have at least one such specialized service. In 2000, just a few countries had a retinopathy of prematurity (ROP) program (*302*); currently, 18 countries have ROP programs at different stages of development. Several programs for refractive defects in schoolchildren have been organized, along with the sustainable production of low-cost spectacles. Successful communication

programs to detect glaucoma in high-risk groups have being implemented and evaluated in the Caribbean (*303*); the production of low-cost eyedrops improved accessibility of glaucoma medications in the same subregion.

Several pilot programs on diabetic retinopathy have being initiated to create models of screening and treatment, assessing feasibility and cost-effectiveness. During 2006 and 2007 OEPA is conducting ophthalmologic evaluations in the different foci to assess the elimination of ocular morbidity related to that disease.

Partnerships

The Pan American Health Organization has had long-standing partnerships with Sight Savers, the Caribbean Council for the Blind, the Christoffel Blindenmission (CBM), the Fundación Once para America Latina (FOAL), and others. Vision 2020: The Right to Sight was launched in 1999 by the World Health Organization and the International Agency for the Prevention of Blindness to provide technical and resource support to Member Countries. Other organizations (Lions Club International, Rotary International) and countries (Venezuela and Cuba, through *Operación Milagro* [Operation Miracle]) also are providing technical and financial support to Latin American and Caribbean countries to help them reduce avoidable blindness.

The Future

Efforts should continue to increase coverage of cataract surgery in order to control the leading cause of blindness. Implementation should give priority to underserved groups (ethnic, gender, minorities, rural residents, and the poor). It also is necessary to expand programs to address low vision, childhood blindness, and refractive defects; develop model programs for diabetic retinopathy; and promote research in glaucoma detection and treatment.

SEXUAL AND REPRODUCTIVE HEALTH

In spite of advances made in the years after the International Conference on Population and Development in Cairo in 1994 (*304*) and the Fourth World Conference on Women in Beijing in 1995 (*305*), the impact of actions to improve sexual and reproductive health (SRH) has been very weak, inasmuch as it has not yet been determined how to narrow the inequity gap or provide support to countries, their leaders, and the community in correcting the disparities in access to information and services that will lead to a more equitable distribution of health-care goods. In considering sexual and reproductive health, the International Conference issued pronouncements on several key issues (*304*). First, everyone has the right to the enjoyment of physical , mental, and social well-being, not merely to the absence of disease or infirmity in all matters relating to the reproductive system and to its functions and processes. Reproductive health, therefore, implies that people are able to have a satisfying and safe sex life and have the capability to reproduce as well as the freedom to decide if, when, and how often to do so. Implicit in this last condition is the right of men and women to be informed and to have access to safe, effective, affordable, and acceptable methods of family planning of their choice; the right to access appropriate health-care services that will ensure safe pregnancy and childbirth; the right to medical care for sexually transmitted infections, including HIV/ AIDS; and the prevention of cancer of the female reproductive system, menopause-related disabilities, and sexual violence.

Although advances are being made in defining policies and programs, which in turn have brought about improvements in aspects of sexual and reproductive health in the Region, a Regional strategy has yet to be developed.

Action must be focused at political, social, and administrative levels, where effective strategic plans should be formulated, the capacity to define priorities in the field of sexual and reproductive health developed, legal and political constraints eliminated, political will mobilized, and the visibility of the problem and accountability of the various actors enhanced. Activities also must focus on sexual and reproductive health promotion and services, in which utilization of human resources must be improved; the adoption of good practices at the national and regional levels must be fostered; and the barriers preventing or limiting the use of services by individuals, families, and the community must be eliminated.

Status of Sexual and Reproductive Health in the Region's Countries

The total estimated population of the Region in 2005 was 892 million, with 561 million (63%) living in Latin America and the Caribbean. Each year, slightly more than 16.2 million children are born in the Region, 11.7 million of them in Latin America. Although the population continues to increase (*306*), birth and fertility rates are clearly declining, which in conjunction with falling mortality rates has meant that 10 countries in the Region have completed or have nearly completed their demographic transition. For example, the overall estimated fertility rate in Cuba is 1.6 children per woman. At the other extreme is Guatemala, however, with a fertility rate of 4.3 children per woman.

This decline in the birth rate, along with changes in mortality, translates into a slowing of the natural growth rate of the Region, but also into major growth of the population of adolescents and young people owing to demographic inertia, as well as to a clear trend towards the aging of the population in most countries. This situation, combined with the increase in the absolute number of poor people in Latin America and the Caribbean (currently estimated at more than 150 million persons), the feminization of poverty, and a sharp increase in unemployment in most countries, translates into a widening of inequity gaps for large popula-

tion groups, an increase in poverty transmitted from generation to generation, and an ever-increasing shift of major population groups to urban peripheries and to nearby or distant countries. The conditions described impose additional burdens on health-care systems in general and adversely affect sexual and reproductive health in particular.

Sexual and reproductive health accounts for approximately 20% of the total illness burden among women and 14% among men, revealing a clear-cut gender gap. Individual countries and the Region as a whole have advanced in some aspects of sexual and reproductive health, but there is a very marked contrast between the health indicators of the Region's most developed countries (Canada and United States) and those of Latin American and Caribbean countries. This disparity can be partly explained by the sharp economic adjustment these countries have undergone, which has widened existing inequity gaps between countries and within countries.

Contraceptive use in the Region exceeds 60%, although Bolivia, the Dominican Republic, Guatemala, Haiti, Honduras, Mexico, Paraguay, and Venezuela still see limited progress (*306*). Emergency contraception and condom use for preventing sexually transmitted infections and unwanted pregnancies are barely practiced by users or in the health care services in the Region.

Women's Health and Maternal Health

Maternal health can be regarded as a summary gauge of reproductive health and can be used as an indicator, for lack of a more accurate one, of the status of maternal health. Estimates published in the annual yearbook of health statistics (*307*) show 22,680 maternal deaths (circa 2003) and 16.2 million births (same year) in the Region; accordingly, the maternal mortality rate is around 140 per 100,000 live births. Yet PAHO basic indicators informed by reports from the countries' ministries of health for the same year show a maternal mortality rate of 71.9 per 100,000 live births (11,652 deaths due to maternity-related causes).

If the risk of maternal death in Latin America and the Caribbean is compared with the risk in Canada, the average in the former is 21 times greater than that in the latter. Moreover, when national averages of maternal death rates are examined, a broad range is seen, ranging from 523 per 100,000 live births in Haiti to 13.4 in Chile (*306*). Another way to analyze these differences is by the time lag of the indicator, which can be measured by comparing the current rate in one country with a time series in another. For example, if the current rate of maternal mortality in Haiti is compared with a time series of the same rate in the United States, the former corresponds to the 1930 rate in the United States; in other words, a lag of more than 75 years. If the current rate in Haiti is compared with the time series for Chile, the former corresponds to the 1980 rate in the latter, or a lag time of more than 25 years.

TABLE 24. Leading causes of maternal mortality, by mortality rate and availability of reproductive services, groups of countries, Region of the Americas, 2004.

Service coverage	Maternal mortality rate per 100,000 live births			
	<20	20–49	50–100	>100
Contraception, 70%–75% Prenatal care, 100% Delivery, 100%	**Group A countries** 1. Indirect 2. Preeclampsia 3. Infections			
Contraception, 45%–69% Prenatal care, 90%–100% Delivery 90%–100%		**Group B countries** 1. Abortion 2. Preeclampsia 3. Hemorrhage		
Contraception, 45%–66% Prenatal care, 45%–96% Delivery 83%–97%			**Group C countries** 1. Preeclampsia-eclampsia 2. Hemorrhage 3. Abortion	
Contraception 28%–58% Prenatal 53%–86% Delivery 24%–86%				**Group D countries** 1. Hemorrhage 2. Preeclampsia-eclampsia 3. Obstructed delivery

Note: Group A countries: Canada, United States, Puerto Rico; Group B countries: Argentina, Brazil, Chile, Costa Rica, Cuba, Mexico, and Uruguay; Group C countries: Colombia, Ecuador, Panama, Nicaragua, and Venezuela; Group D countries: Bolivia, El Salvador, Guatemala, Haiti, Honduras, Jamaica, Paraguay, and Peru.

Source: Based on Schwarcz R, Fescina R. Maternal Mortality in Latin America and the Caribbean. Lancet 2000; 356 (suppl.) S11:3245–67. (Figures updated to 2004).

An analysis of the indicators in several countries of the Americas (accounting for approximately 98% of the total population), in terms of their maternal mortality rates (less than 20, 20–49, 50–100, and over 100 per 100,000 live births), their prenatal and delivery care coverages, and the prevalence of contraception use (Table 24), shows that the basic causes of death are almost the same in the four groups, although their rank order differs (*308*).

This type of analysis enables more specific interventions to be proposed. For example, a recommendation for group A would be to strengthen care in pre-pregnancy for the most vulnerable populations; for group B, the recommendation would be to intensify sex education and family planning programs, including emergency contraception; for group C, prenatal monitoring coverage should be broadened; and for group D, access to care should be guaranteed through the elimination of economic and cultural barriers, the establishment of birthing homes near health-care services, and improvements to services.

Prenatal care coverage of at least one office visit averaged higher than 85%. However, an analysis by income quintile shows that in Bolivia, Brazil, Colombia, Guatemala, Haiti, Nicaragua, Paraguay, and Peru, 90% or more of pregnant women in the highest-income quintile had prenatal check-ups, compared to just 35%–68% in the lowest-income quintile (*309*). It bears noting that this level of coverage is not a measure of the real prenatal care situation. Prenatal care should consist of at least four or five duly scheduled office visits, with early enrollment and a well-defined procedure. If these standards were applied, actual coverage figures would be much lower.

In terms of delivery care by trained personnel, an increase of 11% between 1999 and 2002 was observed; as a result this indicator averages above 88% in Latin America (*309*). Nonetheless, there are still nine countries with below-average figures, with coverage ranging from 24% (Haiti) to 84% (Guatemala). An analysis of qualified delivery care by income quintiles shows that it exceeds 90% among the wealthiest in countries such as Brazil, Bolivia, Colombia, Guatemala, Haiti, Nicaragua, Paraguay, Peru, and the Dominican Republic. Yet among lower-income quintiles it stands at just 20% in Bolivia, Guatemala, Haiti, and Peru; between 30% and 40% in Nicaragua and Paraguay; and between 60% and 85% in Brazil, Colombia, and the Dominican Republic (*309*).

The incidence of cesarean section is an indicator of the quality of perinatal care. A WHO recent study in different regions found an overall cesarean section rate of 35% in Latin America. Data from the 2006 World Yearbook of Health Statistics (*307*) show wide variations between countries, from 2% in Haiti and 8% in Belize, to 36% in Brazil and 37% in Chile. WHO has indicated that the optimal rate of cesarean section is between 15% and 20%.

The prevalence of modern contraceptive use in Latin America and the Caribbean averaged 65%, with a range from 28% in Haiti to 84% in Uruguay.

A serious public health problem is unsafe abortion, one of the three leading causes of maternal deaths in all countries (except Canada and the United States). Estimates are that more than four million abortions are performed every year in Latin America, 2.2 million of them in three countries (Brazil, 1.2 million; Argentina, 500,000; and Mexico, 500,000) (*310*). In addition, one-quarter of maternal deaths in Chile were the result of an abortion, and in Argentina, Jamaica, and Trinidad and Tobago the proportion exceeds 30%.

The rate of HIV infection among pregnant women and newborns has increased in recent years. The rate of HIV seroprevalence among pregnant women, which is an approximate measure of the extent of infection among the population at large, is as high as 13% in Haiti as a whole, 10% among urban adults, and 4% in rural areas (*311*). In several regions of the Dominican Republic, 1 of every 12 women receiving prenatal care was infected, with rates of 7.1% in Guyana, 3.6% in the Bahamas, 2.5% in Belize, 1.5% in Jamaica, and 1.4% in Honduras (*311*).

Perinatal Health

Several indicators provide a comprehensive assessment of perinatal health, including fetal, neonatal, and perinatal mortality rates. However, due in part to significant underreporting and because countries continue to use different cutoff points for these indicators, the magnitude of fetal and perinatal mortality is not well known Regionwide. Despite reporting-related difficulties, in 2006 WHO estimated a total of 280,000 perinatal deaths (a rate of 17.3 per 1,000) in the Americas, around 45% of which were late stillbirths and 55% (152,000) early neonatal deaths (*312*). The risk of perinatal death in Latin America and the Caribbean is, on average, three times higher than that in Canada and the United States (*312*).

Moreover, 85% of all neonatal deaths are associated with low birthweight (<2500 g); the most common causes are preterm births and fetal growth retardation. In the Region, the proportion of low-birthweight children ranges from 5.7% in Canada to 12% in Guatemala. The neonatal component accounts for the highest proportion of infant mortality (61%) in Latin America and the Caribbean. The infant mortality rate in Latin America and the Caribbean circa 2003 averaged 24.8 per 1,000 live births, or an approximate 290,000 infant deaths, 177,000 of them associated with the perinatal period (*306*).

Sexual and Reproductive Health of Adolescents

Every year there are some 54,000 births to mothers under age 15 and two million to mothers between 15–19 years old. The specific birthrate among mothers 15–19 years old ranges from 23.4 per 1,000 live births in Chile to 136 per 1,000 in Honduras. Among 10–14-year-olds, the rate ranges from approximately 1% in Uruguay and Cuba to 4% in Brazil and Haiti (*302, 313*). In the latter age group the rate of maternal mortality doubles that of the 15–19-year-olds (Table 25).

Adolescents tend to be sexually active at early ages in the Region, where the average age at which both sexes start having sexual relations is 16; the lower end is 14 in the Caribbean and the higher end, 17 in Paraguay. In the United States, 77% of adolescent girls have had their first sexual relationship, but only 17%

TABLE 25. Maternal mortality rate (per 100,000 live births) by age of adolescents, selected countries, Region of the Americas, circa 2003.

Country	10–14 years old	15–19 years old
Mexico	131	37
Argentina	190	23
Chile	42	20
Brazil	65	38

Source: Statistics from the countries:

Mexico: Secretaría de Salud. http://www.salud.gob.mx/.

Argentina: Instituto Nacional de Estadísticas y Censos http://www.indec.mecon.gov.ar/.

Chile: Instituto Nacional de Estadística http://www.ine.cl/ine/canales/chile estadistico/home.php.

Brazil: Ministério da Saúde. Datasus http://w3.datasus.gov.br/datasus/datasus.php. (Accessed 6 November 2006).

become pregnant; in contrast, in Latin America and the Caribbean, only 56% have started having sex, but 34% have had a child before age 19. This situation could be explained by the difference in education, especially with regard to sexual and reproductive health, and differences in access to contraception between the two subregions (*304*). Besides the repercussions of pregnancy for adolescent mothers themselves, neonatal and infant mortality is twice as high among mothers in that age group than among 20–24-years-olds. Fetal mortality is not substantially different.

Sexual and reproductive health in the Region requires safeguarding advances already made and addressing unresolved issues (unfinished business) and any new challenges. The framework for technical cooperation to cope with the future is presented in Figure 29.

PREVENTING RISKS

Food and Nutrition for a Healthier Life

In the Region, 12.5 million disability-adjusted life years (DALYs) are lost to nutrition-related noncommunicable chronic diseases such as hypertension, cardiovascular disease, and type 2 diabetes; in addition, 4.6 million are lost because of malnutrition in mothers and young children (*314*). As does malnutrition in children, the burden of noncommunicable diseases disproportionately affects the poor in both relative and absolute terms. Yet, whereas child malnutrition affects some countries in the Region more than others, depending on a given country's level of poverty and relative equity in income distribution, chronic noncommunicable diseases are a problem in all the countries. Micronutrient deficiencies also are widespread. Some, such as iodine deficiency and vitamin A deficiency, overlap considerably with child malnutrition. Others, such as iron, zinc, and folate deficiencies, are highly prevalent in infants and young children and in women of reproductive age in all income groups.

145

FIGURE 29. Conceptual framework for technical cooperation in sexual and reproductive health.

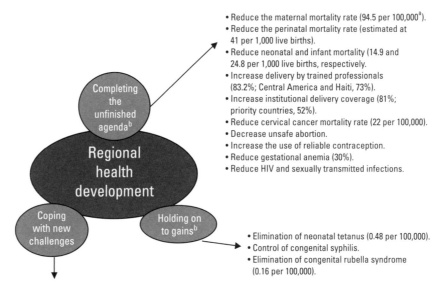

- Reduce the maternal mortality rate (94.5 per 100,000[a]).
- Reduce the perinatal mortality rate (estimated at 41 per 1,000 live births).
- Reduce neonatal and infant mortality (14.9 and 24.8 per 1,000 live births, respectively.
- Increase delivery by trained professionals (83.2%; Central America and Haiti, 73%).
- Increase institutional delivery coverage (81%; priority countries, 52%).
- Reduce cervical cancer mortality rate (22 per 100,000).
- Decrease unsafe abortion.
- Increase the use of reliable contraception.
- Reduce gestational anemia (30%).
- Reduce HIV and sexually transmitted infections.

- Elimination of neonatal tetanus (0.48 per 100,000).
- Control of congenital syphilis.
- Elimination of congenital rubella syndrome (0.16 per 100,000).

- Involvement of men in sexual and reproductive health.
- Addressing sexual, family, and gender violence.
- Addressing teenage pregnancy.
- Preventing vertical transmission of HIV.
- Vaccinating against human papillomavirus.
- Addressing complications of menopause.
- Implementing evidence-based norms and standards.

[a]Estimated rate: 190 per 100,000 (UNICEF/UNFPA/WHO, 2002) and 140 per 100,000 (World Health Statistics, 2006).
[b]The latest available figures are given in parentheses.

The quality of the food consumed is a greater problem than the amount of food consumed. Poor dietary quality, coupled with diarrhea and acute respiratory infections in infants and young children, causes growth failure early in life. Micronutrient deficiencies throughout the life cycle, coupled with sedentary lifestyles, are causing an epidemic of chronic noncommunicable diseases in adults. These factors translate into overweight and obese parents sharing the household with stunted and anemic children in both rural and urban areas.

Growth Patterns of Infants and Young Children

Linear growth retardation (stunting) is the most prevalent form of growth failure worldwide. Linear growth faltering begins at birth and continues through the first two years of life (*315*). Failure to adequately gain weight also begins at birth, but is less pronounced compared to height, and continues for a shorter period of time. Once growth faltering in height and weight ceases, children begin to gain weight and height at about the reference standard. Height deficits are permanent, however. As a result of the greater loss of linear growth compared to weight gain, most children tend to have weight-for-height ratios that are above the median of the reference standard, indicating a tendency toward overweight. This tendency puts such children at later risk of chronic diseases. The age-specific risk patterns for stunting are similar in all the Region's countries, despite widely varying levels of stunting. This confirms that the first two years of life represent a critical window of opportunity for improving nutrition.

The prevalence of stunting in the Americas is about three to four times greater than that of underweight. The fact that children are much more likely to gain weight adequately, as compared to growing in length adequately, illustrates that dietary quality is a much greater problem than energy sufficiency. Micronutrient deficiencies, particularly iron, zinc, and calcium deficiencies, are known to be widespread in the complementary feeding diets of young children (*316*). High prevalence of diarrhea early in life also causes linear growth retardation.

The prevalence of growth retardation is declining in countries for which trend data are available (Table 26); nonetheless, more than one in four children are stunted in Bolivia, Ecuador, Honduras, and Peru, and one in every two is stunted in Guatemala. It should be noted that national-level data mask increasingly wide

TABLE 26. National prevalence of low height-for-age, weight-for-age, and weight-for-height, selected countries, Region of the Americas.

Country	Year	Height-for-age[a] (%)	Weight-for-age[a] (%)	Weight-for-height[a] (%)	Source of Information
Argentina	1996	13.0	5.4	2.9	MOH, 1999
Bolivia	1989	38.3	13.3	1.6	DHS, 1989
	1993–1994	28.3	15.7	4.4	DHS, 1994
	1998	26.8	9.4	1.8	DHS, 1998
	2003	26.5	8.0	1.3	DHS, 2003
Brazil	1986	27.7	13.2	1.0	DHS, 1986
	1996	10.5	5.7	2.3	DHS, 1997
Chile	2003	NA	0.9	0.4	MOH, 2003
Colombia	1986	22.7	11.9	1.0	DHS, 1986
	1995	15.0	8.4	1.4	DHS, 1995
	2000	13.5	6.7	0.8	DHS, 2000
	2005	12.0	7.0	1.3	DHS, 2005
Costa Rica	1996	6.1	5.1	2.3	Encuesta Nacional de Nutrición, MOH
Dominican Republic	1991	19.4	10.4	1.1	DHS, 1991
	1996	10.7	5.9	1.2	DHS, 1996
	2002	8.9	5.3	1.8	DHS, 2002
Ecuador	1986	34.0	16.5	1.7	Freire et al., 1988
	1998	26.4	14.3	2.4	LSMS, 1998
El Salvador	1993	22.8	11.2	1.3	CDC, 1994
	1998	23.3	11.1	1.1	CDC, 1998
	2002–2003	18.9	10.3	1.4	CDC, 2004
Guatemala	1987	69.7 (12–23 months)	41.5 (12–23 months)	21.8 (12–23 months)	DHS, 1996
	1995	68.7 (24–35 months)	41.5 (24–35 months)	10.0 (24–35 months)	DHS, 1996
	1998–1999	49.7	26.6	3.3	DHS, 1995
	2002	46.4	24.2	2.5	DHS, 2003
		49.3	22.7	1.6	
Honduras	1987	43.8	24.1	1.9	CDC, 1987
	1991	42.4	21.4	1.8	CDC, 1991
	1996	37.8	24.3	1.4	CDC, 1996
	2001	29.2	16.6	1.0	CDC, 2002
Haiti	1978	39.6	37.4	8.9	DHS, 1995
	1990	33.9	26.8	4.7	DHS, 1994/1995
	1994–1995	31.9	27.5	7.8	DHS, 1994/1995
	2000	22.7	17.3	4.5	DHS, 2000
Mexico	1988	22.8	14.2	6.0	Sepulveda, 2000
	1999	17.7	7.5	2.0	Rivera et al., 2001
Nicaragua	1998	24.9	12.2	2.2	DHS, 1999
	2001	20.0	9.6	2.0	DHS, 2002
Paraguay	1990	16.6	3.7	0.1	DHS, 1990
	1995–1996	NA	NA	NA	CDC, 1995/1996
	1998	NA	NA	NA	CDC, 1999
Peru	1991–1992	36.5	10.8	1.4	DHS, 1991/1992
	1996	25.8	7.8	1.1	DHS, 1996
	2000	25.4	7.1	0.9	DHS, 2000
Uruguay	2002	10.6	4.9	1.8	MOH, 2002

Notes:

[a] < − 2 standard deviations from the growth reference point set by WHO and the United States National Center for Health Statistics.

NA = not available.

Argentina: Encuesta Antropométrica en menores de 6 años bajo Programa Materno Infantil, Ministry of Health, 1999. Note that this is the only data included in the table that is not representative nationally. Rather it is representative of the Province of Buenos Aires, which has one-third to one-half of the total population.

Chile: Ministerio de Salud, 2003.

Costa Rica: Ministerio de Salud, 1996.

Ecuador: Freire W, Dirren H, Mora JO, Arenales P, Granda E, Breih J, Campaña A, Páez R, Darquea L, Molina E. Diagnóstico de la situación alimentaría, nutricional y de salud de la población Ecuatoriana menor de cinco años (DANS). Quito: CONADE, Ministerio de Salud Publica, 1988; Life Standards Measurement Survey, World Bank, 1998.

Mexico: Sepúlveda-Amor J, Lezana MA, Tapia-Conyer R, Valdespino JL, Madrigal H, Kumate J. Estado nutricional de preescolares y mujeres en México: resultados de una encuesta probabilística nacional. Gac Med Mex 1990;126:207–244; Rivera Dommarco J, Shamah Levy T, Villapando Hernández S, González de Cossio T, Hernández Prado B, Sepúlveda J. Encuesta Nacional de Nutrición 1999. Estado nutricio de niños y mujeres en México. Cuernavaca, Morelos, México: Instituto Nacional de Salud Pública, 2001.

Uruguay: Children seen in the health services, 2002.

Data from all other countries is from the Demographic and Health Surveys (DHS) conducted by Macro International or by the Centers for Disease Control and Prevention (CDC).

TABLE 27. Prevalence of breast-feeding initiation and median duration of exclusive and any breast-feeding, selected countries, Region of the Americas.

Country	Year	Breast-feeding initiation (%)	Median duration (months)	
			Exclusive breast-feeding	Any breast-feeding
Bolivia	2003	97.1	4.0	19.6
Brazil	1996	92.5	1.1	7.0
Colombia	2005	97.1	3.7	16..3
Dominican Republic	2002	92.0	0.5	6.6
Ecuador	1999	97.0	2.2	15.5
El Salvador	2002–2003	94.4	1.4	19.2
Guatemala	2002	96.1	3.5	20.5
Haiti	2000	97.4	0.4	18.5
Honduras	2001	96.6	2.3	17.6
Mexico	1999	92.3	NA	9.0
Nicaragua	2001	94.5	2.5	17.6
Paraguay	2004	95.0	Not reported	Not reported
Peru	2005	97.9	3.9	19.6

Source: Nationally representative data. All data from Demographic and Health Surveys, except for Mexico, which is from the Mexican National Institute of Public Health.

disparities within the countries, based on income, rural or urban residence, and ethnicity.

Breast-feeding

Although most women in Latin America breast-feed and do so for a relatively long period of time, breast-feeding practices are far from optimal (Table 27). The duration of exclusive breast-feeding, which is the behavior most closely linked to reductions in infant morbidity and mortality, is well below the six months recommended by WHO (*317*). National programs in support of breast-feeding have been successful, and the WHO/UNICEF Baby-friendly Hospital Initiative has been widely implemented in the Region. Several countries still do not have in place enforceable legislation on the International Code of Marketing of Breast-milk Substitutes. Only Argentina, Bolivia, Brazil, Costa Rica, the Dominican Republic, Guatemala, Honduras, Panama, Peru, and Uruguay have enacted legislation covering all or nearly all of the Code's provisions. Colombia, Mexico, and Nicaragua have enacted legislation with many of the provisions. Most of the remaining countries have adopted a voluntary health policy code encompassing all or nearly all the Code's provisions, but with no enforcement mechanism.

HIV and Infant Feeding

Mother-to-child transmission of HIV is a growing problem in Latin America and the Caribbean and the main cause of pediatric HIV. Recognizing that breast-feeding is a significant and preventable mode of HIV transmission, UNAIDS, working with WHO and UNICEF, issued new guidelines on HIV and infant feeding in 2003 (*318*). The guidelines state that, in order to reduce the risk of HIV transmission to infants while minimizing the risk of other causes of morbidity and mortality, "when replacement feeding is acceptable, feasible, affordable, sustainable, and safe, avoidance of all breast-feeding by HIV-infected mothers is recommended. Otherwise, exclusive breast-feeding is recommended for the first months of life," but should be discontinued as soon as it is feasible. When a woman is HIV-negative or of unknown status, the recommendation is that she should breast-feed.

Micronutrients

It is estimated that the prevalence of iron deficiency anemia in the Region is 35% in pregnant women and 19% in school-age children. In 19 of 35 countries, iodine deficiency disorders continue to be a public health problem, as 10% of households lack iodinated salt (*319*). A 1995 report from WHO estimates vitamin A deficiency among preschoolers in the Region at 20% (*320*). It is estimated that 20% to 30% of the population in the Americas suffers from zinc deficiency (*321*). Although data are lacking, vitamin B12 and folate deficiency also are likely to be important.

The prevalence of anemia is higher during early infancy and childhood than at any other time in the life cycle. Nationally data from more than eight of the Region's countries show that between 48% and 63% of infants and young children are anemic, and the figure rises to 75% or more among infants 6 to 12 months old. This high prevalence is consistent with data showing dietary iron to be inadequate and of low bioavailability in most complementary feeding diets and a lack of successful iron supplementation programs in this age group. It also agrees with the extremely high dietary requirement of iron per kg body weight and the low amount of food needed in this age group to meet energy needs (*317*).

Recent randomized trials showing the effect of iron supplements on motor and language development suggest that improving iron status in iron-deficient populations is likely to yield significant benefits (*322, 323*). Translating these efficacy studies into successful public health programs remains a challenge. The current emphasis on fortifying staple food with iron will not address the problem of anemia in infants and young children because of the small amounts they consume relative to their high requirements. Moreover, distribution of iron supplements through the health system does not appear to be effective in reducing anemia, most likely because of problems with supply, distribution, and compliance. Therefore, other strategies must be pursued to address this pressing public health problem, including the use of complementary foods fortified with iron and other vitamins and minerals, as well as home fortification.

Night blindness and ocular injuries are the most frequent clinical manifestations of vitamin A deficiency; however, increases in morbidity and mortality in infants and mothers occur at subclinical levels of deficiency. According to WHO's global database, mean serum retinol levels in the Region vary from 0.6 µmol/L to 1.49 µmol/L in children aged 6 months to 7 years (1996–2004). If 10%–20% of the population has serum retinol levels at or below 0.70 µmol/L, it is indicative of a moderate public health problem. Using this cutoff, several of the Region's countries have mild or moderate vitamin A deficiencies, and some regions of Brazil, Mexico, and Venezuela present severe deficiencies. Several countries have adopted sugar fortification with vitamin A as a public health strategy for preventing and controlling vitamin A deficiency, others have explored the fortification of oils, and still others use vitamin A delivered through their immunization programs.

A dose of 400 µg/day of folic acid during the three months prior to conception and through the first trimester of pregnancy reduces the incidence of neural tube defects. Wheat flour fortification programs have been adopted by most countries of the Americas to ensure that women of childbearing age receive adequate amounts of folic acid. Such fortification programs have successfully reduced the incidence of neural tube defects in Canada, the United States, Costa Rica, and Chile.

Iodine deficiency disorder is the most common cause of preventable brain damage, cretinism, and mental retardation, as well as endemic goiter and hypothyroidism (*324*). There are three internationally recognized indicators to monitor iodine nutrition: fraction of homes consuming adequately iodized salt, concentration of iodine in representative urine samples, and the prevalence of goiter (*325, 326*). Since 2002, 75.1 million persons—10% of the population in the Americas—have been identified as having urinary levels of iodine below the recommended minimum (<100 µg/L) (*327*). The prevalence of urinary iodine excretion <100 µg/L is 21.9% in Guyana, 22% in Mexico, and 13.4% in

Nicaragua. The median urinary iodine excretion for Guatemala, Haiti, and Bolivia is 72 µg/L, 43.4 µg/L, and 100 µg/L, respectively. At the same time, Chile, Brazil, and Ecuador have urinary excretion of iodine in excess of recommended levels (>300 µg/L), which is also considered a health hazard (*328*). Universal iodization of salt has been recommended by different international organizations as a public health strategy to prevent iodine deficiency disorders. Although many countries approved legislation for the fortification of salt with iodine in the 1950s and 1960s, a lack of funding for ongoing quality control systems and inadequate equipment used by small entrepreneurs have delayed the execution or limited the sustainability of these efforts over time.

Although zinc deficiency is difficult to diagnose, using intake estimates and the prevalence of growth retardation it has been estimated that 20% of the population in the Americas is zinc deficient. Based on these Regional estimates, Guatemala, Ecuador, and Honduras have the highest prevalence of zinc deficiency (≥30%), followed by Nicaragua, Peru, and Bolivia, with prevalence rates around 20% and 30% (*321*).

Tackling the Epidemic of Nutrition-related Chronic Diseases in the Americas

Noncommunicable diseases are the leading cause of ill health and death in the Americas. Obesity stands as the most visible and serious risk factor for developing other noncommunicable diseases. Several national surveys in Latin America (*329–331*) and the Caribbean (*332*) show that about 50% to 60% of adult men and women are overweight and obese, similar to the levels seen in the United States (*333*). Moreover, 7% to 12% of children under 5 years old are obese, which represents six times the current percentage of acute malnutrition for that age group. In Mexico and Chile, recent national surveys show that about 15% of adolescents are obese.

Most Latin American and Caribbean countries are experiencing a significant shift in their dietary patterns characterized by a decreased consumption of fruits, vegetables, whole grains, cereals, and legumes and a parallel increased consumption of foods rich in saturated fat, sugars, and salt, such as milk, meats, refined cereals, and processed foods (*334*). These dietary pattern changes have occurred alongside a decrease in levels of physical activity in the population. Between 30% and 60% of the Region's population does not engage in the minimum recommended level of physical activity (*335*). Physical inactivity increases with urbanization and age, and is most prevalent among women. Physical inactivity not only contributes to the development of noncommunicable diseases, but also can lead to mental illness, stress accumulation, lower school achievement, and poor social interactions.

A decreased consumption of fruits, vegetables, whole grains, cereals, and legumes, and an increased consumption of energy-dense foods, are influenced by several factors, including urbanization, as well as cost and availability of various foods and taste preferences. These factors, coupled with intense and highly targeted marketing and advertising, have contributed to a mass consumption of pre-packaged foods and soft drinks, and to eating out, so common in most cities today. In fact, changing food preferences are part of a larger phenomenon, labeled as "diet transition," which is fueled by higher salaries in cities, time constraints, changes in prices, and ongoing innovations in food technology and distribution systems (*336*). At the same time the production, availability, and cost of fruits, legumes, vegetables, and cereals have been harmed by this diet transition.

Environmental factors are a powerful influence on individual behaviors, and economic, marketing, and cultural dynamics strongly shape population eating patterns and preferences. Urban design, motorized transportation, and safety influence physical activity patterns and, therefore, must be addressed to ensure that healthy choices become the easiest choices. An environmental approach is becoming a pillar in current public health efforts to tackle the epidemic of noncommunicable diseases (*336–339*).

Human behavior responds to a variety of factors, not merely to good information or education. Individuals generally consider health issues as one of many factors in deciding what to eat, whether to exercise, or whether to quit smoking. Competing factors include short-term ones such as convenience, time, and price (*340*). Considering this, the goal is to create enabling environments, so that it is easy to make healthy choices. Enabling environments include institutional set-ups in the workplace and in school, regulations, social norms, prices, taxation, and various incentives. Therefore, public health strategists must consider all factors that lead people to make healthy choices. An enabling environment is all the more important given that impoverished populations in the Americas are the ones who bear the greatest burden of noncommunicable diseases and the ones with the lowest rates of good dietary and physical activity practices. This is true among less developed (*341*) and among developed countries in the Region (*342*).

COPING WITH DISASTERS

The years between 2001 and 2005 were characterized by many disasters worldwide: the 2005 hurricane season that buffeted the Caribbean, Central America, and North America, and the tsunami and earthquake in South Asia, are examples of some of the most devastating disasters in the period.

The Americas constitutes one of the world's regions most exposed to natural disasters, and this vulnerability increases the potential risk of destructive effects caused by events of any nature. It is estimated that every year an average of 130 natural disasters of varying degrees of magnitude occur in the Region, and the impact of these destructive phenomena in 2001–2005 has left a toll of some 20,000 deaths, 28 million victims, and US$ 210 billion in property losses in the Americas (*343*).

At-risk Populations: Damages and Death Rates

In 2005, approximately 78.8% of the population in the Region lived in large urban centers (*344, 345*) characterized by a lack of appropriate urban planning and a meager capacity in both public and private institutions for risk reduction and management. In the case of poverty stricken or socially excluded populations, their levels of vulnerability increase on a day-to-day basis due to a scarcity of resources, a lack of suitable locations for their dwellings— which are frequently poorly built or do not follow appropriate construction standards—as well as a lack of access to basic health care services.

The exposure levels of the population to threats are increasingly more difficult to determine. Nevertheless, it is estimated that approximately 73% of the population[15] and 67% of health clinics and hospitals[16] in 18 of the Region's countries[17] are located in high risk areas. This means that in the event of a disaster, millions of people and thousands of health care facilities will be exposed to potential destruction. This, in turn, could create obstacles that prevent the flow of services in disaster situations, increasing the population's vulnerability.

In 2001–2005 the estimated damages attributed to disasters in the Region exceeded US$ 216 billion, or several times the total gross domestic product of many of the Region's countries.[18] Based on this estimate, 90% of the figure[19] represented estimated damages from disasters in countries such as Canada and the United States, and 10% represented damages in developing countries. The economic impact from each disaster event is proportionate to infrastructure losses in the affected countries. In 2005, for example, hurricanes were responsible for 2,900 deaths, 3 million victims, and approximately US$ 180 billion in economic losses in the Region. Hurricanes Stan and Wilma together struck Cuba, Guatemala, Honduras, Jamaica, Mexico, Nicaragua, and South Florida in the United States, with losses totaling US$ 3.6 billion. Hurricane Katrina, which only affected the United States, caused US$ 176.4 billion in losses, or 98% of total economic losses attributed to hurricanes that year.

Taken together, natural disasters in the Americas in 2001– 2005 resulted in 21,500 deaths. It is estimated that hurricanes ac-

---

[15] **Source:** Relevamiento acerca del Estado de Mitigación y Preparativos para Desastres en el Sector Salud. Área de Preparativos en Caso de Emergencias y Desastres de OPS/OMS – March to July 2006.

[16] **Source:** Relevamiento acerca del Estado de Mitigación y Preparativos para Desastres en el Sector Salud. Área de Preparativos en Caso de Emergencias y Desastres de OPS/OMS – March to July 2006.

[17] The countries included are: Anguilla, Argentina, the Bahamas, Belize, Chile, Colombia, Costa Rica, the Dominican Republic, Ecuador, El Salvador, French Guiana, Guadeloupe, Guatemala, Haiti, Honduras, Martinique, Nicaragua, and the Turks and Caicos Islands.

[18] This amount represents 22 times Bolivia's gross domestic product and 27 times Honduras'.

[19] **Source:** EM-DAT (CRED) – www.em-dat.net.

counted for 25.7% of the total number of natural disasters for the period, affecting 56%[20] of the countries of the Region and causing 28.5% of the total number of deaths attributed to natural disasters (6,131 deaths). The destructive power of this force became evident during the 2005 hurricane season in the Caribbean and the United States. Floods followed as the next leading cause of fatalities (5,281 deaths), with their maximum impact in Haiti; and earthquakes (1,381 deaths), with the largest number of victims occurring in two disasters in El Salvador (2001) and one in Peru (2001).

Other disasters in the period that together were responsible for 1,328 deaths included droughts (Guatemala, 2001; Paraguay, 2002); extreme temperatures (cold waves in Argentina, 2001; Mexico, 2002, 2003, 2004; Peru, 2003–2004; heat waves in the United States, 2001, 2002, 2005); and mudslides (in Bolivia, 2003; Brazil, 2002; Colombia, 2001, 2002, 2003; Ecuador, 2002; the United States, 2003; Guatemala, 2002, 2003, 2005; Mexico, 2003; Nicaragua, 2004; and Peru, 2001, 2004).

Elsewhere, transport accidents[21] accounted for 21.6% of the total for disasters and caused approximately 16.5% of the total 3,560 deaths attributed to disasters in the Region. Industrial accidents and those linked to urban fires and explosions resulted in 2,310 fatalities in 2001–2005. Several disasters of various and of lesser intensity resulted in 1,509 additional deaths.

Impact of Natural Disasters

Hurricanes

In 2001–2005 there were 175 tropical storms in the Caribbean, Central America, and North America, representing the most frequent disaster event in the period. In 2005 alone there were 28 tropical storms, 14 of which became hurricanes, 4 of them category 5 storms. This was considered the most active hurricane season in history.

The destructive force of Hurricane Ivan (affecting Barbados, the United States, Grenada, Haiti, the Cayman Islands, Jamaica, the Dominican Republic, Trinidad and Tobago, and Venezuela) and Hurricane Jeanne (which struck the United States, Haiti, Puerto Rico, and the Dominican Republic) in 2004 was an indication that these kinds of events were increasing not only in number, as reflected in patterns seen in the last 30 years, but also in intensity. This became evident in 2005 with hurricanes Stan, Katrina, and Wilma.

In the Americas, hurricanes left a toll of 6,131 dead, 3,172 injured, more than 14 million homeless, and approximately US$ 189 billion in losses in 2001–2005. The greatest devastation was recorded in Haiti, with 2,809 deaths and economic losses of approximately US$ 21 million. These figures are even more devastating when seen in the context of the country's current vulnerability and risk level.

Disasters occurred in areas previously stricken, such as when Wilma devastated Cancún and struck the Maya Riviera in Mexico after Hurricane Emily already had hit those areas in July 2005. Similarly, Hurricane Stan exacerbated damages already caused in El Salvador, Guatemala, Mexico, and, to a lesser extent, in Honduras and Nicaragua. The two latter countries also were affected weeks later by hurricanes Alfa and Beta. Grenada was devastated by hurricanes Ivan (2004) and Emily (2005), with 40 deaths and approximately 60,000 victims.

The Extraordinary Impact of Katrina

Hurricane Katrina (346), which made landfall on the Gulf Coast of North America on August 29, 2005, packing 128 km/hour winds, became the most devastating and costly natural disaster in United States history. The damage inflicted on the city of New Orleans alone amounted to US$ 176 billion in economic losses and severe damages to the social and economic infrastructures. The National Flood Insurance Program paid out more than US$ 15.3 billion to hurricane victims who had flood insurance. This amount exceeded the combined total for the 37 years that the program has been in existence.

After an initial delayed response, the weeks-long recovery mobilization was unprecedented in the country. In the aftermath of Hurricane Katrina, some 275,000 citizens in the states of Alabama, Louisiana, Mississippi, and Texas required housing in temporary shelters. The Federal Emergency Management Agency (FEMA) relocated tens of thousands of homeless persons to hotel and motel rooms, while attempts were made to find better housing arrangements for the victims. The official death toll reported was 1,322, but investigations by the U.S. Congress indicated that the toll could have been even higher given the lack of planning and initiative, and a meager capacity to respond to large scale and devastating events.

The health care system in the affected areas was seriously overburdened as demand suddenly spiked and equipment, supplies, and the health services network sustained damages or were disabled. At least 215 people died in extended care facilities and patients with special health care needs were not able to get adequate medical attention. The health sector further deteriorated when several hospitals and health care facilities, including Southeast Louisiana Veterans Hospital, had to be completely evacuated because they were located in areas at high risk for flooding or lacked the necessary resources to provide adequate care for their patients.

---

[20]The countries affected by hurricanes in 2001–2005 were: Bahamas, Barbados, Belize, Bermuda, Brazil, Canada, Cayman Islands, Colombia, Costa Rica, Cuba, Dominica, Dominican Republic, El Salvador, Grenada, Guatemala, Haiti, Honduras, Jamaica, Mexico, Nicaragua, Puerto Rico, Saint Lucia, Saint Vincent and the Grenadines, Trinidad and Tobago, Turks and Caicos Islands, the United States, and Venezuela.

[21]Includes land, air, and sea transport accidents that resulted in a massive number of victims.

Flooding and Related Consequences

Floods were the second most frequent disaster to strike the Region in 2001–2005—171 floods, or 25.1% of all the events in the period. In the Americas, 85% of the countries and territories were affected, with 5,283 deaths and more than 260,000 persons left homeless; 90% of the floods occurred after heavy and sustained rains in areas made vulnerable by poor land use, areas close to riverbeds, or because of weak levees, as occurred in New Orleans (United States, 2005) and Santa Fe (Argentina, 2003).

Torrential rains also led to other kinds of events. In 2004, for example, the border area between Haiti and the Dominican Republic was devastated by mud- and rockslides after 10 days of heavy rains. In the Dominican Republic the disaster left a death toll of 688, while in Mapou, a city in Haiti located in a valley surrounded by deforested mountains, the rains produced a river of mud and rock that swept away everything in its path. According to authorities 2,665 people perished. Haiti's long history of natural disasters and its humanitarian and political crises have hindered its development and this in turn has stalled improvements in its population's health conditions.

Earthquakes and Volcanoes

Much of the Americas is located in areas with significant earthquake activity and sporadic volcanic eruptions. In 2001–2005, earthquakes were recorded in Chile, the United States, and Mexico, but the greatest damage was reported in El Salvador and Peru.

At the beginning of 2001, El Salvador suffered two large-scale earthquakes in the span of a few weeks, which left 1,259 dead and 8,122 injured, according to figures compiled by the country's National Emergency Committee. The most damage occurred in the poorest areas of the departments of Cuscatlán, La Paz, Morazán, San Salvador, and San Vicente, and in Las Colinas development in the department of La Libertad.

In Peru, an earthquake measuring 8 points on the Richter Scale, with its epicenter on the country's southern coast, shook a large portion of the Andean region. Despite its magnitude, the earthquake generated comparatively less damage than the one in El Salvador. In the Peruvian cities of Arequipa, Moquegua, Tacna, and Ayacucho 145 people lost their lives; 11 more died in two other earthquakes that struck Peru that same year.

Chile, one of the most earthquake-prone countries on the planet, recorded only one earthquake during the period (in 2005), which measured 7 points on the Richter Scale and whose epicenter was in the province of Taracapá, where 11 people perished.

In the state of Colima, Mexico, a volcano with the same name erupted in 2002, leaving 300 victims. The following year, a violent earthquake shook the same area, destroying hundreds of homes and public facilities, including hospitals, and leaving 29 dead. In Ecuador, the Tungurahua volcano became more active in 2002; it remains active, with phases marked by intense eruptions that by the end of 2005 had affected 174,650 people. Other volcanoes

showing increased activity, although with less damage to the population, were the Fuego (Guatemala, 2002) and Galeras volcanoes (Colombia, 2005). In El Salvador, the Santa Ana volcano spewed incandescent material, gases, and ash that resulted in 2 deaths, 2,000 homeless victims, and several thousands of evacuees in 2005.

Other Disaster Events

Bolivia, Brazil, Cuba, El Salvador, Haiti, Honduras, Mexico, Nicaragua Peru, and the United States experienced droughts during the period. In Guatemala, a prolonged drought affected tens of thousands of people and left a death toll of 42 in 2001. The next year, a large area of Paraguay sustained a drought that resulted in at least 12 deaths. The 2001 drought was attributed to an unusual drop in trade winds that normally arrive at the beginning of April and bring moisture and precipitation from the Pacific Ocean. According to experts, this shift was associated with global atmospheric events, different from those associated with El Niño. The 2001–2002 droughts worsened already difficult conditions in the Region due to the crash in the world price of coffee and other Central American and South American export crops.

For several years, the increasing frequency of extreme temperatures has resulted in hundreds of victims throughout the Americas. Peru was severely affected by cold waves that caused at least 429 deaths in late 2003 and early 2004. In Mexico, 85 deaths between 2002 and 2004 were caused by extreme cold temperatures, whereas in the United States 103 people died from heat waves in 2001, 2002, and 2005.

Impact of Manmade Disasters

The damages resulting from manmade disasters have taken a high toll in human suffering, loss of life, and long-term damage. Fires in urban areas were responsible for 1,557 deaths and thousands of injuries in 2001–2005, including many fires in shopping centers, discothèques, prisons, and hospitals in South America and Central America.

One of the largest fires recorded in the period occurred in Peru on December 29, 2001, at a shopping center in downtown Lima. The conflagration was caused by a chain reaction when tons of fireworks were set off, spreading flames across hundreds of vendor stalls packed together. In a few minutes the fire had engulfed four city blocks in the shopping area, making it impossible for hundreds of vendors and customers to escape. First responders, physicians, nurses, and emergency response teams carried out rescue operations, stabilized the burn victims, and transported the wounded to hospitals, which had been put on red alert by the Ministry of Health. The fire lasted seven hours; 277 bodies were recovered, 117 human remains were taken to the Institute of Forensic Medicine to be identified; 247 victims were hospitalized for burns, asphyxia, and multiple traumas; and the Civil Defense Agency reported 180 missing.

On August 1, 2004, a raging fire broke out in a supermarket in Asunción, Paraguay, spreading quickly and generating panic; the doors in the facility were locked and more than 1,000 people were trapped. Paraguayan authorities reported that in 364 bodies had been found, as well as 42 unidentified human remains; 48 persons were missing and 298 were hospitalized. The leading cause of death in the fire was smoke inhalation, followed by burns.

On December 30, 2004, in Buenos Aires, Argentina, 48 ambulances, 8 firefighting units, 110 Civil Defense teams, and more than 600 personnel including medical staff, paramedics, and volunteers mobilized to rescue, treat, and transport hundreds of victims of a fire at a discothèque where 2,000 young people had gathered. Authorities confirmed that 194 people died and 714 were injured.

In the early morning of July 12, 2005, a fire broke out at a hospital in San José, Costa Rica; 19 people lost their lives, monetary losses reached US$ 17 million, and the hospital (which contained highly sophisticated equipment and 522 beds) was forced to shut down, except for the emergency medical facility that served as a temporary hospital for evacuating patients.

Five fires broke out in prisons in Argentina, the Dominican Republic, and Honduras, leaving a death toll of 387. The two most deadly took place at the prison in Higuey, Dominican Republic, in 2005, with 136 dead, followed by the fire at the prison in San Pedro Sula, Honduras, in 2004, with a toll of 104. During the reporting period several coal mine explosions occurred in Argentina (2004), Colombia (2001), Mexico (2002), and the United States (2001). Two explosions followed by fires occurred at the oil refineries in Campos, Brazil, and in Houston, Texas (United States), in 2001 and 2005, respectively, which caused the deaths of 65 people.

Transport-related accidents[22] accounted for 145 incidents and constituted the third most frequent disaster event in the Region. On September 11, 2001, terrorism was responsible for the attacks on the World Trade Center in New York; the Pentagon in Washington, D.C.; and a rural Pennsylvania area. This event resulted in 2,973 deaths and led to the formulation of policies and international agreements aimed at intensifying security measures, including closely monitoring and restricting financial flows.

Impact of Disasters on the Health Care System

Impact on Health

The damage and disruption produced by catastrophic events can increase the risk of infectious diseases, mainly due to population displacements, overcrowding, a drop in the amount or quality of clean water, disruptions in wastewater and solid waste disposal, inadequate handling of food products, and the health

services network's reduced response capability. Fortunately, no outbreaks of epidemics have resulted from the disasters reported in the Region; overall, the countries have responded, particularly their health sectors, and they have succeeded in adequately controlling potential risk factors.

One of the priorities established was to attend to the health needs of the victim population, particularly by providing care, early detection, and timely treatment for cases of dengue, typhoid fever, malaria, cholera, gastroenteritis, leptospirosis, Chagas' disease, and hepatitis A, mainly to flood stricken communities (*347*) and in endemic areas in Belize and Nicaragua.

The damaging effects on mental health were evident in every disaster. In El Salvador, the two closely spaced, large earthquakes and the scores of aftershocks that followed affected the population's mental health. In the ensuing weeks, more than 8,000 medical consultations for depression and anxiety disorders were reported in the country.

Impact on the Health Services Infrastructure

Many health care facilities sustained structural damage and damage to their equipment and operations. In addition to their direct damages, many health care facilities had great difficulty in providing medical treatment because of the disruption of public utilities, including electricity, water, communications, sewage, solid waste management, and hospital care services; damaged roads also impaired access in some cases. The increased demand for medical treatment in a catastrophic event's aftermath had to be diverted to hospitals or other health care facilities in unaffected areas, and this, in turn, had medium- and long-term consequences for the health care services networks (*348*).

In 2001–2005, more than 100 hospitals and at least 1,000 health care centers in the Region suffered damages as a result of natural disasters. For example, in El Salvador 19 hospitals (63% of the national capacity) were damaged during the 2001 earthquakes, 4 of which had to be completely evacuated; after several years, medical services were still being provided in makeshift facilities and tents. Other earthquakes in Costa Rica's southern Pacific (Golfito) and central Pacific (Parrita) regions in 2003 and 2004, respectively, damaged two clinics and various child nutrition centers. In the region of Siquirres, Costa Rica (2005), at least 16 clinics and some primary care centers suffered equipment losses as well as various other kinds of damage.

In Jamaica, during Hurricane Ivan (2004), 124 (36%) of the approximately 343 health care centers suffered various kinds of damages. The Ministry of Health kept 93% (319) of the medical centers operating, while the remaining 7% (24) of the centers and 35% of the public hospitals were shut down either because they were severely damaged or because the access roads to them were damaged.

As hurricanes Frances, Ivan, and Jeanne swept through the city of Gonaïves, on Haiti's northern coast, parts of the city were subjected to a torrential mudslide and flooding that raised the

---

[22]Includes land, air, and sea transport accidents with a massive number of victims.

water level to 3 m, which put the main hospital in the city of La Providence out of service. All health care facilities in Grenada were unable to operate after Hurricane Ivan in 2004. In May 2004, in the city of Santa Fe, Argentina, the Dr. Orlando Alassia Children's Hospital and the Vera Candioti Rehabilitation Hospital sustained the most severe damage, remaining submerged for several days. Shutting down these two specialized hospitals lost 170 beds (13% of the available beds in the affected area). In addition, 14 other primary health care facilities were partially flooded.

Disasters and large-scale medical emergencies can create chaos in a country's health care system; they also can create opportunities for implementing risk-reduction measures and improving disaster preparedness, however. Such was the case with the Benjamín Bloom Children's Hospital in El Salvador, which, after suffering damages from a severe earthquake in 1986, was repaired in accordance with earthquake-resistant construction standards. In 2001, the hospital suffered only minor damage, and was operating at its maximum capacity immediately after the earthquakes struck that year, serving as a referral center and treating patients from more than 19 other damaged facilities.

Overall Risk Patterns

Indiscriminate and intense exploitation of natural resources, pronounced land degradation, and deforestation have adversely affected the capabilities of ecosystems to regenerate and offset direct and indirect human activity (*349*). Moreover, such factors as inadequate urban planning, increased migration from rural areas to large cities, poor handling of hazardous substances, and the increase in the number of poor populations have brought low-income populations to live in at-risk areas. As a result, adverse events wreaked greater destruction in 2001–2005.

Hurricane-related disasters increased 80%, although the number of destructive hurricanes only increased by 14% in 2001–2005 (25 hurricanes and 88 disasters) compared with 1996–2000 (22 hurricanes and 49 disasters). Floods increased by 48%, from 113 (1996–2000) to 168 (2001–2005). Manmade disasters (technological and transportation-related accidents) showed a slight increase, continuing with the trend of the last 30 years.

There is international consensus that the increase in the number of disasters presents a challenge that nations must face with additional and better tools, if they are to reduce risks and improve response capabilities. More than a decade after the International Conference on Disaster Mitigation for Health Care Facilities was held in Mexico in 1996, at least 21 countries in the Americas have conducted risk assessments, while many others have implemented risk-reduction measures in health care facilities to address natural disasters.

The ministers of health assessed the damage inflicted by the disasters on health services and agreed, in September 2004, that all hospitals currently in operation needed to be structurally reinforced, while new facilities would have to be designed and built in a way that would ensure that they could remain operational during disasters. This agreement signaled the beginning of a Regional policy initiative of "safe hospitals" that was ratified and supported by more than 169 countries at the Global Conference on Disaster Reduction in 2005. The agreement stipulates that each country should maintain a national safe hospitals policy, and a target date of 2015 was set to ensure that newly built hospitals be disaster proof and that current health care facilities be structurally reinforced, especially those that provide primary care.

Conclusions

The Region's population as a civic society needs to address its own vulnerabilities as it grapples with an increasing number of disasters (*350, 351*).

Evidence gathered in the last few years related to disasters shows an increasing pattern of natural events and those caused by human activity. Some of the leading causes of this pattern include climate change, technology development, inappropriate exploitation of natural resources, and an increase in low-income human settlements in areas considered at risk.

Addressing risk is a complicated issue that requires complex and comprehensive measures. Managing disaster risks in the Americas should include measures that range from political and economic issues to biodiversity and environmental protection. Risk management, the determination of threats, and risk assessments are crucial steps for developing the policies, strategies, plans, and programs required for managing risks and coping with disasters that involve a wider participation of public and private institutions and the voice of the affected communities. In addressing current risks, the nations and territories of the Americas should review and update their multisectoral and sectoral plans, train the population and response teams located in the areas potentially at risk, and ensure the availability of financial and material resources required to implement risk-reduction measures, humanitarian assistance, and early recovery.

The vast experience within the Region in coping with natural and human-caused disasters has shown that there are no shortcuts that can lead to successful disaster reduction. Rather, this long process is linked to sustainable development. Countries must follow an approach in which the progress in disaster reduction is attained when it is understood that managing disasters requires taking responsibility for development and planning. This, in turn, requires interdisciplinary efforts and a shared commitment by all of civil society.

In a framework of Pan-American solidarity, almost every country and ministry of health of the Americas has adopted formal measures aimed at continuously improving risk-reduction and disaster-preparedness measures. As a result, countries have generated the capabilities to respond to minor and moderate disasters. It will be necessary to constantly reinforce that capability, however, and obtain the necessary political commitment to coordinate the health care sector and other key actors and, thus, be

TABLE 28. Estimates of the indigenous population, total and as a percentage of the total population, selected countries, Region of the Americas.

Percentage of total population	Total indigenous population		
	<100,000	100,000 to 500,000	>500,000
More than 40			Peru Guatemala Bolivia Ecuador
5–40	Guyana Belize Suriname	El Salvador Nicaragua Panama	Mexico Chile Honduras
Under 5	Costa Rica French Guiana Jamaica Dominica	Argentina Brazil Paraguay Venezuela	Canada Colombia United States of America

Note: The table refers to official national statistics showing indigenous peoples as majorities " or "minorities"; however, there may be pockets within countries where indigenous populations comprise a majority in that area that are not reflected in the national figures.

Sources: Reports on the Evaluation of the International Decade of the Indigenous Peoples of the World, PAHO, 2004. Hall G, Patrinos AH. Indigenous Peoples, Poverty and Human Development in Latin America: 1994–2004. Washington, DC: World Bank, 2005. Montenegro R, Stephens C. Indigenous Health in Latin America and the Caribbean [Indigenous Health 2]. Lancet 2006;367:1859–69.

able to address unforeseen circumstances and large scale disasters. In this way not only will they be able to respond and provide humanitarian assistance, but also to reduce the potential risk of emergencies and disasters.

HEALTH OF SPECIAL GROUPS

INDIGENOUS PEOPLES

Between 45 million and 50 million indigenous people belonging to more than 600 ethnic groups live in the Americas today,[23] comprising almost 10% of the total population and 40% of the rural population of Latin America and the Caribbean (*352–355*). Indigenous peoples add much vitality and diversity to the 24 countries of the Region in which they live, and are the repositories of much of the Americas' cultural heritage and biodiversity (Table 28) (*352*). Despite their historic presence and invaluable contributions, indigenous peoples are highly vulnerable in the countries where they live, and their human rights, as well as their

[23] ILO Convention 169, Article 1, concerning Indigenous and Tribal Peoples in Independent Countries (1989), recognizes as indigenous that distinct section of the national community which is understood to consist of: "... peoples in independent countries who are regarded as indigenous on account of their descent from the populations which inhabited the country, or a geographical region to which the country belongs, at the time of conquest or colonization or the establishment of present state boundaries and who, irrespective of their legal status, retain some or all of their own social, economic, cultural, and political institutions." The concept of a *people* refers to the set of traits that characterize a human group in territorial, historical, cultural, and ethnic terms and give it a sense of identity.

social, political, and economic equality, are often compromised or denied. As a result, pervasive inequities exist in the living conditions, health status, and health service coverage of indigenous peoples as compared to the rest of the population (Table 29) (*352–356*).

The incidence of poverty and extreme poverty is much higher among indigenous peoples in the Americas than among non-indigenous groups. In Bolivia and Guatemala, for instance, more than half of the total population is poor, but almost three-quarters of the indigenous population is poor. Of all poor households in Peru, 43% are indigenous (*353*). Poverty is intertwined with other compounding factors, such as significantly higher illiteracy and unemployment rates, lack of access to or availability of social services, violations of human rights, displacements due to armed conflicts, and environmental degradation. In indigenous municipalities in Mexico, the rate of illiteracy is 43%, more than three-fold that of the national average; the rate is more than 60% among indigenous women (*353, 357*). High levels of toxic contaminants have been recorded in several indigenous communities. In Canada's Arctic regions, studies of infant development among the Nunavik have linked deficits in immune function, an increase in childhood respiratory infections, and low birthweight to prenatal exposure to organochlorides (*358, 359*).

Traditionally, indigenous populations have suffered from disproportionately high rates of maternal and infant mortality, malnutrition, and infectious diseases. The maternal mortality ratio in Guatemala, a country with 42% indigenous population, is among the highest in Latin America, and it is higher still among

155

TABLE 29. Inequities affecting indigenous populations in terms of the Millennium Development Goals, selected countries, Region of the Americas.

Issue	Country	Indigenous	Nonindigenous
1. Poverty	Canada Chile	34% (2004) 32.2% (2000)	16% (2004) 20.1% (2000)
2. Illiteracy	Bolivia	19.61% (2001)	4.5% (2001) (2001 census)
3. Gender equity and women's independence	Guatemala	Illiteracy among indigenous women is between 50% and 90%, and only 43% finish elementary school, 5.8% finish high school, and 1% get a higher education (2001).	
4. Infant mortality	Panama	Bocas del Toro 37.6; Darién 29.2; Comarca Nögbe-Buglé 27.9/1,000 live births (2003)	15.2/1,000 live births 2003
5. Maternal mortality	Honduras	255/100,000 live births (Intibuca)	147/100,000 live births (data from the 2004 Honduras report)
6. Fight against malaria, HIV/AIDS, and other diseases	Nicaragua	90% of the cases of malaria by *P. falciparum* are concentrated in 24 municipalities with indigenous populations.	
7. Environmental sustainability and nutritional status	El Salvador	95% of surface water sources are contaminated; malnutrition in children and adults is associated with parasites; 40% of indigenous children suffer malnutrition, compared to 20% nationally.	
8. Fostering of a global partnership for development		The presence of similar problems among indigenous peoples (i.e., similar epidemiological profiles, refugees' status, lifestyle changes, acculturation, lags in development, loss of territory), particularly those living in border areas, makes it critical to coordinate work towards development and application of international and subregional agreements.	

Note: This table responds to the need for applying the content of the Millennium Development Goals to the realities of indigenous peoples and shows the burden of disease and inequity that affects them in the Americas. Real compliance with these statements, as is called for by the indigenous leaders, will require that indigenous peoples' views, such as those about poverty, alliance, and development, be taken into consideration.

Source: Data provided by the countries participating in the national evaluation of health achievements within the framework of the International Decade of Indigenous Peoples of the World, PAHO, 2004.

indigenous women. Actually, the latter is three times (211 per 100,000 live births) the rate of non-indigenous mothers (70 per 100,000 live births), according to the Baseline Maternal Mortality study for 2000 (*360, 361*). In Bolivia, the average infant mortality rate is 102 per 1,000 live births in 51 rural municipalities with more than 50% native monolingual women, or more than twice the rate of 54 per 1,000 live births for the general population (*362*). Malnutrition among indigenous children in the northern part of Argentina is the leading cause of morbidity and mortality; 80% of the cases of child malnutrition are due to parasitosis linked to precarious environmental sanitation conditions (*352*). In Mexico, mortality rates from pulmonary tuberculosis among the indigenous population are twice those in the general population (*363*), and in Canada, the tuberculosis rate is 8 to 10 times higher than the national average (*352*).

In Nicaragua 90% of the cases of malaria by *Plasmodium falciparum* are concentrated in 24 municipalities with indigenous populations. In 2002, in Brazil's Special Indigenous Health Districts, respiratory diseases were the second leading cause of health services demand. Moreover, 81.5% of deaths from pneumonia affected children under 5 years of age and 48.2%, children under 1 year of age, showing the importance of this disease in infant mortality among Brazil's indigenous population (*352*).

As these populations become increasingly more mobile, less isolated, more urban, and more likely to reside in border areas, chronic disease and such issues as drug and alcohol use, suicide, sexually transmitted diseases, and the loss of influence of traditional health practices become increasingly important. In 1999, a study that included data from population censuses, interviews, clinical data, and biochemical evaluations was conducted among

80 men and 71 women in selected Guaraní-Mbyá communities (Sapukai, Paraty-Mirim, and Araponga) in the state of Rio de Janeiro, Brazil; the prevalence of selected risk factors in the overall sample was as follows for the three communities, respectively: hypertension (4.8%, 2.6%, and 7.4%); overweight (26.7%, 19.5%, and 34.8%); high total cholesterol levels (2.8%, 2.7%, and 2.9%); and increased triglyceride levels (12.6%, 9.5%, and 15.9%). All prevalence rates were higher among women and at older ages. Results suggest that Guaraní communities have a moderate risk of chronic diseases and that measures to reduce these risk factors should be adopted (*364*). Furthermore, although the prevalence of cardiovascular diseases has been declining in Canada, there are data to suggest that the cardiovascular disease rates are increasing among aboriginal people in that country. In a study conducted among randomly selected participants from a comprehensive list of 301 Six Nations Band members and 326 people of European origin, it was reported that aboriginal people had significantly more carotid atherosclerosis than individuals of European descent. These problems were linked to higher rates of smoking, glucose intolerance, obesity, abdominal obesity, and substantially higher concentrations of fibrinogen and plasminogen activator inhibitor-1, and to significantly higher rates of unemployment and a lower annual household income (*365*).

Available data on alcohol consumption among indigenous peoples in Latin America and the Caribbean are limited, but sufficient to show the severity of the problem. In Peru, a 2000 study conducted in several Aymara altiplano communities of Puno and Shipibo Amazonian communities reported that alcohol consumption was predominant among males, and associated with aggressive behavior towards their wives, children, and other close relatives (*366*). Several reports suggest growing alcohol consumption among the urban indigenous population. Particularly troubling is the increase in alcoholism among indigenous women in special situations, such as widowhood, abandonment, uprooting, and solitude (*367–369*).

In recent decades, the Garífunas' search for work has increasingly taken them to the Honduran cities of La Ceiba or San Pedro Sula, and even to New York, Los Angeles, and New Orleans; even London now has a Garífuna community. This diaspora intensified in the 1990s, as foreign and domestic investors bought up Garífuna property for tourism development. The cumulative rate of AIDS among the Garífunas in Honduras is nearly 15 times the national rate. More than 8% of adult Garífunas test HIV positive, four times higher than the national average (*370*).

The increasing number of suicides among young indigenous people in Colombia's northwest is generating much concern in the United Nations Refugee Agency (UNHCR) and indigenous people organizations. In a little over a year, 17 young Embera and Wounaan people 12 to 24 years old committed suicide or attempted to commit suicide. According to the indigenous organization CAMIZBA (Asociación de Cabildos Mayores Indígenas del Bajo Atrato, composed of 25 communities of the Wounaan, Embera, Katío, Tule, and Chamí peoples), young indigenous peo-

ple are losing "the desire for life" due to the effect that the Colombian conflict has had on their communities (*371*).

Approximately 30 years ago, lobster and shrimp commercial fishing began in the Atlantic Coast of Honduras and Nicaragua (*372–374*). The endeavor is performed under precarious conditions without proper diving gear, and it has resulted in a high rate of disability and death among adolescent and young adult Miskitos, and in social problems and an ecological imbalance created by indiscriminate lobster fishing (*373–375*). The age of those suffering from decompression disease was found to be 20–41 years (*376*).

Although the burden of disease and the transitional-stage epidemiological profile of indigenous peoples are similar to those of other disadvantaged groups in the Region, the poor health status of the former is compounded by discrimination and inequity within the health system. Part of the challenge in offsetting these disparities is to better link the indigenous health system and its multiple health agents and practices with public health services offered by the governments. These communities depend upon traditional and spiritual healers to promote health, prevent illness, and provide treatment for common conditions; they are often the only health care provider available on a continuing basis (*352*).

Gender inequalities also are present, and indigenous women in particular face challenges in obtaining quality health care for reproductive health. For example, the prevalence rate of contraceptive use among indigenous women in Guatemala is 10%, whereas the national average is 40%. In that same country, 41% of deliveries are assisted by trained health personnel at the national level; the rates are 57% among non-indigenous women and 16.4% among indigenous women (*360, 361, 377*).

Although low-quality health services are present in many developing country contexts, the weaknesses are more acute in areas inhabited by indigenous peoples. Persistent issues of poor quality in service provision, such as limited staff competency, noncompliance with evidence-based treatment protocols, medication shortages, and low staff retention rates, are common in many of the remote locations in which indigenous peoples live. Additionally, geographic barriers prevent these populations from gaining access to health care, due to distance, means and affordability of transportation, and seasonal geographic isolation. Although health care services are largely free to indigenous peoples, the real cost of care, including out-of-pocket expenses related to transportation, food, accommodation, family care, medication, and loss of workdays, pose a challenge to their access to health care (*352, 378–380*).

Cultural barriers are the most complicated challenge, since there is little understanding of the social and cultural factors deriving from the knowledge, attitudes, and practices in health of indigenous peoples. The bias of Western medicine and intervention can be offensive or inappropriate for traditional medicine practitioners. Finding health staff that speak and understand indigenous languages is difficult, and poor communication between providers and clients at all levels compromises access to quality

BOX 5. International Labor Organization Convention (No. 169) Concerning Indigenous and Tribal Peoples in Independent Countries

Part V. Social and Health Security

Article 24

Social security schemes shall be extended progressively to cover the peoples concerned, and applied without discrimination against them.

Article 25

1. Governments shall ensure that adequate health services are made available to the peoples concerned, or shall provide them with resources to allow them to design and deliver such services under their own responsibility and control, so that they may enjoy the highest attainable standard of physical and mental health.

2. Health services shall, to the extent possible, be community-based. These services shall be planned and administered in co-operation with the peoples concerned and take into account their economic, geographic, social and cultural conditions as well as their traditional preventive care, healing practices and medicines.

3. The health care system shall give preference to the training and employment of local community health workers, and focus on primary health care while maintaining strong links with other levels of health care services.

4. The provision of such health services shall be co-coordinated with other social, economic and cultural measures in the country.

Source: International Labor Organization. International Labor Norms. C169 Indigenous and Tribal Peoples Convention, 1989 [Internet site]. Available at http://www.ilo.org/ilolex/cgi.lex/convde.pl?C169.

care. Moreover, indigenous people are often discriminated against in health centers by non-indigenous staff, and both fear and distrust caused by the attitudes and behaviors of health care workers prevent indigenous people from seeking the health care they need (*381, 382*). For example, traditional beliefs and practices related to childbirth are frequently not respected in institutional settings (*383, 384*). At the policy level, lack of vital statistics or breakdown by ethnic groups, gender, and age makes the generation of evidence-based policies and managerial processes more difficult. An analysis presented by the Economic Commission for Latin America and the Caribbean indicates that 13 out of the 24 countries with indigenous populations that have conducted population censuses in recent years have incorporated questions designed to identify indigenous populations. Furthermore, 10 countries of the Region have already processed their most recent censuses, and relevant studies on indigenous populations are being carried out (*385*). In terms of vital and service coverage statistics, although studies and estimates have been carried out, there is not an adequate characterization of the indigenous peoples of the Region, and certainly not a reliable system of information, monitoring, and evaluation of their health conditions (*352*).

National policies and international agreements guide some countries in their development of indigenous-focused programs and designate funding specifically for indigenous social services.

Argentina, Bolivia, Brazil, Colombia, Costa Rica, Chile, Ecuador, Guatemala, Guyana, Mexico, Nicaragua, Panama, Paraguay, Peru, and Venezuela have included an acknowledgment of diversity in their Constitutions. The promotion of indigenous people's health and the incorporation of indigenous traditional medicine into national health systems is part of the national legislation of Argentina, Bolivia, Brazil, Colombia, Ecuador, Mexico, Nicaragua, Panama, Peru, and Venezuela (*386*). Most countries report that they have technical units devoted to indigenous health affairs within their ministries of health and that they have national programs or projects in place regarding the health of indigenous peoples. However, the implementation of these policies and experiences is largely uncoordinated and does not include consistent indigenous participation in the formation or implementation of these efforts as stated, for instance, by Convention 169 of the International Labor Organization (Box 5) (*369*). A lack of communication, as well as the fragmentation or duplication of efforts at every level, impedes the dissemination of lessons learned and restricts the systematization and use of information to deliver end products to society. In addition, issues such as collective property rights, patents, biodiversity protection, and conservation have not been adequately addressed (*352*).

Aware of health disparities, in 2000, the Region's countries committed themselves to reducing gaps through the achievement

BOX 6. Objectives of the Second International Decade of the World's Indigenous Peoples

(1) Promoting nondiscrimination and inclusion of indigenous peoples in the design, implementation, and evaluation of international, regional, and national processes regarding laws, policies, resources, programs, and projects.

(2) Promoting full and effective participation of indigenous peoples in decisions which directly or indirectly affect their lifestyles, traditional lands, and territories, their cultural integrity as indigenous peoples with collective rights or any other aspect of their lives, considering the principle of free, prior, and informed consent.

(3) Redefining development policies that depart from a vision of equity and that are culturally appropriate, including respect for the cultural and linguistic diversity of indigenous peoples.

(4) Adopting targeted policies, programs, projects, and budgets for the development of indigenous peoples, including concrete benchmarks, with particular emphasis on indigenous women, children, and youth.

(5) Developing strong monitoring mechanisms and enhancing accountability at the international, regional, and particularly the national level, regarding the implementation of legal, policy, and operational frameworks for the protection of indigenous peoples and the improvement of their lives.

Source: United Nations Permanent Forum on Indigenous Issues. Second International Decade of the World's Indigenous People [Internet site]. Available at: http://www.un.org/esa/socdev/unpfii/en/second.html.

of the Millennium Development Goals (MDGs). However, evaluations in the Americas and recent projections show that although there have been some gains in the health sector, expected results will not be reached in time nor in form, especially among indigenous populations, unless certain current strategies are reoriented. For instance, poverty reduction and economic development strategies do not consider indigenous identities, world views, and cultures; the right to self-determination; the right of indigenous peoples to control their territories and resources; and the indigenous peoples' holistic perspective of health. Currently, the assessment of progress toward the MDGs is based on averages, not on disaggregated data; progress (or lack thereof) of indigenous populations is, therefore, lost in the calculations (*387*).

In December 2004, the General Assembly of the United Nations Permanent Forum of Indigenous Issues adopted a resolution for a Second International Decade of the World's Indigenous Peoples (2005–2015). The decade's goal is to further strengthen international cooperation for solving problems faced by indigenous peoples in such areas as culture, education, health, human rights, the environment, and economic and social development, through action-oriented programs and specific projects, increased technical assistance, and relevant standard-setting activities (Box 6) (*388*).

In acknowledging the priorities of indigenous peoples, PAHO and the Member Countries have recognized the urgent need to move forward with innovative and respectful ways of working with indigenous representatives and to show clear results that can demonstrate the reduction of the burden of disease and disability, and of barriers of access to quality health care for indigenous communities. This process will adhere to along the following 2007–2011 strategic lines of action (*389*): 1) to ensure that indigenous perspectives will be incorporated into the attainment of the MDGs and national health policies; 2) to improve information and knowledge management on indigenous health issues to strengthen regional and national evidence-based decision-making and monitoring capabilities; 3) to integrate the intercultural approach into the national health systems of the Region as part of the primary health care strategy; and 4) to develop strategic alliances with indigenous peoples and other key stakeholders to further advance the health of indigenous peoples.

AFRO-DESCENDANT POPULATIONS

The Region of the Americas is enriched by its great ethnic and cultural diversity, inherited from its sociological and historic processes of conquest, colonialism, and immigration. In addition to the indigenous populations analyzed in the previous section, an estimated 250 million Afro-descendants live in the Americas. Afro-descendants make up more than 45% of the population of the English-speaking Caribbean, Brazil, Haiti, and the Dominican Republic. Brazil has the largest Afro-descendant population in the Region, with an official count of roughly 75 million persons; the United States is home to 36 million Afro-descendants (12.9% of the population); and Colombia has approximately 8 million (23%).

TABLE 30. Household type, by ethnic group and sex of household head, Brazil, 2001.

Type of household	Households headed by an Afro-descendant (%)			Other households (%)		
	Males	Females	Total	Males	Females	Total
Single-person homes	6.8	15.6	8.9	6.0	23.4	10.3
Two-parent nuclear families	71.8	7.2	56.2	76.7	7.8	59.8
Single-parent nuclear families	1.8	39.0	10.8	1.7	38.7	10.8
Extended and mixed families	19.5	38.1	24.0	15.7	30.1	19.2
Total	100	100	100	100	100	100

Source: Data from Pesquisa Nacional por Amostra de Domicilios (household survey) 2001. Developed by PAHO.

Despite its size, this segment of the population has been socially invisible since the independence era, due to characteristics such as its high rate of urbanization and the loss, in most countries, of a linguistic identity. Most countries have not had specific data on their Afro-descendant populations. Thanks to efforts launched at the beginning of the 1990s with the support of financial institutions and United Nations agencies, a handful of countries (Brazil, Costa Rica, Colombia,[24] Ecuador, Guatemala, Honduras, and Trinidad and Tobago) have designated Afro-descendants as an ethnic category in statistical sources. Disaggregated information from the aforementioned countries' censuses and household surveys can be used to analyze the living and health conditions of this population group. In the future, this will make it possible to monitor the extent to which policies improve the quality of life of Afro-descendants.

PAHO's analysis of the aforementioned statistical information confirms that Afro-descendants in South America live in high-risk conditions similar to those affecting indigenous communities. In Ecuador, for example, 52% of Afro-descendants live in poverty, which is similar to poverty rates in the indigenous population. In Brazil, 52% of Afro-Brazilians are poor, compared to 26% of the general population. In Colombia, indigenous people suffer the highest rates of poverty and indigence, followed by the Afro-Colombian population (*390*). Importantly, the poverty distribution by ethnicity is coupled with gender-based differences in household structure. Female-headed extended families are overrepresented in the Afro-descendant population (Table 30).

This situation, which is common to this population group in several countries, points up the great social exclusion that Afro-descendants have endured for centuries, which affects all aspects of life, and is manifested in other indicators. For example, in Ecuador, 78% of Afro-descendant males and 80% of females 15–19 years old have completed six years of schooling, compared to 87% of their peers in non-ethnic groups. In Brazil, this gap is even wider. For the same age group, only 56.2% and 66% of Afro-descendant males and females, respectively, have completed six

years of school, compared to 80.9% of males and 85.2% of females in the rest of the population.

The situation of Afro-descendants in Central America is not quite so dire. In Honduras, Afro-descendants[25] account for 5% of the total population; they live primarily in cities along the Atlantic Coast, including Tela, La Ceiba, Puerto Cortes, and Puerto Castilla. In Honduras, poverty, as measured by unmet basic needs, is less severe among Afro-descendants than indigenous people: 42% of Afro-Hondurans have one or more unmet basic needs, compared to 78% among the indigenous population. Educational attainment, as measured by the percentage of youth 15–19 years old who have completed six years of school, is also higher in the Afro-descendant population than in the indigenous population or the rest of the population (Figure 30).

There is a lack of data in regard to health indicators, because up until very recently the countries' health information systems did not record the ethnic origin of Afro-descendants. As a result, the data cannot be disaggregated. Studies that draw on other sources reveal significant disparities in living conditions and access to services to the detriment of Afro-descendants.[26]

With regard to infant mortality, the rate in the Afro-descendant population in Ecuador is higher (32.6 deaths per 1,000 live births) than that in the non-ethnic population (25.8), according to data from the 2001 census. The gap remains even when data are disaggregated by urban area (29.3 among Afro-descendants and 21.3 among non-ethnic groups) and rural area (39.4 and 32.9, respectively). In Brazil, according to the 2000 census, the infant mortality rate in the Afro-descendant population is higher (37.6 deaths per 1,000 live births) than that in the rest of the population (25.0). Colombia's infant mortality rate is close to the Latin American average. In the department of Chocó, however, where Afro-descendants are the majority of the population (70%), male infant mortality rates are three times higher than the national average (98.6 deaths per 1,000 live births) and female infant mortality rates are four times higher (80.9) (Figure

---

[24] As information from Colombia's 2005 Census is not yet available, data was taken from the following publication: Situación de salud en Colombia. Indicadores Básicos 2003, Instituto Nacional de Salud Ministerio de Promoción Social y OPS. Bogotá, Colombia, 2003.

[25] The Afro-Honduran population descends from Africans who came to the country from Saint Vincent and the Grenadines and mixed with indigenous Caribs and Arawaks.

[26] For more information on this topic, see PAHO, *Health in the Americas, 2002 edition* (pp. 105–106). PAHO, Washington, D.C., 2002.

FIGURE 30. Percentage of the population 15–19 years old that completed six years of schooling, by ethnicity and sex, Honduras, 2001.

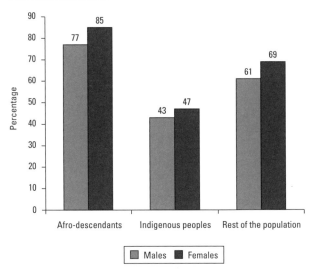

Source: 2001 Population Census, prepared by PAHO.

31); these figures are higher than those in Haiti (79 deaths per 1,000 live births), India (65), and Kenya (68).

In Honduras, the mortality rate for children under 5 is higher in urban Afro-descendant populations (30.7 deaths per 1,000 live births) than in urban indigenous populations (21.3) and non-ethnic populations (25.3).

The risk of dying from HIV-infection and diseases linked to poverty varies by ethnicity and sex. In Honduras, more than 8% of adults in the Garifuna population are HIV-positive, compared with a national average of 2%, and the cumulative rate of HIV infection is nearly 15 times the national average among Garifunas. In Brazil, the Government adopted a policy of universal, free access to antiretroviral therapy in 1998. Since then, in the state of São Paulo, white men have seen their mortality risk fall considerably, but their Afro-descendant counterparts have not seen such an improvement; the mortality risk is similarly higher among women of African descent than among white women (Figure 32).

With regard to water supply, the 2000 censuses indicate that Afro-descendants have less access than does the non-ethnic population. In Brazil, 85.4% of Afro-Brazilians have adequate access to drinking water, compared to 92% in the non-ethnic population. In Ecuador, 66% of Afro-Ecuadorians have access to drinking water, compared to 69% of the non-ethnic population. Afro-Hondurans have nearly the same access as the non-ethnic population (74% vs. 73%).

In 2004, Brazil's Special Secretariat for Policies for the Promotion of Racial Equality convened the regional workshop, "Working to Achieve Ethnic Equity in Health," under the auspices of the Office of the United Nations High Commissioner for Human Rights and PAHO. Delegations from 24 countries attended, with representatives from the health ministries, civil society, and the foreign ministries responsible for monitoring summits. Delegates acknowledged that indicators for the Millennium Development Goals for Afro-descendants were lagging (Box 7) and declared that "efforts should redouble to ensure that the Millennium Development Goals benefit the groups that are victims of racism, racial discrimination, xenophobia, and related intolerance" (*391*).

Although Afro-descendants make up nearly half of Brazil's total population, they account for just 10% of its physicians. The percentage of female doctors of African descent is even lower (Table 31). In Ecuador, the percentage of Afro-descendant physi-

FIGURE 31. Infant mortality rate (per 1,000 live births), by sex, various departments, Bogotá, and national average, Colombia, 2003.

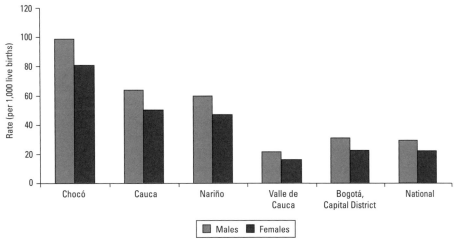

Source: República de Colombia, Ministerio de Protección Social, Instituto Nacional de Salud, Situación de Salud en Colombia. Pan American Health Organization, Basic Indicators, 2003.

FIGURE 32. Risk of dying from AIDS, by sex and ethnicity, trends in the *municipio* of São Paulo, Brazil, 1998–2005.

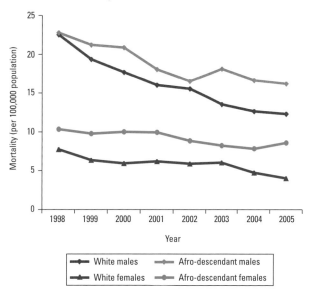

Source: Proaim, São Paulo, Brazil, with PAHO collaboration.

TABLE 31. Percentage of health workers of African descent, by profession and sex, Brazil, 2002.

Profession	Total	Males	Females
Physicians	10	11	8
Oral surgeons	9	11	8
Veterinarians	15	14	16
Pharmacists	8	12	5
First-level nurses and related personnel	20	38	18
Physiotherapists and related personnel	11	12	11
Nutritionists	31	0	32
Total	12	12	12

Source: Household survey, 2001.

cians (1.5%) is much lower than for the population as a whole. In Honduras, of the 17,320 people identified in the census as working in health-related professions, including categories such as midwifery and naturopathy, fewer than 2% (336) were identified as Afro-descendants, which is below the Afro-descendant percentage of the total population (approximately 5%).

To achieve greater equity for ethnic and racial groups in the Region during the "Decade of Human Resources for Health" (2006–3015), efforts by educational institutions to provide training and education with a multicultural focus will be critical, as will those of the health care system to provide updated training to its officials.

FAMILY AND COMMUNITY HEALTH

In order to ensure full access to health care services and change the situations and factors that affect the health of persons and communities, it is necessary to resort to strategies that combine programs, services, and activities and also obtain effective results as a consequence of a conjunction of efforts. One of the proposed approaches relates to family and community health, where families and communities are the key actors in managing health and are not simply relegated to receive comprehensive care and health promoting measures. In summary, the family and community health approach attempts to combine actions and participatory interventions of proven success, that through mutual empowerment increase each one's effectiveness and allow for access to the health objectives and goals throughout the life cycle

(*392*). For example, reducing infant mortality can become an attainable goal if comprehensive care incorporates the promotion and preservation of health, the prevention of exposure to risk factors, the early detection and restoration of functions impaired by disease, as well as curative and palliative interventions focused on individuals and families.

In Brazil, for example, evidence shows that the family health program has been successful in reducing infant mortality, and it is estimated that a 10% increase in the program's coverage could reduce infant mortality by 4.5% (*393*). In theory, significant progress could be made in improving the quality of life of children and reducing child morbidity and mortality rates through a family health program that includes care for pregnant women from the onset of gestation and even earlier, to prevent complications and fetal development problems (*394*) and the spread of infections in utero; delivery by trained professionals; immunization of newborns and children; the prevention of respiratory infections and treatment of diarrhea and parasitosis; and nutritional guidance, early stimulation, development, and reductions in risks in the home. There also is evidence that shows that programs that stress skill development among fathers and mothers to be able to talk to their teenage children about risks associated with having unprotected sexual relations are highly effective in generating an understanding about the risks and behavior patterns of self-protection (*395*).

Although it is still necessary to compile information that can conclusively show how integrating programs geared to families can lead to a more efficient use of services and a greater participation by people in the management of their own health, preliminary evidence shows that this strategy is not only advisable, but absolutely necessary for achieving the Millennium Development Goals and expanding the coverage of services. Throughout their lives, individuals maintain associations with their families and communities through various links. Consequently, the use of these social structures is conducive to ensuring an expansion of coverage, as well as an improved efficiency of services and a greater level of participation by families and the community. Similarly, the constant implementation of the actions of the pro-

BOX 7. Reducing the Ethnic and Racial Gap to Meet the Millennium Development Goals

In countries where Afro-descendants make up a large segment of the population, the infant mortality rate must be reduced to meet the Millennium Development Goals with greater equity.

The case of Brazil, where people of African descent make up 46% of the population, illustrates the point. The infant mortality rate in Brazil fell by nearly 40% in one decade, dropping from 49.4 deaths per 1,000 live births in 1990 to 30.8 deaths per 1,000 live births in 2000. In terms of ethnicity, the following table shows that in 2000, the mortality risk for Afro-Brazilian infants was double the risk for infants in the rest of the population.

Infant mortality rate and mortality rate in children under 5, by area and ethnicity, Brazil, 2000.

Ethnic group	Infant mortality rate (per 1,000 live births)			Mortality rate in children under 5 (per 1,000 live births)		
	Total	Urban	Rural	Total	Urban	Rural
Afro-descendant population	37.6	35.1	45.0	46.7	43.3	57.6
Rest of population	25.0	23.3	32.7	29.8	27.5	40.0
Total	30.8			37.6		

Source: Data from Brazil's 2000 Population Census, available from the ECLAC/CELADE database.

To achieve the goal of reducing the infant mortality rate to 16.5 deaths per 1,000 live births by 2015, different strategies for closing the gap between segments of the population should be considered. Under a first scenario, the goal would be met by maintaining the gap at 50%, which would require rates of approximately 19.5 deaths per 1,000 live births among Afro-descendants and 13 deaths per 1,000 live births among the rest of the population. If the infant mortality rate for the general population fell to 16.5, with no drop in the Afro-descendant population, the gap would grow, causing adverse social effects.

Another possible scenario is to attempt to reach the goal while also narrowing the gap. This would require reducing the mortality rate to 18.5 deaths per 1,000 live births for Afro-Brazilian infants, and to 14 deaths per 1,000 live births for the rest of the population. In this case, the goal would be met as in the other scenarios, but with the added value of a 25% reduction in the gap in the infant mortality rate. As illustrated in the table, the same approach could be taken for reducing mortality in children under 5 years old.

The implementation of strategies for achieving these results will require considerable coordination between sectors. For example, the positive impact that maternal education has on infant mortality has already been amply demonstrated. In addition, successful coordination between government programs and the support of civil society will be necessary.

grams and initiatives prevents the neglect and marginalization that can have an impact on persons during critical points in their lives, especially during adolescence and old age. Finally, these kinds of programs encourage older persons to contribute to the well-being of their children and grandchildren (*396*).

CHILDREN

Infant Mortality and Mortality in Children under 5 Years Old

Approximately 12 million children are born each year in Latin America and the Caribbean. According to estimates, close to 400,000 die before reaching their fifth birthday; 270,000 die before their first year and, of these, 180,000 die during their first month of life (*397*). This steady loss of life is mainly due to causes that can be prevented, or treated if detected early, such as malnutrition and many infectious and respiratory diseases that together are responsible for one of every four deaths among children under 5 years old. In Latin American countries, the average infant mortality rate dropped from 43 per 1,000 live births to 25 between 1990 and 2003 (*398*).

Nevertheless, despite this reduction and some progress attained, in many Latin American and Caribbean countries, the high mortality rate among newborns has not dropped as expected. Between 1989 and 1998, the infant mortality rate in Bolivia dropped 29%, but during the same period, the neonatal mortality rate in the country only fell by 7% (*397*).

Low birthweight, asphyxia, and sepsis are responsible for some 40% of the deaths attributed to perineonatal causes, and together are responsible for 80,000 deaths annually. Most of these deaths could have been prevented by improving prenatal care and ensuring adequate care is given during childbirth and for the newborn. A varying percentage of deaths due to problems during pregnancy and childbirth also could be avoided if women reaching childbearing age were in better health (especially in terms of nutrition and being disease-free), received appropriate prenatal care, and qualified care during delivery (*399*).

Rates of childhood malnutrition in terms of weight-for-age, weight-for-height, and height-for-age have decreased, although high rates of micronutrient deficit persist in countries with the highest infant mortality rates. Low height-for-age reflects chronic malnutrition, the most frequent kind of malnutrition in the Americas, with a regional average of 16% in 2003 (*400*), although this figure masks disparities in some areas within countries. Low weight-for-age in boys and girls under 5 years old is increasing, on average, by 7% (*400*). Although information has been published about the benefits of exclusive breast-feeding during the first 6 months of life on infant morbidity and mortality (*401*), in 21 countries of the Region only 29% of infants benefit from this practice (*402*).

Poverty and Inequity

Poverty remains as the leading obstacle to achieving good health, adequate development, and quality of life in childhood. In Latin America in 2004, 36.7% of the urban population and 58.1% of the rural was considered poor; 45% lived in extreme poverty, 55% of whom were children (*400*). Poor families tend to have more children, and they are raised in adverse conditions. In 2000, it was estimated that 36% of all children under 2 years old in Latin America were at high risk in terms of nutrition; in rural areas the percentage rose to 46%, given precarious health conditions and the great difficulties in gaining access to public health services (*400*).

In 2002, only 69% of Latin America's rural population had access to drinking water and only 44% had access to basic sanitation. Approximately 30% of children under the age of 6 lived in homes without access to drinking water systems and, therefore, were at high health risk associated with the quality of water used for housework and food preparation. In addition, 40% of these children were at high risk for contracting diseases, owing to a lack of systems for excreta disposal and the presence of waste around the home (*400*).

Integrated Management of Childhood Illnesses

In 1996, the World Health Organization (WHO) and the United Nations Children's Fund (UNICEF) designed the Integrated Man-

agement of Childhood Illnesses (IMCI) strategy as a way to help reduce infant mortality and morbidity caused by easily preventable diseases and thus foster healthy growth and development of children under 5 years old, especially among the most vulnerable population groups. IMCI's neonatal component, which targets the first week of life, was recently formulated and is considered crucial to further reduce infant mortality (*397*). PAHO promotes the implementation of IMCI in the Americas; in 2001, 18 countries, comprising 52% of the population under the age of 5 and accounting for 75% of the deaths that occur annually in this age group, adopted the strategy. The IMCI implementation process consists of the following three fundamental components:

- The *clinical component* aims to enhance the skills of health care workers in managing cases through training, supervision, the provision guidelines for the comprehensive treatment of childhood diseases tailored to local needs, and activities focused on promoting the use of guides for expanding training coverage.
- The *health care systems component* aims to improve the health systems that are necessary for providing good care.
- The *community component* focuses on incorporating family and community practices that are key factors for childhood survival and sound growth and development by enlisting the participation of actors in society and the community.

Through the clinical component, IMCI addresses the evaluation, classification, and treatment of the most frequently seen problems, including aspects dealing with detection, treatment, disease prevention, and health promotion. In this way, IMCI incorporates the treatment of the main reason for the medical consultation and the overall state of health of the child in a comprehensive approach. To this end, IMCI emphasizes the identification of signs and symptoms of other diseases and problems and takes into account the epidemiological profile of each location (*403*). The community component focuses on community mobilization and participation, based on an analysis of the local circumstances, and enlists the commitment of stakeholders to foster sound health care practices in families and in the community. In other words, it promotes behavior patterns that are essential for preventing disease, improving the physical and mental development of children, providing adequate care in the home, and seeking medical assistance outside the home (*404*).

IMCI also incorporates a systematic evaluation of children's current state of nutrition, the food they are given, and their immunization schedule. In so doing, nutritional disorders or problems related to diet that can serve to prevent malnutrition or stunted growth can be detected early. Finally, the implementation of the IMCI strategy also encompasses basic child care in the home by strengthening the role of health care personnel in informing and educating parents about how to improve their knowledge and behavioral practices associated with their children's health.

In 2004, a WHO team conducted an in-depth national evaluation of the activities associated with the clinical and community components of the IMCI in Peru. The country was selected because IMCI has broad coverage there, in that every department had received training as part of the strategy (*405*). In Chao, Peru, the benefits perceived by the society stakeholders and by the mothers consisted of: 1) a better awareness by families of key family practices, and 2) changes in the behavioral practices of families, especially in relation to cleanliness in the home, hand washing, caring for children with diarrhea at home, identifying dangerous warning signs, and seeking medical assistance (*406*).

Child Development within the Framework of the Millennium Development Goals (MDGs)

The specific goal agreed upon by countries in relation to infant mortality stipulates that by the end of 2015, infant mortality levels would have been reduced by two-thirds of the 1990 figures (MDG 4). The estimates for the Region of the Americas show that achieving this goal will require accelerating the rate of decrease of mortality levels of children under the age of 5, a reduction rate that during the 1990s averaged nearly 2.4% annually. In order to achieve by 2015 a mortality rate that is one-third the earlier figure, the rate of decrease in the mortality levels of children under the age 5 will have to more than double, to 5.6% annually. If this goal were achieved, the number of annual deaths in children under 5 years old would be around 250,000, fewer than half the number that, according to estimates, occurred in 2000 and one-third the number estimated in 1990.

The assessment of the IMCI strategy implementation showed an improvement in the rate of reduction of cases of diarrhea, from 29% annually in 1975 to 50% annually in 2000. In respiratory diseases, the annual reduction in 1975 was 33%, increasing to 50% annually in 2000. This shows that the IMCI strategy has a good potential for reducing the burden from these diseases when it is broadly implemented in national, regional, and international programs (*404*).

HEALTH AND DEVELOPMENT OF ADOLESCENTS AND YOUTHS

The 2000 Millennium Declaration reaffirmed the commitment to the principles of equality, equity, and human dignity, including as they apply to adolescents and youths. Furthermore, the United Nations General Assembly Special Session on HIV/AIDS (UNGASS) pressed for a reduction in the prevalence of HIV in the population 15–24 years old (2001) (*407, 408*), while the UN General Assembly Special Session on Children (*409*) called for the design and implementation of national adolescent health policies and programs (2002). Most countries in the Region of the Americas have already met this latter goal, placing the issue of adolescent and youth health and development on their political agenda.

> ❝*The most important new health problem confronting the Americas is the acquired immune deficiency syndrome (AIDS). The number of reported cases in the countries of the Region by the end of December 1987 was 56,368—approximately 74% of the world's reported cases.*❞
>
> Carlyle Guerra de Macedo, 1987

Demographic Factors

Young people between the ages of 10 and 24 made up 28% of the total population of Latin America and the Caribbean (161 million individuals) in 2006, with the population 10–19 years old representing 20% (*410*). Youths 10–24 years old account for a large share of the total population of the Region's poorest countries, such as Haiti and Nicaragua, where they represent 35% of the general population. Youths account for 30% to 35% of the population of the Dominican Republic, Guatemala, Honduras, and Paraguay, compared with a figure of 23% in Cuba, Puerto Rico, and Uruguay. A breakdown of the population structure of English-speaking Caribbean nations, by country, puts the share of adolescents (young people between 10 and 19 years old) at only 11% in Bermuda, 13% in Aruba, and 24% in the Cayman Islands and Grenada (*410*).

The growing numbers of young people are putting pressure on education, health, employment, legal, and recreational systems.

Indigenous populations include an even larger share of youths, who make up 24% of the indigenous population of Panama, for example, compared with 18% of the general population. According to data for 2000, the countries with the largest indigenous youth populations as a share of the general population were Bolivia (62%), Guatemala (48%), Ecuador (25%–40%), Belize (16%), Honduras (12%), Suriname (10%), and Guyana (6.3%) (*411*).

In general, the Region's youth is the group hardest hit by poverty, as defined by household income level (*412*). More specifically, 41% of youths between 15 and 29 years of age are living in poverty and 15% are living in extreme poverty (*413*). More than 50% of youths in Bolivia, Guatemala, Honduras, Nicaragua, Paraguay, and Peru live in poverty. However, there are large disparities between urban and rural areas. Thus, in 2002, one in three youths residing in urban areas was poor, compared with half of all youths in rural areas. Moreover, the likelihood of rural youths being poor is 64% greater than that of youths living in cities around the Region (*413*).

Adolescent and young women and indigenous youths are among the most vulnerable populations. Females are at a higher risk than males of experiencing a sexual assault or early marriage and/or pregnancy and of dropping out of school (*414*). Indigenous peoples are one of the poorest and most socially excluded population groups, with 75% to 85% of the indigenous population living in poverty (*415*), with low levels of education, high dropout rates, poor-quality jobs, low incomes, poor health and nutrition, and limited access to goods and services (*416*).

There is more migration by adolescents and young adults (between the ages of 15 and 29) than by children and older adults (*413*), which heightens this group's health risks in general and their risk of contracting HIV and sexually transmitted infections, in particular. Most migration involves youths between the ages of 17 and 22 (*417*), who face greater social vulnerability and disadvantages in terms of education, employment, language skills, and legal protection (*413*). One of the leading forms of migration is rural-to-urban migration. In 2000 in Mexico, for example, 53% of males and 34% of females between 20 and 24 years of age moved to urban areas in search of employment, and 23% of females moved for purposes of marriage or consensual unions. That same year, 73% of residents of rural areas of Brazil between the ages of 15 and 24 moved to an urban area (*418*).

The rate of international migration by youths between Latin American and Caribbean countries in 2004 was estimated at 17%. There are large concentrations of immigrants in countries such as Argentina, Costa Rica, and Venezuela, consisting mostly of female domestic workers (*413*). That same year, the rate of out-migration to the United States was 9% in Colombia, 7.7% in the Dominican Republic, 8.8% in El Salvador, and 5.5% in Mexico; the average age of these immigrants was 25.6 (*419*).

Education

There was progress at all levels of education in Latin American countries in 2001–2005 (*412*). Most countries have achieved universal primary education coverage and have closed the gender gap. However, only 39.8% of Latin American youths complete their secondary education, compared with 85% of their peers in Organization for Economic Cooperation and Development member countries. The figure is even lower in the Region's poorest countries, at 12%. At higher education levels, only 6.5% of the college-age population graduates, compared with a mere 0.9% in the Region's poorest countries (*413*).

There are stubborn socioeconomic and rural-urban disparities in the Region. According to data for 2000, 48% of youths in the poorest quintile completed primary school and only 12% of this group completed secondary education, compared with rates of 80% and 58%, respectively, in the richest quintile (*420*). The dropout rate at the primary education level in rural areas (54%) was double that in urban areas (22%) (*413*). The indigenous youth population is even more severely affected by these exclusions. In Guatemala, for example, the repeater rate for indigenous students at the primary education level was 90%, while in Bolivia, the probability of a non-Spanish-speaking indigenous child repeating a grade was twice that of a Spanish-speaking child (*420*). Data for 2001 shows indigenous adolescents in Panama with higher dropout rates and less access to secondary and higher education (*421*). There is little or no gender gap with re-

spect to access to education, and females reportedly outperform males, particularly in the English-speaking Caribbean countries. Countries like Bolivia, Guatemala, and Peru, however, do not have this same gender equality (*407*).

Education is a key variable associated with lower pregnancy rates, lower rates of HIV and other sexually transmitted infections, better physical and mental health, and a lower probability of substance abuse, social exclusion, and violence. Improvements in access to and quality of secondary education are crucial for the achievement of positive health outcomes.

Employment

The employment status of the youth population is marked by high job turnover, low pay, and limited social security coverage (*412*). According to data for 2005, the percentage of the economically active population between the ages of 15 and 19 ranged from 55% in Brazil, to 42.5% in Guatemala, to 14% in Puerto Rico (*410*), averaging out to 54.2% for the Region as a whole (63.8% for males and 44.5% for females) (*422*). Since 1995, employment rates for 15-to-19-year-olds have come down by 6.6% in males and edged upwards by 2.2% in females (*422*).

The unemployment rate for the Region's youth population is 16.6%, 2.8 times higher than the adult rate (*422*). Of each 100 new employment contracts in the Region's countries, 93 involve adults; the 7 involving youths are mostly for part-time jobs (*420*). There are clear socioeconomic disparities in employment status, with the Regionwide average unemployment rate for youths in the richest quintile at 8.7%, compared with a rate of 28.1% for youths in the poorest quintile (*412*). In addition to high unemployment, there are growing numbers of youths in low-paying jobs as street vendors or domestic workers and miscellaneous jobs in the informal sector. More specifically, 69% of working youths between 15 and 19 years of age and 49% of working youths between the ages of 20 and 24 held these types of low-paying jobs (*420*). According to data for 2000, Haiti had a total of 25,000 female domestic workers, of whom 75% were between the ages of 7 and 14 and 85% were from the countryside (*423*). An estimated 21% of 15-to-24-year-old poor youths in Latin America and the Caribbean were out of school and out of work (*424*).

Family Structure and Dynamics

Family structure and dynamics are crucial to healthy adolescent development, and nurturing family relationships can help protect against early sexual initiation, substance abuse, and depression (*425*). The share of two-parent households in which the mother stayed at home dropped from 46% to 36% between 1990 and 2002, while the share of two-parent households with working mothers rose from 27% to 33% over the same reference period (*426*). According to data for 2002, 26% of urban households were headed by women. This figure ranged from 21.4% in Mexico and

Ecuador to 35.3% in El Salvador (*427*). The share of fatherless families with female heads of household increased from 13% to 16% between 1990 and 2002 (*426*). The percentage of youths living at home with their original families is inversely correlated with their age. In Chile, for example, 98.6% of 15-to-19-year-old adolescents still lived at home with their parents, compared with only 68.4% of youths between 25 and 29 years of age (*413*). Still, this latter figure suggests a growing trend for children to live at home longer which, in turn, reflects how difficult it is for youths to make it on their own (*428*).

Youths living in poverty, with little education, and scant employment prospects are at greater risk of having adverse health and development outcomes. They particularly need support that embraces human rights, gender, and equity perspectives.

Mortality and Morbidity

The mortality rate for 15-to-24-year-old youths in the Region in 2003 was approximately 130 per 100,000 population (*429*). Argentina, Barbados, Bermuda, Canada, Chile, Costa Rica, Cuba, Dominica, Paraguay, the United States, and Uruguay had the lowest rates (<100 per 100,000), while Colombia, Haiti, Honduras, and Peru all had rates of over 200 per 100,000 (*429*). A breakdown of adolescent and youth mortality rates shows males and youths aged 15 to 24 with comparatively higher rates. The mortality gender gap has widened everywhere, except in Colombia, Cuba, and El Salvador (*413*).

Table 32 breaks down mortality rates by cause for 15-to-24-year-old males and females in selected countries in the Americas. In or around 2000, so-called "external" causes—including accidents, homicides, suicides, etc.—were the leading cause of death, followed by communicable diseases, noncommunicable diseases, and complications of pregnancy, childbirth, and the puerperium. In Colombia, homicides accounted for 62.5% of male fatalities in this age group, compared with rates of 46.1% in El Salvador, 42.0% in Brazil, and 38.3% in Venezuela (*430*). During this same period, suicide was the leading cause of death for females in the same age group in Ecuador, El Salvador, and Nicaragua and among the five leading causes of death in another 16 countries.

Complications of pregnancy, childbirth and the puerperium were the main cause of death for 15-to-24-year-old females in Haiti, Honduras, and Paraguay and are still among the five leading causes of death in 18 countries in the Region. In Haiti, complications of pregnancy were the leading cause of death for 15-to-24-year-old females between 2001 and 2003 (*429*). In the Caribbean, AIDS is already among the five leading causes of death for youths in this age group and, in Jamaica, was one of the three leading causes of death for 15-to-19-year-olds in 2005 (*431*).

According to morbidity data, obstetric conditions were the most common cause of hospitalization for 10-to-19-year-old females (accounting for 27% and 31%, respectively, of hospital stays in the Caribbean and Central America), followed by trauma

and violence and diseases of the respiratory tract in both males and females. HIV infection was the fourth most common cause of hospitalization in Honduras (*430*). Tuberculosis is a stubborn problem among 15-to-24-year-olds in the Region, affecting males more than females (*432*). This age group accounted for 60% of diagnosed cases of tuberculosis in Peru, 40% in Ecuador, 30% in Argentina and Paraguay, and 7% in Uruguay.

Around half of all preventable premature adult deaths are attributable to acquired risk factors dating back to adolescence, such as smoking, poor eating habits, and a lack of physical exercise. Adolescent obesity is on the rise, with a current prevalence rate of between 8% and 22% (*433*). Half of all obese adolescents continue to suffer from this condition in adulthood. Obese adolescents between the ages of 10 and 15 are at the greatest risk (*433, 434*). According to data for 2003, 12.7% of females (between 12 and 19 years of age) and 14.6% of their male counterparts in the United States were overweight. The share of overweight adolescents of Latin American descent was as high as 24.7% among females and 19.9% in males (*435*).

Sexual and Reproductive Health

There are close ties between adolescent sexual and reproductive health and achievement of the Millennium Development Goals (MDGs) (*409–412*).

Sexual Initiation

Most youths first become sexually active in adolescence, and youths in many countries in the Region are sexually active at an increasingly early age. Over 50% of 15-to-24-year-old females in some Central American countries had had sexual relations by the age of 15 (*436*); the percentage is even higher in rural areas. In Brazil, according to data for 2006, 36% of young men and women between 15 and 24 years of age reported having been sexually active since the age of 15, and 1 in 5 reported having had sexual intercourse with more than 10 partners during their lifetime (*437*). In the Dominican Republic, 44% of the female adolescent population had had sexual intercourse before age 15 and 78% had gotten pregnant (*438*). In Peru, 62% of females who had had sexual relations before the age of 14 were coerced into doing so (*407*). In Jamaica, 46% of 15-year-old males and 21% of 15-year-old females were sexually active, compared with 90% of 19-to-20-year-old youths (*439*).

Contraceptive Use

According to a 2002 report by the Economic Commission for Latin America and the Caribbean (ECLAC), nearly 90% of Latin American and Caribbean adolescents were familiar with at least one method of contraception, except in Bolivia (74%), Guatemala (68%), and Paraguay (89%) (*416*). In the 2004 ECLAC report, 7% of sexually active Honduran females between the ages of 15 and 24 reported having used some form of contraception in their first

TABLE 32. Percentage breakdown of mortality among 15-to-24-year-old youths, by sex and selected broad groups of causes, Latin America and the Caribbean, circa 2000.[a]

Country	Sex	Communicable diseases		Noncommunicable diseases			External causes		
		All	HIV/AIDS	Malignant neoplasms	Diseases of the circulatory system	Pregnancy, childbirth, and the puerperium	All	Homicide	Suicide
Latin America and the Caribbean (14 countries)	Female	13.3	2.9	9.9	9.1	7.9	37.6	9.4	5.7
	Male	6.3	1.9	4.9	3.8	—	76.8	36.3	4.6
Argentina (1997)	Female	12.8	4.0	13.2	8.8	4.8	41.0	2.7	6.9
	Male	6.9	3.2	7.0	5.3	—	72.0	10.2	6.5
Brazil (1998)	Female	14.6	3.7	8.9	10.6	7.9	37.7	11.2	3.7
	Male	6.4	1.9	4.0	4.4	—	78.3	42.0	3.1
Chile (1999)	Female	9.1	0.5	18.4	5.5	3.3	39.8	1.9	8.0
	Male	4.2	1.4	9.6	2.1	—	73.6	6.9	11.3
Colombia (1998)	Female	9.1	1.4	8.2	7.4	10.0	51.1	20.9	9.5
	Male	3.0	0.8	3.0	2.1	—	89.5	62.5	4.2
Costa Rica (2001)	Female	5.5	0.0	20.6	9.9	3.2	28.8	9.3	7.0
	Male	2.4	0.5	9.7	3.2	—	73.0	12.7	8.5
Dominican Republic (1998)	Female	25.7	14.9	7.3	12.8	6.6	27.4	3.8	2.6
	Male	10.7	3.1	3.1	7.0	—	69.7	17.0	2.1
Ecuador (2000)	Female	16.9	0.6	9.8	11.1	8.7	30.0	4.8	7.7
	Male	11.8	1.5	4.9	7.6	—	64.6	24.8	5.8
El Salvador (1999)	Female	10.9	1.6	8.3	8.9	2.1	43.5	10.6	20.0
	Male	7.7	2.4	2.7	3.3	—	75.5	46.1	7.1
Mexico (2000)	Female	10.0	1.9	12.1	7.2	8.9	31.9	5.8	4.7
	Male	6.2	2.5	7.2	3.6	—	69.5	18.1	7.0
Nicaragua (2000)	Female	11.5	1.1	6.6	5.6	12.8	41.4	5.5	22.9
	Male	5.6	0.5	7.6	3.6	—	71.2	17.9	16.8
Panama (2000)	Female	24.0	12.0	12.0	1.7	8.8	29.8	2.8	5.6
	Male	10.0	5.8	5.7	2.1	—	69.8	26.8	6.6
Peru (2000)	Female	21.5	2.1	9.4	8.1	6.4	28.8	1.2	3.3
	Male	18.8	3.8	9.6	5.8	—	45.6	3.2	1.9
Uruguay (2000)	Female	7.2	3.2	15.6	10.4	12.2	42.5	7.2	11.5
	Male	5.4	2.0	6.8	3.4	—	73.9	9.8	19.0
Venezuela (2000)	Female	8.5	1.5	11.3	8.2	7.8	43.5	10.1	4.4
	Male	3.3	1.4	3.3	2.0	—	85.8	38.3	3.9

[a]As a percentage of total deaths.

Source: Pan American Health Organization (PAHO) database, Health Statistics from the Americas, 2003 Edition.

sexual encounter, compared with 7.3% of this same group in Guatemala, 17.8% in El Salvador, and 23.6% in Paraguay (*413*). According to a Jamaican survey, the rate of contraceptive use by young women in their first sexual encounter rose from 42.7% to 67.3% between 1993 and 2002, while the rate of contraceptive use by male youths went from 21.6% to 43% during the same time frame (*440*). The same survey found a link between delaying sexual activity until after 18 years of age and a higher likelihood of contraceptive use in the first sexual encounter (77%, compared with 42% for those choosing not to delay sexual initiation) (*439*). The unmet need for contraception among young women in 2006 was 48% in Honduras, 38% in Guatemala, and 36% in Nicaragua (*440–442*).

The launching of programs aimed at providing youths with access to contraceptives to reduce the number of unwanted children and prevent deaths due to unsafe abortions should be a priority for the Region's countries.

Pregnancy

Half the countries in the Americas have adolescent fertility rates higher than 72 per 1,000 live births. Honduras (137), Nicaragua (119), Guatemala (114), El Salvador (104), and the Dominican Republic (96) have the highest rates (*440–442*). Figure 33 shows fertility rates for 15-to-19-year-old girls for 2000–2005.

According to data for 2001, approximately 33% of young women in Nicaragua between the ages of 20 and 24 had had a child before age 18, and nearly half this group had had a child before the age of 20. The figures for Guatemala and Honduras were 44% and 50%, respectively (*440–442*).

Adolescents account for 15% of the burden of disease attributable to maternal conditions and 13% of all maternal mortality (*443*). According to a 2005 study in El Salvador, 52% of maternal deaths involved young women between 15 and 24 years of age (*444*). Adolescents run a higher risk of adverse pregnancy outcomes such as postpartum hemorrhages, puerperal endometriosis, low-birthweight-for-gestational-age babies, and preterm deliveries. A comparison of mothers under the age of 20 with 20-to-24-year-old mothers shows the former twice as likely to have eclampsia and episiotomies and more likely to have a forceps delivery and to experience postpartum hemorrhaging (*445*). According to the same study, adolescent girls under the age of 15 were at a four times higher risk of maternal mortality than young women between the ages of 20 and 24 (*445, 446*).

An estimated 40% of pregnancies are unplanned and a result of no contraceptive use, improper contraceptive use, or contraceptive failure. Available data shows 45% of children born to mothers between the ages of 15 and 19 in Nicaragua to have been unplanned pregnancies (*440*), compared with figures of 40% in Honduras (*441*) and 29% in Guatemala (*442*). These young girls are also less likely to get prenatal care or to have their deliveries attended by a health care professional.

FIGURE 33. Age-specific fertility rate for 15–19-year-old adolescents, selected countries, Region of the Americas, 2000–2005.

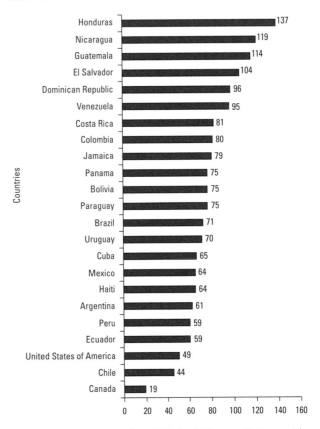

Annual births (per 1,000 women 15–19 years old)

Sources:
Corrales G et al. Honduras: encuesta nacional de epidemiología y salud familiar—2001 (ENESF-01, Informe Final). Tegucigalpa, Honduras: ASHONPLAFA; and Atlanta, GA, USA: Centers for Disease Control and Prevention (CDC); 2002.
Blandón LF et al. Encuesta Nicaragüense de demografía y salud 2001 (ENDESA- 01, Informe Final). Managua, Nicaragua: Instituto Nacional de Estadísticas y Censos; 2002.
Stupp P et al. Guatemala: encuesta nacional de salud materno infantil 2002 (ENSMI-2002). Volumen I: Mujeres. Ciudad de Guatemala, Guatemala: Universidad del Valle; 2003.
Monteith RS, Stupp PW, McCracken SD. Reproductive, maternal, and child health in Central America: trends and challenges facing women and children. Atlanta, GA, USA: CDC Division of Reproductive Health and U.S. Agency for International Development (USAID); 2005.
Central Statistical Office (CSO). 1999 Belize family health survey, females. Belize City, Belize: CSO; 2001.
United Nations, Department of Economic and Social Affairs. World population prospects: the 2004 revision. Acessed 8 February 2007. Available at: http://esa.un.org/unpp.
CDC. Knowledge and Outcomes for Young Adults in Jamaica/Gender Differences in Reproductive Health. 2006
UNICEF, UNICEF Statistics. Fertility and Contraceptive Use. Acessed 8 February 2007. Available at: http://www.childinfo.org/eddb/fertility/dbadol.htm.

An estimated 1 in 270 women in developing countries undergoing an abortion are at risk of dying, and 15% of all unsafe abortions are performed on 15-to-19-year-old girls and 29% on young women between the ages of 20 and 24. Abortions are responsible for 13% of all pregnancy-related deaths (*447*).

"All countries have shown declines in infant and childhood mortality and increases in life expectancy at birth, primarily as a result of the control of infectious diseases in the early years of life. As populations have aged and concentrated in large urban areas, chronic and degenerative diseases, particularly cardiovascular disease and cancer, have become more important as causes of morbidity and mortality."

George A. O. Alleyne, 1995

The prevention of pregnancy in young adolescents is vital for achieving the MDGs and reducing the intergenerational transmission of poverty.

HIV/AIDS and Sexually Transmitted Infections

An estimated 1.6% of Caribbean females (an average of the lowest estimate of 0.9% and the highest estimate of 2.3%) and 0.7% of Caribbean males (low estimate of 0.4%, high estimate of 1.5%) between the ages of 15 and 24 were infected with HIV in 2004. The figures for Latin America were 0.3% (low estimate of 0.2%, high estimate of 0.8%) for females and 0.5% (low estimate of 0.4%, high estimate of 1.5%) for males (437). Adolescent girls between 15 and 19 years of age were six times more likely to be infected with HIV than adolescent males in the same age group in Trinidad and Tobago, compared with a ratio of 2.5 in Jamaica. The AIDS mortality rate for Latin American youths was 2.9 per 100,000 and was the leading cause of death among young women between the ages of 15 and 24 in Belize, Guyana, and Trinidad and Tobago. In general, estimated AIDS mortality rates in Latin America for 2001–2003 were higher for males than for females. However, figures for 15-to-24-year-old females in the Dominican Republic, El Salvador, Paraguay, and Puerto Rico outstripped male rates for the same age group (437).

The increasing feminization and youthfulness of the AIDS epidemic require stepping up AIDS prevention efforts targeted at these population groups.

Sexually transmitted infections affect 1 in 20 adolescents a year. The most common sexually transmitted infections are chlamydiosis, gonorrhea, syphilis, and trichomoniasis. In pregnant adolescent girls, they increase the risk of delivering premature and low-birthweight infants. Moreover, if left untreated, over the long term, these infections heighten the risk of infertility (accounting for half of all cases of infertility), cancer, and HIV infection (407).

Violence

Africa and Latin America have the world's highest rates of youth violence. There are studies which show that, for every youth homicide, there are anywhere from 20 to 40 victims of attempted homicides in this same age group requiring hospital care (448). In Colombia and Peru, 6 out of 10 adolescents report having suffered psychological and physical abuse in the home (449). Colombia's 2005 National Population and Health Survey found 44% of women reporting an incident of physical abuse by their spouse to be between the ages of 15 and 29. In Central America, between 3% (Honduras) and 10% (Costa Rica) of male respondents between the ages of 15 and 44 reported having been sexually abused, with the abuse occurring between the ages of 10 and 13 in 30% to 46% of these cases (450). Another cause of violence is gang activity. The current number of gang members in Central America is estimated at somewhere between 30,000 and 285,000, mostly in El Salvador, Guatemala, and Honduras, with another estimated 50,000 gang sympathizers counted among area youths (451).

Substance Abuse

A survey of seven countries in the Region by the Inter-American Drug Abuse Control Commission, an agency of the Organization of American States (CICAD-OAS), found that approximately 10% of 13-to-17-year-old adolescents in school had used illegal drugs sometime in their lives (452). Rates of reported drug use in the month immediately prior to the survey ranged from 1% in El Salvador and the Dominican Republic, to 4% in Uruguay, and 8% in Paraguay (452). Approximately 40% of the students surveyed indicated that it was easy to get hold of drugs in their country, and one in four reported having been offered some type of illegal drug at some point (452). Dependency rates for marijuana and inhalants among Brazilian adolescents were 6.9% and 5.8%, respectively (433).

Rates of tobacco use by 13-to-18-year-old adolescent male and female respondents in the month immediately prior to the survey ranged from 9.7% for Venezuelan males to 37.0% for Uruguayan females (452). Rates of exposure to tobacco advertising for 14-to-17-year-old adolescents in Latin American and Caribbean countries run extremely high, exceeding 90% in Argentina, Bolivia, Costa Rica, Mexico, and Uruguay. In Uruguay, 35% of male and female students between the ages of 11 and 15 reported having already tried their first cigarette, and 21.6% of adolescents had received a free offer of cigarettes from some tobacco company sometime between 1999 and 2001. In Argentina, 35% of 12-to-15-year-old adolescents reported having used tobacco in the last 30 days. Argentina has the world's highest percentage of adolescents exposed to tobacco smoke in public places (at 86.7%). Ironically, 70.4% of adolescents in Argentina feel that smoking should be banned in public places, which is almost the exact number of adolescent non-smokers in that country (433).

According to a number of studies, alcohol consumption is on the rise in Brazil, Chile, Costa Rica, and Mexico, particularly among young women (433). A study of adolescent health in the Caribbean found 40% of females and 50% of males between the ages of 12 and 18 to have consumed alcohol and 1 in 10 youths between the ages of 16 and 18 to have consumed four or more alcoholic drinks at a time. In Brazil, 25% of 6-to-18-year-olds spending all day on the street used alcohol regularly (*433*).

PAHO is helping the Region's countries strengthen adolescent health and development through a child development, rights, gender, and equity-based approach. Given the links between different types of high-risk behavior, the Organization is recommending use of the so-called Integrated Management of Adolescent Needs (IMAN) strategy, which coordinates country efforts in the area of primary health care, mainly at the first level of care, focusing on the health sector, with cross-sector integration.

The IMAN strategy is designed to consolidate health promotion, prevention, and treatment efforts through the following components: 1) assistance in improving information systems for gathering disaggregated data by age group (10–14, 15–19, and 20–24), gender, and ethnic origin; 2) assistance in framing youth policies, including health policies; and 3) in-country cooperation for the delivery of high-quality services with universal service coverage for adolescents and youths. It also helps train necessary human resources for addressing prevailing health needs and problems. The family and community-based component is geared to promoting interventions for strengthening the families of adolescent girls, addressing gender issues by empowering adolescents and developing a more equitable social construct of masculinity, and coordinating youth involvement. Strategic alliances with organizations such as the United Nations, the Swedish International Development Agency, and the Norwegian International Development Agency have optimized the effort's effect. There are still many challenges, such as improving program monitoring and evaluation capacity at the country level, mounting evidence-based interventions, generating data in key areas, and mobilizing necessary resources at the country and regional levels.

The inter-program initiative for the promotion of child development and violence prevention mounted by PAHO and the German Technical Cooperation Agency with funding from the German Government is a good example of this kind of partnership. It has produced hard data on the subject, has organized classroom and online distance training courses, has helped establish a conceptual framework, and has strengthened the monitoring of results and evaluation systems.

OLDER ADULTS

The aging of the population varies a great deal from subregion to subregion in the Americas. In Bolivia, for example, there are 17 persons 60 years old and older for every 100 adolescents under 15 years old, while in Uruguay, there are 70 older persons for every 100 children, and in Canada, there are 88 for every 100. With the exception of Bolivia, Haiti, Guatemala, Honduras, and Nicaragua, every country of the Region will have at least as many or more persons aged 60 than children under the age of 15 by the middle of the 21st century. In Cuba, Barbados, and Puerto Rico, there will be 200 older persons for every 100 adolescents under the age of 15 (*453*).

In the last 25 years, life expectancy at birth in the Americas has increased by 17 years, and the current average exceeds 70 years of age, with a seven-year difference in averages between figures for North America and those for Latin America and the Caribbean. Of Latin American and Caribbean persons born today, 78.6% are expected to live beyond age 60, and 4 of every 10 will live beyond 80 years. On average, older adults in the Region are living increasingly longer lives: while in the 1950s they lived 9.9 additional years after age 60, the data for 2006 shows that today they live an average of 20.5 years after age 60 and 7.1 years after age 80.

A Decrease in Premature Deaths before Age 85

Increases in longevity beginning in the 1940s mainly have been due to reductions in the number of cases of infectious diseases and to success in reducing mortality rates during infancy and other early live stages. Since the 1980s, the absolute risk of dying has dropped by 10% among those aged 60 and older; as a result, the life expectancy at age 60 increased an average of 1.5 years.

An analysis of the burden of mortality on the population older than 60 years old to determine the gap between ages 60 and 85 (years of life lost or years of life to be gained) since the 1980s showed that there are still between six and nine years of life that can be potentially gained by reducing mortality at these ages (Figure 34). Therefore, an important challenge for the public health sector is to reduce the difference between life expectancy observed at the beginning of the 21st century in persons 60 years old and older, and a theoretical projected life expectancy of 85 years (*454*).

The standardized mortality rates from specific causes and their contribution to potential years of life lost (PYLL) underscore the priorities for improving life expectancy in the Region. Between the 1980s and the 1990s, mortality rates from infectious diseases dropped 16% among men and 19% among women age 60 and older. The risk of dying from these causes currently contributes 0.5 PYLL, with respiratory infections being responsible for half. There was, for example, a reduction in the number of deaths from tuberculosis by more than 50%. The standardized mortality rate attributed to malignant neoplasms increased slightly among men (4%) and dropped among women (5%), with an increase in mortality from prostate cancer of 52% among men and of cancer of the lung (25%), stomach (34%), breast (15%), and uterus (14%) among women.

Malignant neoplasms contributed to a 1.7-year loss in life expectancy among men and 1.2 years among women older than 60. In addition, there was a drop in the risk of dying from cardiovascular diseases of 21% in men and 29% in women, despite the fact that these diseases continue to be among the leading causes contributing to PYLL among the population 60 years and older: 3.5

FIGURE 34. Years of life expectancy to be gained up to age 85 years in the population 60 years old and older, by cause of death, Latin America and the Caribbean, beginning of the 1980s to end of the 1990s.

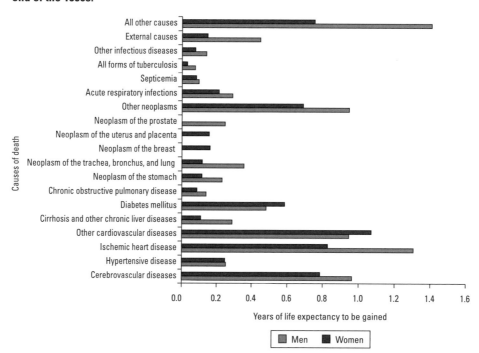

Source: Pan American Health Organization, Washington, D.C. Mortality burden in adults (DPM/GPP/Pg and AD/THS/MH), 2003.

years among men and 2.9 among women, with a greater specific weight of deaths associated with ischemic heart disease. There also was a drop in the risk of dying from external causes (women, 19% and men, 16%). It is worth mentioning that suicide is six times more prevalent among older men than among women in the Region. The risk of dying from other causes increased, and underscores an increase in mortality rates attributed to diabetes mellitus of 57% in men and 38% in women. Among the latter, this disease is a greater contributor to PYLL (0.58) than all of the negative inputs from infectious (0.39) and external causes (0.14) together; in men, diabetes contributes to 0.48 PYLL.

With an increasingly aging population in Latin America and the Caribbean, older persons' mortality burden also grows in weight and relevance, given changes in the risk profiles of falling ill and dying, the real or potential impact of mortality on life expectancy, and inequities in the quality and access to health care services. The efficacy of health policies and the performance levels of health care systems targeted to the older population should be evaluated based on assigning priority to reducing premature death, and the effectiveness of actions aimed at increasing the number of years of life without disability after age 60.

Increasing Health and Functionality in Years Gained

Four population studies have been conducted in Latin America and the Caribbean on the health and welfare of older persons:

the Health, Well-being, and Aging Survey conducted in seven Latin American and Caribbean cities (SABE, 2000) (*455*); the National Study on Health and Aging of Mexico (ENASEM, 2001 and 2003) (*456*); the survey on the Health Conditions of Older Persons in Puerto Rico (PREHCO, 2004–2006) (*457*); and the Study of Longevity and Healthy Aging in Costa Rica (CRELES, 2004–2008) (*458*). In the United States (*459*) and Canada (*460*) longitudinal and representative population studies have been conducted, which facilitate the study of health patterns among the older population and help to systematically assess policies and programs. The results of these studies have served to enhance the understanding of the health situation and the epidemiological features of the older population, mainly in the Region's urban areas and more developed countries. Nevertheless, there is a need to conduct studies that will measure the health and well-being of older populations living in rural areas, as well as of older indigenous adults, in order to identify inequalities in health among the Americas' diverse groups.

In all the available studies, a majority of older adults indicated they had been diagnosed with hypertension (48.7% in selected Latin American and Caribbean cities; 56.7% in Puerto Rico; 37.2% in Mexico; 51.9% in the United States; and 32% in Canada). In the SABE survey, only 61.3% of persons diagnosed with hypertension reported that they had received outpatient services in the 12 months immediately prior to the survey; 72.2% took some medication for hypertension, but one of every two had to pay all or partial costs; 65% reported they were not in good health; and 20.6% exhibited symptoms of depression. In addition, one out of five persons with hypertension reported suffering from at least two chronic ailments.

The prevalence of diabetes mellitus is increasing worldwide. In the PREHCO study, the prevalence rate among persons aged 60 years and older in Puerto Rico was 28%, a rate similar to that in Mexico City and in Bridgetown, Barbados, where 22% reported having been diagnosed with diabetes mellitus. The prevalence rates of diabetes found in the SABE studies and in the PREHCO study underestimate the actual prevalence of the disease, in that it entails diagnoses carried out by medical and nursing staff. In Mexico City, the SABE survey conducted there reported that the prevalence of diabetes doubled when the interviewer also conducted a fasting glucose test of all those questioned in the survey. It is well known that diabetes complications can be serious, and that proper care in dealing with the disease is vital. Diabetes also is known as one of the main causes of blindness among older persons. It is alarming to note that among persons aged 60 to 74 that reported that they suffered from diabetes in the SABE and PREHCO surveys, at least 60% and 58%, respectively, also reported that they had vision problems, both with and without glasses; 20% in the SABE survey and 16% in the PREHCO survey reported having difficulty performing at least one basic activity in their daily lives.

The predominant risk factor associated with living with disabilities in old age is being female. In the SABE survey, three out of every four women reported suffering from at least one of three disabling conditions: arthritis, incontinence, and poor vision (this last factor contributes to falls, hip fractures, and depression among older persons). And yet, most elderly persons cannot afford to pay for ophthalmologic treatments. Chronic pain due to arthritis and isolation due to urinary incontinence contribute to inactivity and the loss of functions in this age group, although there is evidence showing that the proper management of these chronic afflictions leads to improved health and increases the number of years of life free from disability. Nevertheless, most older persons in Latin America and the Caribbean do not have access to treatment needed to deal with their chronic ailments, either because of a lack of skilled personnel in geriatrics or a lack of access to medicines.

Regional Strategy for the Implementation of the Madrid International Action Plan on Aging

The adoption of the Madrid International Action Plan on Aging (PAIME) (*461*), in April 2002, represents a historic marker in addressing the demographics of aging worldwide. Subsequently, in November 2003, the Economic Commission for Latin America and the Caribbean (ECLAC), together with the other organizations of the Inter-Agency Group on Aging—the United Nations Population Fund, PAHO, the International Labor Organization, the Inter-American Development Bank, the World Bank,

and the United Nations Program on Aging—held a Regional intergovernmental conference on aging in which the implementation of the PAIME strategy for Latin America and the Caribbean was agreed upon. The Region's countries agreed to establish, tailored to their particular circumstances, specific goals for completing the Regional strategy objectives and follow-up mechanisms to assess national goals. In 2004–2005 three intergovernmental sub-regional meetings were held to promote the development of national goals.

The process of establishing national goals and determining follow-up mechanisms has been extremely difficult and is not yet completed. If any significant progress was made, it was when the Region's countries identified a focal point to follow up on the PAIME commitments, although only 8 of 20 countries in Latin America and 2 of 22 countries and territories in the Caribbean have created national multisectoral committees charged with establishing goals for three of the PAIME priority areas: 1) older persons and development, 2) promoting health and well-being among the elderly, and 3) creating a conducive and favorable environment.

Regional Commitment to Promote Health and Welfare among the Elderly

According to PAIME, older persons should have access to comprehensive health care that is appropriate to their needs, that ensures a better quality of life in their old age, and that preserves their functionality and autonomy. To this end, the Regional strategy has set out four objectives (*462*):

1. Promote universal health service coverage of older persons and incorporate aging as an essential component of national health legislation and policies.
2. Establish a comprehensive health plan that responds to the needs of older adults, reinforcing and reorienting existing services and creating new ones that are needed.
3. Promote healthy behaviors and environments by formulating legislation, policies, programs, and actions at the national and community levels.
4. Create appropriate legal frameworks and mechanisms to protect the rights of older persons who use long-term care services.

In regard to the first two objectives, social protection related to the health of older persons in Latin America and the Caribbean is carried out through three systems: a free-access public system, a social security system that includes enrollee contributions and government subsidies, and private insurance plans. No country in the Region specifically guarantees a comprehensive health care plan for older persons. In most health benefit systems there are no evidence-based standards or protocols dealing with care provided for chronic and age-related diseases and specifically designed for older persons. In terms of objective 3 despite WHO's global dissemination of the "active aging" concept (463), the countries that have developed national health promotion plans have left out specific goals for changing behavior patterns of persons 60 years old and older. In response to objective 4, countries have made significant advances in developing legal frameworks to protect the rights of older persons, although no programs or protocols have been developed to monitor the rights of those using long-term care services.

Technical Cooperation Strategies

PAHO promotes the following strategies for improving access and quality of health services provided to older persons:

1. Develop, define, and promote preventive medicine and specific disease management strategies for older persons as part of the effort to strengthen primary health care in all of the countries of the Region.
2. Establish, in cooperation with the Region's countries, quality and access to health service indicators that can measure progress in the Regional strategy for implementing PAIME.
3. Cooperate with human resource training programs and with the Latin American Academy of Medicine for Older Adults (ALMA) to implement training programs for health care personnel and in managing the health of older persons.
4. Develop standards and follow-up protocols to protect the human rights of persons who use long-term care services.

PERSONS WITH DISABILITIES

Analyzing the conditions of persons with disabilities in the Region is a difficult and complex endeavor, given such factors as the scattered nature of the data, a lack of standardized technical language that can articulate the issue's various aspects, and a lack of an intersectoral approach. Providing care to people with disabilities is one of the greatest challenges for the health sector and for society in general in the 21st century. This care must be able to prevent disability and provide rehabilitation; improve the quality of life and foster independence of people with disabilities; and promote the integration and inclusion in society of persons with disabilities under conditions of equal opportunity and respect for their rights and dignity. To achieve this, efforts must be pursued within an intersectoral and interdisciplinary framework and with the community's active participation (464). The *International Classification of Functioning, Disability, and Health* states that disability (465):

> [...] is a generic term that includes impairments in body functions and structures, activity limitations (capacity) and participation restrictions (performance). It indicates the negative aspects of the interaction between an individual (with a "health condition") and his context (environmental and per-

sonal factors). In this approach, disability is the result of the interaction between a person's functioning and environment, always related to a health condition.

Disability is a multidimensional, multifactor phenomenon in which poverty plays an important role because of its ability to generate or perpetuate disabilities. In the Americas, the prevalence rate of disability varies considerably, given the wide range of methods used to measure it and a lack of standardization and harmonization in the technical criteria used to define it. To assess the magnitude of the problem, several countries have used population censuses conducted around 2000. Data revealed widely varying rates: 14.4% in Brazil; 5.3% in Costa Rica; 6.4% in Colombia; 4.7% in the Dominican Republic; 2.6% in Honduras; 1.8% in Mexico and Panama; 1.1% in Paraguay; and 3.9% in Venezuela. In most cases, these percentages reflect only the most serious or permanent disabilities. Other countries have used specific surveys on prevalence, as has Argentina, or household surveys, as has Uruguay, which had prevalence rates of 7.1% and 7.6%, respectively.

Relying on the *International Classification of Functioning, Disability, and Health* (ICF), national studies were conducted between 2003 and 2005 in Chile, Ecuador, Nicaragua, and Panama, and, more recently, in Colombia, using the disability module of the Population Census (466, 467) (Table 33). Some of the survey results are described below.

Nicaragua recorded a disability prevalence rate of 10.3%, with women accounting for 56% of the total, and urban dwellers accounting for 60%. The age group that was most affected were persons 20–59 years old, who accounted for 47% of the total. Of persons with disabilities, 45% had never attended school. The most common disabilities were associated with mobility, communication, and participation in society, and the most commonly identified causes included age-related degenerative disorders, chronic disease, accidents of all kinds, complications related to pregnancy and childbirth, and work-related diseases (468).

In Chile, the national prevalence rate, based on the ICF, was 12.9%, with 2.5% of the population suffering a serious disability. Women accounted for 58.2% of the total population of persons with disabilities, and urban dwellers accounted for 83.3%. The most affected age group were persons 30–64 years old (51%). The prevalence rate was twice as high in the low-income population, where one in two people with a disability had not completed basic education. The most common impairments were physical (structures and functions related to movement, neuromusculoskeletal functions), accounting for 31.2% of the total, followed by visual impairments (18.9%) and bodily function impairments (13.9%). All created problems related to activity, such as seeing, moving, hearing, and personal care. The survey found that the main causes of disability were chronic disease, age-related degenerative problems, accidents of all kinds, and newborns' complications related to pregnancy and childbirth (469).

TABLE 33. Disability prevalence (%), by data source, selected countries, Latin America, 2000–2006.

Country	Census[a] (2000)	Household surveys (2003)	Prevalence studies (using ICF) (2002–2006)	Others
Argentina			7.1[d]	
Brazil	14.4			
Chile	2.2	5.3	12.9	
Colombia[c]	6.4			
Costa Rica	5.3			
Cuba[b]				3.2
Dominican Republic[a]	4.7			
Ecuador	4.6		12.1	
El Salvador		1.5		
Honduras	2.6			
Mexico	1.8			
Nicaragua			10.3	
Panama	1.8		11.6	
Paraguay	1.1			
Uruguay[c]		7.6		
Venezuela	3.9			

[a]Moderate or severe impairment.
[b]Severe impairment, excluding mental problems.
[c]Used ICF (International Classification of Functioning, Disability, and Health) as a technical basis.
[d]No ICF.
Source: Technical document CD47715, Disability: Prevention and Rehabilitation in the Context of the Right to the Enjoyment of the Highest Attainable Standard of Health and Other Related Rights.

In Ecuador, the national disability prevalence rate, based on the ICF, was 12.1%, with women accounting for 50.3% of the total and persons 20–64 years old accounting for 51%. In the survey, 80% of respondents reported the cause of their disability as related to a health condition. The remainder indicated that their disabilities were the result of accidents or other causes. In all, 56% of people with disabilities were unemployed, and the main impairments noted were related to mobility, learning, communication, and interaction with others (*470*).

In Panama, the prevalence rate was 11.6%, with women accounting for 52.4% of the total, and men, 47.6%. The survey found that 77.6% of people with disabilities did not work, and only one in ten attended school. The most common impairments were multiple impairments (23.5%), followed by motor (23.8%), visual (15.7%), and mental (13.3%) impairments (*471*).

Data from the 2005 census in Colombia, which used the ICF, indicate that, of the total number of people identified as having a permanent impairment, 71.2% had just one impairment, 14.5% had two, 5.7% had three, and 8.7% had four or more. Of the total number of people reporting some type of disability, 29% had impairments in moving or walking; 14.6% had impairments in the use of arms and hands; 43.2% had visual impairments, even with corrective lenses; 17.3% had hearing impairments, even with hearing aids; 12.8% had speaking impairments; 11.9% had learning or comprehension impairments; 9.9% had problems relating to others, due to mental or emotional problems; 9.4% had diffi-

culty bathing, dressing, or feeding themselves; and 19.4% had some other limitation (*472*).

All the studies provided extremely important data for assessing the situation of people with disabilities in Latin America and the Caribbean: 25% are children and adolescents; between 2% and 3% have access to rehabilitation programs and services; half of all people with injuries from traffic accidents are young people between 15 and 34 years of age; the population with disabilities older than 65 represents a high percentage of the total population with disabilities; 50% of people with disabilities in the Region are working age; between 2% and 3% of newborns have serious disabilities; and between 6% and 8% of children (2–6 years of age) have a high risk of disability. Of children with disabilities between the ages of 2 and 12, between 20% and 30% attend school, but only 5% complete their primary education; they suffer more discrimination, violence, and mistreatment than other children and are often confined to institutions (*467, 468*).

Access to the health care system, and particularly to rehabilitation services, for persons with disabilities continues to be a problem, as does inequality in the provision of these services. For example, in Chile, 1 in 15 people with disabilities used rehabilitation services in 2004, but people living in urban areas had better access than their rural counterparts. An analysis of the data from Chile's study reveals that 1 in 9 people with disabilities in high-income groups had received rehabilitation services, compared to 1 in 20 persons in low-income groups. Of the latter group, 9 of 10

175

BOX 8. Strategic Guidelines for Technical Cooperation in the Field of Rehabilitation and Participating Countries, Region of the Americas

Guideline	Countries
Early detection of disability in children 0–6 years old in the primary care network.	Argentina, Cuba, El Salvador, Guatemala, Honduras, Mexico, Nicaragua, and Venezuela.
Community-based rehabilitation incorporated into the health care system.	Argentina, Bolivia, Colombia, El Salvador, Guatemala, Guyana, Honduras, Nicaragua, Panama, Paraguay, Peru, and Venezuela.
Strengthening of rehabilitation activities at the intermediate- and high-complexity levels.	Argentina, Chile, Costa Rica, Cuba, El Salvador, Guatemala, Honduras, Nicaragua, Panama, Peru, and Venezuela.
Conduct of disability prevalence studies.	Chile, Colombia, Nicaragua, and Panama.
Uses and applications of the International Classification of Functioning, Disability, and Health (ICF). Analysis of the situation of people with disabilities.	Argentina, Chile, Costa Rica, Cuba, Dominican Republic, El Salvador, Nicaragua, Panama, Paraguay, and Venezuela.
Epidemiological surveillance of disability.	Argentina, Chile, Colombia, Mexico, Peru, and Venezuela.
Safe access to the physical environment and information.	Argentina, Cuba, Dominican Republic, Guatemala, Honduras, Mexico, Nicaragua, Panama, and Venezuela.

Source: Technical Document CD47715, Disability: Prevention and Rehabilitation in the Context of the Right to the Enjoyment of the Highest Attainable Standard of Health and Other Related Rights.

---

people were seen in public facilities, whereas 3 of 4 people in high-income groups were treated in private facilities (*469*).

In Nicaragua, 60% of people with disabilities in urban areas received health care, compared to 48% in rural areas. Of the total population with disabilities, 87% reported having at least one unmet basic need in the area of health care; 43% lacked prescription medication; 20% were in need of auxiliary aids; and 18% were in need of specialized services. As of 2003, 56% of Nicaraguans with disabilities had used a health care service and 2% had attended a rehabilitation center (*468*).

In Panama, 1 in 8 people with disabilities used rehabilitation services in 2005 (*471*), and in Argentina, 60.3% of the population with disabilities had health-care coverage through a government, private, or mutual plan. However, public and private plans did not always cover rehabilitation treatment (*473, 474*). Overall, there are inequalities in the care people with disabilities receive through the Region's health care systems. Furthermore, the health care systems do not make sustained, systematic efforts to prevent disability or reduce risk factors; provide care for all types of disabilities; develop rehabilitation services by degree of complexity; or meet the needs of the population with disabilities. Health and access to disability-related services is now considered to be a

human right and, as such, society should approach the issue from an intersectoral perspective (*475*). To this end, in 2001–2005, PAHO established a series of strategic guidelines for technical cooperation with the Region's countries in the field of rehabilitation (Box 8).

In conclusion, the multiple causes of disability and the complexity of the factors that interact to produce disabilities compel us to search for and identify approaches and strategies that will facilitate an integrated response, through programs and public policies that respond to the needs of people with disabilities and promote their rehabilitation and social integration.

NEW PUBLIC HEALTH CHALLENGES

NEGLECTED DISEASES IN LATIN AMERICA AND THE CARIBBEAN

The Problem

More than 209 million persons in Latin America and the Caribbean live below the poverty line (*476*), and they bear the burden of several infectious parasitic diseases. PAHO has grouped

---

BOX 9. List of Common Neglected Diseases in Latin America and the Caribbean

Common in shantytowns and slums:
- Lymphatic filariasis (elephantiasis).
- Leptospirosis (Weil's disease).

Common in rural and agricultural areas of several countries:
- Schistosomiasis (snail fever or blood fluke).
- Fascioliasis.
- Leishmaniasis (cutaneous and visceral).
- Chagas' disease (American trypanosomiasis).
- Cysticercosis and trichinosis.
- Plague.

Common in some indigenous communities:
- Onchocerciasis (river blindness).
- Parasitic skin diseases (scabies, sandfleas, and tinea fungal mycoses).

Common in most impoverished populations:
- Roundworms, hookworms, and whipworms (soil-transmitted helminths).

Source: PAHO/HDM/CD/P 2006.

---

some of these diseases under the category of "neglected diseases of neglected populations," and they require urgent attention because of their extraordinary contribution to poverty, malnutrition, interrupted schooling, and reduced employment opportunities. Neglected diseases result from the interactions between biological determinants of health, ecosystems, and human social systems, which have come to be out of balance because of poverty and environmental degradation. Neglected diseases are termed as such because they are continually overlooked for health and development funding and are not subject to regular reporting. Funding is more heavily focused on HIV/AIDS, tuberculosis, and malaria, which have higher mortality rates in comparison to neglected diseases. However, neglected diseases cause the suffering of millions, and are responsible for high rates of morbidity and drastic reductions in income for the most marginalized and poverty-stricken members of communities. Where neglected diseases overlap geographically, they often produce a high cumulative disease burden, since many individuals and communities are infected with more than one type of parasite simultaneously (coinfections).

Many persons affected by neglected diseases are indigenous peoples, minority ethnic groups, marginalized urban populations living in shantytowns and slums, isolated rural populations, or seasonal migrant workers. This makes addressing neglected diseases a question of human rights and equity, as well as a significant public health issue (see Box 9). Certain neglected diseases also carry with them much stigmatization in that they involve physical deformities or disabilities, further marginalizing affected individuals. As a result, the issue of neglected diseases in neglected populations is emerging as an important one and one that needs to be supported and tackled as a part of the current global debate on health inequalities and burden of disease. Neglected diseases also impede countries from reaching the health objectives of United Nations Millennium Development Goals.

Neglected Diseases in Neglected Populations

Neglected diseases such as intestinal helminthiasis disproportionately affect the poor, particularly poor children, cause anemia, and adversely affect children's growth and development, which contributes significantly to cognitive problems (learning), school absenteeism, and poor scholastic performance. Ultimately, they lead to overall poor health status and a poor quality of life, thus making it difficult for future generations to escape the cycle of poverty.

Disease Burden

Neglected diseases can cause high rates of morbidity among those infected, although mortality rates associated with their infection are often low. Soil-transmitted helminths, an important group of neglected diseases, are widespread throughout the Region; PAHO and WHO estimate that 20%–30% of persons living in the Americas are infected with one of several helminthiases (*477*). Intestinal helminth infections in slums can often reach 50%; they can reach up to 95% in some indigenous tribes (*478*). These infections are known to lower the work capacity of adults (*479, 480*) and are among the main causes of anemia among women of childbearing age (*481, 482*). Schistosomiasis, another helminth infection transmitted by water contact, occurs in seven of the Region's countries, mostly in small geographic foci and at low prevalence (*483*). This suggests that the elimination of this disease from some foci is possible, such as those in the Caribbean.

Other neglected diseases such as lymphatic filariasis (elephantiasis), leprosy, and Chagas' disease also cause severe chronic disease or debilitation if not treated, are often accompanied by prejudice and stigma, and prevent adults from assuming their full economic and social potential in the workplace, in the home, and in society. Leishmaniasis and onchocerciasis are two neglected diseases that cause disfiguring skin lesions, and, in the case of onchocerciasis, infection can lead to blindness.

Despite the enormous cumulative toll that neglected diseases have on the health and productivity of marginalized populations, many of them can be effectively controlled or even eliminated through large-scale preventive chemotherapy and health-promotion activities such as school-based health education campaigns and community efforts that promote healthy behaviors and teach people how to avoid certain risks. These should be coupled with the provision of clean household water, street drainage, and basic sanitation systems. Certain neglected diseases cost only pennies to treat with medicines; in the case of schistosomiasis and intestinal helminths, US$ 1 will buy one annual treatment for 5 and 50 infected children, respectively.

PAHO's strategy to combat neglected diseases takes a holistic approach to disease prevention, treatment, and elimination that recognizes the range of social, economic, and environmental factors that influence health and well-being. PAHO is developing an intersectoral and integrated approach to neglected diseases that is expected to have a positive effect in the battle against neglected diseases, and to be cost-effective; it will need demonstration and testing in the field, however. This approach takes advantage of the geographic overlap of some neglected diseases, their common risk and protective factors, and the presence of local-level disease prevention and control programs. PAHO's approach provides innovative and cost-effective opportunities for one disease control intervention as it is combined with another (i.e., "piggybacking"). An example includes using combined therapies to control soil-transmitted helminths and schistosomiasis by jointly administering albendazole and praziquantel in the same interval. Another involves taking advantage of synergies by packaging together deworming, vitamin A supplementation, and childhood immunization.

PAHO's neglected disease strategy goes beyond these opportunities for improved service delivery by the health sector. The strategy involves local community- and family-focused activities with other sectors, utilizing field-tested, development-based interventions that have proven to be successful. The combination |of integration, intersectoral partnering, and interprogrammatic approaches to health is emerging as an increasingly important strategy in the face of current development trends, which include a decline in international development funding and the growing interest in corporate responsibility towards social issues. In the future, the fight against neglected diseases will seek to take full advantage of the synergies and efficiencies created by these approaches.

Leishmaniasis

Leishmaniasis is a group of parasitic diseases distributed worldwide and transmitted to humans by the bite of approximately 30 species of sandfleas infected by protozoa of the genus *Leishmania*. It is estimated that two million new cases occur every year throughout the world, of which 1.5 million cases are cutaneous leishmaniasis. There are more than 12 million persons estimated to be infected. Official data underestimate the reality of the human affliction by these protozoa, because much of the official data is obtained exclusively through passive detection; there are many undiagnosed cases; many persons are asymptomatic; and only 32 of the 88 countries where the disease is endemic require compulsory reporting. With the exception of Chile and Uruguay, cases in the Americas have been reported from northern Argentina to southern Texas. Based on 2005 data on cutaneous leishmaniasis, the countries reporting the greatest number of cases were Bolivia, Brazil, Colombia, Ecuador, Panama, Paraguay, Peru, and Venezuela. Brazil had the most cases of visceral leishmaniasis.

The leading factors that contribute to leishmaniasis morbidity are inaccessibility to patient care, limited or no organized social participation, insufficient use of information in decision-making, lack of treatment, and human interaction with the vector.

With support from PAHO and Brazil's Ministry of Health, in November 2005, a meeting of experts was convened in Brasilia to discuss ways to strengthen systems for the prevention of visceral leishmaniasis in the countries of the Americas. The experts mainly concluded that leishmaniasis in all forms is an important disease in the Region, and that the incidence of visceral leishmaniasis has increased in recent years. They also concluded that surveillance systems are insufficient and there are no human resources trained to perform diagnostic and treatment activities or implement control measures. The lack of medication for timely treatment is another obstacle.

The Leishmaniasis Control Program, in conjunction with the Global Program, prepared an action plan for 2007–2009 that proposes the following: determine the burden of disease from leishmaniasis; standardize diagnostic techniques for the Region's countries with the greatest burden of disease (Brazil, Colombia, Ecuador, Panama, Paraguay, and Venezuela); and strengthen

TABLE 34. Population at risk of lymphatic filariasis and estimated number of infected persons, Region of the Americas.

Country	Population	Population at risk	Population at risk (%)	Estimated number of infected persons
Brazil	186,405,000	1,500,000	0.8	60,000
Costa Rica	4,327,000	10,000	0.2	0
Dominican Republic	8,895,000	740,000	8.3	50,000
Guyana	751,000	630,000	83.9	50,000
Haiti	8,528,000	6,000,000	70.4	560,000
Suriname	449,000	35,000	7.8	0
Trinidad and Tobago	1,305,000	0	0	0
Total	210,660,000	8,915,000	4.2	720,000

Notes: Population data is derived from PAHO Basic Indicators 2005. Data for the population at risk and estimated number of infected persons for Brazil, the Dominican Republic, Haiti, and Guyana are derived from the Weekly Epidemiological Record, No. 22, 81, pp. 221–232, 2006. Data for the population at risk and estimated number of infected persons for Suriname, Trinidad and Tobago, and Costa Rica come from 2002 figures presented in the 2004 Report of the Regional Review Program Group, Region of the Americas, to the Third Meeting of the Global Alliance for the Elimination of Lymphatic Filariasis (GAELF-III).

human resources and epidemiological surveillance of the disease. The action plan emphasizes the need to promote decentralized leishmaniasis prevention and control activities from national programs into the primary care network, empower the community, and form strategic partnerships to fight the disease.

Lymphatic Filariasis

Lymphatic filariasis is the second largest cause of disability worldwide, affecting over 120 million people in 80 countries. In the Americas an estimated 8.8 million people are at risk for lymphatic filariasis, with 720,000 persons estimated to be infected (Table 34). Lymphatic filariasis in the Americas is caused by *Wuchereria bancrofti* and is transmitted by the night-biting mosquito *Culex quinquefasciatus.* As a result of mass drug administration, and, to a lesser extent, selective treatment of individual microfilaria carriers and vector control, there has been a marked decrease in the prevalence of lymphatic filariasis in the Americas.

Lymphatic filariasis is disfiguring and painful, and affects a person's ability to work and lead a normal life. Infection is usually acquired in childhood, but the worst clinical problems (elephantiasis and genital damage) are seen in adults during their most productive years, thus imposing a significant social and economic burden. The disease typically affects the poorest people in the world's poorest countries. In the Americas, most cases are concentrated in and around urban and periurban slums.

Subsequent to the 50th World Health Assembly in 1997, which called for the elimination of lymphatic filariasis as a public health problem by the year 2020, significant progress has been made in the Region. According to consensus reached as a result of the resolution emanating out of that World Health Assembly, elimination of lymphatic filariasis would be achieved when the five-year

cumulative incidence rate is reduced to less than 1 new infection per 1,000 individuals. The focalized nature of the infection and the relatively small number of cases in the Americas suggest that this goal could be met before 2020.

Since 1981, there have been reports of transmission in seven countries: Brazil, Costa Rica, the Dominican Republic, Guyana, Haiti, Suriname, and Trinidad and Tobago. Currently, only Brazil, the Dominican Republic, Guyana, and Haiti report active transmission, with epidemiological and entomological studies indicating interruption of transmission in the other three countries.

Governments of endemic countries have been initiating programs to eliminate lymphatic filariasis primarily by mass drug administration coupled with interventions to alleviate the suffering of affected individuals. Two drugs are currently used in the Region for treating the disease, albendazole and diethylcarbamazine (DEC). Albendazole, which is donated by Glaxo Smith Kline, also acts against soil-transmitted helminths, one of the major underlying causes of malnutrition and anemia in poor children. Albendazole is usually administered in combination with DEC tablets or DEC-fortified salt. A total of 1,754,146 persons in the Region were estimated to have been treated with either DEC salt or DEC tablets plus albendazole for lymphatic filariasis in 2005 (*484*).

In addition, national programs in the four endemic countries are focusing their attention on the alleviation of the physical, social, and economic hardship caused by the disease. Patient education, promotion of regular hygiene, and community education and awareness programs have had an effect on reducing the morbidity associated with infection, such as swollen limbs and episodes of pain.

Haiti bears the greatest burden of lymphatic filariasis in the Americas, with an estimated at-risk population of six million, approximately 70% of the total population at risk in the Region. The largest concentration of infection is found in the country's western region. Based on current population figures and mapping results, approximately 560,000 persons are estimated to be infected (see Table 34). In 2006, mass drug administration did not proceed due to a lack of funds, but funding has been secured for 2007 and the Haitian campaign to eliminate lymphatic filariasis will continue to build on past successes. In 2005, more than 1.2 million persons were treated with DEC and albendazole, achieving a coverage of 70% in the targeted areas. In Leogane, where mass drug administration began in 2000, microfilaria prevalence below 1% was reached in all four sentinel sites, demonstrating the positive impact of the intervention. Support groups to provide care for persons affected by lymphedema are now operating in at least three communities.

The Dominican Republic has an estimated 740,000 people at risk for lymphatic filariasis infection and an estimated 50,000 infected. Recent studies revealed prevalence rates ranging from 2% to 14% using nocturnal blood films and 9% to 35% using immunochromatographic test (ICT) cards. Mapping of the principal areas has been carried out, but needs to be completed in some areas in the east and north of the country. In 2005 there was a significant increase in mass drug administration coverage in the National District, from 82% to 92.5%. The current program is based on multidisciplinary activities, and is integrated into primary health care in the province of Barahona.

Guyana has 630,000 individuals, or more than 80% of its population, at risk; 50,000 are estimated to be infected. The at-risk population is located in various regions throughout the country. In response to this, a program of DEC-fortified salt was initiated in 2003. Guyana is the only country in the Region using DEC-fortified salt as the basis of its lymphatic filariasis elimination strategy and is working to improve coverage.

In Brazil, active transmission of lymphatic filariasis exists in two foci, primarily in the metropolitan area of Recife (Pernambuco), where the entire population of nearly 1,500,000 is considered to be at risk. The second focus for active transmission is Maceió (Alagoas); however, it is considered to be in a stage of pre-elimination. Epidemiological mapping of active foci in Brazil is almost complete, with only the area of Recife remaining. The intervention strategy traditionally followed in Brazil has been that of blood surveys and selective treatment of individuals. Since 2003, part of the metropolitan area of Recife has adopted a mass drug administration strategy using DEC tablets alone, which has expanded from 18,000 initial annual treatments to just over 55,000 annual treatments in 2005. This reflects coverage of approximately 87% of the 63,800 individuals who are eligible for treatment in those areas.

Studies in Trinidad and Tobago demonstrate an absence of transmission; however, it is necessary to maintain rigorous monitoring due to the flow of tourists and migrants from endemic countries. Recent studies in Suriname also suggest an absence of transmission, but intense surveillance along the Guyana border is required to monitor prevalence of the infection and risk of renewed transmission. Monitoring and surveillance activities in Costa Rica demonstrate there is no transmission, suggesting that lymphatic filariasis is no longer a public health problem. In addition, transmission also appears to be interrupted in the focus area of Belém, Brazil.

Despite challenges faced by some programs, including the lack of human and financial resources and, at times, political commitment, in 2007 an estimated 2.4 million persons at risk in the region will be covered by mass drug administration. Some of the determinants of this disease and its complications lie outside the purview of the health sector, including inadequate infrastructure, especially basic sanitation, water supply, drainage and waste removal, and precarious housing. Intersectoral partnerships are encouraged in order to ensure sustainability of the lymphatic filariasis elimination programs. PAHO actively encourages cooperation between the ministries of health of the seven countries where the disease is endemic, and coordinates partnerships with the U.S. Centers for Disease Control and Prevention, bilateral agencies, other United Nations agencies, the private sector, and NGOs to eliminate lymphatic filariasis in the Region.

Onchocerciasis

Infection caused by the filarial nematode worm *Onchocerca volvulus* can lead to eye lesions, including blindness, as well as severe itching and disfiguring skin lesions, known as onchocerciasis and onchocercal skin disease, respectively. Because the vectors, black flies in the genus *Simulium*, are insects whose immature stages breed in fast-flowing rivers and streams and where adult flies bite humans near these sites, the disease is also known as river blindness.

Onchocerciasis was first recognized in the Region in Venezuela in 1948, in Colombia in 1965, in Brazil in 1967, and in Ecuador in 1982. However, since 1985, there has been no convincing evidence of any expansion of existing foci in these countries. Based on historical data and estimates obtained prior to the 1990s, the total number of infected persons in the Region is estimated to be 150,000 to 200,000, while the estimated population at risk for the disease in the six countries of the Americas where it is endemic (Brazil, Colombia, Ecuador, Guatemala, Mexico, and Venezuela) was 4,700,000 persons in 1995. More data have been obtained as a result of rapid epidemiological and entomological assessments undertaken by the countries since 1995. As a result of these assessments the at-risk population estimates for 2005 dropped to a little over one-tenth, or 515,675, of the number in 1995 (Table 35). The total population at risk in the Americas now lives in only 13 restricted endemic foci in 1,950 villages, of which 232 are considered to be hyperendemic and at a higher risk of developing ocular disease. The areas at highest risk are those inhabited principally by indigenous peoples or isolated rural communities.

TABLE 35. Population at risk of onchocerciasis, communities at risk and at high risk of the disease, and endemic foci, countries of the Americas, 2004–2005.

Country	Population at risk[a]	Communities at risk[b]	Communities at high risk (hyperendemic)[b]	Endemic foci[b]
Mexico	168,819	670	39	• Oaxaca • Northern Chiapas • Southern Chiapas
Guatemala	199,558	518	42	• Huehuetenango • Sololá/Suchitepéquez/Chimaltenango • Escuintla • Santa Rosa
Colombia	1,410	1	0	• López de Micay
Ecuador	23,386	119	42	• Esmeraldas
Venezuela	113,019	625	104	• North-central: Aragua, Carabobo, Cojedes, Guárico, Miranda, and Yaracuy • Northeast: Anzoátegui, Monagas, and Sucre • Southern: Amazonas (Yanomami Area)
Brazil	9,483	17	5	• Amazonas—Roraima (Yanomami Area)
TOTAL	515,675	1,950	232	

[a]OEPA data for 2005, via e-mail correspondence from Dr. Mauricio Sauerbrey, OEPA Director, received on July 21, 2006.

[b]2004 Program Review for the Lions-Carter Center SightFirst River Blindness Programs, Cameroon, Ethiopia, Nigeria, OEPA, Sudan, and Uganda, 3–5 March 2005. The Carter Center, Atlanta, GA.

Massive drug administration of the anti-filarial drug ivermectin (Mectizan®) to the total population at risk is the core activity of the Regional initiative in each country; this is referred to as the ultimate treatment goal (UTG) (eligible population treated twice a year). The Pan American Health Foundation and the Mectizan® Donation Program in Atlanta coordinate the delivery of the drug, which is donated for free by Merck Inc. The national elimination programs coordinate regionally with the Onchocerciasis Elimination Program in the Americas or OEPA. PAHO is a member of OEPA's technical coordinating committee. National programs are monitored in terms of the percentage of the UTG attained every year in each of the endemic countries.

In Brazil, onchocerciasis is limited to one focus located in the northern part of Amazonas state and in the western part of Roraima state, bordering Venezuela. The eligible at-risk population was estimated at 7,522 individuals in 2005. The disease primarily affects Amerindians of the Yanomami and the Yek'wana ethnic groups, although immigration by miners could put other areas of Brazil at risk if competent local vectors are encountered in the miners' main residence. Brazil managed to attain 90% of its UTG in 2005, a noteworthy effort given the extreme difficulties of physical access to undeveloped forest and mountainous area. The alliance between the Ministry of Health and the nongovernmental sector to date has proven invaluable to the program as it attempts to cover all of the endemic villages.

The only known focus in Colombia is in and around the community of López de Micay, Cauca, on the Pacific coast. This community is classified as mesoendemic. Only 70 cases were identified between 1965 and 1991. The eligible population was estimated at 1,179 persons in 2005. The program attained 94% of its UTG in 2005, the seventh year in a row, and could well be approaching the interruption of transmission.

In Ecuador, the main onchocerciasis focus is located in the northwestern coastal province of Esmeraldas (the Esmeraldas/Pichincha focus) in the Santiago River basin, which has been divided into six operational areas. Satellite foci have been detected and can be traced to the migration of Chachi Amerindians from this area. The eligible at-risk population was estimated at 20,021 individuals in 2005. In that same year the program exceeded its treatment goal of 85%, achieving 98% of its UTG.

There are four foci in Guatemala, and the eligible population was estimated at 174,812 persons in 2005. The program attained 94% of its UTG in 2005, a marked improvement over previous years. In 2006 OEPA's technical coordinating committee recommended to the Government of Guatemala that ivermectin mass treatments be suspended in the Santa Rosa focus due to evidence of absence of transmission; a three-year epidemiological surveillance system was recommended to accompany any cessation of mass treatment in this focus. By the end of 2006 the Ministry of Health of Guatemala had taken the decision to end mass treatment in Santa Rosa, and monitoring is under way. However, elsewhere in the country, migrants crossing the Mexico-Guatemala border could pose a challenge in securing high treatment coverage in the remaining foci in both countries.

In Mexico, the population eligible for treatment was estimated at 152,303 in 2005. The country has managed to achieve high levels of treatment coverage in the three endemic foci: in 2004 and 2005 the program attained 95% of the country's UTG. The Oaxaca focus may be approaching interruption of transmission. Mexico also has been providing ivermectin four times a year (quarterly) in 50 of its most endemic communities in the Southern Chiapas focus since 2003, in a trial aimed at hastening onchocerciasis elimination; results are pending.

Three main foci have been detected in Venezuela. Significant efforts have been made in recent years to increase coverage in its three endemic foci, the Northeastern, North-central, and Southern foci. The Southern focus is still poorly accessible (access is by boat or helicopter, the latter being very costly). Those primarily infected are Amerindians of the Yanomami, Sanema, and Yek'wana groups. In 2005 94% of its UTG was achieved. In 2006 Venezuela attained the 85% treatment goal for the first time in the Southern focus. Studies conducted in Amazonas state in Venezuela have found that the geographical distribution of competent vectors is considerably larger than that of the disease. This means new foci could be created by the migration of individuals, especially miners. This issue, as well as the migration of Amerindians across the border to and from Brazil, requires added attention and needs to be placed in the wider context of improving access of these migratory populations to general primary health care services on both sides of the border.

In summary, onchocerciasis has been recognized as a problem for which there is now a relatively easy and economical solution. With the advent of ivermectin in 1987 and the Mectizan® Donation Program, the disease can be suppressed and controlled globally with chemotherapy. Morbidity and transmission rates in the countries have dropped significantly in response to the Regional initiative. It is probable that the Americas will be the first region in the world where ocular morbidity from onchocerciasis will cease to be a public health problem (OEPA's target: end of 2007) and where transmission will be interrupted in most if not all endemic foci. Mexico and Colombia are approaching this stage, followed by Ecuador and Guatemala. Currently, the hard to reach areas of Venezuela and Brazil continue to pose the greatest challenge to the elimination of onchocerciasis from the Region.

EMERGING AND REEMERGING INFECTIOUS DISEASES

The international spread of infectious diseases continues to pose a problem for global health security due to factors associated with today's interconnected and interdependent world—population movements through tourism, migration, or as a result of disasters; growth in international trade in food and biological products; social and environmental changes linked with urban-

ization, deforestation, and climate change; and shifts in the methods of food processing, distribution, and patterns of consumption. These factors have reaffirmed that infectious disease events in one country or region are of potential concern for the entire world (485).

An additional concern is the possibility of outbreaks resulting from the intentional or accidental release of biological agents. Epidemics that might occur naturally and those due to the release of biological agents both present a threat to global health security. Recent examples of these are the deliberate release of anthrax in the United States; the severe acute respiratory syndrome (SARS) epidemic; and the emergence of a new highly pathogenic strain of avian influenza H5N1 that has alerted the world to the possible emergence of a new pandemic influenza strain.

In the Americas, there were significant infectious disease outbreaks in 2001–2006 that required international collaboration and collective action in detection, confirmation, and/or public health intervention. In Martinique, chikungunya was imported from the Island of Reunion; in Belize, for the first time, West Nile virus was detected in a horse; in Bolivia, a chickenpox case being misreported through informal channels as a smallpox case resulted in an international rapid response; in Guatemala, a cluster of acute respiratory infections of unknown etiology in a health care setting prompted national and international rapid response teams to deploy and contain the outbreak in fear that a new influenza strain had emerged; a Rocky Mountain spotted fever outbreak was described for the first time in Urubá, Colombia, requiring international assistance in implementing prevention measures; and E. coli O157:H7 outbreaks affected tourism and food trade in Mexico and the United States.

Factors relating to the management of epidemics can also escalate an epidemic into a public health emergency of international concern. Some such factors include the absence of correct information, misinformation, or inconsistent information available to national governments, which can result in overreaction to media coverage and subsequent internal pressure on the governments to respond; insufficient capacity at the country level to recognize disease events in a timely manner and to contain them; fear of costly repercussions if disease events are notified; and lack of appropriate international response mechanisms, both legal and technical (485). Given all these factors, the need for international cooperation in the detection and response to epidemics has become critical. Such cooperation has been pursued by PAHO and WHO, using the 1969 International Health Regulations and the revised and version adopted in 2005 as a legal framework.

The 2005 revised International Health Regulations, IHR (2005), adopted by the 58th World Health Assembly, have been redesigned so as to provide a new international legal framework for the control of transborder infectious diseases (485). The IHR (2005) also has set out country core capacities for the detection and response to health threats—early warning and surveillance systems, epidemiological and outbreak investigation capabilities, laboratory expertise and infrastructure, information and communication mechanisms, and management systems (*486*). Their purpose and scope is to prevent, protect against, control, and provide a public health response to the international spread of disease in ways that are commensurate with and restricted to public health risks, while avoiding unnecessary interference with international traffic and trade (*487*).

Moreover, countries need to develop core capacities to respond to the political and administrative decentralization and health sector reform processes, which are profoundly changing the management, organization, delivery, and financing of Latin America's and the Caribbean's health services. These processes are redefining the functions of central, regional, and local governments in managing both individual and population-based health care services. Therefore, countries need to strengthen their health service infrastructure and establish an ongoing process for building institutional capacity to detect and intervene in a timely, effective, efficient, and sustainable manner in public health emergencies caused by epidemics (*488*).

The Subregional Surveillance Networks of Emerging and Reemerging Infectious Diseases (Southern Cone, Amazon Basin, Central America, and the Caribbean) were created under the principle of interaction between laboratory services and epidemiology. The networks provide fora in which countries can collaborate with one another to monitor, prevent, and control communicable diseases that represent common threats to the countries in each subregion; coordinate surveillance and control standards or protocols; exchange and optimize human, material, and financial resources; and create systematic coordinated mechanisms of action among all countries.

Influenza Pandemic Preparedness in the Americas

Influenza is a viral disease that affects both animals and humans. When a new strain of influenza virus emerges and adapts to enable transmission from person to person, the disease can quickly spread far and wide, resulting in a pandemic. Although the disruption caused by influenza pandemics is often compared to natural disasters, a pandemic is more likely to affect a larger portion of the population with widespread and sustained effects, overstretching the resources of every country, state, and municipality. Such a strain will challenge the possibility of shifting resources, emphasizing the need for all countries to develop pandemic preparedness plans.

The 56th World Health Assembly and the 44th Directing Council of the Pan American Health Organization, held in 2003, issued resolutions urging countries to strengthen their capacity to prevent, detect, and diagnose influenza virus infection, and to be prepared to respond to a pandemic situation (*489, 490*). These contingency plans must be put in place now, during the interpandemic period, to better respond to this threat with potentially catastrophic consequences worldwide.

In 2006, some 130 million people (23% of the total population) lived in rural areas of Latin America and the Caribbean

(*491*), most of them coming in direct contact with chickens and pigs. The Food and Agriculture Organization of the United Nations (FAO) reports that poultry accounts for approximately 70% of the animal protein consumed in Latin America and the Caribbean (*492*). Also, the expanding poultry industry has become a major source of income and employment, contributing to urban and periurban development. The impact of a pandemic in the Region would represent not only a public health problem, but also a food security threat and an economic disaster for the poorest population in rural areas and for national economies.

Considering the threat posed by a possible influenza pandemic, in 2005 a multidisciplinary task force on epidemic alert and response was created within PAHO to advise, coordinate, and monitor all activities of the Organization related to the planning and implementation of influenza pandemic preparedness and response, within the framework of the new mandates set forth by IHR (2005) (*493*). These stipulate that countries develop, strengthen, and maintain core capacities to detect, assess, and intervene to control events of international public health importance. The interprogrammatic nature of the task force allows it to better tackle the complex process involved in IHR implementation and better plan for an influenza pandemic, which requires highly coordinated efforts from a variety of sectors.

The focus of PAHO's technical cooperation has been initially to assist Member States in drafting National Influenza Pandemic Preparedness Plans (NIPPPs), taking into account the recommendations for national measures before and during pandemics presented in WHO's Global Influenza Preparedness Plan (*494*). Box 10 summarizes key steps in the development and assessment of NIPPPs.

These multisectoral plans must integrate human and veterinary health and be flexible enough to consider multiple scenarios of potential pandemic impact according to different levels of viral pathogenicity and availability of resources. Subregional workshops have been carried out to train those charged with preparing NIPPPs in the use of modeling software, tools that the U.S. Centers for Disease Control and Prevention (CDC) have developed to estimate the potential impact of a given pandemic (*495–497*). This enables countries to ensure that their national plans are flexible by considering many contingencies, including a worst-case scenario where there are neither available vaccines nor antiviral medications. Table 36 summarizes estimates of potential pandemic impact in Latin America and the Caribbean for a 1968-like and a 1918-like scenario that were prepared by country teams during those workshops.

After Member Countries provided draft plans, a series of self-assessment exercises were carried out, in which NIPPPs were evaluated using a PAHO-developed tool based on WHO's checklist for influenza pandemic preparedness planning (*498*). The tool covers the seven core components in WHO's checklist: emergency preparedness; surveillance; case investigation and treatment; preventing spread of the disease in the community; maintaining essential services; research and evaluation; and implementation,

---

BOX 10. PAHO Strategy in Support of Member States for the Development and Assessment of National Influenza Pandemic Preparedness Plans (NIPPPs)

1. Development of draft NIPPPs:
   a. Introduction of WHO guidelines for pandemic preparedness planning.
   b. Introduction and application of modeling tools such as FluAid, FluSurge, and FluWorkloss in order to estimate the potential impact of a pandemic.
   c. Development of national action plans that adequately incorporate the drafting of NIPPPs.

2. Assessment and testing of draft NIPPPs:
   a. Self-assessment of NIPPPs.
   b. Table-top exercises to highlight issues of chain of command and need for multisectoral integration and coordination.
   c. Development of action plans to address remaining gaps identified during the self-assessment and simulation exercises.

3. Local implementation of NIPPPs:
   a. Development of simulation drills and table-top exercises to test local preparedness and put local contingency plans into practice.
   b. Promotion of subnational, multisectoral training to promote the development of local contingency plans in the event of a pandemic that adequately incorporate all pertinent areas, including surveillance, health services, disaster management, and social communication.
   c. Carrying out of table-top exercises to test the completeness of local plans, taking into account subnational realities.

4. Monitoring and strengthening of NIPPPs:
   a. Promotion of the use of subnational drills to assist in the monitoring of "suitability" of local contingency plans.
   b. Promotion of any necessary changes in order to update plans.

---

testing, and revision of the national plan. These core components are further divided into 44 main categories, comprising a total of 368 checkpoints for assessment. One of the major achievements of this interaction was the generation of multisectoral discussions about the required steps for completing the national plans, promoting joint work, and integrating the contingency planning process. Table 37 presents the average compliance (%) of the Region's four subregions with WHO guidelines for each of the seven core components of a NIPPP.

Influenza pandemics have historically taken the world by surprise, leaving minimal time for health services to prepare for the surge in cases and deaths that characterize these events and make them so disruptive (499). The current situation is markedly different, as the world has been warned in advance, providing an unprecedented opportunity, especially in the Americas, to prepare for a pandemic and develop ways to mitigate its effects even in areas with problems of access to basic health services.

Evidence suggests that an influenza pandemic will be most intensely felt at the community level, especially among the young, the poor, and other vulnerable groups (500). Despite tremendous strides in advocating for influenza pandemic preparedness at the national level, a significant challenge lies in bringing preparedness to local policymakers, practitioners, and concerned citizens who will be called on to implement national plans. In order to bridge the current gap between planning and implementation, local counterparts must be encouraged and enlisted to take part in the national planning process. Such local implementation of NIPPPs will be tested through simulation drills and table-top exercises to test local preparedness and to put local contingency plans into practice.

Current global threats, including an influenza pandemic, require a concerted effort by all those capable of effective action. Moreover, the intersectoral effort must harness the participation of the private sector, nongovernmental organizations, and academia. Undoubtedly, more resources will be needed to stimulate counterpart support by the countries, to piggy-back on and expand existing surveillance systems to become population-based, and to scale up the preparedness and rapid response at the local level. Access to drugs, vaccines, and other supplies is as yet an unresolved issue.

The threat of an influenza pandemic has revealed the weaknesses of some systems in the Americas, but it once again has highlighted the strong determination among the countries of the

TABLE 36. Potential impact of an influenza pandemic with a 25% clinical attack rate, by main health impact and severity scenario, Latin America and the Caribbean, 2006.

	Pandemic scenario	
Potential health impact	1968 (moderate)	1918 (severe)
Deaths	334,163	2,418,469
	(131,630–654,960)	(627,367–5,401,035)
Hospitalizations	1,461,401	11,798,613
	(459,051–1,937,503)	(3,189,747–16,418,254)
Outpatient visits	76,187,593	68,470,386
	(59,738,730–109,207,769)	(58,114,124–92,227,761)

Source: Pan American Health Organization, Washington, D.C.

TABLE 37. Current compliance (%) with WHO checklist for influenza pandemic preparedness planning, by core component and subregion, Latin America and the Caribbean, mid-2006.

Core component	Andean Area	Central America	Caribbean	Southern Cone
1. Emergency preparedness	38.6	34.6	56.7	58.5
2. Epidemiological surveillance	37.0	34.8	56.5	54.4
3. Case management	52.3	54.5	48.9	60.9
4. Population containment	20.0	38.0	37.0	64.0
5. Essential services continuity	24.5	33.3	45.2	41.9
6. Research and evaluation	10.0	40.0	15.0	30.2
7. Implementation of the national plan	40.0	60.0	30.0	50.0

Source: Pan American Health Organization, Washington, D.C.

Region to work together quickly to overcome disparities and to share information (Box 11). Technical cooperation has served to further strengthen public health in the countries, which represents an extraordinary global contribution and, ultimately, could save many lives.

Severe Acute Respiratory Syndrome

Severe acute respiratory syndrome (SARS) was first recognized at the end of February 2003 in Hanoi, Vietnam. It is believed to have originated in southern China in November 2002; by February 2003, it had crossed into Hong Kong (China). Shortly after, in mid-March, WHO considered it a global threat. As of 5 July 2003, when the last human chain of transmission had been broken, 26 countries had been affected, resulting in 8,096 probable cases and 774 deaths (*501*).

Canada and the United States were the only two countries in the Americas that reported probable SARS cases. After China and Hong Kong, Toronto, Canada, was the Region's hardest hit area by SARS, with 438 probable/suspected cases, including 44 deaths. The toll on health care workers was especially high: more than 100 fell ill and 3 died. In the United States, 27 cases were reported and no deaths (*502*).

The etiological agent, SARS coronavirus (SARS-CoV), is thought to be an animal virus that crossed the species barrier from animal to humans and adapted itself, enabling human-to-human transmission (*503*). Although the natural reservoir of SARS-CoV has not been identified, several animal species are potentially involved, since a variety of animals, including the Himalayan masked palm civet (*Paguma larvata*), the Chinese ferret badger (*Melogale moschata*), the raccoon dog (*Nyctereutes procyonoides*), ferrets (*Mustela furo*), and domestic cats (*Felis domesticus*), have tested positive for SARS-CoV infection (*502*). Investigations of modes and routes of transmission from animals to humans or other animal species are still being conducted.

The most probable sources of recent infection are exposures in laboratories that handle the virus for research purposes or from animal reservoirs. Since July 2003, there have been four events of SARS reemergence. Three of them were attributed to breaches in laboratory biosafety and resulted in one or more cases (Singapore, Taipei, and Beijing) (*504, 505*). The fourth event resulted in four sporadic, community-acquired cases arising over a six-week period in Guangzhou, Guangdong province of China. Three of the cases were attributed to exposure to animal or environmental sources, while in the other case the source of exposure remains unknown (*504*).

These events demonstrate the possibility of a resurgence of a SARS outbreak, thereby stressing the need for all countries to remain vigilant and maintain their capacity to detect and respond to the disease.

The WHO Guidelines for the Global Surveillance of Severe Acute Respiratory Syndrome (SARS); Updated Recommenda-

BOX 11. Achievements of PAHO Member States in Developing and Assessing NIPPPs

- Professionals from various sectors are working together, often for the first time, on building national capacity to cope with a pandemic.
- Countries are creating, analyzing, and refining their NIPPPs in an integrated and coordinated fashion.
- Pandemic influenza preparedness is included in the health agendas of the Regional Integration Systems (MERCOSUR, CARICOM, CAN, SISCA).
- The public health infrastructure is bolstered, targeted to a possible influenza pandemic but applicable to an array of public health emergencies.
- A regional cadre of professionals is trained in multiple aspects of influenza preparedness—health services delivery, surveillance, risk and social communication, and disaster and emergency management.
- There are professionals who are able to replicate training to associates and colleagues at the subnational levels.
- Trained professionals are committed to continue to pursue influenza preparedness activities.

TABLE 38. Cases of hantavirus pulmonary syndrome, Region of the Americas, 1993–2005.

	1993	1994	1995	1996	1997	1998	1999	2000	2001	2002	2003	2004	2005	Total
Argentina														
Cases	21	10	10	42	51	67	81	68	92	86	54	61	...	643
Deaths						11				...	...	...	...	11
Bolivia														
Cases	3		1	1	7	6	2	1	5	8	11	7	18	70
Deaths										...		2	3	5
Brazil														
Cases	3		1	3		11	28	56	77	75	84	159	167	664
Deaths	2		1	3		7	12	19	24	...	...	53	...	121
Canada														
Cases		8	3	3	7	6	2	1	...	44	14	...	...	88
Deaths										...	...	...	...	...
Chile														
Cases			1	3	30	35	26	31	81	65	60	56	67	455
Deaths			...	...	18	20	11	12	30	19	18	18	21	149
Panama														
Cases							3	21	5	2	4	...	...	35
Deaths									1		2	...	...	3
Paraguay														
Cases		16	15	5	4	5	4	15	27	4	4	...	...	99
Deaths			2	1	1	0	2	2	5	...	...	...	...	13
Uruguay														
Cases					2	3	12	8	4	9	10	...	...	48
Deaths					1	2	1	1	0	3	5	...	...	13
United States														
Cases	21	20	14	15	18	24	30	35	8	13	22	19	27	266
Deaths	27	12	10	7	5	9	13	11	3	10	9	7	9	132
Venezuela														
Cases										2	...	...	...	...	2
Deaths										...	...	...	...	...
Total cases	48	54	45	72	119	157	188	236	299	308	263	302	279	2,370
Total deaths	29	12	13	11	25	49	39	45	63	32	34	80	33	465

TABLE 39. Cholera cases, Region of the Americas, 1991–2005.

Country/territory	1991	1992	1993	1994	1995	1996	1997	1998	1999	2000	2001	2002	2003	2004	2005
Region of the Americas	**396,536**	**358,174**	**210,972**	**127,187**	**75,690**	**21,028**	**17,923**	**57,312**	**9,683**	**2,703**	**534**	**23**	**32**	**36**	**24**
Argentina	—	553	2,080	889	188	474	637	12	1	1	—	—	—	—	—
Belize	—	159	135	6	19	26	2	28	12	—	—	—	—	—	—
Bermuda	…	…	…	…	…	…	—	—	—	—	—	—	—	—	—
Bolivia	206	22,260	10,134	2,710	3,136	2,847	1,632	466	—	750	7	—	—	21	5
Brazil	2,103	37,572	60,340	51,324	4,954	1,017	3,044	2,745	4,717	5[d]	6[e]	4	5[e]	3	7
Canada	3	5	7	2	5	3	—	3	3	—	—	4	—	—	—
Chile	41	73	32	1	—	1	4	24	—	1	—	—	—	2	—
Colombia	16,800	13,287	609	996	1,922	4,428	1,508	442	20	1	—	—	—	—	—
Costa Rica	—	12	14	37	24	19	1[a]	—	—	—	—	—	—	—	—
Ecuador	46,284	31,870	6,883	1,785	2,160	1,059	65	3,755	171	27	9	…	25	5	—
El Salvador	947	8,106	6,573	11,739	2,923	182	—	8	134	63[d]	—	—	—	—	—
Guayana	1	16	2	…	…	…	…	—	—	—	—	—	—	—	—
Guatemala	3,664	15,861	30,821	16,779	7,970	1,568	1,263	5,970	2,077	178	13	1	—	—	—
French Guiana	—	556	66	—	—	—	…	—	—	—	—	—	—	—	—
Honduras	17	407	4,013	5,049	4,717	708	90	306	56	15	1	—	—	—	—
Mexico	2,690	8,162	10,712	4,059	16,430	1,088	2,356	71	9	5	1	—	—	—	—
Nicaragua	1	3,067	6,631	7,881	8,825	2,813	1,283	1,437	545	12	—	—	—	—	—
Panama	1,178	2,416	42	9	—	4	—	—	—	—	—	—	—	—	—
Paraguay	—	—	3	—	—	—	—	—	—	—	—	—	—	—	—
Peru	322,562	210,836	71,448	23,887	22,397	4,518	3,483	41,717	1,546	934	494	16	—	—	—
Suriname	—	12	—	—	—	—	—	—	—	—	—	—	—	—	—
United States	26	102	18	34	20	5	4[b]	15[c]	6[b]	4[a]	3	2[d]	2[d]	5	12[e]
Venezuela	13	2,842	409	—	—	268	2,551	313	386	140	—	—	—	—	—

[a] One imported case.
[b] Three imported cases.
[c] Eight imported cases.
[d] Two imported cases.
[e] Five imported cases; one unknown.
— No cases reported.
… Data not available.
Source: Ministries of health.
Updated in October 2006.

tions October 2004 and WHO SARS Risk Assessment and Preparedness Framework are two documents intended to be used together by the countries. The latter introduces important changes to the global risk assessment and case definitions for SARS, thus replacing all previous WHO guidance on SARS surveillance and response. The former sets out a framework for national and international levels to assess the risk of SARS reemergence and prepare appropriate contingency plans.

Hantavirus Pulmonary Syndrome

In the Americas, hantavirus pulmonary syndrome (HPS) was first described in North America in 1993. Since then, up to 2004, the number of HPS cases totals 2,196. The average annual number of cases reported from 1993 to 1999 was 108. Since 2000, the average number of annual cases increased to 281. Argentina, Bolivia, Brazil, Canada, Chile, Panama, Paraguay, the United States, Uruguay, and Venezuela have reported cases (Table 38).

No new viruses have been identified other than the ones previously described in the Region, namely, Oran, Lechiguanas, Hu39694, Andes virus, Rio Mamore virus, Laguna Negra, Sin Nombre, New York, Bayou, Black Creek Canal, Choclo, and Calabazo.

Even though the severity of cases relates to the specific viral strain and the patient's immunological response, in general case fatality rates from HPS consistently decreased from approximately 50% in 1996–2000 to 30% in 2001–2005 in countries with the highest rates (*506*).

Cholera

Since the cholera pandemic of 1991, the Region of the Americas has observed a steady decline in the number of reported cases (Table 39). A marked decrease was observed in 2002, with only 23 cholera cases reported to WHO from Peru (16), Canada (4), the United States (2), and Guatemala (1). From 2003 through 2005, the total number of cases reported in the Region was similarly low, with 32, 36, and 24 cases, respectively. It should be noted that in analyzing the data, Brazil, Canada, and the United States have consistently reported cases and in some years they have made the distinction between indigenous and imported cases. In the Region, the occurrence of cholera cases was characteristically limited to clusters that were rapidly contained with very low public health impact. Many countries continue to implement passive and active surveillance to detect circulating *Vibrio cholerae*.

References

1. Comisión Económica para América Latina y el Caribe, Centro Latinoamericano y Caribeño de Demografía. Dinámica demográfica y desarrollo en América Latina y el Caribe. Serie Desarrollo y Población Nº 58. Santiago de Chile: CELADE; Fondo de Población de las Naciones Unidas; 2005.

2. Economic Commission for Latin America and the Caribbean. Demographic inequalities and social inequality: recent trends, associated factors and policy lessons. In: Social Panorama of Latin America 2005. Santiago, Chile: ECLAC; 2005.

3. Economic Commission for Latin America and the Caribbean. Demographic changes in Latin America and the Caribbean and their policy implications. In: Social Panorama of Latin America 2004. Santiago, Chile: ECLAC; 2004.

4. Chackiel J. La dinámica demográfica en América Latina. Serie Población y Desarrollo Nº 52. Santiago de Chile: CELADE/CEPAL; 2004.

5. Bloom D, Canning D, Weston M. The value of vaccination. World Economics. 2005;6(3):15–39.

6. Pan American Health Organization. Disease prevention. In: Health in the Americas. Washington, DC: PAHO; 2002. (Scientific publication No. 587; 2 vols).

7. Andrus JK, Fitzimmons J, de Quadros CA. Introduction of New and Under-utilized Vaccines: Perspectives from the Americas. In: Andrus JK, de Quadros CA (eds.). Recent Advances in Immunization. 2nd edition. Washington, DC: Pan American Health Organization; 2006.

8. Pan American Health Organization. Taylor Commission. The Impact of the Expanded Program on Immunization and the Polio Eradication Initiative on Health Systems in the Americas. Washington, DC: PAHO; 1995.

9. Pan American Health Organization. Resolution CD31.R22. Expanded Program for Immunization in the Americas. 31st Directing Council. Washington, DC: PAHO; 1985.

10. de Quadros CA, Andrus JK, Olivé JM, Macedo CG de, Henderson DA. Polio eradication from the Western Hemisphere. Annu Rev Public Health. 1992;12:239–52.

11. World Health Organization. Global Polio Eradication Initiative 2005. Annual Report. Geneva: WHO; 2006.

12. World Health Organization. Resurgence of wild poliovirus type 1 transmission and effect of importation into polio-free countries, 2000–2005. Wkly Epidemiol Rec. 2006;81:61–8.

13. Kew O, Morris-Glasgow V, Landaverde M, Burns C, Shaw J, Garib Z, et al. Outbreak of poliomyelitis in Hispaniola associated with circulating type 1 vaccine-derived poliovirus. Science. 2002;296(5566):356–59.

14. United States, Centers for Disease Control and Prevention. Public Health Dispatch: Acute Flaccid Paralysis Associated with Circulating Vaccine-Derived Poliovirus—Philippines, 2001. Morb Mortal Wkly Rep. 2001;50(40):874–75.

15. United States, Centers for Disease Control and Prevention. Poliovirus Infections in Four Unvaccinated Children—Minnesota, August–October 2005. Morb Mortal Wkly Rep. 2005;54:1–3.

16. Pan American Health Organization. Polio Weekly Bulletin. 2004;19(30).

17. Pan American Health Organization. Final Report. XVII Technical Advisory Group (TAG) Meeting on Vaccine-Preventable Diseases, Guatemala City, Guatemala, 25–27 July 2006.

18. Pan American Health Organization. Resolution CD37.R13. Expanded Program for Immunization in the Americas. 37th Directing Council. Washington, DC: PAHO; 1994.

19. de Quadros CA, Izurieta H, Venczel L, Carrasco P. Measles eradication in the Americas: progress to date. J Infect Dis. 2004;189(Suppl 1):227–35.

20. de Quadros CA, Olivé JM, Hersh BS, et al. Measles elimination in the Americas: evolving strategies. JAMA. 1996;275:224–29.

21. Pan American Health Organization. Measles Elimination Field Guide. Washington, DC: PAHO; 2005. (Scientific publication No. 605; 2nd edition).

22. Organización Panamericana de la Salud. ¡19 semanas sin notificación de transmisión del virus del sarampión en el continente americano! Bol PAI. 2003;25:1. Available from: http://www.paho.org/spanish/ad/fch/im/sns2501.pdf. Accessed 15 September 2006.

23. de Quadros CA, Izurieta H, Carrasco P, Brana M, Tambini G. Progress toward measles eradication in the region of the Americas. J Infect Dis. 2003;187(Suppl 1):102–10.

24. Andrus JK, Vicari A, Tambini G, Periago MR. The global inter-relatedness of disease control. Lancet Infect Dis. 2007;7(3):176.

25. Narváez B, Barrezueta O. La experiencia de Venezuela en la eliminación del sarampión. Pan American Health Organization. The Culture of Prevention: A Model for Control of Vaccine-Preventable Diseases. XVI Technical Advisory Group (TAG) Meeting on Vaccine-Preventable Diseases, Mexico City, Mexico, 3–5 November 2004.

26. Pan American Health Organization. Final Report. The Culture of Prevention: A Model for Control of Vaccine-preventable Diseases. XVI Technical Advisory Group (TAG) Meeting on Vaccine-Preventable Diseases, Mexico City, Mexico, 3–5 November 2004.

27. United Nations Children's Fund. Maternal and Neonatal Tetanus Elimination by 2005: Strategies for Achieving and Maintaining Elimination. New York: UNICEF; 2000.

28. Pan American Health Organization. Elimination of Neonatal Tetanus. Field Guide. Washington, DC: PAHO; 2005. (Scientific publication No. 602; 2nd edition).

29 Pan American Health Organization. Final Report. XIII Technical Advisory Group (TAG) Meeting on Vaccine-Preventable Diseases, Quebec, Canada, 12–16 April 1999.

30. Pan American Health Organization. Final Report. XVIII Technical Advisory Group (TAG) Meeting on Vaccine-Preventable Diseases in the Regions of Central America, Mexico and the Hispanic Caribbean, Antigua, Guatemala, 6–7 June 2005.

31. United States, Centers for Disease Control and Prevention. Epidemiology and Prevention of Vaccine-preventable Diseases. 9th edition. Washington, DC: Public Health Foundation; 2006.

32. United States, Centers for Disease Control and Prevention. Preventing Tetanus, Diphtheria, and Pertussis among Adolescents: Use of Tetanus Toxoid, Reduced Diphtheria Toxoid and Acellular Pertussis Vaccines. Recommendations of the Advisory Committee on Immunization Practices (ACIP). Morb Mortal Wkly Rep. 2006;55:1–34.

33. Landazabal N, Burgos M, Pastor D. Brote de difteria en Cali (Valle), Colombia, agosto–octubre 2000. Bol Epidemiol. 2001;22(3):13–15.

34. Pan American Health Organization. Control of Diphtheria, Pertussis, Tetanus, Haemophilus influenzae type b, and Hepatitis B: Field Guide. Washington, DC: OPS; 2005. (Scientific and technical publication No. 604).

35. Haiti, Ministry of Public Health and Population. Expanded Program on Immunization. Port-au-Prince; 2005. Unpublished.

36. Cochi SL, O'Mara D, Preblud SR. Progress in Haemophilus type b polysaccharide vaccine use in the United States. Pediatrics. 1988;81:166–68.

37. Peltola H. Haemophilus influenzae type b disease and vaccination in Latin America and the Caribbean. Pediatr Infect Dis J. 1997;16(8):780–87.

38. World Health Organization. Haemophilus influenzae type b (Hib) meningitis in the pre-vaccine era: a global review of incidence, age distributions, and case-fatality rates. Geneva: WHO; 2002. (WHO/V&B/02.18).

39. Dominican Republic, Secretaría de Estado de Salud Pública y Asistencia Social. República Dominicana: vigilancia epidemiológica de las meningitis y neumonías bacterianas. (Presented at the PAHO Subregional Meeting on Surveillance of Bacterial Meningitis and Pneumonia in the Americas, Mexico City, Mexico, 6–8 March 2000).

40. Schlech WF, Ward JI, Bard JD. Bacterial meningitis in the United States. J Infect Dis. 1986;153:8–16.

41. Pan American Health Organization. Final Report. XII Technical Advisory Group (TAG) Meeting on Vaccine-Preventable Diseases, Guatemala City, Guatemala, 3–5 September 1997. Washington, DC: PAHO; 1997.

42. Ropero AM, Danovaro-Holliday MC, Andrus JK. Progress in vaccination against Haemophilus Influenzae type b in the Americas. J Clin Virol. 2005 Dec;34 Suppl 2:S14–9.

43. Pan American Health Organization. Final Report. XVI Technical Advisory Group (TAG) Meeting on Vaccine-Preventable Diseases, Foz de Iguaçu, Brazil, 2–5 October 2000.

44. Ropero AM, Danovaro-Holliday MC, Andrus JK. Progress in vaccination against *Haemophilus influenzae* type b in the Americas. J Clin Virol. 2005 Dec;34 Suppl 2:S14–9.

45. Fay OH. Hepatitis B in Latin America: epidemiological patterns and eradication strategy. The Latin American Regional Study Group. Vaccine. 1990;8(Suppl):82–92.

46. de la Hoz F, Martinez M, Iglesias A, Rojas M. Factores de riesgo en la transmisión de hepatitis B en la Amazonia Colombiana. Biomédica. 1992;12:5–9.

47. Leon P, Venegas E, Bengoechea L, Rojas E, Lopez JA, Elola C. Prevalencia de las infecciones por virus de las hepatitis B, C, D y E en Bolivia. Rev Panam Salud Publica. 1999;5:144–51.

48. Silveira TR, da Fonseca JC, Rivera L, Fay OH, Tapia R, Santos JI, et al. Hepatitis B seroprevalence in Latin America. Rev Panam Salud Publica. 1999;6:378–383.

49. Tanaka J. Hepatitis B epidemiology in Latin America. Vaccine. 2000;18(Suppl 1):7–9.

50. Castillo-Solórzano C, Andrus JK. Rubella elimination and improving health care for women. Emerg Infect Dis. 2004;10(11):2017–21.

51. Danovaro-Holliday MC, LeBaron CW, Allensworth C, Raymond R, Borden TG, Murray AB, et al. A large rubella outbreak with spread from the workplace to the community. JAMA. 2000;284:2733–39.

52. Pan American Health Organization. Measles and Rubella Surveillance Integration in the Americas. EPI Newsletter. 2000;22:2. Available from: http://www.ops-oms.org/english/ad/fch/im/nlrubella_MRSurveillanceIntegration_April2000.pdf. Accessed 15 September 2006.

53. Irons B, Lewis MJ, Dahl-Regis M, Castillo-Solórzano C, Carrasco P, de Quadros CA. Strategies to eradicate rubella in the English-speaking Caribbean. Am J Pub Health. 2000; 90(10):1545–49.

54. Caribbean Community, Council for Human and Social Development. Resolution on the elimination of rubella. In: Report of the First Meeting of the Council for Human and Social Development, Kingston, Jamaica, 20–21 April 1998. Georgetown (Guyana): Council for Human and Social Development; 1998. pp. 21–22. (Report 98/1/53).

55. Pan American Health Organization. Rubella/CRS Elimination Strategy: Contributing to PHC Renewal. Immunization Newsletter. 2005 August; 27(5):4. Available from: http://www.paho.org/english/ad/fch/im/sne2704.pdf. Accessed 15 September 2006.

56. United States, Centers for Disease Control and Prevention. Achievements in public health: elimination of rubella and congenital rubella syndrome—United States, 1969–2004. Morb Mortal Wkly Rep. 2005;54(11):279–82.

57. Pan American Health Organization. XVII TAG Meeting. Protecting the Health of the Americas: Moving from Child to Family Immunization. Immunization Newsletter. 2006;

28:4. Available from: http://www.paho.org/English/AD/FCH/IM/sne2804.pdf. Accessed 6 July 2007.

58. Pan American Health Organization. Ad-hoc Meeting of Experts to Establish Best Practices in CRS Surveillance. Immunization Newsletter. 2006;28:4. Available from: http://www.paho.org/English/AD/FCH/IM/sne2804.pdf. Accessed 6 July 2007.

59. Icenogle J. Nomenclature and molecular epidemiology of rubella virus in the Americas and the world. (Presented at the 16th meeting of the Technical Advisory Group on Vaccine-Preventable Disease, Mexico City, Mexico, November 2004.)

60. Andrus JK, Periago MR. Elimination of rubella and congenital rubella syndrome in the Americas: another opportunity to address inequities in health. Pan Am J Public Health. 2004;15(3):145–46.

61. Pan American Health Organization. Resolution CE126.R4. Vaccines and Immunization. 42nd Directing Council. Washington, DC: PAHO; 2000.

62. Pan American Health Organization. Immunization in the Americas: 2006 Summary. Washington, DC: PAHO; 2006.

63. Andrus JK. Immunization: The Unfinished Agenda and Achieving the Millennium Development Goals. (Presented at the 46th Directing Council, PAHO, Washington, DC, 28 September 2005.)

64. Pan American Health Organization. Resolution CD44.R1. 44th Directing Council. Sustaining Immunization Programs—Elimination of Rubella and Congenital Rubella Syndrome (CRS). Washington, DC: PAHO; 2003.

65. World Health Organization. Global Immunization Vision and Strategy 2006–2015. Geneva: WHO; 2005. (WHO/IVB/05.05).

66. World Health Organization. Global Burden of Disease 2002 Estimates (Web page). Available from: http://www.who.int/healthinfo/bodgbd2002/en/index.html. Accessed 19 September 2006.

67. Pan American Health Organization. Influenza Vaccination among Risk Groups in Costa Rica: An Evidence-based Decision. EPI Newsletter. 2004;26:32–4. Available from: http://www.paho.org/english/ad/fch/im/sne2603.pdf. Accessed 15 September 2006.

68. Pan American Health Organization. Influenza control in El Salvador. Immunization Newsletter. 2006;28:2. http://www.paho.org/english/ad/fch/im/sne2802.pdf. Accessed 15 September 2006.

69. United States, Centers for Disease Control and Prevention. Prevention and control of influenza: recommendations of the Advisory Committee on Immunization Practices (ACIP). Morb Mortal Wkly Rep. 2006;55:RR–10.

70. Parashar UD, Hummelman EG, Bresee JS, Miller MA, Glass RI. Global illness and deaths caused by rotavirus disease in children. Emerg Infect Dis. 2003;9(5):565–72.

71. Vesikari T, Matson DO, Dennehy P, Van Damme P, Santosham M, Rodriguez Z, et al. Safety and efficacy of a pentavalent human-bovine (WC3) reassortant rotavirus vaccine. N Engl J Med. 2006;354:23–33.

72. United States, Centers for Disease Control and Prevention. Withdrawal of rotavirus vaccine recommendation. Morb Mortal Wkly Rep. 1999;48:1007.

73. Danovaro-Holliday MC, Wood AL, LeBaron CW. Rotavirus vaccine and the news media, 1987–2001. JAMA. 2002; 287(11):1455.

74. Pan American Health Organization. Experts meet in Mexico City to discuss rotavirus. EPI Newsletter. 2004;26:5. Available from: http://www.paho.org/english/ad/fch/im/sne 2605.pdf. Accessed 15 September 2006.

75. Carmona RC, Timenetsky MC, Morillo SG, Richtzenhain LJ. Human rotavirus serotype G9, Sao Paulo, Brazil, 1996–2003. Emerg Infect Dis. 2006;12(6):963–68.

76. Gentsch JR, Laird AR, Bielfelt B, Griffin DD, Bányai K, Ramachandran M, et al. Serotype diversity and reassortment between human and animal rotavirus strains: implications for rotavirus vaccine programs. J Infect Dis. 2005;192: S146–59.

77. Castello AA, Arvay ML, Glass RI, Gentsch J. Rotavirus strain surveillance in Latin America. A review of the last nine years. Pediatr Infect Dis J. 2004;23:168–72.

78. Urbina D, Rodriguez JG, Arzuza O, Parra E, Young G, Castro R. G and P genotypes of rotavirus circulating among children with diarrhea in the Colombian northern coast. Int Microbiol. 2004;7:113–20.

79. World Health Organization. World Health Report 2005: Make Every Mother and Child Count. Geneva: WHO; 2005.

80. Garcia S, Levine OS, Cherian T, Gabastou JM, Andrus J. Pneumococcal disease and vaccination in the Americas: an agenda for accelerated vaccine introduction. Pan Am J Public Health. 2006;19(5):340–48.

81. World Health Organization. Pneumococcal vaccines. Wkly Epidemiol Record. 2003;14:110–19.

82. World Health Organization, International Agency for Research on Cancer. GLOBOCAN 2002: Cancer Incidence, Mortality and Prevalence Worldwide. IARC CancerBase No. 5, version 2.0. Lyon: IARC Press; 2004. Available from: www-depdb.iarc.fr/globocan/GLOBOframe.htm. Accessed 15 September 2006.

83. Harper DM, Franco EL, Wheeler C, Ferris DG, Jenkins D, Schuind A, et al. Efficacy of a bivalent L1 virus-like particle vaccine in prevention of infection with human papillomavirus types 16 and 18 in young women: a randomised controlled trial. Lancet. 2004;364(9447):1757–65.

84. Harper DM, Franco EL, Wheeler CM, Moscicki AB, Romanowski B, Roteli-Martins CM, et al. Sustained efficacy up to 4–5 years of a bivalent L1 virus-like particle vaccine against human papillomavirus types 16 and 18: follow-up from a randomized control trial. Lancet. 2006;367(9518): 1247–55.

85. Villa LL, Costa RL, Petta CA, Andrade RP, Ault KA, Giuliano AR, et al. Prophylactic quadrivalent human papillomavirus (types 6, 11, 16, and 18) L1 virus-like particle vaccine in young women: a randomized double-blind placebo-controlled multicentre phase II efficacy trial. Lancet Oncology. 2005;6(5):271–78.

86. Paavonen J. Efficacy of a quadrivalent HPV (types 6/11/18) L1 virus-like particle (VLP) vaccine against vaginal and vulvar precancerous lesions: a combined analysis. (Presented at the American Society of Clinical Oncology Annual Meeting, Atlanta, Georgia, 2–6 June 2006.)

87. Pan American Health Organization. Sustaining National Immunization Programs in the Context of Introducing New Vaccines and Achieving the Millennium Development Goals. Immunization Newsletter. 2005;27(5):1–3. Available from: http://www.paho.org/english/ad/fch/im/sne2705 .pdf. Accessed 19 September 2006.

88. Pan American Health Organization. Analysis of Vaccination-related Legislation. Immunization Newsletter. 2006;28(2):5. Available from: http://www.paho.org/ english/ad/fch/im/sne2802.pdf. Accessed 19 September 2006.

89. Pan American Health Organization. Malaria in the Countries and Region of the Americas: Time Series Epidemiological Data, 1998–2004. Available from: http://www.paho .org/English/AD/DPC/CD/mal-2005.htm. Accessed 20 July 2006.

90. Carter KH, Escalada RP. Malaria in the Americas 2006: Regional Situation, Challenges, and Strategies. Epidemiol Bull. March 2006. (In press).

91. Pan American Health Organization. Regional Strategic Plan for Malaria in the Americas, 2006–2010. Washington, DC: PAHO; 2006. Available from: http://www.paho.org/ English/AD/DPC/CD/mal-reg-strat-plan-06.pdf. Accessed 30 October 2006.

92. Pan American Health Organization. 2007 Malaria in the Americas Report. Washington DC: PAHO; 2007. (In press).

93. Pan American Health Organization. Health Situation in the Americas: Basic Indicators 2006. Available from: http://www.paho.org/english/dd/ais/BI-brochure-2006.pdf. Accessed 15 December 2006.

94. Najera JA, Zaim M. Malaria Vector Control: Decision Making Criteria and Procedures for Judicious Use of Insecticides. Geneva: WHO/CDS/WHOPES; 2003. Available from: http://whqlibdoc.who.int/hq/2003/WHO_CDS_WHOPES_ 2002.5_Rev.1.pdf. Accessed 20 July 2006.

95. Pan American Health Organization. Report on the Status of Malaria Programs in the Americas. (Based on 2001 data). Washington, DC: PAHO; 2002. (COLL/WC750.O68S En).

96. Pan American Health Organization. Report on the Status of Malaria Programs in the Americas. (Based on 2000 data). Washington, DC: PAHO; 2001. (COLL/CD43/INF/1 En).

97. Pan American Health Organization. Report on the Status of Malaria Programs in the Americas. (Based on 1999 data). Washington, DC: PAHO; 2000. (COLL/CD42/INF/1 En).

98. Pan American Health Organization. Report on the Status of Malaria Programs in the Americas. (Based on 1998 data). Washington, DC: PAHO; 1999. (COLL/CD41/INF/1 En).

99. Pan American Health Organization. Resolution CD42.R15. Roll Back Malaria in the Region of the Americas. Final Report. 42nd Directing Council. Washington, DC: PAHO; 2000. Available from: http://www.paho.org/english/gov/cd/cd42_fr-e.pdf. Accessed 20 July 2006.

100. Pan American Health Organization. Population Living in Malaria-Endemic Areas in the Americas, 1994–2004 [table]. Available from: http://www.paho.org/english/ad/dpc/cd/mal-status-2004.pdf. Accessed 20 July 2006.

101. Pan American Health Organization. Resolution CD46.R13. Malaria and the Internationally Agreed-Upon Development Goals Including Those Contained in the Millennium Declaration. 46th Directing Council. Washington, DC: PAHO; 2005. Available from: http://www.paho.org/english/gov/cd/CD46.r13-e.pdf. Accessed 20 July 2006.

102. Guha-Sapir D, Schimmer B. Dengue fever: new paradigms for a changing epidemiology. Emerg Themes Epidemiol. 2005 Mar 2;2(1):1–10.

103. Meltzer MI, Rigau-Perez JG, Clark GG, Reiter P, Gubler DJ. Using disability-adjusted life years to assess the economic impact of dengue in Puerto Rico: 1984–1994. Am J Trop Med Hyg. 1998 Aug;59(2):265–71.

104. Pan American Health Organization. Number of Reported Cases of Dengue and Dengue Hemorrhagic Fever (DHF), Region of the Americas (by country and subregion). Available from: http://www.paho.org/english/ad/dpc/cd/dengue.htm. Accessed November 2006.

105. Halstead SB, Streit TG, Lafontant JG, Putvatana R, Russell K, Sun W, et al. Haiti: absence of dengue hemorrhagic fever despite hyperendemic dengue virus transmission. Am J Trop Med Hyg. 2001 Sep;65(3):180–83.

106. Rodríguez Cruz R. Estrategias para el control del dengue y del *Aedes aegypti* en las Américas. Rev Cubana Med Trop. 2002 sep–dic;54(3).

107. Pan American Health Organization. Framework: New Generation of Dengue Prevention and Control Programs in the Americas. Washington, DC: PAHO; 2001. Available from: http://www.paho.org/english/hcp/hct/vbd/dengue-nueva-generacion.htm. Accessed October 2006.

108. San Martin JL, Prado M. Risk perception and strategies for mass communication on dengue in the Americas. Rev Panam Salud Publica. 2004 Feb;15(2):135–39.

109. World Health Organization. Communication-for-Behavioural-Impact (COMBI). In: Parks W, Lloyd L. Planning Social Mobilization and Communication for Dengue Fever Prevention and Control: A Step-by-Step Guide. Geneva: WHO; 2004. (WHO/CDS/WMC/2004.2).

110. Parks W, Lloyd L. Planning Social Mobilization and Communication for Dengue Fever Prevention and Control: A Step-by-Step Guide. Geneva: WHO; 2004. (WHO/CDS/WMC/2004.2).

111. World Health Organization. Global Strategic Framework for Integrated Vector Management. Geneva: WHO; 2004.

112. World Health Organization. Strategic Plan for Integrated Vector Management in the Americas. Proposal to support implementation of IVM as a Regional Strategy in the Americas. Draft 6.0. Unpublished.

113. World Health Organization, Pan American Health Organization. DengueNet implementation in the Americas. Geneva: WHO; 2003. (WHO/CDS/CSR/GAR/2003.8).

114. Ecoclubs International. Available from: http://www.ecoclubs.org/DENGUE/ingles/dengue.asp. Accessed October 2006.

115. World Health Organization, Special Program for Research and Training in Tropical Diseases (TDR). Strategic Direction for Research. Available from: http://www.who.int/tdr/diseases/dengue/direction.htm. Accessed July 2006.

116. Corea del Sur, International Vaccine Institute. Pediatric Dengue Vaccine Initiative (PDVI). Available from: http://www.pdvi.org/. Accessed August 2006.

117. Blaney JE Jr, Durbin AP, Murphy BR, Whitehead SS. Development of a live attenuated dengue virus vaccine using reverse genetics. Viral Immunol. 2006 Spring;19(1):10–32.

118. Shepard DS, Suaya JA, Halstead SB, Nathan MB, Gubler DJ, Mahoney RT, et al. Cost-effectiveness of a pediatric dengue vaccine. Vaccine. 2004;22:1275–80.

119. Kroeger A, Lenhart A, Ochoa M, Villegas E, Levy M, Alexander N, et al. Effective control of dengue vectors with curtains and water container covers treated with insecticide in Mexico and Venezuela: cluster randomised trials. BMJ. 2006 May 27;332(7552):1247–52.

120. Briceño-León R. La casa enferma: sociología de la enfermedad de Chagas. Caracas: Acta Científica Venezolana; 1990.

121. Organización Panamericana de la Salud. Informe de un grupo de estudio sobre estrategias de control de la enfermedad de Chagas. (PNSP/87.03). Washington, DC: OPS; 1987.

122. World Health Organization. Chagas Disease Control. Geneva: WHO; 2000.

123. World Bank. Human Development Report 1993. Investing in Health. Washington, DC: World Bank; 1993.

124. Pan American Health Organization. Análise de Custo-Efetividade do Programa de Controle da Doenca de Chagas no Brasil. Brasilia: PAHO; 2000.

125. Organización Panamericana de la Salud. El control de la enfermedad de Chagas en los países del Cono Sur de América. Historia de una iniciativa internacional. 1991/2001. Washington, DC: OPS; 2002. Available from: http://www.paho.org/Spanish/AD/DPC/CD/dch-historia-incosur.PDF.

126. Organización Panamericana de la Salud; Centro Internacional de Investigaciones para el Desarrollo; Fundación Oswaldo Cruz. Memorias de la 2ª Reunión de la Iniciativa Intergubernamental de Vigilancia y Prevención de la Enfermedad de Chagas en la Amazonia, Cayena, Guayana Francesa, 2–4 de noviembre de 2005. Montevideo: IDRC; 2006.

127. Salvatella R, Schofield CJ. Enfermedad de Chagas. Iniciativas para el control de la enfermedad en Latinoamérica. Biomedicina. 2006;1(2):48–55.

128. Uranga N, Herranz E. Chagas: enfermedad silenciosa y silenciada. Barcelona: Médicos sin Fronteras; 2002.

129. Taylor LH, Latham SM, Woolhouse ME. Risk factors for human disease emergence. Philos Trans R Soc Lond B Biol Sci. 2001;359(1411):983–99.

130. Organización Panamericana de la Salud, Centro Panamericano de Fiebre Aftosa. Sistema de Información Regional de la Rabia en las Américas. Available from: http://siepi.panaftosa.org.br/Painel.aspx.

131. Pan American Health Organization. Regional Core Health Data Initiative. Available from: http://www.paho.org/english/dd/ais/coredata.htm. Accessed 25 May 2005.

132. World Organization for Animal Health. Handistatus II. OIE; 2006. Available from: http://www.oie.int/hs2/report.asp?lang=en. Accessed 6 November 2006.

133. Pan American Health Organization. Elimination of Dog-Transmitted Human Rabies in Latin America: Situation Analysis. Washington, DC: PAHO; 2005.

134. Schneider MC, Belotto A, Ade MP, Hendrickx S, Leanes LF, Rodrigues MJ, et al. Status of dog-transmitted human rabies in Latin America. Cad Saude Publica. (In press).

135. Belotto A, Leanes LF, Schneider MC, Tamayo H, Correa E. Overview of rabies in the Americas. Virus Research. 2005;111:5–12.

136. Schneider MC, Belotto A, Adé MP, Leanes LF, Correa E, Tamayo H, et al. Epidemiologic Situation of Human Rabies in Latin America in 2004. Epidemiol Bull. 2005;26(1):2–4. Available from: http://www.paho.org/english/dd/ais/be_v26n1-en-rabia_humana_al_2004.htm.

137. Schneider MC, Burgoa CS. Algunas consideraciones sobre la rabia humana transmitida por murciélago. Rev Salud Publica Mex. 1995;37(4).

138. Acha PN, Szyfres B. Zoonosis y enfermedades transmisibles comunes al hombre y a los animales, 3ª edición. Washington, DC: OPS; 2001.

139. Brazil, Ministério da Saúde, Secretaria de Vigilância em Saúde, Departamento de Vigilância Epidemiológica. Available from: http://portal.saude.gov.br/portal/svs/area.cfm?id_area=451. Accessed 28 July 2006.

140. Organización Panamericana de la Salud. Reunión constitutiva proyecto subregional Cono Sur de control y vigilancia de la hidatidosis, Argentina, Brasil, Chile y Uruguay. Informe final. 2005. Available from: http://www.panaftosa.org.br/inst/zoonosis/HIDATIDOSIS/informe_final_hid.doc. Accessed 3 November 2006.

141. United States, Department of Agriculture, Animal and Plant Health Inspection Service. Cooperative State/Federal Brucellosis Eradication Program Status Report, Fiscal Year 2005. USDA; 2005. Available from: http://www.aphis.usda.gov/vs/nahps/brucellosis/yearly_report/yearly-report.html Accessed 3 November 2006.

142. Organización Panamericana de la Salud, Centro Panamericano de Fiebre Aftosa. Brucelosis y tuberculosis *M. bovis*. Situación de los programas en las Américas, 2000. Available from: www.panaftosa.org.br/inst/texto_brucelosis.htm. Accessed 3 November 2006.

143. Pan American Health Organization. Action plan for the eradication of bovine tuberculosis in the Americas, Phase I. Washington, DC: PAHO; 2000. (HPV/TUB/113/92).

144. Joint United Nations Program on HIV/AIDS. 2006 Report on the Global AIDS Epidemic. Geneva: UNAIDS; 2006.

145. Pan American Health Organization; World Health Organization; Joint United Nations Program on HIV/AIDS. HIV and AIDS in Latin America and the Caribbean: the evolving epidemic and response and the challenges ahead. Unpublished report, December 2005.

146. Pan American Health Organization, World Health Organization. Regional HIV/STI Plan for the Health Sector, 2006–2015. PAHO; 2006.

147. Adams OP, Carter AO. Feasibility of a population based survey on HIV prevalence in Barbados, and population preference for sample identification method. University of the West Indies, Barbados/Caribbean Health Research Council; 2005.

148. United States, Department of Health and Human Services, Centers for Disease Control and Prevention. Sexually Transmitted Disease Surveillance 2004 Supplement. Syphilis Surveillance Report. Atlanta: U.S. Department of Health and Human Services; 2005. Available from: http://www.cdc.gov/std/Syphilis2004/SyphSurvSupp2004.pdf.

149. Pan American Health Organization, World Health Organization. Adolescent Health in the Caribbean. PAHO; 2007.

150. Clark S, Bruce J, Dude A. Protecting young women from HIV/AIDS: the case against child and adolescent marriage. International Family Planning Perspectives. 2006;32(2).

151. Joint United Nations Program on HIV/AIDS. 2004 Report on the Global AIDS Epidemic. Geneva: UNAIDS; 2004.

152. Lloyd C (ed.). Growing up Global: The Changing Transition to Adulthood in Developing Countries. Washington, DC: Na-

tional Academies Press; 2005. Available from: http://www
.nap.edu.

153. World Health Organization. 3 by 5 Initiative: AIDS treatment in children. 2005. Available from: http://www.who.int/3by5/paediatric/en/.

154. United States, Population Council. Power in sexual relationships: an opening dialogue among reproductive health professionals. New York; 2001. Available from: http://www.popcouncil.org.

155. Bill & Melinda Gates Foundation; Henry J. Kaiser Family Foundation, Global HIV Prevention Group. New approaches to HIV Prevention: Accelerating Research and Ensuring Future Access. 2006. Available from: http://www.gates foundation.org; http://www.kff.org.

156. United Nations Millennium Project Task Force on HIV/AIDS, Malaria, TB and Access to Essential Medicines. Combating AIDS in the Developing World. London: Earthscan; 2005.

157. Velzeboer M, Ellsberg MC, Garcia Moreno A. Violence against Women: The Health Sector Responds. Washington, DC: PAHO; 2003.

158. Marthur S, Greene M, Malhotra A. Too Young to Wed: The Lives, Rights, and Health of Young Married Girls. Washington, DC: International Center for Research on Women; 2003.

159. Yeager J, Fogel J. Male disclosure of sexual abuse and rape. Topics in Advanced Practice Nursing Ejournal. 2006;6(1). Available from: http://www.medscape.com/viewarticle/558821.

160. Frasca T. Men and women–still far apart on HIV/AIDS. Reproductive Health Matters. 2003;11(22):12–20.

161. Boender C, Santana D, Santillan D, Hardee K, Greene ME, Schuler S. The 'So What?' Report: A Look at Whether Integrating Gender Focus into Programs Makes a Difference to Outcomes. Interagency Gender Working Group Task Force Report. Washington, DC: Population Reference Bureau; 2004. Available from: www.prb.org.

162. Gupta G. Vulnerability and Resilience: Gender and HIV/AIDS in Latin America and the Caribbean. Sustainable Development Technical Papers Series. Washington, DC: Inter-American Development Bank; 2003.

163. Voluntary HIV-1 Counseling and Testing Efficacy Study Group. Efficacy of voluntary HIV-1 counseling and testing in individuals and couples in Kenya, Tanzania and Trinidad: a randomized trial. Lancet. 2000;356:103–12.

164. Okie S. Fighting HIV: lessons from Brazil. New Engl J Med. 2006;354(19):1977–81.

165. Kirby D, Laris BA, Rolleri L. Impact of sex and HIV education programs on sexual behaviors of youth in developing and developed countries. Research Triangle Park: Family Health International; 2005.

166. United States, National Academy of Sciences, Institute of Medicine. No Time to Lose: Getting More from HIV Prevention. Washington, DC: National Academy; 2001. p. 118.

167. O'Reilly KR, Medley A, Dennison J, Sweat MD. Systematic review of the impact of abstinence-only programmes on risk behavior in developing countries (1990–2005). Toronto, International AIDS Conference, 2006.

168. World Health Organization. Global Tuberculosis Control: surveillance, planning, financing. WHO report 2005. Geneva: OMS; 2006. (WHO/HTM/TB/2006.362).

169. World Health Organization; STOP TB Partnership. The Stop TB Strategy. Building on and Enhancing DOTS to Meet the TB-related Millennium Development Goals. Geneva: WHO; 2006. (WHO/HTM/TB/2006.368).

170. STOP TB Partnership; World Health Organization. The Global Plan to Stop TB 2006–2015. Geneva: WHO; 2006. (WHO/HTM/STB/2006.35).

171. Pan American Health Organization. TB Regional Plan 2006–2015. Washington, DC: PAHO; 2006.

172. World Health Organization. Interim Policy on Collaborative TB/HIV Activities. Geneva: WHO; 2004. (WHO/HTM/TB/2004.330).

173. Tupasi TE, Gupta R, Quelapio MID, Orillaza RB, Mira NR, et al. Feasibility and cost-effectiveness of treating multi-drug-resistant tuberculosis: a cohort study in the Philippines. PLoS Medicine. 2006 September;3(9):e352.

174. World Health Organization. A Primary Health Care Strategy for the Integrated Management of Respiratory Conditions in People of Five Years of Age and Over. Geneva: WHO; 2005. (WHO/HTM/TB/2005.351).

175. World Health Organization. Practical Approach to Lung Health: Respiratory Care in Primary Care Settings. A Survey in 9 Countries. Geneva: WHO; 2004. (WHO/HTM/TB/2004.333).

176. World Health Organization. Global Strategy for Further Reducing the Leprosy Burden and Sustaining Leprosy Control Activities Plan 2006–2010. Geneva: WHO; 2005. (WHO/CDS/CPE/CEE/2005.53).

177. World Bank. Global Burden of Disease and Risk Factors. Washington, DC: World Bank; 2006.

178. World Health Organization. Preventing Chronic Diseases: A Vital Investment. WHO Global Report. Geneva: WHO; 2005.

179. Pan American Health Organization. Resolution CE130.R13. Public Health Response to Chronic Diseases. 26th Pan American Sanitary Conference. Washington, DC: PAHO; 2002. (CSP26/15).

180. Barceló A, Aedo C, Swapnil R, Robles S. The cost of diabetes in Latin America and the Caribbean. Bull World Health Organ. 2003;81(1):19–27.

181. United States, Department of Health and Human Services, Centers for Disease Control and Prevention. The Burden of Chronic Diseases and Their Risk Factors. National and State Perspectives. Atlanta: U.S. Department of Health and Human Services; 2004.

182. Arredondo A, Zúñiga A, Parada I. Health care costs and financial consequences of epidemiological changes in

chronic diseases in Latin America: evidence from Mexico. Public Health. 2005;119:711–20.

183. Caribbean Commission on Health and Development. Report of the Caribbean Commission on Health and Development. Kingston: Ian Randle Publishers; 2006.

184. McKay J, Mensah G. The Atlas of Heart Disease and Stroke. Geneva: WHO; 2004.

185. Pan American Health Organization, Health Analysis and Information Systems. Regional Mortality Database. Washington, DC: PAHO; 2006.

186. Rodríguez T, Malvezzi M, Chatenoud L, Bosetti C, Levi F, Negri E, et al. Trends in mortality from coronary heart and cerebrovascular diseases in the Americas: 1970–2000. Heart. 2006;92:453–60.

187. Ciruzzi M, Schargrodsky H, Pramparo P, Rivas Estany E, Rodriguez Naude L, de la Noval Garcia R, et al. Attributable risk for acute myocardial infarction in four countries of Latin America. Medicina. 2003;63(6):697–703.

188. Bosetti C, Malvezzi M, Chatenoud L, Negri E, Levi F, La Vecchia C. Trends in cancer mortality in the Americas, 1970–2000. Ann Oncol. 2005;16:489–511.

189. World Health Organization. WHO Mortality Database [updated in July of 2006]. Available from: http://www-dep.iarc.fr/. Accessed 14 September 2006.

190. World Health Organization, International Agency for Research on Cancer, Biostatistics and Epidemiology Cluster, Descriptive Epidemiology Group. GLOBOCAN, 2002. [Database updated in 2002]. Lyon: IARC. Available from: http://www-dep.iarc.fr/. Accessed 14 September 2006.

191. Robles S, Galanis E. Breast cancer in Latin America and the Caribbean: Raising awareness of the options. Washington, DC: PAHO; 2001.

192. Wild S, Roglic G, Green A, Sicree R, King H. Global prevalence of diabetes. Estimates for the year 2000 and projections for 2030. Diabetes Care. 2004;27(5):1047–53.

193. Gregg EW, Cadwell BL, Cheng YJ, Cowie CC, Williams DE, Geiss L, et al. Trends in the prevalence and ratio of diagnosed to undiagnosed diabetes according to obesity levels in the US. Diabetes Care. 2004;27:2806–12.

194. United States, American Diabetes Association. Diagnosis and classification of diabetes mellitus. Diabetes Care. 2006; Suppl1:S43–S48.

195. Imperatore G, Cheng YJ, Williams DE, Fulton J, Gregg EW. Physical activity, cardiovascular fitness, and insulin sensitivity among U.S. adolescents: the National Health and Nutrition Examination Survey 1999–2002. Diabetes Care. 2006;29(7):1567–72.

196. del Rio-Navarro BE, Velazquez-Monroy O, Sanchez-Castillo CP, Lara-Esqueda A, Berber A, Fanghanel G, et al. The high prevalence of overweight and obesity in Mexican children. Obes Res. 2004;12(2):215–23.

197. United States, Centers for Disease Control and Prevention. Sensitivity of Death Certificate Data for Monitoring Dia-

betes Mortality. Diabetes Eye Disease Follow-up Study, 1985–1990. Morb Mortal Wkly Rep. 1991;40:739–41.

198. Barceló A, Peláez M, Rodriguez-Wong L, Pastor-Valero M. The prevalence of diagnosed diabetes among the elderly of seven cities in Latin America and the Caribbean. J Aging Health. 2006;18(2):224–39.

199. Hennis A, Wu SY, Nemesure B, Li X, Leske MC, Barbados Eye Study Group. Diabetes in a Caribbean population: epidemiological profile and implications. Int J Epidemiol. 2002; 31(1):234–39.

200. Belize, Ministry of Health; Pan American Health Organization. Central American Diabetes Initiative (CAMDI). Survey of Diabetes, Hypertension, and Chronic Disease Risk Factors, Belize City, Belize. Washington, DC: PAHO/WHO; 2007.

201. Klein-Geltink JE, Choi BCK, Fry RN. Multiple exposures to smoking, alcohol, physical inactivity and overweight: prevalences according to the Canadian Community Health Survey Cycle 1.1. Chronic Dis Can. 2006;27(1):25–33.

202. Ferreccio C, Margozziini P, Gonzalez Psic C, Gederlini Stat A, et al. High prevalence and inequity of chronic diseases: The First National Health Survey of Chile. 2007. Unpublished.

203. Costa Rica, Ministerio de Salud; Pan American Health Organization. Central American Diabetes Initiative (CAMDI). Survey of Diabetes, Hypertension, and Chronic Disease Risk Factors, San José, Costa Rica. Washington, DC: PAHO/WHO; 2007. (In press).

204. El Salvador, Ministerio de Salud; Pan American Health Organization. Central American Diabetes Initiative (CAMDI). Survey of Diabetes, Hypertension, and Chronic Disease Risk Factors, San Salvador, El Salvador. Washington, DC: PAHO/WHO; 2007. (In press).

205. Cowie CC, Rust KF, Byrd-Holt DD, Eberhardt MS, Flegal KM, Engelgau MM, et al. Prevalence of diabetes and impaired fasting glucose in adults in the U.S. population. National Health and Nutrition Examination Survey 1999–2002. Diabetes Care. 2006;29(6):1263–68.

206. National Center for Health Statistics. Health, United States, 2005, with chartbook on trends in the health of Americans. Hyattsville: U.S. Department of Health and Human Services; 2005.

207. Ogden CL, Carroll MD, Curtin LR, McDowell MA, et al. Prevalence of overweight and obesity in the United States, 1999–2004. JAMA. 2006;295(13):1549–55.

208. Guatemala, Ministerio de Salud; Pan American Health Organization. Central American Diabetes Initiative (CAMDI). Survey of Diabetes, Hypertension, and Chronic Disease Risk Factors, Villa Nueva, Guatemala. Washington, DC: PAHO/WHO; 2007. (In press).

209. Jean-Baptiste ED, Larco P, Charles-Larco N, Vilgrain C, Simon D, Charles R. Glucose intolerance and other cardiovascular risk factors in Haiti. Prevalence of diabetes and hypertension in Haiti. Diabetes Metab. 2006;32(5):443–51.

210. Honduras, Secretaría de Salud; Pan American Health Organization. Central American Diabetes Initiative (CAMDI). Survey of Diabetes, Hypertension, and Chronic Disease Risk Factors, Tegucigalpa, Honduras. Washington, DC: PAHO/WHO; 2007. (In press).

211. Aguilar-Salinas CA, Velazquez Monroy O, Gómez-Pérez FJ, Gonzalez Chávez A, Esqueda AL, Molina Cuevas V, et al. Characteristics of patients with type 2 diabetes in Mexico. Results from a large population-based nationwide survey. Diabetes Care. 2003;26(7):2021–26.

212. Velázquez Monroy O, Rosas Peralta M, Lara Esqueda A, Pastelón Hernández G, Attie F, Tapia-Conyer R. Grupo Encuesta Nacional de Salud 2000. Hipertensión arterial en México: Resultados de la Encuesta Nacional de Salud (ENSA) 2000. Archivos de Cardiología de México. 2002; 72(1):71–84.

213. Sanchez-Castillo CP, Velazquez-Monroy O, Berber A, Lara-Esqueda A, Tapia-Conyer R, James WP. Anthropometric cut-off points for predicting chronic diseases in the Mexican National Health Survey 2000. Obes Res. 2003;11(3):442–51.

214. Nicaragua, Ministerio de Salud; Pan American Health Organization. Central American Diabetes Initiative (CAMDI). Survey of Diabetes, Hypertension, and Chronic Disease Risk Factors, Managua, Nicaragua. Washington, DC: PAHO/WHO; 2007. (In press).

215. Pan American Health Organization. The U.S.-Mexico border diabetes prevention and control project. First report of results. Available from: http://www.fep.paho.org/english/publicaciones/Diabetes/Diabetes%20first%20report%20of%20Results.pdf. Accessed 21 February 2007.

216. Hennis A, Wu SY, Nemesure B, Leske MC; Barbados Eye Studies Group. Hypertension prevalence, control and survivorship in an Afro-Caribbean population. J Hypertens. 2002;20(12):2363–69.

217. Mexico, Secretaría de Salud. Encuesta Nacional de Enfermedades Crónicas. Tercera edición. Mexico City: SSA; 1996.

218. Velazquez-Monroy O, Rosas Peralta M, Lara Esqueda A, Pastelin Hernandez G, Sanchez-Castillo C, Attie F, et al. Prevalence and interrelations of noncommunicable chronic diseases and cardiovascular risk factors in Mexico. Final outcomes from the National Health Survey 2000. Arch Cardiol Mex. 2003;73(1):62–77.

219. Ordunez P, Munoz JL, Espinosa-Brito A, Silva LC, Cooper RS. Ethnicity, education, and blood pressure in Cuba. Am J Epidemiol. 2005;162(1):49–56.

220. Rosas Peralta M, Lara Esqueda A, Pastelin Hernandez G, Velazquez Monroy O, Martinez Reding J, Mendez Ortiz A, et al. National re-survey of arterial hypertension (RENAHTA). Mexican consolidation of the cardiovascular risk factors. National follow-up cohort. Arch Cardiol Mex. 2005;75(1): 96–111.

221. Yusuf S, Hawken S, Ôunpuu S, Dans T, Avezum A, Lanas F, et al. Effect of potentially modifiable risk factors associated with myocardical infarction in 52 countries (the INTERHEART study): case-control study. Lancet. 2004;364: 937–52.

222. Pan American Health Organization, World Health Organization. Actions for the Multifactorial Reduction of Noncommunicable Diseases (CARMEN). Washington, DC: PAHO/WHO; 2003.

223. Banegas J, Rodríguez F, Graciani A. Interacción de los factores de riesgo en las enfermedades crónicas. Rev Esp Salud Publica. 2002;76:1–5.

224. Baena JM, Álvarez B, Piñol P, Martín R, Nicolau M, Altès A. Asociación entre la agrupación (clustering) de factores de riesgo cardiovascular y el riesgo de enfermedad cardiovascular. Rev Esp Salud Publica. 2002;76:7–15.

225. Gómez LF, Lucumí DI, Girón SL, Espinosa G. Conglomeración de factores de riesgo de comportamiento asociados a enfermedades crónicas en adultos jóvenes de dos localidades de Bogotá, Colombia: importancia de las diferencias de género. Rev Esp Salud Publica. 2004;78:493–504.

226. Warner KE, MacKay J. The global tobacco disease pandemic: nature, causes, and cures. Global Public Health. 2006;1(1):65–86.

227. United States, Department of Health and Human Services, Centers for Disease Control and Prevention. The Burden of Chronic Diseases and Their Risk Factors. National and State Perspectives. Atlanta: U.S. Department of Health and Human Services; 2002.

228. Mackay J, Eriksen M, Shafey O. The Tobacco Atlas. Atlanta: American Cancer Society; 2006.

229. Jacoby E, Bull F, Neiman A. Cambios acelerados del estilo de vida obligan a fomentar la actividad física como prioridad en la Región de las Américas [editorial]. Rev Panam Salud Publica. 2003;14(4):223–25.

230. World Health Organization. Diet, Nutrition and the Prevention of Chronic Diseases. Report of a Joint WHO/FAO Expert Consultation. Geneva: WHO; 2003.

231. World Health Organization. Global InfoBase. Geneva: WHO. Available from: http://infobase.who.int. Accessed 10 September 2006.

232. Lara A, Rosas M, Pastelín G, Aguilar C, Attie F, Velásquez O. Hipercolesterolemia e hipertensión arterial en México. Consolidación urbana actual con obesidad, diabetes y tabaquismo. Arch Cardiol de Mex. 2004;74(3):231–45.

233. Argentina, Ministerio de Salud y Ambiente. Encuesta Nacional de Factores de Riesgo 2005. Buenos Aires: Ministerio de Salud y Ambiente; 2006.

234. Chile, Ministerio de Salud. Resultados Encuesta de Salud, Chile 2003. Santiago: Ministerio de Salud; 2004.

235. Miranda M, Landmann C, Borges PR. Socio-demographic characteristics, treatment coverage, and self-rated health of

individuals who reported six chronic diseases in Brazil, 2003. Cad Saude Publica. 2005;21(Suppl):S43–S53.

236. Jacoby E, Goldstein J, López A, Núñez E, López T. Social class, family, and life-style factors associated with overweight and obesity among adults in Peruvian cities. Prev Med. 2003;37:396–405.

237. Goldstein J, Jacoby E, del Agila R, López A. Poverty is a predictor of non-communicable disease among adults in Peruvian cities. Prev Med. 2005;41:800–6.

238. Pan American Health Organization. A Situational Analysis of Cervical Cancer. Latin America and the Caribbean. Washington, DC: PAHO/WHO; 2004.

239. World Health Organization. The Preliminary Report of the Global Survey on Assessing the Progress in National Chronic Diseases Prevention and Control. Geneva: WHO; 2006.

240. United States, Harvard School of Public Health, Center for Population and Development Studies. The Global Burden of Disease: A Comprehensive Assessment of Mortality and Disability from Diseases, Injuries and Risk Factors in 1990 and Projected to 2020. Cambridge: Harvard University Press; 1990.

241. Kohn R, Levav I, Caldas de Almeida JM, Vicente B, Andrade L, Caraveo-Anduaga JJ, et al. Los trastornos mentales en América Latina y el Caribe: asunto prioritario para la salud publica. Rev Panam Salud Publica. 2005;18(4/5):229–40.

242. Andrade LH, Lolio CA, Gentil V, Laurenti R. Epidemiologia dos transtornos mentais em uma área definida de captação da cidade de São Paulo, Brasil. Rev Psiquiatr Clin. 1999; 26:257–62.

243. Saldivia S, Vicente B, Kohn R, Rioseco P, Torres S. Use of mental health services in Chile. Psychiatr Serv. 2004;55: 71–6.

244. Bonander J, Kohn R, Arana B, Levav I. An anthropological and epidemiological overview of mental health in Belize. Transcult Psychiatry. 2000;37:57–72.

245. Kohn R, Levav I, Donair I, Machuca M, Tamashiro R. Psychological and psychopathological reactions in Honduras following Hurricane Mitch: implications for service planning. Rev Panam Salud Publica. 2005;18(4/5):287–95.

246. Rodríguez J, Barret T, Saxena S, Narvaez S, Levav I. Los servicios de salud mental en El Salvador, Guatemala y Nicaragua. Unpublished.

247. World Health Organization. Mental Health Atlas 2005. Geneva: WHO; 2005.

248. Caldas de Almeida JM. Estrategias de cooperación técnica de la Organización Panamericana de la Salud en la nueva fase de la reforma de los servicios de salud mental en América Latina y el Caribe. Rev Panam Salud Publica. 2005;18(4/5):314–26.

249. World Health Organization. World Health Report 2001. Mental Health: New Understanding, New Hope. Geneva: WHO; 2001.

250. Pan American Health Organization. Proposed 10-year Regional Strategy and Action Plan on Oral Health (2005–2015). Report to the Directing Council-Regional Committee. Washington, DC: PAHO; 2006.

251. Petersen PE. The World Oral Health Report 2003: continuous improvement of oral health in the 21st century—the approach of the WHO Global Oral Health Programme. Community Dent Oral Epidemiol. 2003;31(Suppl 1):3–24.

252. Organización Panamericana de la Salud. Promoviendo la salud oral en la Región. Reunión Regional de Jefes de Salud Oral, Havana, OPS, 2004.

253. Pan American Health Organization. Strategic and Programmatic Orientations 1999–2002. Washington, DC: PAHO; 1999.

254. World Health Organization. Oral Health Surveys: Basic Methods. 4th edition. Geneva: WHO; 1997.

255. Estupiñán-Day S. Promoting Oral Health: The Use of Salt Fluoridation to Prevent Dental Caries. Washington, DC: PAHO; 2005. (Scientific and technical publication No. 615).

256. de Crouzas P, Marthaler TM, Wiesner V, Bandi A, Steiner M, Robert A, Meyer R. Caries prevalence in children after 12 years of salt fluoridation in a canton of Switzerland. Schweiz Monatsschr Zahnhelik. 1985;95(9):805–15.

257. Toth K. Ten years of domestic salt fluoridation in Hungary. Acta Paediatr Acad Sci Hung. 1978;19(4):319–27.

258. Estupiñán-Day SR, Baez R, Horowitz H, Warpeha R, Sutherland B, Thamer M. Salt fluoridation and dental caries in Jamaica. Community Dent Oral Epidemiol. 2001;29:247–52.

259. Dean HT, Arnold FA Jr, Jay P, Knutson JW. Studies on mass control of dental caries through fluoridation of the public water supply. Public Health Rep. 1950;65:1403–8.

260. Estupiñán-Day S. Overview of salt fluoridation in the Region of the Americas. Part I: Strategies, cost-benefit analysis, and legal mechanisms utilized in the National Programs of Salt Fluoridation. In: Geertman RM (ed.). Salt 2000, 8th World Salt Symposium. Amsterdam: Elsevier Science; 2000.

261. Estupiñán-Day S. The Success of Salt Fluoridation in the Region of the Americas after a Decade. Abstract 52080. 128th Annual Meeting of APHA, Boston, 2000.

262. Estupiñán-Day S. Improving oral health in Latin America. Oral Care Report/Harvard. 1999;9(3).

263. Marino RJ, Villa AE, Weitz A, Guerrero S. Caries prevalence in a rural Chilean community after cessation of a powdered milk fluoridation program. J Public Health Dent. 2004; 64(2):101–5.

264. Sanchez H, Parra JH, Cardona Dora. Dental fluorosis in primary school students of the department of Caldas, Colombia. Biomédica. 2005;25(1):46–54.

265. Beltran-Aguilar ED, Barker LK, Canto MT, Dye BA, Gooch BF, Griffin SO, et al. Surveillance for dental caries, dental sealants, tooth retention, edentulism, and enamel fluoro-

sis—United States, 1988–1994 and 1999–2002. Morb Mortal Wkly Rep. Surveillance Summaries. 2005;54(3):1–43.

266. Beltran-Valladares PR, Cocom-Tun H, Casanova-Rosado JF, Vallejos-Sánchez AA, Medina-Solís CE, Maupomé G. Prevalence of dental fluorosis and additional sources of exposure to fluoride as risk factors to dental fluorosis in schoolchildren of Campeche, Mexico. Rev Invest Clin. 2005 Jul–Aug; 57(4):532–39.

267. Soto-Rojas AE, Urena-Cirett JL, Martinez-Mier E. A review of the prevalence of dental fluorosis in Mexico. Pan Am J Public Health. 2004;15(1):9–18.

268. Frencken JE, Makoni F, Sithole WD. ART restorations and glass ionomer sealants in Zimbabwe: survival after 3 years. Community Dent Oral Epidemiol. 1998;26:372–81.

269. Holmgren CJ, Lo EC, Hu D, Wan H. ART restorations and sealants placed in Chinese school children—results after three years. Community Dent Oral Epidemiol. 2000;28: 314–20.

270. Phantumvanit P, Songpaisan Y, Pilot T, Frencken JE. Atraumatic Restorative Treatment (ART): a three-year community field trial in Thailand. Survival of one-surface restorations in the permanent dentition. J Public Health Dent. 1996;56:141–45.

271. Horowitz AM. Introduction to the symposium on minimal intervention techniques for caries. J Public Health Dent. 1996;56(3):133–34; discussion 161–63.

272. Estupiñán-Day S, Millner T, Tellez M. Oral Health of Low Income Children: Procedures for Atraumatic Restorative Treatment (PRAT). Washington, DC: PAHO; 2006.

273. Petersen PE, Ogawa H. Strengthening the prevention of periodontal disease: the WHO approach. J Periodontol. 2005; 76(12):2187–93.

274. Gjermo P, Rosing CK, Susin C, Oppermann R. Periodontal diseases in Central and South America. Periodontol 2000. 2002;29:70–8.

275. Taylor GW. Bidirectional interrelationships between diabetes and periodontal diseases: An epidemiological perspective. Ann Periodontol. 2001;6:99–112.

276. Dortbudak O, Eberhardt R, Ulm M, Persson GR. Periodontitis, a marker of risk in pregnancy for preterm birth. J Clin Periodontol. 2005;32:45–52.

277. Williams CE, Davenport ES, Sterne JA, Sivapathasundaram V, Fearne JM, Curtis MA. Mechanisms of risk in preterm low birthweight infants. Periodontol 2000. 2000;23:142–50.

278. Lopez NJ, Smith PC, Gutierrez J. Periodontal therapy may reduce the risk of preterm low birth weight in women with periodontal disease: a randomized controlled trial. J Periodontol. 2002;73:911–24.

279. Lopez NJ, Da SI, Ipinza J, Gutierrez J. Periodontal therapy reduces the rate of preterm low birth weight in women with pregnancy-associated gingivitis. J Periodontol. 2005; 76:2144–53.

280. Pascolini D, Mariotti SP, Pokharel GP, Pararajasegaram R, Etya'ale D, Negrel AD, et al. 2002 global update of available data on visual impairment: a compilation of population-based prevalence studies. Ophthalmic Epidemiol. 2004 Apr;11(2):67–115.

281. Resnikoff S, Pascolini D, Etya'ale D, Kocur I, Pararajasegaram R, Pokharel GP, et al. Global data on visual impairment in the year 2002. Bull World Health Organ. 2004 Nov;82(11):844–51.

282. World Health Organization. State of the World Sight Vision 2020: The Right to Sight: 1999–2005. Geneva: WHO; 2005. pp. 1–110.

283. Silva JC. Limburg H. Rapid assessment of cataract surgical services in Latin America. IAPB News. 2006 Apr;49.

284. Nano ME, Nano HD, Mugica JM, Silva JC, Montana G, Limburg H. Rapid assessment of visual impairment due to cataract and cataract surgical services in urban Argentina. Ophthalmic Epidemiol. 2006;13(3):191–97.

285. Pongo Aguila L, Carrión R, Luna W, Silva JC, Limburg H. Ceguera por catarata en personas mayores de 50 años en una zona semirural del norte del Perú. Rev Panam Salud Publica. 2005;17(5/6):387–93.

286. Pan American Health Organization, Technology and Health Services Delivery. Health Services Organization Series. Eye Diseases in People 40–84. The Barbados Eye Studies: A Summary Report. Washington, DC: PAHO; 2006. (THS/OS/06/8).

287. Morales E, Angeles M, Batlle J, et al. Primera Encuesta de Diabetes y Ceguera en la República Dominicana. Santo Domingo: Editora Colores; 1997. pp. 1–36.

288. Leske MC, Wu SY, Hyman L, Li X, Hennis A, Connell AM, Schachat AP. Diabetic retinopathy in a black population: the Barbados Eye Study. Ophthalmology. 1999;106(10):1893–99.

289. Weih LM, VanNewkirk MR, McCarty CA, Taylor HR. Age-specific causes of bilateral visual impairment. Arch Ophthalmol. 2000;118(2):264–69.

290. Wu SY, Nemesure B, Leske MC. Refractive errors in a black adult population: the Barbados Eye Study. Invest Ophthalmol Vis Sci. 1999;40(10):2179–84.

291. Maul E, Barroso S, Munoz SR, Sperduto RD, Ellwein LB. Refractive error study in children: results from La Florida, Chile. Am J Ophthalmol. 2000;129(4):445–54.

292. Guatemala, Onchocersiasis Elimination Program in the Americas. ¿Cómo vamos en coberturas de tratamiento con Mectizan®? Reporte de tratamiento 2005, en la Región, por país y foco endémico. Guatemala City: OEPA; 2006.

293. Mora JO, Gueri M, Mora OL. Vitamin A deficiency in Latin America and the Caribbean: an overview. Rev Panam Salud Publica. 1998;4(3):178–86.

294. Laine A. Activities for the prevention of xerophthalmia and vitamin A deficiency in the communities served by Project HOPE, Haiti. Sight and Life Newsletter. 1999;1:20.

295. World Health Organization. Report of the Global Scientific Meeting on Future Approaches to Trachoma Control. Geneva: WHO; 1996. pp. 4–7. (WHO/PBL/96.56).

296. World Health Organization. Report of the ninth meeting of the WHO Alliance for the Global Elimination of Blinding Trachoma. Geneva: WHO; 2005. pp. 1–58 (WHO/PBD/GET 05.1).

297. Pan American Health Organization. Guidelines for Development of Eye Care Programs and Services in the Caribbean. Washington, DC: PAHO; 1998. pp. 1–26.

298. Gilbert C, Judnoo R, Eckstein M, O'Sullivan J, Foster A. Retinopathy of prematurity in middle-income countries. Lancet. 1997;350(9070):12–24.

299. Frick KD, Foster A. The magnitude and cost of global blindness: an increasing problem that can be alleviated. Am J Ophthalmol. 2003 Apr;135(4):471–76.

300. Frick KD, Kymes SM. The calculation and use of economic burden data. Br J Ophthalmol. 2006 Mar;90(3):255–57.

301. Silva JC, Bateman JB, Contreras F. Eye disease and care in Latin America and the Caribbean. Surv Ophthalmol. 2002; 47(3):267–74.

302. Silva JC. Eye care situation in Latin America and the Caribbean: an update year 2000. Bogotá: PAHO; 2000. pp. 1–9. (PAHO/PBL/2000.1).

303. Musa J, Silva JC, Cambell F, Graham R, Wormald R, Dineen B, et al. The use of an eye care communication program to detect those with glaucoma and other blinding conditions in Belize. IAPB News. 2004 Apr;42:4–5.

304. Pan American Health Organization. Resolution CE122.R5. Population and Reproductive Health. 25th Pan American Sanitary Conference. Washington, DC; PAHO: 1998. Available from: http://www.paho.org/English/GOV/CSP/csp25_ 15.pdf. Accessed 6 November 2006.

305. World Health Organization, Department of Reproductive Health and Research. Reproductive health strategy to accelerate progress towards the attainment of international development goals and targets. Strategy adopted by the 57th World Health Assembly, May 2004. Available from: http://www.who.int/reproductive-health/publications/ strategy.pdf#search=%22who%20strategy%20for%20 accelerating%20progress%20towards%20the%20 attainment%22. Accessed 6 November 2006.

306. United Nations, Department of Economic and Social Affairs, Population Division. World Population Prospects: The 2004 Revision. Population database. Available from: http://esa.un.org/unpp/index.asp?panel=6. Accessed 6 November 2006.

307. World Health Organization. World Health Statistics 2006. Available from: http://www.who.int/whosis/en/. Accessed 6 November 2006.

308. Schwarcz R, Fescina R. Maternal mortality in Latin America and the Caribbean. Lancet. 2000;356(Suppl S11):3245–67.

309. Kunst A, Houweling T. A global picture of poor-rich differences in the utilization of delivery care. In: De Brouwere V, Van Lebergne W (eds.). Safe motherhood strategies: a review of the evidence. Stud Health Serv Organ Policy. 2001; 17:297–316. Available from: http://www.eldis.org/static/ DOC12420.htm. Accessed 6 November 2006.

310. World Health Organization, Department of Reproductive Health and Research. Safe Abortion: Technical and Policy Guidance for Health Systems. Geneva: WHO; 2003. Available from: http://whqlibdoc.who.int/publications/2003/ 9241590343.pdf. Accessed 6 November 2006.

311. World Health Organization. World Report on Violence and Health. Geneva: WHO; 2002. Available from: http://www.who.int/violence_injury_prevention/violence/world_report/en/full_en.pdf. Accessed 6 November 2006.

312. World Health Organization. Neonatal and perinatal mortality 2006. Country, regional and global estimates. Available from: http://whqlibdoc.who.int/publications/2006/ 9241563206_eng.pdf. Accessed 6 November 2006.

313. Argentina, Instituto Nacional de Estadísticas y Censos, http://www.indec.mecon.gov.ar/. Brazil, Ministério da Saúde, http://w3.datasus.gov.br/datasus/datasus.php. Chile, Instituto Nacional de Estadística, http://www.ine.cl/ ine/canales/chile estadistico/home.php. Mexico, Secretaría de Salud, http://www.salud.gob.mx/. Accessed 6 November 2006.

314. Jacoby E. Diet, physical activity and health in the Americas: a call to action. Food Nutr Bull. 2004;25(2):172–74.

315. Shrimpton R, Victora C, de Onis M, Lima RC, Blossner M, Clugston G. The worldwide timing of growth faltering: implications for nutritional interventions. Pediatrics. 2001; 107:e75.

316. Lutter CK, Rivera JA. Nutritional status of infants and young children and characteristics of their diets. J Nutr. 2003; 133(9S):2941S–49S.

317. World Health Organization. Resolution WHA54.2. Infant and young child nutrition. Fifty-fourth World Health Assembly. Geneva: WHO; 2001.

318. World Health Organization. HIV and Infant Feeding: Framework for Priority Action. Geneva: WHO; 2003.

319. United Nations, Administrative Committee on Coordination Sub-Committee on Nutrition. Fourth Report on the World Nutrition Situation. Geneva: UN; 2000.

320. World Health Organization. Global Prevalence of Vitamin A Deficiency. Geneva: WHO; 1995.

321. Hotz CH, Brown KH. Assessment of the risk of zinc deficiency in populations and options for its control. Food Nutr Bull. 2004;25:130–62.

322. Logan S, Martins S, Gilbert R. Iron therapy for improving psychomotor development and cognitive function in chil-

dren under the age of three with iron deficiency anemia. Cochrane Database Sys Rev. 2001;3:CD0001444.

323. Lozoff B, Jimenez E, Smith JB. Double burden of iron deficiency in infancy and low socioeconomic status. Arch Pediatr Adolesc Med. 2006;160:1109–13.

324. World Health Organization. Global Database on Iodine Deficiency. Iodine Status Worldwide. Geneva: WHO; 2004.

325. World Health Organization; United Nations Children's Fund; International Council for the Control of Iodine Deficiency Disorders. Indicators for assessing iodine deficiency disorders and their control through salt iodization. Geneva: WHO; 1994. (WHO/NUT/94.6).

326. World Health Organization; United Nations Children's Fund; International Council for the Control of Iodine Deficiency Disorders. Assessment of Iodine Deficiency Disorders and Monitoring their Elimination. Geneva: WHO; 2001. (WHO/NHD/01.1).

327. World Health Organization. Global Database on Iodine Deficiency. Iodine Status Worldwide. Geneva: WHO; 2004.

328. Pretell EA, Delange F, Hostalek U, Corigliano S, Barreda L, Higa AM. Iodine nutrition improves in Latin America. Thyroid. 2004;14(8):590–99.

329. Rivera J, Barquera S, Campirano F, Campos I, Safdie M, Tovar V. Epidemiological and nutritional transition in Mexico: rapid increase of non-communicable chronic diseases and obesity. Public Health Nutr. 2002;5(1A):113–22.

330. Vio F, Uauy R. The public policy response to epidemiological and nutritional transition: The case of Chile. In: Freire W (ed.). Nutrition and Active Life: From Knowledge to Action. Washington, DC: PAHO; 2006. pp. 205–219.

331. Cortez R, Jacoby E. Determinantes de la obesidad y sobrepeso en el Perú. In: Cortez R (ed.). Salud, Equidad y Pobreza en el Perú. Lima: Universidad del Pacífico; 2002.

332. World Health Organization. Global Database on Body Mass Index. Available from: http://www.who.int/bmi/index.jsp. Accessed July 2006.

333. United States, Centers for Disease Control and Prevention. U.S. Obesity Trends 1985–2006. Available from: http://www.cdc.gov/nccdphp/dnpa/obesity/trend/maps/index.htm. Accessed July 2006.

334. Uauy R, Monteiro CA. The challenge of improving food and nutrition in Latin America. Food Nutr Bull. 2004; 25(2): 175–82.

335. World Health Organization. Sedentary Lifestyle: A Global Public Health Problem. Geneva: WHO; 2002.

336. Uauy R, Monteiro CA. The challenge of improving food and nutrition in Latin America. Food Nutr Bull. 2004;25(2): 175–82.

337. Glasgow RE, Lichtenstein E, Marcus AC. Why don't we see more translation of health promotion research to practice? Rethinking the efficacy-to-effectiveness transition. Am J Public Health. 2003;93(8):1261–67.

338. Forrester T. Report to Caribbean Commission on Health and Development: Cardiovascular Disease and Cancer. Jamaica; 2003.

339. World Health Organization. Global Strategy on Diet, Physical Activity and Health. Geneva: WHO; 2004.

340. Hill JO, Wyatt HR, Reed GW, Peters JC. Obesity and the environment: Where do we go from here? Science. 2003; 299:853–56.

341. World Health Organization. World Health Report 2002. Geneva: WHO; 2002.

342. Eyre H, Robertson RM, Kahn R. Preventing cancer, cardiovascular disease, and diabetes. Diabetes Care. 2004;7: 1812–24.

343. World Health Organization, Center for Research on the Epidemiology of Disasters. Emergency Disasters Database. Available from: http://www.em-dat.net. Accessed July 2006.

344. Pan American Health Organization, Emergency Preparedness and Disaster Relief. State of Mitigation and Disaster Preparedness in the Health Sector. PAHO; 2006.

345. Pan American Health Organization. Progress Report on National and Regional Health Disaster Preparedness and Response. 47th Directing Council. Washington, DC: PAHO; 2006.

346. United States, House of Representatives. A Failure of Initiative. Final Report of the Select Bipartisan Committee to Investigate the Preparation for and Response to Hurricane Katrina. 109th Congress, 2nd Session, February 2006.

347. Organización Panamericana de la Salud. Impacto de los desastres en la salud. Bogotá: OPS; 2000.

348. Centro Regional de Información sobre Desastres de América Latina y el Caribe. Available from: http://www.crid.or.cr. Accessed July 2006.

349. Cardona O. La necesidad de repensar de manera holística los conceptos de vulnerabilidad y riesgo: una crítica y una visión necesaria para la Gestión. Centro de Estudios sobre Desastres y Riesgos, Universidad Nacional de Los Andes, Bogotá, Colombia.

350. United Nations Development Program. Reducing Disaster Risk: A Challenge for Development. A Global Report. New York: UNDP; 2004.

351. Lavell A. Decision making and risk management. Science Faculty (FLACSO) and La Red de Estudios Sociales en la Prevención de Desastres en América Latina. (Presented at Furthering Cooperation in Science and Technology for Caribbean Development, Port of Spain, Trinidad, September 1998).

352. Pan American Health Organization. Evaluation of the International Decade of the World's Indigenous Peoples: Health of indigenous peoples in the Americas. Washington, DC: PAHO; 2004.

353. Hall G, Patrinos AH. Indigenous Peoples, Poverty and Human Development in Latin America: 1994–2004. Washington, DC: World Bank; 2005.

354. Montenegro R, Stephens C. Indigenous health in Latin America and the Caribbean. (Indigenous Health Series no. 2). Lancet. 2006;367:1859–69.

355. Stephens C, Porter J, Nettleton C, Willis R. Disappearing, displaced, and undervalued: a call to action for indigenous health worldwide. (Indigenous Health Series no. 4). Lancet. 2006;367:2019–28.

356. Stephens C, Nettleton C, Porter J, Willis S. Indigenous people's health—why are they behind everyone, everywhere? Lancet. 2005 July;366.

357. Mexico, Comisión Nacional para el Desarrollo de los Pueblos Indígenas. La situación de los pueblos indígenas. ¿Dónde estamos? [Web page]. Available from: http://cdi.gob.mx/index.php?id_seccion=176. Accessed 25 May 2006.

358. Webster P. Health in the Arctic Circle. Lancet. 2005; 365:741–42.

359. Oostdama J, Donaldson A S, Feeley C M, Arnold D, Ayotted P, Bondy C G, et al. Contaminants in Canadian Arctic Biota and Implications for Human Health. Sci Total Environ. 2005 December;351–2:165–246.

360. Alonso C, Miranda L, Hughes S, Fauveau L. Reducing maternal mortality among repatriated populations along the Guatemala-Mexico border. In: Reproductive Health for Displaced People: Investing in the Future. Forced Migration Review. 2004 January;19:13–16.

361. Guatemala, Ministerio de Salud Pública y Asistencia Social. Lineamientos estratégicos para reducir la mortalidad materna. Guatemala City: Secretaría Presidencial de la Mujer; 2003.

362. Calvo A. Situación de salud: Sub-Región Andina [PowerPoint presentation]. Montevideo: Reunión Subregional de Representantes de la OPS/OMS y Directores de Centro del Cono Sur y Área Andina; 2006.

363. Zolla C. La salud de los pueblos indígenas de México [PowerPoint presentation]. Comisión Nacional para el Desarrollo de los Pueblos Indígenas de México; 2004.

364. Cardoso A, Mattos I, Koifman, R. Prevalence of risk factors for cardiovascular disease in the Guaraní-Mbyá population of the State of Rio de Janeiro. Cad Saude Publica. 2001 Mar/Apr;17(2):345–54.

365. Anand S, Yusuf S, Jacobs R, Davis D, Yi Q, Gerstein H, et al. Risk factors, atherosclerosis, and cardiovascular disease among aboriginal people in Canada: the Study of Health Assessment and Risk Evaluation in Aboriginal Peoples (SHARE-AP). Lancet. 2001;358:1147–53.

366. Organización Panamericana de la Salud. Salud de los pueblos indígenas: patrones de consumo de alcohol en los Shipibo y Aymara de Perú. Washington, DC: OPS; 2001.

367. Organización Panamericana de la Salud. Salud de los pueblos indígenas: una aproximación a los patrones de consumo de alcohol. Washington, DC: OPS; 2006.

368. Mexico, Secretariado Técnico del Consejo Nacional contra las Adiciones. Retos para la atención del alcoholismo en pueblos indígenas. 2006. Bonilla A. Drogas y alcohol en Kuna Yala. La Prensa. Panama, 10 December 2005. Available from: http://mensual.prensa.com/mensual/contenido/2005/12/10/hoy/nacionales/430486.html. Accessed 4 March 2006.

369. Ecuador, Ministerio de Salud. Pueblos indígenas en el Ecuador y consumo de bebidas alcohólicas: cosmovisión, conocimientos, actitudes y prácticas, causas y consecuencias. Quito; 2000.

370. Jackson J. Facing the music. Perspectives. 2002;7(1).

371. Naciones Unidas Colombia. Creciente preocupación por los indígenas colombianos. Boletín de las Naciones Unidas, 2004. Available from: http://www.nacionesunidas.org.co/noticia1.asp?Id=143. Accessed 2 February 2006.

372. Dodds D. Lobster in the rain forest: The political ecology of Miskito wage labor and agricultural deforestation. J Polit Ecology. 1998;5:83–108.

373. Organización Panamericana de la Salud. Derechos humanos y discapacidad entre los pueblos indígenas. Atención integral de los Buzos Miskito de Honduras. Washington, DC: OPS; 2004. Available from: http://www.paho.org/spanish/dd/pin/MISKITO_Derechos.doc.

374. Von Gleich U, Gálvez E. Pobreza étnica en Honduras. Washington, DC: Banco Interamericano de Desarrollo; 1999.

375. Naborre M. Atendiendo la discapacidad en la Mosquitia hondureña. Washington, DC: Banco Interamericano de Desarrollo; 2004.

376. Kaplan J, Eidenberg M. Barotrauma. Emedicine. 11 November 2004. Available from: http://www.emedicine.com/emerg/topic53.htm. Accessed 3 June 2004.

377. Guatemala, Ministerio de Salud y Asistencia Social; Instituto Nacional de Estadística. Encuesta Nacional de Salud Materno Infantil 2002: Mujeres. Guatemala City; 2003.

378. Colombia, Ministerio de la Protección Social; Organización Panamericana de la Salud. Insumos para la conceptualización y discusión de una política de protección social en salud para los grupos étnicos de Colombia. Ministerio de la Protección Social; OPS; 2004.

379. Ramírez S. Donde el viento llega cansado: sistemas y prácticas de salud en la ciudad de Potosí. La Paz: Cooperación Italiana; 2005.

380. Chile, Ministerio de Salud; Fondo Nacional de Salud. Política de Salud y Pueblos Indígenas. Ministerio de Salud; 2006.

381. Yánez del Pozo J. Allikai: La salud y la enfermedad desde la perspectiva indígena. 1ª edición. Quito: Editorial Abya Yala; 2005.

382. Organización Panamericana de la Salud. Abya-Yala Kuyarinakui: Promoción de la salud sexual y prevención del VIH/sida y de las ITS en los pueblos indígenas de las Américas. Washington, DC: OPS; 2005.

383. Knipper M, Mamallacta G, Narváez M, Santi S. Mal aire entre los Naporuna: enfermedades por viento entre la gente que vivimos a la orilla del río Napo. Quito: 1999.

384. Rojas R. Crecer sanitos. Estrategias, metodologías e instrumentos para investigar y comprender la salud de los niños indígenas. Washington, DC: OPS; 2003.

385. Comisión Económica para América Latina y el Caribe. Pueblos indígenas y afrodescendientes de América Latina y el Caribe: información sociodemográfica para políticas y programas. Santiago de Chile: CEPAL; 2006.

386. Inter-American Development Bank. Databank on Indigenous Legislation. Available from: http://www.iadb.org/sds/IND/site_3152_e.htm.

387. Tauli-Corpuz V. Indigenous peoples and the Millennium Development Goals. (Paper submitted to the 4th Session of the UN Permanent Forum on Indigenous Issues, New York, 16–27 May 2005). New York; 2005.

388. United Nations Permanent Forum on Indigenous Issues. Second International Decade of the World's Indigenous People. (General Assembly Resolution A/RES/59/174, adopted 12 December 2004.) Available from: http://www.un.org/esa/socdev/unpfii/en/second.html. Accessed 12 July 2006.

389. Pan American Health Organization. 138th Session of the Executive Committee. Health of the Indigenous Population in the Americas. Washington, DC: PAHO; 2006. (CE138/13, Rev. 1).

390. Urrea F. La población afrodescendiente en Colombia. Los pueblos indígenas y afrodescendientes en América Latina y el Caribe. Santiago de Chile: CEPAL; 2006.

391. Organización Panamericana de la Salud. Trabajando para alcanzar la equidad étnica en salud. Taller Regional para América Latina y el Caribe. Washington, DC: OPS; 2004.

392. Pan American Health Organization. Progress Report on Family and Health. 46th Directing Council. Washington, DC: PAHO; 2005. (CD46/21).

393. Mackino J, Guanais FC, Souza MFM. An evaluation of impact of the Family Health Program on infant mortality in Brazil, 1990–2002. J Epidemiol Comm Health. 2006;60:13–19.

394. Johnson K, Posner SF, Bierman J, Cordero JF, Atrash HK, Parker CS, et al. Recommendations to Improve Preconception Health and Health Care, United States. A Report of the CDC/ATSDR Preconception Care Work Group and the Select Panel on Preconception Care. MMWR Recommendations and Reports. 2006 April;55(RR06):1–23.

395. Baptiste DR, Bhana A, Petersen I, Mc Kay, Voisin D, Bell C, et al. Community-collaborative youth focused HIV/AIDS prevention in South Africa and Trinidad: preliminary findings. J Ped Psyc. 2006;31(9):905–16.

396. Pan American Health Organization. Family and Health. 44th Directing Council. Washington, DC: PAHO; 2003. (CD44/10).

397. Pan American Health Organization. Neonatal Health in the Context of Maternal, Newborn and Child Health for the Attainment of the Millennium Development Goals of the United Nations Millennium Declaration. 47th Directing Council. Washington, DC: PAHO; 2006.

398. Economic Commission for Latin America and the Caribbean. Social Panorama of Latin America 2005. Santiago, Chile; ECLAC; 2005.

399. Organización Panamericana de la Salud. Estimaciones de mortalidad en menores de 5 años e infantil en la región de las Américas. Washington, DC: OPS; 2005. Unpublished.

400. Economic Commission for Latin America and the Caribbean. Statistical yearbook for Latin America and the Caribbean, 2005. Santiago, Chile: ECLAC; 2006. (LC/G.2311-P/B).

401. Jones G, Steketee RW, Black RE, Bhutta ZA, Morris SS, Bellagio Child Survival Study Group. ¿Cuántas muertes infantiles se pueden evitar este año? Lancet. 2003;362:65–71.

402. United Nations Children's Fund. State of the World's Children. New York: UNICEF; 2005.

403. Organización Panamericana de la Salud. La mortalidad por enfermedades transmisibles en la infancia en los países de la Región de las Américas. Bol AIEPI. 2000 junio; No. 4.

404. World Health Organization; Pan American Health Organization; United Nations Children's Fund, Integrated Attention to Prevalent Childhood Diseases. Key Family Practices for Healthy Growth and Development. PAHO; 2001. Available from: http://www.paho.org/english/ad/fch/ca/GSIYCF_keyfam_practices.pdf.

405. Huicho L, Davila M, Gonzales F, Drasbek C, Bryce J, Victora CG. Implementation of the Integrated Management of Childhood Illness Strategy in Peru and its association with health indicators: an ecological analysis. Health Policy Plan. 2005;20:33–41.

406. Quijano AM, Drasbek C. Informe de evaluación de participación y movilización social, Distrito de Chao, Perú. Informe del proyecto. Washington, DC: OPS; 2007. Unpublished.

407. Global Health Council. Commitments: youth reproductive health, the World Bank, and the Millennium Development Goals. Washington, DC: Global Health Council; 2004.

408. United Nations. Declaration of Commitment on HIV/AIDS. United Nations General Assembly 26th Special Session, 25–27 June 2001. New York: UN; 2001.

409. United Nations. A World Fit for Children. United Nations General Assembly 27th Special Session, 8–10 May 2002. New York: UN; 2002.

410. United States, Population Reference Bureau. The World's Youth, 2006 datasheet. Washington, DC: PRB; 2006. Available from: http://www.prb.org/pdf06/WorldsYouth2006DataSheet.pdf.

411. United States, Georgetown University, School of Foreign Service, Center for Latin American Studies. Pueblos indígenas, democracia y participación política. Accessed Septem-

ber 2006. Available from: http://pdba.georgetown.edu/IndigenousPeoples/demographics.html.

412. Economic Commission for Latin America and the Caribbean. Social Panorama of Latin America 2004. Santiago, Chile: ECLAC; 2004.

413. Economic Commission for Latin America and the Caribbean. Youth in Ibero-America: Trends and Urgencies. Santiago, Chile: ECLAC; 2004.

414. United Nations Population Fund. State of world population 2005 report: the promise of equality gender equity, reproductive health and the Millennium Development Goals. New York: UNFPA; 2005.

415. United Nations Population Fund. Overcoming gender disparities [Web page]. Available from: http://www.unfpa.org/adolescents/gender.htm. Accessed July 2006.

416. Comisión Económica para América Latina y el Caribe. La vulnerabilidad reinterpretada, asimetrías, cruces y fantasmas. Santiago de Chile: CEPAL; 2002.

417. Rodríguez J. Migración interna en América Latina y el Caribe: estudio regional del período 1980–2000. Santiago de Chile: CELADE; 2004.

418. United States, National Academies, National Research Council, Institute of Medicine. Growing up global: the changing transitions to adulthood in developing countries. Washington, DC: National Academy Press; 2005.

419. Kalmanovitz S. Emigración colombiana a los Estados Unidos: trasterritorialización de la participación política y socioeconómica. In: Macroeconomía y gasto público en economías de desarrollo intermedio: esquemas de reproducción kaleckianos y marxistas. August 2006. Available from: http://www.lablaa.org/blaavirtual/sociologia/guarniz-1/perfil.html.

420. Kliksberg B. O contexto da juventude na América Latina e no Caribe: as grandes interrogações. In: Thompson A (ed.). Associando-se á juventude para construir o futuro. Sao Paulo: Fundación W. K. Kellogg; 2006. pp. 21–58. Available from: http://www.wkkf.org.

421. Stanley J. Situación de la juventud indígena en Panamá [Web page]. Available from: http://www.gobernabilidad.cl. Accessed October 2006.

422. International Labor Organization. Global Employment Trends for Youth. Geneva: ILO; 2004.

423. United States Agency for International Development. Country profile Caribbean region (April 2003). Accessed June 2003. Available from: http://www.synergyaids.com/summaries.asp.

424. International Labor Organization, Inter-American Research and Documentation Center on Vocational Training. [Web page]. Available from: http://www.ilo.org/public/english/region/ampro/cinterfor/index.htm. Accessed July 2006.

425. World Health Organization, Family and Community Health; Department of Child and Adolescent Health and Develop-

ment. Broadening the horizon: balancing risk and protection for adolescents. Geneva: WHO; 2002.

426. Machinea JL. Panorama social de América Latina 2004 [PowerPoint presentation]. CEPAL. Available from: http://www.eclac.cl/publicaciones/xml/6/20386/Presentacion_ps04_JLM.pdf.

427. Economic Commission for Latin America and the Caribbean. Social Panorama of Latin America 2002–2003. Santiago, Chile: ECLAC; 2003.

428. Jelin E, Díaz-Muñoz A. Major Trends Affecting Families: South America in Perspective. United Nations; 2003.

429. Pan American Health Organization. Health Statistics in the Americas. 2006 edition. Washington, DC: PAHO; 2006.

430. Pan American Health Organization, Health Analysis Area. Regional Core Health Data Initiative. Washington, DC: OPS; 2005.

431. Jamaica, Ministry of Health. National HIV/STI Prevention and Control Program 2005. HIV/AIDS epidemic update: January to December 2004. Kingston: Ministry of Health; 2005.

432. World Health Organization. Global Tuberculosis Control: Surveillance, Planning, Financing. WHO Report 2003. Geneva: WHO; 2003.

433. Breinabuer C, Maddaleno M. Youth: choices and change: promoting healthy behavior in adolescents. Washington, DC: PAHO; 2005. (Scientific and technical publication No. 594).

434. Dietz WH. Childhood weights affect adult morbidity and mortality. J Nutr. 1998;128(2 suppl 2):411–14.

435. United States, Robert Wood Johnson Foundation; American Heart Association. Nation at Risk: Obesity in the US: A Statistical Sourcebook. 2005.

436. United States, Centers for Disease Control and Prevention, Division of Reproductive Health; United States Agency for International Development. Reproductive, maternal, and child health in Central America: trends and challenges facing women and children: El Salvador, Guatemala, Honduras, Nicaragua. Atlanta: CDC/USAID; 2005.

437. Joint United Nations Program on HIV/AIDS. 2006 Report on the Global AIDS Epidemic. A UNAIDS 10th anniversary special edition. Geneva: UNAIDS; 2006.

438. Calderon V. Foro nacional de prevención y atención de prevención y atención de adolescentes embarazadas. República Dominicana, Ministerio de Salud Pública; 2002.

439. Jamaica, National Family Planning Board. Reproductive Health Survey 2002. Kingston: NFPB; 2005.

440. United States, Guttmacher Institute. Early Childbearing in Nicaragua: A Continuing Challenge. In Brief, 2006 Series, No. 3.

441. United States, Guttmacher Institute. Early Childbearing in Honduras: A Continuing Challenge. In Brief, 2006 Series, No. 4.

442. United States, Guttmacher Institute. Early Childbearing in Guatemala: A Continuing Challenge. In Brief, 2006 Series, No. 5. Available from: http://www.guttmacher.org/pubs/2006/11/09/rib-Guatemala-en.pdf.

443. World Health Organization, Family and Community Health, Department of Child and Adolescent Health and Development. Pregnant Adolescents: Delivering on Global Promises of Hope. Geneva: WHO; 2006.

444. El Salvador, Ministerio de Salud Pública. Estudio de línea de base de mortalidad materna. El Salvador: OPS; 2005.

445. Conde-Agudelo A, Belizan JM, Lammers C. Maternal-perinatal morbidity and mortality associated with adolescent pregnancy in Latin America: cross-sectional study. Am J Obstet Gynecol. 2005 Feb;192(2):342–49.

446. Halcon L, Blum RW, Beuhring T, Pate E, Campbell-Forrester S, Venema A. Adolescent health in the Caribbean: a regional portrait. Am J Public Health. 2005; Nov;93(11):1851–57.

447. World Health Organization. Unsafe abortion: global and regional estimates of incidence of unsafe abortion and associated mortality in 2000. 4th edition. Geneva: WHO; 2004.

448. World Health Organization. World Report on Violence and Health. Geneva: WHO; 2003. Available from: http://www.who.int/violence_injury_prevention/violence/world_report/en/introduction.pdf.

449. Palacio M. Violencia que afecta a los jóvenes: la magnitud en Colombia. In: Curso teoría enfoques y herramientas para la prevención de la violencia que afecta a los jóvenes. Bogotá: OPS; 2006.

450. Organización Panamericana de la Salud. La salud sexual y reproductiva: también un asunto de hombres. Buenos Aires: OPS; 2005.

451. Guatemala, Centro de Estudios de Guatemala. Las maras: ¿amenazas a la seguridad? Informe especial 2005. Accessed August 2006. Available from: http://www.laneta.apc.org/ceg.

452. Organization of American States, Inter-American Drug Abuse Control Commission. Comparative Report on Nationwide School Surveys in Seven Countries: El Salvador, Guatemala, Nicaragua, Panama, Paraguay, Dominican Republic, and Uruguay 2003. Washington, DC: OAS/CICAD; 2004.

453. United Nations, Department of Economic and Social Affairs, Population Division. World Populations Prospects: The 2004 Revision. New York: UN; 2005.

454. Pan American Health Organization, Area of Technology and Health Services Delivery, Mental Health and Specialized Programs Unit. Older Adults. Washington, DC: PAHO; 2003. Unpublished.

455. Albala C, Lebrao ML, León EM, Ham-Chande R, Hennis A, Palloni A, Pelaez M, Pratts O. Encuesta Salud, Bienestar y Envejecimiento (SABE): metodología de la encuesta y perfil de la población estudiada. Rev Panam Salud Publica. 2005;17(5/6):307–22.

456. Mexico, Instituto Nacional de Estadística Geográfica e Informática; United States, Universities of Pennsylvania, Maryland, and Wisconsin. Mexican Health and Aging Study (MHAS). Available from: http://www.mhas.pop.upenn.edu/. Accessed 17 January 2006.

457. Puerto Rico, Universidad de Puerto Rico. Puerto Rican Elderly: Health Conditions (PREHCO). Universidad de Puerto Rico; University of Wisconsin-Madison; 2006. Available from: http://prehco.rcm.upr.edu. Accessed 17 January 2006.

458. Costa Rica, Universidad de Costa Rica, Centro Centroamericano de Población. Estudio de Longevidad y Envejecimiento Saludable (CRELES). Available from: http://ccp.ucr.ac.cr/creles/. Accessed 17 January 2006.

459. United States, Federal Interagency Forum on Aging-Related Statistics. Older Americans Update 2006: Key Indicators of Well-Being. Washington, DC: U.S. Government Printing Office; 2006. Available from: http://www.agingstats.gov. Accessed 17 January 2006.

460. Canada, Canadian Longitudinal Study on Aging. Available from: http://www.clsa-elcv.ca/. Accessed 17 January 2006.

461. United Nations. Second World Assembly on Ageing. Madrid International Plan of Action on Ageing 2002. Available from: http://www.un.org/esa/socdev/ageing/waa/a-conf-197-9b.htm. Accessed 17 January 2006.

462. Economic Commission for Latin America and the Caribbean. Report of the Regional Intergovernmental Conference on Ageing: Towards a Regional Strategy for the Implementation in Latin America and the Caribbean of the Madrid International Plan of Action on Ageing (LC/L.2079). Santiago, Chile, 19–21 November 2003.

463. World Health Organization. Active Ageing: A Policy Framework. Geneva: WHO; 2002. Available from: http://whqlibdoc.who.int/hq/2002/WHO_NMH_NPH_02.8.pdf. Accessed 17 January 2006.

464. Organización Panamericana de la Salud. Seminario Políticas Sociales y Rehabilitación Integral en los Países del Cono Sur. Montevideo: OPS; 2002.

465. World Health Organaization. International Classification of Functioning, Disability and Health. Geneva: WHO; 2001.

466. Organización Panamericana de la Salud. Atención Primaria en Salud y Rehabilitación. Programa Regional de Rehabilitación OPS/OMS. Documento de trabajo. Managua: OPS; 2005.

467. Organización Panamericana de la Salud. Situación de la discapacidad en las Américas. Programa Regional de Regional de Rehabilitación OPS/OMS. Documento de trabajo. Managua: OPS; 2004.

468. Organización Panamericana de la Salud. La discapacidad en Nicaragua: situación actual y perspectivas. Managua: OPS; 2005.

469. Chile, Fondo Nacional de la Discapacidad. Discapacidad en Chile. Pasos hacia un modelo integral de funcionamiento humano. Santiago de Chile; 2006.

470. Ecuador, Instituto Nacional de Estadísticas y Censos; Consejo Nacional de Discapacidad. Ecuador: La discapacidad en cifras. Quito; 2005.

471. Organización Panamericana de la Salud. La discapacidad en Panamá: situación actual y perspectivas. Panama City: OPS; 2005.

472. Colombia, Departamento Administrativo Nacional de Estadística. Censo Nacional de Población de. Informe preliminar cifras de población con discapacidad. Bogotá: DANE; 2006.

473. Argentina, Fundación Par. La discapacidad en Argentina. Un diagnóstico de situación y políticas públicas vigentes al 2005. Buenos Aires: Fundación Par; 2005.

474. Argentina, Instituto Nacional de Estadísticas y Censos. La población con discapacidad en Argentina. Encuesta Nacional de Personas con Discapacidad (ENDI). 2005.

475. Montero F. Right to Health and Rehabilitation for Persons with Disabilities. Geneva: Disability and Rehabilitation/WHO; 2006.

476. Economic Commission for Latin America and the Caribbean. Social Panorama of Latin America. Santiago: ECLAC; 2006. Available from: http://www.cepal.org/cgi-bin/getProd.asp?xml=/publicaciones/xml/4/27484/P27484.xml&xsl=/dds/tpl-i/p9f.xsl&base=/tpl-i/top-bottom.xsl. Accessed 8 December 2006.

477. Pan American Health Organization. Meeting on control of the intestinal helminth infections in the context of IMCI: report. Washington, DC: PAHO; 2000.

478. Hurtado AM, Lambourne CA, James P, Hill K, Cheman K, Baca K. Human rights, biomedical science, and infectious diseases among South American indigenous groups. Annu Rev Anthropol. 2005 Oct;34:639–65.

479. Guyatt H. Do intestinal nematodes affect productivity in adulthood? Parasitol Today. 2000 Apr;16(4):153–58.

480. Crompton DW, Nesheim MC. Nutritional impact of intestinal helminthiasis during the human life cycle. Annu Rev Nutr. 2002;22:35–59.

481. Gyorkos, TW, Larocque R, Casapia M, Gotuzzo E. Lack of risk of adverse birth outcomes after deworming in pregnant women. Pediatr Infect Dis J. 2006 Sept;25(9):791–94.

482. Larocque R, Casapia M, Gotuzzo E, Gyorkos TW. Relationship between intensity of soil-transmitted helminth infections and anemia during pregnancy. Am J Trop Med Hyg. 2005 Oct;73(4):783–89.

483. Ehrenberg JP, de Merida AM, Sentz J. An epidemiological overview of geohelminth and schistosomiasis in the Caribbean. Washington, DC: PAHO; 2003.

484. World Health Organization. Global Programme to Eliminate Lymphatic Filariasis. Wkly Epidemiol Rec. 2006 June;22: 221–32. Available from: http://www.filariasis.org/pdfs/WER_81_2006_221-232.pdf.

485. World Health Organization. Fifty-fourth World Health Assembly Resolution, Provisional agenda item 13.3. Geneva: WHO; April 2001.

486. Merianos A, Peiris M. International Health Regulations (2005). Lancet. 2005 Oct;366.

487. World Health Organization. Resolution WHA58.3. Revision of the International Health Regulations. Fifty-eighth World Health Assembly. Geneva: WHO; 2005. Available from: http://www.who.int/gb/ebwha/pdf_files/WHA58/WHA58_3en.pdf. Accessed 24 October 2006.

488. Pan American Health Organization. Regional Strategic Plan for Technical Cooperation in Epidemic Alert and Response. 21 September 2006.

489. World Health Organization. Resolution WHA56.19. Prevention and control of influenza pandemics and annual epidemics. Fifty-sixth World Health Assembly, Geneva, 2003. Available from: http://www.who.int/gb/e/e_wha56.html/#Resolutions/. Accessed 15 January 2007.

490. Pan American Health Organization. Resolution CD44.R8. Influenza Pandemic: Preparation in the Hemisphere. 44th Directing Council. Washington, DC: PAHO; 2003. Available from: http://www.paho.org /english/gov/cd/cd44index-e.htm#resolutions. Accessed 15 January 2007.

491. United Nations. World Urbanization Prospects: The 2005 Revision. New York: UN; 2006. Available from: http://www.un.org/esa/population/publications/WUP2005/2005wup.htm. Accessed 17 January 2007.

492. Food and Agriculture Organization of the United Nations. Helping Prevent Avian Influenza in Latin America and the Caribbean. Rome: FAO; 2006. Available from: http://www.fao.org /newsroom/en/news/2006/1000381/index.html. Accessed 11 January 2007.

493. World Health Organization. Resolution WHA58.3. Revision of the International Health Regulations. Fifty-eighth World Health Assembly. Geneva: WHO; 2005.

494. World Health Organization, Global Influenza Program. Global Influenza Preparedness Plan: the role of WHO and recommendations for national measures before and during pandemics. Geneva: WHO; 2005. (WHO/CDS/CSR/GIP/2005.5). Available from: http://www.who.int/csr/resources/publications/influenza/WHO_CDS_CSR_GIP_2005_5/en/index.html. Accessed 16 January 2007.

495. Meltzer MI, Shoemake HA, Kownaski M, Crosby R. FluAid 2.0. Software and Manual to Aid State and Local-Level Health Officials Plan, Prepare and Practice for the Next Influenza Pandemic. Atlanta: CDC; 2000. Available from: http://www.cdc.gov/flu/tools/fluaid/.

496. Zhang X, Meltzer MI, Wortley P. FluSurge 2.0. Software to Estimate the Impact of an Influenza Pandemic on Hospital

Surge Capacity. Atlanta: CDC; 2005. Available from: http://www.cdc.gov/flu/tools/flusurge/.

497. Praveen Dhankhar, Zhang X, Meltzer MI, Bridges CB. Flu-WorkLoss 1.0. Software and Manual to Aid State and Local Public Health Officials Estimating the Impact of an Influenza Pandemic on Work Day Loss. Atlanta: CDC; 2006. Available from: http://www.cdc.gov/flu/tools/fluworkloss/.

498. World Health Organization. Checklist for Influenza Pandemic Preparedness Planning. Geneva: WHO; 2005. (WHO/CDS/CSR/GIP/2005.4). Available from: http://www.who.int/csr/resources/publications/influenza/WHO_CDS_CSR_GIP_2005_4/en/index.html. Accessed 16 January 2007.

499. Glezen WP. Emerging Infections: Pandemic Influenza. Epidemiologic Reviews. 1996;18(1):64–76.

500. Knobler SL, Mack A, Mahmoud A, Lemon SM (eds.). The Threat of Pandemic Influenza: Are We Ready? Washington, DC: National Academies Press; 2005.

501. World Health Organization. Outbreak News–Severe acute respiratory syndrome (SARS). Wkly Epidemiol Rec. 78(12); 81–8.

502. Canada, Public Health Agency of Canada. Learning from SARS–Renewal of Public Health in Canada. Ottawa: Public Health Agency of Canada; 2003. Available from: http://www.phac-aspc.gc.ca/publicat/sars-sras/naylor/. Accessed 15 February 2007.

503. World Health Organization. Consensus document on the epidemiology of severe acute respiratory syndrome (SARS). Geneva: WHO; 2003. (WHO/CDC/CSR/GAR/2003.11). Available from: http://www.who.int/csr/sars/guidelines/en/index.html. Accessed 15 February 2007.

504. World Health Organization. China's latest SARS outbreak has been contained but biosafety concerns remain–Update 18 May 2004. Available from: http://www.who.int/csr/don/2004_05_18a/en/index.html. Accessed 15 February 2007.

505. Singapore, Ministry of Health. Biosafety and SARS Incident in Singapore September 2003. Report of the Review Panel on New SARS Case and Biosafety. Available from: http://www.moh.gov.sg/corp/sars/pdf/Report_SARS_Biosafety.pdf. Accessed 15 February 2007.

506. Pan American Health Organization. EID Updates: Emerging and Reemerging Infectious Diseases, Region of the Americas. Washington, DC: PAHO; 2004. Available from: http://www.paho.org/english/AD/DPC/CD/eid-eer-2004-oct-06.htm. Accessed 15 February 2007.

APPENDIX. List of the Leading Causes of Death (ICD-10/LC)

Total	A00–R99, V01–Y89
LC-01	Intestinal infectious diseases (A00–A09)
LC-02	Tuberculosis (A15–A19)
LC-03	Vector-borne diseases and rabies (A20, A44, A75–A79, A82–A84, A85, A90–A96, A98.0–A98.2, A98.8, B50–B57)
LC-04	Vaccine-preventable diseases (A33, A37, A80, B01, B05, B06, B15, B16, B17.0, B18.0, B18.1, B18.9, B19, B26)
LC-05	Meningitis (A39, A87, G00–G03)
LC-06	Septicemia (A40–A41)
LC-07	Human immunodeficiency virus (HIV) disease (B20–B24)
LC-08	Malignant neoplasm of esophagus (C15)
LC-09	Malignant neoplasm of stomach (C16)
LC-10	Malignant neoplasm of colon, sigmoid, rectum, and anus (C18–C21)
LC-11	Malignant neoplasm of liver and intrahepatic bile ducts (C22)
LC-12	Malignant neoplasm of gallbladder or of other unspecified parts of the biliary tract (C23, C24)
LC-13	Malignant neoplasm of pancreas (C25)
LC-14	Malignant neoplasm of larynx (C32)
LC-15	Malignant neoplasm of trachea, bronchus, and lung (C33, C34)
LC-16	Melanoma and other malignant neoplasms of skin (C43, C44)
LC-17	Malignant neoplasm of female breast (C50)
LC-18	Malignant neoplasms of the uterus (C53–C55)
LC-19	Malignant neoplasm of ovary (C56)
LC-20	Malignant neoplasm of the prostate (C61)
LC-21	Malignant neoplasm of kidney, except renal pelvis (C64)

LC-22	Malignant neoplasm of bladder (C67)
LC-23	Malignant neoplasm of brain (C71)
LC-24	Malignant neoplasms of the hematopoietic and lymphatic systems (C81–C96)
LC-25	In situ neoplasms or of uncertain or unknown behavior (D00–D48)
LC-26	Diabetes mellitus (E10–E14)
LC-27	Malnutrition and nutritional anemias (D50–D53, E40–E64)
LC-28	Volume depletion or other disorders of fluid, electrolyte, and acid-base balance (dehydration) (E86–E87)
LC-29	Dementia and Alzheimer's disease (F01, F03, G30)
LC-30	Mental and behavioral disorders due to psychoactive substance use (F10–F19)
LC-31	Parkinson's disease (G20)
LC-32	Epilepsy and status epilepticus (G40, G41)
LC-33	Chronic rheumatic heart diseases (I05–I09)
LC-34	Hypertensive diseases (I10–I15)
LC-35	Ischemic heart diseases (I20–I25)
LC-36	Pulmonary heart disease and diseases of pulmonary circulation (I26–I28)
LC-37	Nonrheumatic mitral valve disorders (I34–I38)
LC-38	Cardiomyopathy (I42)
LC-39	Cardiac arrest (I46)
LC-40	Cardiac arrhythmias (I47–I49)
LC-41	Heart failure, complications, and ill-defined diseases of the heart (I50–I51)
LC-42	Cerebrovascular diseases (I60–I69)
LC-43	Atherosclerosis (I70)
LC-44	Aortic aneurysm and dissection (I71)
LC-45	Acute upper respiratory infections except influenza and pneumonia (J00–J06, J20–J22)
LC-46	Influenza and pneumonia (J10–J18)
LC-47	Chronic lower respiratory diseases (J40–J47)
LC-48	Pulmonary edema and other respiratory diseases affecting the interstitium (J80–J84)
LC-49	Respiratory failure (J96)
LC-50	Diseases of the appendix, hernia, and intestinal obstruction (K35–K46, K56)
LC-51	Cirrhosis of the liver and other chronic liver diseases (K70–K76)
LC-52	Diseases of the musculoskeletal system and connective tissue (M00–M99)
LC-53	Diseases of the urinary system (N00–N39)
LC-54	Pregnancy, childbirth, and the puerperium (O00–O99)
LC-55	Certain conditions originating with the perinatal period (P00–P96)
LC-56	Congenital malformations, deformations, and chromosomal abnormalities (Q00–Q99)
LC-57	Traffic accidents (terrestrial) (V00–V89)
LC-58	Accidental falls (W00–W19)
LC-59	Handgun discharge (unintentional) (W32–W34)
LC-60	Accidental drowning and submersion (W65–W74)
LC-61	Other accidental threats to breathing (W75–W84)
LC-62	Accidental poisoning (X40–X49)
LC-63	Intentional self-harm (suicides) (X60–X84)
LC-64	Assault (homicides) (X85–Y09)
LC-65	Event of undetermined intent (Y10–Y34)
LC-88	Others
LC-99	Ill-defined causes (R00–R99)

Chapter 3
SUSTAINABLE DEVELOPMENT AND ENVIRONMENTAL HEALTH

Among the principal remits of the health sector is to safeguard the public's well-being by ensuring a sound, healthy physical and social environment, one that enables sustainable human development—understood to mean improvement of material conditions to respond to the needs of the present generation without jeopardizing the ability to respond to those of future generations—and that protects the most vulnerable members of society. Towards that end, the health sector collaborates with other sectors—the environment, labor, agriculture, and education, among others. Moreover, it behooves local communities, countries, and the international alliances, each on its own and all together, to both monitor and counter the many causes of environmental degradation. Inequities—in education, employment, health, and political rights—affect individuals' susceptibility to environmental impacts and can result in significant disease and death. Other influences include globalization, governmental reforms, the privatization of services, the vagaries of the labor market, and uncontrolled urbanization. A consensus prevails that sustainable human development depends on reducing poverty while protecting and promoting health.

In Latin America and the Caribbean, the challenge is to conciliate the objectives of development, health, and the environment with those of social equity, which will require, among other means, the elaboration of effective urban development policies. A case in point is water and sanitation: as urban populations increase, so too does the demand for drinking water and sewage and solid waste disposal services. Disparities between urban-center and urban-periphery populations and between urban and rural populations in access to those services and in exposure to environmental risks compound the vulnerability of the poor.

Accelerated, unplanned growth of the industrial sector is a direct cause of biological, chemical, and physical contamination; it increases transportation and energy consumption, produces more wastes, and renders their disposal inadequate. Industrialization, coupled with the untoward effects attributed in recent years to climate change, is resulting in the deterioration of the environment and of people's quality of life and health. Production processes—the extraction of raw materials, their transformation into products, the consumption of those products, the elimination of industrial wastes, and the use of pesticides in agriculture and forestry—pose direct and indirect physical and chemical risks to populations. Mining, petroleum exploration, agrochemical farming, hospitals, health centers and laboratories, energy plants, and industrial manufacturers are among the biggest producers of dangerous chemical and solid wastes. The consumption of goods and services poses a major challenge to environmental management in terms of controlling risks and promoting health.

Since the home and the workplace are people's primary environments, adequate housing and working conditions are as important to ensure their good health as is the larger environment. A major problem is that of rural communities where the poor are particularly exposed to health risks, especially those living in endemic areas plagued by vector-borne diseases—Chagas', malaria, dengue, and yellow fever. Another set of problems relates to changes in the work profile and in the working population wrought by globalization, regional integration, trade liberalization, structural adjustments and privatization, and social policies—all of which greatly impact the living conditions and health of the working population and lead to increased inequities. Most worrisome in this respect are the increasing proportions of children and elderly in the workforce.

Along with greater poverty, social inequity, and urbanization, the breaking up of family and community structures fosters unhealthy environments that can lead to likewise unhealthy lifestyles and risky behaviors at every stage of life. Aggravating those conditions are the persistence of mortality among mothers and children due to poor nutrition, infections, and lack of access to goods and services. A direct link has been drawn between poor diet and chronic diseases: together, nutritional deficiencies and excesses contribute to a double burden of diseases that affect the population at every age. The increase in risky lifestyles and behaviors—smoking, the consumption of alcohol and drugs, and various forms of violence and accidents—underscore the critical need for health promotion strategies.

The countries of the Region recognize the inextricable relationship between health and the environment. To enhance that relationship—in effect, to prevent and control the adverse effects of the environment on health—they have agreed to concentrate on five main areas: intersectoral collaboration, decentralization of responsibilities, information systems, social participation, and compliance with commitments struck at international conferences. Efforts are under way to monitor and evaluate environmental health, develop healthy policies that can be sustained over the long term, seek alliances, prepare human resources, establish appropriate legislation regarding the consumption of goods and services, and carry out direct interventions. The focus is on strengthening the normative, regulatory, and response capacities of national health authorities; on reinforcing existing environmental institutions and redefining their functions and organizational arrangements; and on setting aside funds to protect the environment and mitigate the adverse effects on health resulting from environmental disturbances. Two major health promotion responses to the population's needs in this area are the regional health-promoting schools initiative and the healthy communities strategy.

HEALTH AND THE ENVIRONMENT

Over the last several decades, inequalities in living and health conditions in the Region of the Americas have become more pronounced, and inequalities in environmental health are no exception to this pattern. Marked inequalities are seen not only in effects on health and access to services, but also in exposure to environmental risks in all of the Region's countries and territories, within each of these, and among the different population groups. It is estimated that 24% of the global burden of disease and 23% of all deaths can be attributed to factors related to the environment (1). In developing countries 25% of mortality is attributable to environmental causes, and in developed countries this percentage reaches 17%.

Environmental health is the result of an interaction of factors operating on different levels of aggregation within a framework of complex processes, which go beyond the environment's traditional biological, physical, and chemical components. In order to gain a better understanding of environmental health, it may be put into context using as a frame of reference determining health factors (Figure 1). According to this framework, a series of determining structural factors of a social, economic, political, environmental, technological, and human biological nature—some of which are interrelated—interact in a significant manner with the health system. These relationships give rise in turn to intermediate determining factors that create inadequate living conditions, environmental risks and hazards, and modifications in lifestyles and behavior whose consequences impact life expectancy; cause disease, injuries, disabilities, and deaths; and affect the population's overall well-being.

The Region's socioeconomic decline, particularly the increase in poverty and inequity, rapid urbanization, and fragmentation and disintegration of family and community structures, help create unhealthy environments that in turn lead to high-risk lifestyles and behaviors lasting throughout the life cycle. These conditions coexist with the long-standing problems of maternal and infant mortality from malnutrition, infections, and lack of access to basic goods and services, as well as problems related to smoking, alcoholism, violence, HIV/AIDS infection, and road safety issues (2).

In the Region of the Americas, inequalities in environmental health have been described at different stages of development, which allows specific groups who are most vulnerable to be identified. Some of these inequalities are seen in rural areas and relatively well-preserved ecosystems where traditional populations reside (for example, indigenous groups, Afro-descendants, gold panners, or fisherman) or in more developed areas populated by agricultural workers. Other inequalities exist in urban areas populated by the poorest and most marginalized groups (e.g., the Brazilian *favelas*), who are generally in closest geographical proximity to the production of hazardous wastes and thus at risk of contamination by such products, as well as among occupational groups employed in industries involving environmental pollutants.

Many health problems will continue worsening due to the degradation of living conditions caused by inadequate road safety, noise pollution, limited drinking water coverage, inadequate sanitation, deficient waste disposal, chemical pollution, smoking, and physical hazards associated with urban overcrowding. Problems that emerge in urban settlements and overcrowded housing facilitate the spread of infectious diseases and contribute to a large extent to an increase in violence and illicit drug use. Urban growth has weakened the capacity of many municipalities and local government to provide basic health services.

Urban growth also means greater reliance on transportation systems, which in turn create more pollution and greater risk of injuries. Both outdoor and indoor air pollution (including in the work environment) will remain the leading cause of respiratory infections, asthma, and acute respiratory infections—especially in children—and of chronic respiratory diseases among women and the elderly. In Latin America, more than 300 million people live in large cities, where exposure to particulate matter and other air pollutants places their lives at risk.

Trade globalization, human displacements, and cultural factors may have both positive and negative effects on health. There is a brisk trade in goods and services that are harmful to the en-

FIGURE 1. Health and its determinants: the interplay between health and the environment.

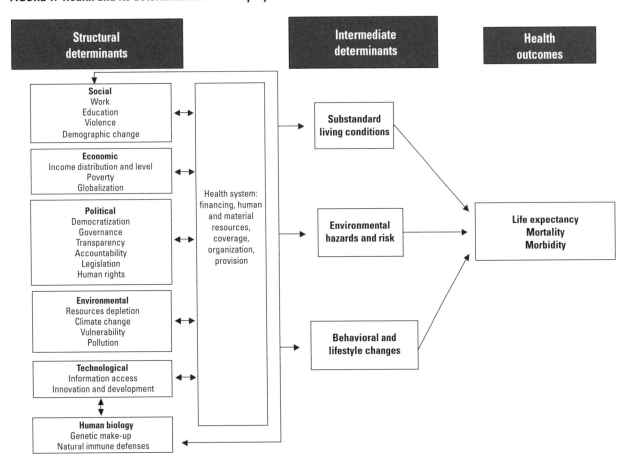

Source: Loyola E. Progress on Children's Environmental Health in the Americas. International Conference for the Evaluation of Global Health Strategies. Florence, Italy; 2006.

vironment and human health, and massive population migrations create additional global threats to health. Communicable diseases such as tuberculosis are increasingly spreading to other developed nations, where they affect the poorest and most vulnerable segments of the population.

There is growing concern about food safety, both in terms of chemical substances and microorganisms. In many parts of the world, the growing incidence of foodborne diseases has become evident over the last decade. The direct and indirect health consequences of biotechnological applications in food production are also of concern. The increase in trade in food has the benefit of ensuring secure and nutritional diets, but at the same time could contribute to a greater spread of food infections and poisoning. Promoting food safety standards and international guidelines can promote health and trade. The World Health Organization (WHO) and the Food and Agriculture Organization of the United Nations (FAO) are working together to improve food surveillance, monitoring, and the risk-assessment methodologies.

In response to the current situation, and bearing in mind the socio-environmental diversity that exists in Latin America and the Caribbean, the Sustainable Development and Environmental Health Area of the Pan American Health Organization (PAHO), the United Nations Environment Program (UNEP), and the Oswaldo Cruz Foundation (FIOCRUZ) of Brazil have designed a methodological strategy called GEO-Salud that is based on the DPSEEA model (the acronym stands for "driving forces-pressures-state-exposure-effects-action"), facilitates environmental health assessment and monitoring, and enables the development of long-term sustainable health policies and the resolution or prevention of problems (*3*). This strategy provides a multi-causal analysis model for the biophysical, temporal-spatial, and social dimensions of the ecosystem to which the assessment is applied.

Breaking the problem down into different stages gives the proposed analysis framework the flexibility to be adapted to the information needs of different management levels. Regardless of the level to which it is applied, this methodological approach should

FIGURE 2. Environmental health management interaction flowchart.

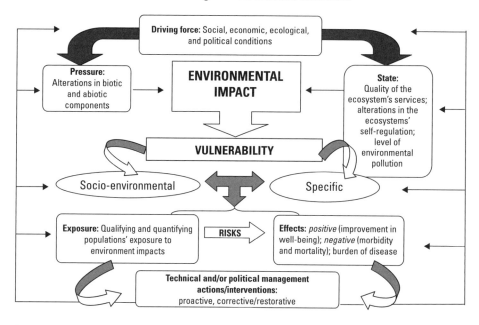

Source: Organización Panamericana de la Salud; Programa de las Naciones Unidas para el Medio Ambiente; Fundación Oswaldo Cruz. Proyecto GEO-Salud. En búsqueda de herramientas y soluciones integrales a los problemas de medio ambiente y salud an América Latina y el Caribe. Mexico City: OPS; PNUMA; FIOCRUZ; 2005.

allow for the identification of environmental changes that are harmful to human health and the mapping of risks and assessment of vulnerabilities in terms of environmental impacts. The information obtained will assist in defining control actions needed to stop the effects of such impacts and reverse them. Finally, if possible, the integral assessment should also envisage what the consequences would be of not taking short- and medium-term measures, so as to make political decision-makers aware of the need to act in an intersectoral fashion, not only in evaluating the problem, but also in seeking solutions to it (Figure 2).

Environmental issues can be addressed by reducing specific risks, such as improving water quality or encouraging alternatives to pesticide use, or by modifying intermediate and structural determinants that impact health (the latter through health promotion strategies, and poverty reduction and sustainable development, aimed at meeting the Millennium Development Goals [MDGs]). Among the specific contributions of the health sector, the Healthy Municipalities Initiative and the Health-Promoting Schools Regional Initiative are noteworthy regional strategies.

Environmental justice is a tool that can be used for addressing inequalities. This term is understood as "a set of principles and practices that ensure that no social group endures a disproportionate burden from negative environmental consequences stemming from economic transactions; political decisions; and federal, state, and local programs, as well as from the lack or absence of such policies, allowing fair and equitable access to national re-

sources and relevant information for affected communities and vulnerable groups, and favoring construction of alternative and democratic development models" (4, 5).

In keeping with these concepts, PAHO and its Member States propose dealing with all environmental and health-related issues through actions guided by this definition of environmental justice, and through public and institutional health and environmental policies that embrace broad intersectoral approaches. Examples of the former include drawing up socio-environmental vulnerability maps that allow target populations to be identified; implementing educational programs, enabling information access, and developing community leadership training programs in vulnerable areas; participating in environmental licensing processes from risk analysis to future scenario design; applying, where pertinent, prevention principles; cleaning up areas contaminated by hazardous products; and drafting master infrastructure plans within the framework of urban ecology and the healthy spaces concept. Examples of the latter are demarcating land and creating healthy environment reserves, adopting incentive policies for agroecological and family agricultural production, implementing human rights and anti-discrimination policy programs, fostering community tourism, and generating and utilizing alternative energies. The future of current generations and those to come will depend on how policy- and decision-makers go about managing and developing a healthy and sustainable environment.

WATER, SANITATION, AND SOLID WASTE DISPOSAL

Sanitation is an integral part of health, development, and poverty-reduction strategies. Basic sanitation is the series of actions taken within the human ecosystem to improve water supply services and sanitary wastewater and excreta disposal, solid waste management, household hygiene, and industrial water use in an institutional, legal, and political context in which diverse players from the national, regional, and local levels participate. This series of actions keeps public health and basic sanitation management in permanent interaction. Several countries from the Region incorporate management of these areas into such sectors as the environment and housing, whose subsequent coordination with the health sector is essential for achieving sustainable development.

The population's access to drinking water supply, sanitation services, and sanitary disposal of solid waste are analyzed here within the context of the MDGs, public health, and the economic benefits accruing from good health through the achievement of sustainable services of acceptable quality. Critical and emergency situations that have arisen in Latin America and the Caribbean are also addressed.

At the Millennium Summit of the United Nations held in September 2000, 189 Member States, 147 of which were represented by Heads of State and Government, adopted the Millennium Declaration that set forth the Millennium Development Goals. The United Nations General Assembly proclaimed the 2005–2015 period as the International Decade for Action under the slogan "Water for Life" (6), which began on 22 March 2005 and coincided with that year's observance of World Water Day. Nations were urged to provide a coordinated response to achieve fulfillment of the MDGs related to water and sanitation and to lay the foundations for going forward in upcoming years, without overlooking the need to enhance equity in access, quality, and sustainability of services, including the protection of water resources.

The International Decade for Action will be instrumental in keeping these worldwide goals focused on measures aimed at improving equitable access to water and sanitation services in order, at the same time, to reach international goals projected for water that are contained in Agenda 21 and its local action plan, the Millennium Declaration, and the Johannesburg Plan of Implementation. This is important for Latin America and the Caribbean, where one out of every four persons lacks access to safe water and basic sanitation services, and in the Region's communities and areas in which socioeconomic inequalities are most acute, this need affects one out of every two persons.

General Comment No. 15, which relates to Articles 11 and 12 of the International Covenant on Economic, Social, and Cultural Rights and pertains to the right to water, was adopted in November 2002, constituting a milestone in the history of human rights. For the first time, access to water is explicitly recognized as a fundamental human right, thereby establishing the obligation of

"In the past, and too frequently today, public water supplies have given rise to much illness and death caused by diseases such as typhoid, dysentery, diarrhea, and cholera. A safe water supply is absolutely essential and should figure among the first permanent measures adopted by communities to protect their health."

Hugh Cumming, 1933

governments to progressively ensure universal and equitable access to safe drinking water without discrimination. In setting the legal basis for the right to water, the Comment states: "the human right to water entitles everyone to sufficient, safe, acceptable, physically accessible, and affordable water for personal and domestic uses." As a result, Member States recognized that water must be treated as a cultural and social good, and not merely an economic one (7), a perspective that marks a radical departure from the focus adopted at different international fora held during the 1990s when water was considered a commodity.

There is a strong social movement that advocates for water as a human right and a common good, which came to the fore at the 4th World Water Forum held in Mexico City at the end of March 2006 (8). Nevertheless, and in spite of the subsequent controversy, the Forum's final declaration does not recognize access to water as a human right, and the Governments of Bolivia, Cuba, Uruguay, and Venezuela issued a separate declaration affirming this access as a fundamental human right. At the same time, social organizations from more than 40 countries organized an alternative forum in which they denounced the idea that many governments and companies consider drinking water just one of many commodities and not a fundamental right that guarantees human survival.

To attain MDG water and sanitation targets, intense pressure must be brought to bear on health authorities. The right to drinking water will not be achieved solely through application of economic approaches; rather it also requires a strong moral conviction for the respect of three fundamental values: freedom, equity, and solidarity with society's most disadvantaged.

Monitoring MDG Targets

The WHO/UNICEF Joint Monitoring Program (JMP) for Water Supply and Sanitation evaluates progress made in fulfilling Target 10 (halving the proportion of people without sustainable access to safe drinking water and basic sanitation by 2015) of MDG 7 (ensuring environmental sustainability). This evaluation is based on household surveys and population censuses conducted in the countries, and its main purpose is to monitor trends and programs, strengthen monitoring capacity, and report on the sectors' situation in terms of international and national policies. Only where this kind of data is unavailable does JMP use information

TABLE 1. Technological options for MDG Target 10 indicators of progress, JMP, 2004.

Drinking water		Sanitation	
Improved	Unimproved	Improved	Unimproved
Piped water into dwelling, plot, or yard	Unprotected dug well	Piped sewer system	Open pit
	Unprotected spring	Septic tank	Pit latrine without slab
	Cart with small tank/drum	Pit latrine with slab	Bucket or hanging latrine
Public tap/standpipe		Pit latrine	
Tube well/borehole	Bottled water	Ventilated improved pit latrine	No facilities or bush or field
Protected dug well	Tanker truck		
Protected spring	Surface water	Composting toilet	
Rainwater collection			

Note: JMP considers that improved technologies are more likely to provide adequate amounts of drinking water, privacy, and hygiene than unimproved technologies. Bottled water is considered an unimproved source if it is the only source available or is used with another unimproved source of water.

Source: WHO/UNICEF Joint Monitoring Program (JMP) for Water Supply and Sanitation. Meeting the MDG Water and Sanitation Target: A Mid-term Assessment of Progress; 2004.

from companies that provide these services in the countries. Given the current difficulty of taking routine, rapid measurements of the quality of drinking water and sanitation services, JMP uses two indicators for access or coverage: the percentage of the population (urban and rural) that uses improved drinking water sources, and the percentage of the population (urban and rural) that uses improved sanitation facilities.

According to the JMP, drinking water is water used for domestic purposes, including water for consumption and hygiene. The Program considers that in rural areas if more than 30 minutes are needed to reach the water source and return home, there is a tendency to use less water than the amount required to cover basic needs. Monitoring instruments for use do not consider costs, services continuity, or water quality at the source or home. The "improved sources of drinking water" could already be contaminated or, given the lack of household connection or service continuity, the water could become contaminated during its transport or from inappropriate storage in the home. For this reason, the population that has safe water available, as required by Target 10 of MDG 7, is probably far less than that which has access to "improved water sources" (Table 1). To overcome these limitations, JMP applies a methodology to rapidly assess water quality in seven countries in different regions of the world, including Nicaragua in Latin America.

In Nicaragua, the drinking water quality rapid assessment study was conducted between 2004 and 2005. The study highlighted the importance of raising awareness among field personnel and communities regarding water quality and how interaction between the two groups contributed to enhancing environmental education. This methodology yielded highly reliable and representative results in terms of the technologies used in supplying water and distributing it throughout the entire country. The most obvious result of the assessment has been to confirm that there is a serious nationwide problem with the quality of water that Nicaraguans consume. The 2005 final report (9) indicates that arsenic contamination of drinking water may be more far reaching

in geographical terms than what was previously assumed and that household fecal contamination is most likely also greater.

JMP monitoring results of Target 10 in other countries of the Region are analyzed more in depth in the section in this chapter entitled "Equity in Sustainable Access to Water and Basic Sanitation Services." It is likely that Target 10 will not be achieved in all the countries of the Americas, particularly in rural areas, and above all as regards access to sanitation services, due to the greater deficit to be covered. Despite commitments assumed by national leaders, the financing needed for its attainment has not been forthcoming as was expected. In most countries many tasks still remain to be done, including readjusting rates so as to ensure the economic and financial sustainability of the entities that provide these services, creating effective subsidy systems for low income groups, and fully applying regulatory frameworks. In addition to macroeconomic instability and the structural deficit in public finances, reforms in this sector to date have not produced the level of success earlier anticipated. The next five-year period, however, may yield more promising conditions.

Development policies for the solid waste sector in Latin America and the Caribbean must incorporate Agenda 21 and MDG targets related to universal coverage by 2025, improvement of 100 million people's living conditions by 2020, the population's right to receive adequate services, as well as the achievement of equity.

"Improving water resources management and development is also a critical factor for meeting the broader set of [Millennium Development] Goals [. . .] reducing child mortality, improving maternal health, combating major diseases."

"Health, dignity and development: what will it take?"

Final report of the United Nations Millennium Task Force on Water and Sanitation

FIGURE 3. Mortality in children under 5 years of age from acute diarrheal diseases, by country or subregion, Region of the Americas, 1995–2005.

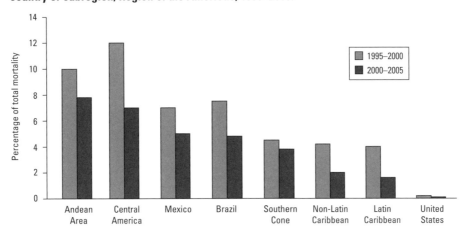

Source: Pan American Health Organization, Area of Sustainable Development and Environmental Health.

Such policies must likewise promote the formal creation of a solid waste disposal sector—alongside currently existing water and sanitation sectors—as well as the restructuring of solid waste management, establishment of laws for the new sector, and strengthening of oversight, regulation, municipal management, institutional coordination, civil society participation and sustainability, and private initiative.

Water, Basic Sanitation, and Public Health

The Global Water, Sanitation, and Hygiene for All (WASH) Forum, held in Dakar, Senegal, in 2004, explicitly links improvements in solid waste management with achievement of MDGs regarding water, sanitation, and human settlements. Fulfillment of Target 10 is central to reaching other targets related to health and development. Access to water and sanitation services also contribute to attaining other MDGs, such as reducing poverty, hunger, and malnutrition; reducing child mortality; and promoting gender equality and empowerment of women, in addition to forming part of MDG 7's emphasis on effective management and protection of natural resources.

Clearly, access to water and sanitation services is an indispensable requisite for improving health conditions in general, but is particularly important in the case of women and children, as well as for groups for whom inequalities in health and services provision constitute a pervasive reality. In the Region's poorest countries, children are the innocent victims in the sense that their right to adequate drinking water and sanitation services goes unprotected. Poverty, characterized by precarious housing conditions and unhealthy physical environments, increases children's exposure to numerous health threats. During the 2000–2005 period, mortality attributable to acute diarrheal diseases among children under 5 years old was 3.7%, and in the Andean subregion, this figure reached 7.8% (Figure 3).

Diarrheal diseases and parasitosis are among the leading causes of morbidity in children under 5 in the Americas and affect three health indicators: life expectancy at birth, as well as the mortality rate and rate of chronic malnutrition among children under age 5. To demonstrate the impact of water and sanitation on health, countries in the Americas have been classified (using the cluster technique in a statistical analysis computer program) in four developmental phases, according to the existing relationship between health (measured by the above-mentioned indicators), water and sanitation, and level of development. Table 2 shows the results of this classification and demonstrates the direct correlation between satisfactory water and sanitation coverage and acceptable levels of human development and health. Haiti, for example, which has the lowest water and sanitation coverage levels, also has the lowest Human Development Index (HDI) values and highest child mortality rates, in contrast to Chile, Costa Rica, Cuba, and Uruguay, among others, which have higher values.

Figure 4 shows the reciprocal relationship between access to water and sanitation and mortality in children under age 5 in the countries of the Region.

Inadequate sanitation infrastructure, discharge of untreated household wastewater into natural water bodies, as well as poorly functioning in situ sanitation systems (septic tanks and latrines), which mainly contaminate groundwater, create enormous problems for public health in the Americas. Using wastewater for irrigation has been associated with the transmission of enteric diseases, such as cholera and typhoid fever, even in areas where these illnesses are not endemic. Other gastrointestinal diseases, such as dysentery, giardiasis, and even infectious hepatitis, can be spread through contaminated vegetables.

In Latin America and the Caribbean there is a high correlation between the HDI and solid waste generation (Figure 5). Nations such as Bolivia, Grenada, Guatemala, Haiti, Honduras and Nicaragua, whose HDI is less than 0.7, generate less than

215

TABLE 2. Countries of the Americas, grouped by level of health development.[a]

Countries in the group	Level of health development	Human Development Index[b]	Life expectancy at birth[c] (years)	Drinking water coverage[d] (%)	Sanitation coverage[d] (%)	Chronic undernutrition in children under 5[c] (%)	Mortality in children under age 5[c] (per 1,000 live births)
Haiti	1	47.5	51.6	71.0	34.0	23.0	117.0
Bolivia, Guyana	2	70.3	63.6	84.0	57.5	19.0	66.5
Honduras, Guatemala	3	66.5	67.5	92.5	64.5	39.0	43.0
Belize, Dominican Republic	4	75.1	69.5	92.0	52.0	12.0	35.5
Argentina, Brazil, Colombia, Ecuador, El Salvador, Jamaica, Mexico, Nicaragua, Panama, Paraguay, Peru, Suriname, Venezuela	5	77.0	72.0	86.4	75.1	15.5	26.8
Antigua and Barbuda, Barbados, Canada, Chile, Costa Rica, Cuba, Dominica, Saint Lucia, Trinidad and Tobago, United States, Uruguay	6	84.3	75.7	96.2	94.7	5.8	11.9

[a]Countries grouped with similar selected indicators, in order from lowest to highest level of health development.
Sources: [b]UNDP. Human Development Report 2004. Values averaged by group of countries.
[c]PAHO. Basic Indicators 2001.
[d]JMP water and sanitation data results for Latin America and the Caribbean, 2002.

0.6 kg/inhabitant/day of solid waste, while Argentina, Uruguay, and the English-speaking Caribbean countries, whose HDI is over 0.8, produce more than 1.0 kg/inhabitant/day. By way of comparison, the per capita generation of solid waste in the Region's industrialized countries is 2.0 kg/inhabitant/day in the United States and 1.9 kg/inhabitant/day in Canada.

Per capita generation of municipal or urban solid waste varies according to the size of the population nucleus. In a large population nucleus (more than 201,000 inhabitants), the weighted regional average for household waste is 0.88 kg/inhabitant/day, and municipal waste generation is 1.09 kg/inhabitant/day. In a medium-sized nucleus (51,000 to 200,000 inhabitants), the corresponding values are 0.58 kg/inhabitant/day (household) and 0.75 kg/inhabitant/day (municipal), while in a small population nucleus (up to 50,000), they are 0.54 kg/inhabitant/day and 0.52 kg/inhabitant/day, respectively. Average values for the Region are 0.79 kg/inhabitant/day (household) and 0.91 kg/inhabitant/day (municipal).

As may be seen in Figure 6, solid waste collection coverage varies a great deal between countries: in Argentina and Chile, for example, nationwide coverage is around 100%, while in the Dominican Republic and Paraguay, these percentages are 70% and 51%, respectively. The English-speaking Caribbean countries typically have collection coverage close to 100%, with the exception of Dominica, where it is 50%.

As Table 3 illustrates, solid waste generation, storage, collection, sorting, recycling, and its inadequate disposal in the Region affect health and the environment. Conditions associated this situation include gastrointestinal, parasitic, respiratory, dermatological, degenerative, infectious, and vector-borne diseases and diseases of the mucous membranes, as well as poisonings, work-related accidents, and mental disorders. The principal groups most exposed are the population that lacks adequate collection and storage systems, workers in the solid waste sector, persons who sort garbage, those who consume meat from swine raised near final waste disposal sites, those who reuse containers, and persons living in close proximity to final disposal or incineration sites for solid waste. The associated environmental effects include hazardous waste exposure; vector proliferation; land, air, and water pollution; food contamination; soil degradation; chemical container reuse; contaminated compost production; drainage systems modifications; and feeding livestock solid waste. In the Region, the percentage of garbage sorters who are women and children exceeds 50% (*10*).

The Economic Benefits of Water and Sanitation Services Access

WHO has conducted studies to estimate the costs and benefits associated with MDG Target 10 and has compared the differences in these based on five separate scenarios (Table 4). These studies

FIGURE 4. Correlation between access to water (A) and sanitation services (B) and child mortality, by country, Region of the Americas.

(A)

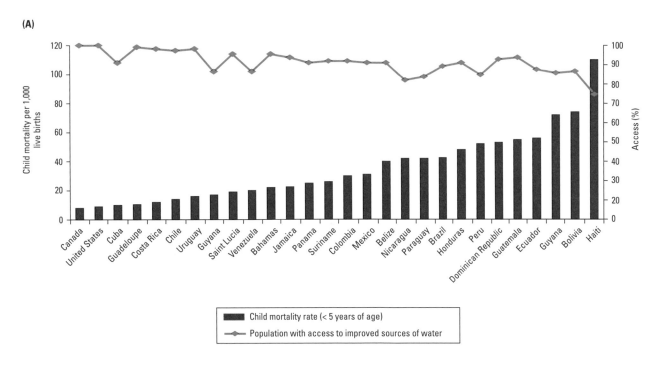

(B)

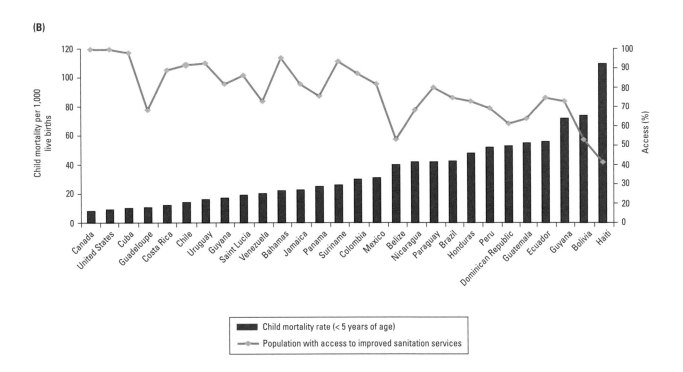

Sources: Adapted from Otterstetter H, Galvão LA, Witt P, Caporali S, Pinto PC. Health Equity in Relation to Safe Drinking Water Supply. In: Pan American Health Organization. Equity and Health: Views from the Pan American Sanitary Bureau (Occasional Publication No. 8), 2001; Pan American Health Organization. Health Statistics from the Americas, 2003 Edition; WHO/UNICEF Joint Monitoring Program for Water Supply and Sanitation. Meeting the MDG Drinking Water and Sanitation Target: A Mid-term Assessment of Progress, 2004.

FIGURE 5. Correlation between the Human Development Index and per capita generation of solid waste in Latin America and the Caribbean.

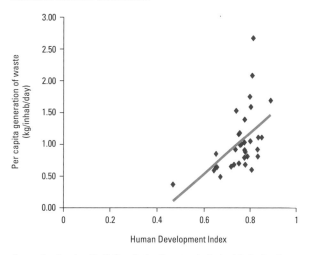

Source: Pan American Health Organization. Report on the Regional Evaluation of Municipal Solid Waste Management Services in Latin America and the Caribbean. Washington, D.C.: PAHO; 2005.

FIGURE 6. Average solid waste collection coverage, by country, Latin America and the Caribbean.

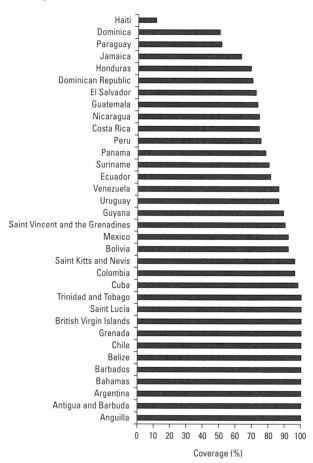

Source: Pan American Health Organization. Report on the Regional Evaluation of Municipal Solid Waste Management Services in Latin America and the Caribbean. Washington, D.C.: PAHO; 2005.

included epidemiological, demographic, and economic data from several international sources, JMP coverage and cost data from 2000, and recurring costs from specialized literature and different projects. The impact of water and sanitation interventions was measured in terms of reductions in incidence of disease and death related to infectious diarrheal diseases and the corresponding savings in treatment for the health sector and patients, values related to death and disabilities that were avoided, and time saved due to not needing medical care or having to carry water, among other factors. Time saved is reflected in productivity, school attendance, and quality of life.

Countries in Latin America and the Caribbean were included in three groups according to their epidemiological characteristics (Table 5).

Reported results have been consolidated in Table 4 and Figure 7, from which the following may be observed:

- Scenario 2 lays out the cost-benefit analysis for achieving Target 10, according to JMP indicators, although a good option would be to include household water quality management (scenario 4), since it has the best cost-benefit ratio and a good additional benefit. This should be done concomitantly without forgoing the quest for universal access to regulated services for treated drinking water and wastewater, in keeping with the need to implement comprehensive water source management and achieve the MDGs as a whole.
- Interventions of this kind yield benefits for the health sector, but the greatest benefit of all is time-savings, which translates into measurable gains in the education, agriculture, industry, and tourism sectors, among others. To better

estimate the value of this time-savings, it would be useful to conduct economic studies at the local and national levels.

- Different sectors may provide financing for such interventions, but the health sector can play a key role in preparing computer programs (for example, on health education for bringing about behavior modification) and contribute with testing and analysis to improve decision-making in other sectors for the benefit of the most vulnerable segments of the population.

Water system privatization was undertaken during the 1990s, within the context of a development model known as the "Washington Consensus." This model—built on the pillars of a free market, fiscal austerity, and public services privatization—argues that the free market, when free from government interference and corruption, can transform developing countries' economies. International lending organizations have advocated this model in

TABLE 3. Environmental health problems related to inadequate management of wastes, Latin American and Caribbean countries.

Solid waste management phase	Environmental problem	Health risks	Exposed population group
Inadequate generation and storage	Environmental hazard due to hazardous or potentially hazardous materials of daily household use. Proliferation of vectors (insects, rats, rodents, and pathogen organisms). Food contamination. Foul odors.	Gastrointestinal diseases. Poisoning of infants and pets. Dengue. Zoonoses.	Population lacking adequate storage and/or collection systems.
Inadequate disposal in public areas	Proliferation of vectors (insects, rats, rodents and pathogen organisms). Air pollution due to open-air burning. Surface water contamination due to dumping of wastes. Food contamination. Foul odors. Landscape deterioration.	Gastrointestinal and respiratory diseases.	Population lacking adequate collection services.
Collection, transportation, storage in transfer stations	Landscape deterioration. Foul odors. Noise pollution.	Gastrointestinal, respiratory, and dermatological diseases. Occupational diseases and accidents (ergonomic disorders, traffic accidents, injuries with sharp objects).	General population. Formal and informal urban sanitation workers.
Sorting and recycling	Reuse of chemical products bottles and containers. Feeding of beef cattle and swine with unhealthy organic wastes. Application of contaminated compost to soil.	Gastrointestinal, respiratory, and dermatological diseases. Occupational diseases and accidents, chronic degenerative diseases, mental health disorders, alcoholism, and drug addiction. Poisonings.	Sorters. Population that acquires products in reused containers. Consumers of beef and pork from animals bred in dumps or fed organic wastes from garbage.
Treatment and final disposal	Soil contamination. Air pollution due to open-air burning. Surface and groundwater contamination. Modification of drainage systems (public sewers, canals, and riverbeds). Landscape deterioration. Fires. Alteration of natural ecosystems.	Infectious and parasitic diseases; allergies; respiratory tract, skin, and mucous membrane diseases. Occupational diseases and accidents, chronic degenerative diseases, mental health disorders, alcoholism, drug addiction, dengue, and emerging diseases.	Population adjacent to final disposal sites. Peri-urban population sectors where wastes are accumulated or burned. Formal or informal workers from this sector.

Source: Pan American Health Organization. Report on the Regional Evaluation of Municipal Solid Waste Management Services in Latin America and the Caribbean. Washington, D.C.: PAHO; 2005.

TABLE 4. Cost-benefit of water and sanitation intervention scenarios, Latin American and the Caribbean countries.

Scenarios (access and level of service by 2015)	Annual cost[a]	Annual benefit[a]	Cost-benefit ratio
1. Reduce by 50% the deficit in water access	171	2,199	12.8
2. Reduce by 50% the deficit in water and sanitation access (in accordance with MDG Target 10 using JMP indicators)	788	9,635	12.2
3. Reduce by 100% the deficit in water and sanitation	1,577	22,532	14.3
4. Universal access to water and sanitation services (scenario 3) plus water disinfection at the point of use	1,937	38,129	19.7
5. Universal access to regulated water and sanitation systems plus water and wastewater treatment	14,085	69,223	4.9

[a]In US$ millions (2000).

Source: Hutton G, Heller L. Evaluation of the Costs and Benefits of Water and Sanitation Improvements at the Global Level. Geneva: WHO; 2004.

TABLE 5. Countries of the Region of the Americas, by mortality stratum.

Mortality stratum	Countries
A[a]	Canada, Cuba, United States
B[b]	Antigua and Barbuda, Argentina, Bahamas, Barbados, Belize, Brazil, Chile, Colombia, Costa Rica, Dominica, El Salvador, Grenada, Guyana, Honduras, Jamaica, Mexico, Panama, Paraguay, Dominican Republic, Saint Kitts and Nevis, Saint Lucia, Saint Vincent and the Grenadines, Suriname, Trinidad and Tobago, Uruguay, Venezuela
D[c]	Bolivia, Ecuador, Guatemala, Haiti, Nicaragua, Peru

[a]Very low child mortality and low adult mortality.
[b]Low adult and child mortality.
[c]High adult and child mortality.
Source: Hutton G, Heller L. Evaluation of the Costs and Benefits of Water and Sanitation Improvements at the Global Level. Geneva: WHO; 2004.

government reforms as a solution to insufficient financing for infrastructure and inefficiency of water and sanitation systems and other public services. On occasions, these organizations have established privatization as a prerequisite for providing loans; until this occurs, affected countries generally suffer from a scarcity of capital in the public sector charged with providing water, which worsens operating capacity of these services.

Almost all countries have implemented or are preparing to implement some modality of private sector participation in their water systems. These privatization schemes vary depending on the country and the specific characteristics of their respective sanitation services, and range from mere operations and maintenance outsourcing to comprehensive water and sanitation man-

agement. Currently, emphasis is placed on service quality, and countries are defining their program policies in this regard.

Equity in Sustainable Access to Water and Basic Sanitation Services

Between 1990 and 2004, the population in Latin America and the Caribbean grew from 441.5 million to 553.7 million. At the same time, the percentage of the population with access to water services increased from 83% to 91%, while access to sanitation services rose from 68% to 77%. In the Assessment of Drinking Water and Sanitation 2000 in the Americas Regional Report, an average production of 600 m³/sec of wastewater is reported, of which 14% is treated and only 6% received adequate treatment. This situation remains unchanged, and according to the 2001 regional assessment of solid waste management, urban centers produced around 369,000 tons of municipal solid waste per day; of this amount, large urban centers generated 56%, medium-sized centers 21%, and small centers 23%.

According to indicators defined and used by the JMP for global monitoring (Table 6), by 2004 the drinking water deficit recorded in 1990 (baseline MDG) decreased by 8%, dropping from 17% in 1990 to 9% in 1994 (a 3% reduction from 7% to 4% in urban areas, and a 15% decrease from 42% to 27% in rural areas). The total reduction required to reach Target 10 of MDG 7 by 2015 is 9%, which would mean a 4% decrease in urban areas, with access rising from 93% in 1990 to 97% by 2015, and a 21% drop in rural areas, with access increasing from 58% in 1990 to 79% by 2015. In keeping with this trend, it is feasible that some countries in the Region would be able to meet this target, while other countries will need to intensify actions (Figure 8).

In general, when comparing urban area drinking water coverage in most Latin American and Caribbean countries in 2004 (*11*)

FIGURE 7. Estimated benefit of water and sanitation interventions envisaged under scenario 2[a], MDG Target 10 in Latin America and the Caribbean, based on JMP indicators.

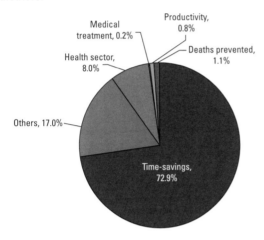

[a]See Table 4.
Source: Hutton G, Heller L. Evaluation of the Costs and Benefits of Water and Sanitation Improvements at Global Level. Geneva: WHO; 2004.

in light of 1990–2015 growth trends, it can be expected that with the exception of Haiti, there will be no serious obstacle in reaching MDG Target 10 by 2015 in terms of the coverage indicator. Efforts must persist, however, in improving and monitoring quality of service indicators as regards continuity, quality, quantity, and cost, and even more so in rural areas of Bolivia, Brazil, Chile, Colombia, El Salvador, Haiti, Nicaragua, Paraguay, and Peru, where inequitable drinking water coverage, both in terms of quality and quantity, is longstanding. According to the JMP report (*11*), some countries did not record data, which therefore are not displayed.

The inequalities between urban and rural areas are well known, and according to the JMP, the vast majority of the 53 million people (more than 68%) who have no drinking water supply live in rural areas. Figure 9 shows deficit distribution by subregion and as can be seen, nearly 66% of the population lacking water lives in Brazil and the Andean countries. The situation is

similar regarding sanitations services, with more than 127 million people having no access to improved facilities.

Although the deficit for basic sanitation coverage is higher than for drinking water coverage, the proportion of the population without access to drinking water is six times greater in rural areas than in urban areas and three-and-a-half times greater with regard to sanitation. The situation is even more critical in light of the fact that in rural areas the conditions under which services are provided do not meet water quality requirements; furthermore, sanitation facilities are often not used as planned. Long distances between rural communities constitute the most significant obstacle to providing services, even more so than potential income level differences between communities. In countries such as Brazil or Peru, for example, even the poorest urban families have higher levels of household connection than the segment of rural families with the highest per capita spending (Figure 10) (*12*).

In Peru, inequality in water and sanitation services provision, particularly sanitation, means that the poorest have the lowest percentage of access to water and sanitation (Figure 11). The sanitation coverage gap between the poorest and the richest quintiles is 68%, while the child malnutrition gap between these same groups is 30%.

It is estimated that more than 127 million people (almost 32% of the urban population) live in informal settlements in underprivileged urban areas of the Region. In general, these are large families who live and carry out their activities in impoverished, overcrowded, and vulnerable conditions (*13*). Lack of access to drinking water services means that this population must resort to unsafe sources of water, such as informal vendors who provide water of questionable quality at higher prices than those paid by individuals who have a connection to the public network.

The sanitation deficit, on average, was reduced by 9% between 1990 and 2004, decreasing from 32% to 23% (13% in rural areas and 9% in urban areas), while the total reduction required to achieve Target 10 by 2015, according to the JPM indicators (Table 7), is 17% (32% in rural areas and 10% in urban areas). Provision of sanitation services lags behind drinking water, such that in most countries actions must be intensified and new

TABLE 6. Access to improved sources of drinking water, Latin American and Caribbean countries.

	Population (in millions)					Proportion of population (%)						
	2004					With access					Access deficit	
	With access		Without access	Total	1990	2004			Projection for 2015[c]	Target for 2015[d]	1990	2004
Area	Home[a]	Others[b]				Home[a]	Others[b]	Total				
Urban	378.7	25.3	16.8	420.8	93	90	6	96	98	97	7	4
Rural	59.8	37.2	35.9	132.9	58	45	28	73	83	79	42	27
Total	438.5	62.5	52.7	553.7	83	80	11	91	97	92	17	9

[a]Access to water service by direct household piped connection.
[b]Other access by means of public taps and fountains and protected wells.
[c]Projected access by 2015, according to 1990–2004 trends.
[d]Projection based on achievement of MDG 7's Target 10, according to JMP indicator.
Source: WHO/UNICEF Joint Monitoring Program for Water Supply and Sanitation database, 2006.

FIGURE 8. Trends in access to drinking water, by country, Latin America and the Caribbean, according to JMP-defined indicators and based on JMP data.

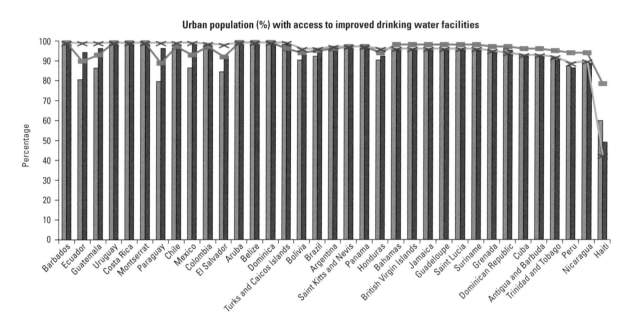

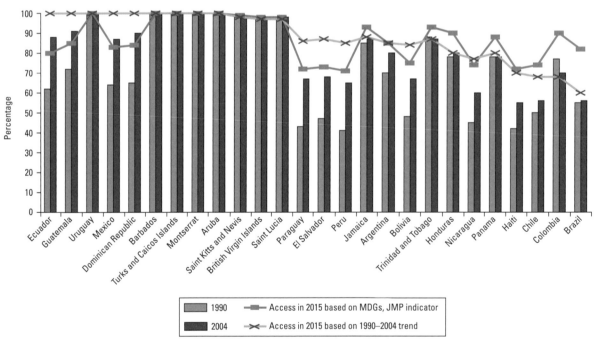

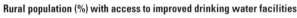

Source: WHO/UNICEF Joint Monitoring Program (JMP) for Water Supply and Sanitation. Meeting the MDG Water and Sanitation Target: A Mid-term Assessment of Progress; 2004.

strategies devised in order to reach sanitation access targets proposed for 2015 (Figures 12 and 16).

Growth trends in sanitation coverage for the 1990–2015 indicate that by 2004, several Latin American and Caribbean countries (*11*), among them Bolivia, Brazil, El Salvador, Nicaragua,

and Peru, began to show signs of having difficulties reaching the Target 10 coverage indicator in urban areas, and would have to redouble efforts to finance construction and maintain infrastructure. The most significant obstacles for fulfilling Target 10 can be found in rural areas, especially in countries such as Bolivia,

FIGURE 9. Population in millions (M) without access to improved drinking water sources, by country or subregion, Latin America and the Caribbean.

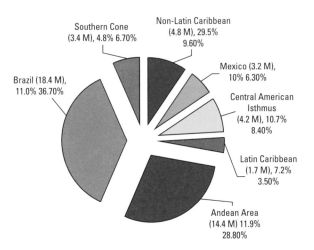

Note: The whole pie represents the 53 million people in Latin America and the Caribbean without access to improved water sources. Population (1st percentage) without access as compared to that subregion's total population. Population (2nd percentage) without access in the subregion as compared to the 53 million people without access in Latin America and the Caribbean.
Source: WHO/UNICEF Joint Monitoring Program for Water Supply and Sanitation database, 2006.

Brazil, Chile, Colombia, El Salvador, Haiti, Jamaica, Nicaragua, Panama, and Peru.

Figure 13 illustrates differences (inequities) in excreta disposal coverage in both urban and rural areas of Latin America and the Caribbean. Mexico has the most marked difference in urban vs. rural coverage (51%), while Barbados, Costa Rica, and Grenada, in contrast, have the greatest differences in rural vs. urban coverage.

Figure 14 depicts the degree of exclusion in rural and urban areas in Latin America and the Caribbean. In the case of Suriname, for every urban inhabitant who lacks sanitation services, there are eight rural dwellers without such services. The situation in Costa Rica and Venezuela is the inverse, with the degree of exclusion being greater in urban areas than rural ones.

By using the Gini coefficient and the Lorenz curve to estimate sanitation coverage inequity in the countries of the Americas (Figure 15), it can be seen that 47.5% of the population accumulates 86.5% of the sanitary deficit, in addition to an unacceptable degree of inequality (Gini coefficient = 0.53).

Despite the progress achieved, limitations to sanitation and water services persist for a significant portion of the population. Indeed, 127 million people (23%) do not have access to improved sanitation facilities. Analysis conducted by subregions highlights the fact that this deficit is most acute in the Andean countries and Brazil, where more than 50% of sanitation coverage shortages are concentrated (Figure 16). In Latin America and the Caribbean, as in most developing countries, the problem of universal access to water and sanitation is found principally in the poorer segments

FIGURE 10. Water coverage in rural and urban areas of Brazil (A) and Peru (B) and its relationship to deciles of expenditure.

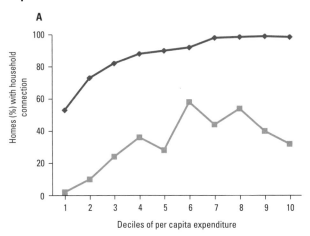

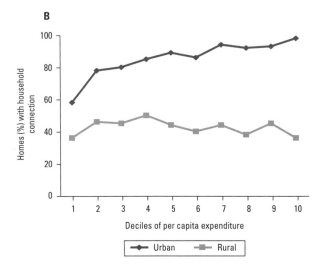

Source: Organización Panamericana de la Salud. Desigualdades en el acceso, uso y gasto del agua potable en América Latina y el Caribe. Serie de informes técnicos no. 2 y no. 11. Washington, D.C.: OPS; 2001.

of the population, which in the case of the Region of the Americas belong to readily identifiable groups. Specifically, the population segments that suffer from the most notable inequities in access to basic services are indigenous peoples and those living in rural and outlying urban areas. Most of these inequalities are linked to geography (given the great distances between rural towns in particular), socioeconomic status (all groups mentioned typically suffer from high levels of poverty or extreme poverty), and ethnic origin.

Quality and Sustainability of Basic Water and Sanitation Services in the Region

Inequalities in drinking water and sanitation are also determined by other service quality indicators, in addition to access or

FIGURE 11. Percentage of population of Peru without water and sanitation coverage; percentage of child malnutrition by quintile of poverty.

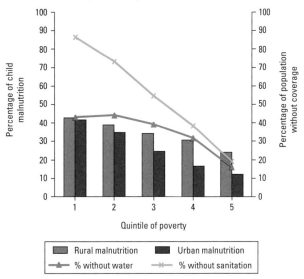

Source: Pan American Health Organization, Area of Sustainable Development and Environmental Health.

fluents from sewage systems in Latin America and the Caribbean receive any kind of treatment before being discharged. Inadequate management of water resources, including wastewater discharges, together with limitations in infrastructure for treating water for human consumption, degrade the quality of water distributed to users.

To ensure sustainability of drinking water and sewerage systems in the countries of the Region and protect progress made in coverage levels, significant challenges must be overcome to guarantee the quality of services, both for drinking water, as well as sanitation in general. In many cases, drinking water and sewerage systems are either totally obsolete or in need of renovations and/or expansion. To make matters worse, in many countries of the Region serious deficiencies persist in equipment and facility operation and maintenance, causing service interruptions, distribution system losses, and disinfection problems, all of which compromise the efficiency of the provision entities and the quality of services rendered to consumers. The Assessment of Drinking Water and Sanitation 2000 in the Americas notes high values of non-metered water, considered to be the ratio between water charged and water produced. In large cities, distribution systems recorded an average of 45% of non-metered water. Although generally speaking, disinfection is applied in large urban centers to 100% of the systems, in rural systems disinfection is insufficient and in many cases nonexistent.

The population that enjoys adequate water quality control and monitoring systems is limited in urban areas and insignificant in rural areas. According to the 2000 Assessment, 52% of the urban population in the Region has effective water quality monitoring systems, with this percentage only reaching 24% in Latin America and the Caribbean. Indeed, in very few of these countries are water quality control and monitoring programs backed by adequate regulation or legislation that determines resources and establishes required responsibilities. PAHO defines a basic monitoring program as one that includes sanitary inspection of system components and, at a minimum, determines levels of residual chlorine, pH, and turbidity.

coverage. In the Assessment of Drinking Water and Sanitation 2000 in the Americas (*14*), 33 countries reported on the continuity of urban water systems; of these, 16 (or nearly half) noted interruptions in service. This intermittence in receipt of services constitutes a public health risk and inefficient use of the existing infrastructure, contributes to a deterioration of public confidence in the service, and compromises its economic viability.

Although the Region's health and environmental authorities share an interest in having more integrated water resources management—expressed in declarations from the Meeting of Health and Environment Ministers of the Americas held in Ottawa in 2002 (*15*) and in Mar del Plata in 2005 (*16*)—only 14% of the ef-

TABLE 7. Access to improved sanitation facilities, Latin American and Caribbean countries.

	Population (in millions)					Proportion of population (%)						
	2004					With access					Access deficit	
	With access		Without access	Total	1990	2004			Projection for 2015[c]	Target for 2015[d]	1990	2004
Area	Home[a]	Others[b]				Home[a]	Others[b]	Total				
Urban	260.9	101.0	58.9	420.8	81	62	24	86	90	91	19	14
Rural	14.6	50.5	67.8	132.9	36	11	38	49	59	68	64	51
Total	275.5	151.5	126.7	553.7	68	51	26	77	84	85	32	23

[a]Access to household sewerage system connection.
[b]Other access to individual sanitation systems in situ, such as septic tanks and latrines.
[c]Projected access by 2015, according to 1990–2004 trends.
[d]Projection based on achievement of MDG 7's Target 10, according to JMP indicator.
Source: WHO/UNICEF Joint Monitoring Program for Water Supply and Sanitation database, 2006.

FIGURE 12. Rural and urban trends in access to sanitation services based on JMP-defined indicators, by country, Latin America and the Caribbean.

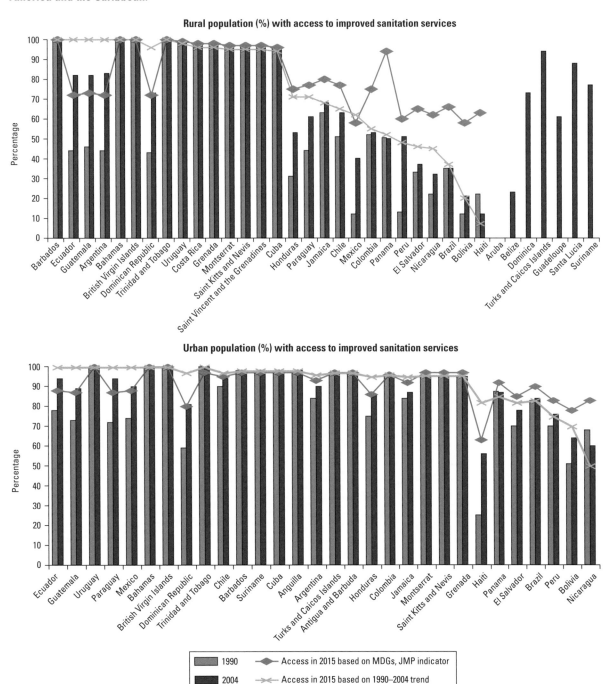

Source: WHO/UNICEF Joint Monitoring Program (JMP) for Water Supply and Sanitation. Meeting the MDG Water and Sanitation Target: A Mid-term Assessment of Progress; 2004.

As part of water services quality assurance, particularly drinking water quality, there must be measurable indicators and reliable data, with an acceptable level of uncertainty in order to adopt needed preventive and corrective measures. The problem lies in the limited capacity of the countries of Latin America and the Caribbean (as compared to developed countries) to take environmental measurements, specifically to determine water quality and the presence of toxic substances in drinking water and wastewaters. Moreover, significant differences can be seen between capitals and large cities, and small cities and rural towns. Countries

225

FIGURE 13. Coverage of excreta disposal, by country, Region of the Americas, 2001.

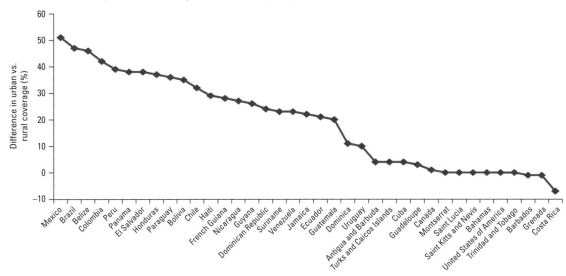

Source: WHO/UNICEF Joint Monitoring Program for Water Supply and Sanitation database, 2002.

FIGURE 14. Rate of exclusion from sanitation in rural and urban areas, by country, Region of the Americas, 2002.

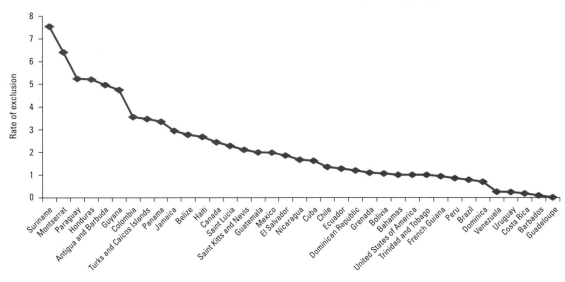

Source: WHO/UNICEF Joint Monitoring Program for Water Supply and Sanitation database, 2002.

such as Argentina, Brazil, Chile, Colombia, Costa Rica, Mexico, and Peru, among others, have the capacity to measure a large number of parameters, but the methods used are not necessarily validated, accredited, or subjected to a permanent quality control program. An assessment study of 40 laboratories conducted by PAHO's Pan American Center for Sanitary Engineering and Environmental Sciences (CEPIS) (*17*) estimated that, on average, measurement capacity is 86% for basic parameters; 37% for nutrients; 68% for toxic metals in general; 46% for lead, 39% for cadmium, 39% for copper, and 30% for mercury; 20% for toxic organic residues and chlorinated pesticides; 11% for phosphorics and other more complex parameters with minimum measurement capacities; 51% for organic matter indicators; and 62% for microbiological quality indicators. The study evaluated laboratories that belong to the Latin American and Caribbean Network of Environmental Laboratories (RELAC), principally laboratories belonging to ministries of health and the environment, water companies, some universities, and other sites. Fifty-eight percent of the laboratories utilized

FIGURE 15. **Lorenz curve for sanitation services, Latin American and Caribbean countries.**

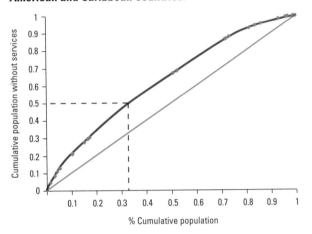

Source: Pan American Health Organization, Area of Sustainable Development and Environmental Health, based on JMP data.

FIGURE 16. **Population in millions (M) without access to improved sanitation facilities, by country or subregion, Latin America and the Caribbean.**

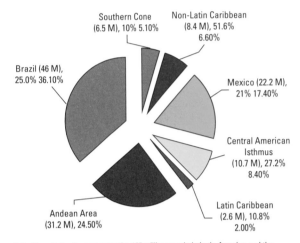

Note: The whole pie represents the 127 million people in Latin America and the Caribbean without access to improved sanitation facilities. Population (1st percentage) without access as compared to that subregion's total population. Population (2nd percentage) without access in the subregion as compared to the 127 million people without access in Latin America and the Caribbean.
Source: WHO/UNICEF Joint Monitoring Program for Water Supply and Sanitation database, 2006.

unvalidated modified methods. According to another inter-laboratory study by CEPIS, PAHO's Sustainable Development and Environmental Health Area, and the International Atomic Energy Agency (*18*), around 25% of the data on water quality have an error exceeding 20%, with variations on the acceptability of data according to the measurement's complexity.

To carry out these activities, measurements of water, biota, sediments, and municipal and hazardous waste are required. Hazardous waste may be household (e.g., batteries, containers for insecticides, pesticides, disinfectants), from medical and hospital centers (e.g., waste from medicines and disinfectants, as well as pathological and radiological waste, among other types), or industrial in nature (from small and medium-sized industry, agribusiness, the metal-working and mining industries, foundries, and factories of different kinds, all of whose hazardous waste materials and discharges can reach water sources and pollute them). Countries need to have reliable laboratories that comply with the respective regulatory frameworks (legislation and technical standards) and public health surveillance, and generate data for purposes of decision-making, research, and control of public health risks and harm. The main problems in this area are related to:

- a lack of knowledge at a local level regarding the environmental risks, both real and potential, related to public health;
- a lack of infrastructure to measure control and monitoring indicators of environmental factors that impact public health, and a dearth of qualified personnel and capital allocated for establishing laboratories;
- inequalities in measurement capacity (programs, training, and technology) between countries, capitals, provinces, and rural areas;
- a need for improvement in environmental analytical quality and capacity and greater participation by authorities in im-

plementing quality management systems to generate reliable primary data; and
- a need for national systems that can certify and accredit environmental laboratories.

CEPIS and PAHO's Sustainable Development and Environmental Health Area promote RELAC's strengthening in order to improve analytical capacity and quality and thus comparative data analysis. To this end, PAHO is promoting a regional strategic plan that includes executing situational analysis programs, training for laboratory professionals and technicians, use of validated and periodically controlled analytical methodologies, performance assessment, laboratory accreditation, research promotion, and development of methodologies to fit specific conditions.

It is recognized that to attain the service quality and coverage levels that the population desires, there must be viable financial systems. This means that rates must at least cover operating and maintenance costs, and, in most cases, investment to expand the systems. Although progress has been observed in some countries of the Region (e.g., Argentina and Chile), in many other countries rates continue to be low and do not even cover operating costs. In general, the sector still depends on the state budget to finance capital investment, and to a lesser extent—albeit to a considerable degree—operating and maintenance costs (*19*).

In several countries in the Americas, decentralization processes of water and sanitation services have taken hold. The common trend is toward transferring responsibility for providing services to the regional, provincial, or municipal levels, or to an autonomous agency that eventually will be managed in accordance

"Since the countries and territories of the Americas are essentially rural, there are increasing needs and opportunities for promotion by health services of satisfactory water supplies and safe disposal of sewage in rural areas."

Fred Lowe Soper, 1954

with commercial and technical criteria. The main difficulty noted is a lack of capacity on the part of many municipalities to effectively manage these services. This situation, in turn, leads to a deterioration of the services, the recovery of which is very costly.

Protection of Water Resources

Protecting sources of drinking water is merely the first line of defense to safeguard water for human consumption from substances and microorganisms that are harmful to human health. For drinking water systems, the raw material is surface and groundwater, and, as such, these should be protected from all types of contamination for the purpose of fostering sustainable development. Underground water resources in the Region have received little attention, and have thus become contaminated from agricultural activities (e.g., nitrates, pesticides), in situ sanitation (e.g., nitrates, microorganisms), solid waste disposal, and industrial activities, among other factors. All of the foregoing suggests that aquifer recovery will be very difficult, if not impossible.

Eutrophication is the process of macrophyte plant and algae overproduction in bodies of water, which can cause problems for drinking water supply due to the alteration of organoleptic properties (smell and taste), and to different disruptions in the water purification treatment process. Although eutrophication may occur gradually from natural causes, today it is essentially cultural in nature and is accelerated by the continuous introduction of nutrients from anthropogenic sources. In some eutrophied lakes and reservoirs, high levels of organic substances, together with the chlorine added to the drinking water supply, could generate substances that are harmful to human health in the long term, through production of chlorinated organic compounds. Furthermore, the harmful impact on human health of toxins produced by different species of cyanobacteria resulting from eutrophication has been documented, both from recreational contact and from their presence in drinking water sources. Indigenous rural populations are particularly exposed to these risks. Eutrophied bodies of water also offer a habitat for some disease vectors, such as mosquitoes. In a CEPIS regional study, more than 75% of the lakes and reservoirs assessed (in Argentina, Brazil, Colombia, Cuba, the Dominican Republic, Ecuador, El Salvador, Guatemala, Honduras, Mexico, Nicaragua, Paraguay, Peru, Puerto Rico, and Venezuela) were classified as eutrophied or undergoing eutrophication.

Sources of water in large Latin American cities will become ever more scarce, both in terms of quality and quantity, and it will be increasingly necessary to resort to increasingly distant sources, thereby increasing competition between different uses and users (e.g., human consumption, agriculture, industry). Economic development in some countries and within specific areas will improve quality of life, increasing the demand for "virtual water," which is defined as water contained in products that are imported by countries or their regions.

Protection of Recreational Waters

In the majority of Latin American and Caribbean coastal cities, raw sewage discharges occur at or very near public recreational beaches. Geometric average levels of total coliforms in excess of 100,000 MPN/100 ml (most probable number/100 ml) have frequently been observed at public recreational beaches, especially during the summer season, with individual measurements at times approaching levels of raw sewage. The problems associated with near-shore discharge of untreated sewage are aesthetic in nature, can cause potential public health and ecological hazards, and often bring economic consequences due to curtailed tourism.

An epidemiological study conducted in 2001 by WHO and the Joint Group of Experts on the Scientific Aspects of Marine Environmental Protection (20) documented the relationship between health and recreational use of waters polluted by urban wastewater discharges. The study estimated that such discharges caused 250 million cases of gastroenteritis and respiratory diseases every year and that the cost to society is approximately US$ 1.6 billion per year. At the XXVIII Congress of the Inter-American Association of Sanitary and Environmental Engineering (AIDIS) held in Cancún, Mexico, in 2002, WHO issued its Guidelines for Safe Recreational Water Environments (21). PAHO is coordinating the adaptation of these Guidelines for Latin America and the Caribbean.

Solid Waste

It is estimated that approximately 78% of the Region's population are urban dwellers. Small and medium-sized urban centers, which face the greatest difficulties in adequately managing solid waste, produce 44% of municipal solid waste. Collection service in outlying areas, where the population is generally poor and access is hampered by inadequate road conditions and infrastructure, is not a high priority.

The Region's solid waste sector and its institutional framework have differing degrees of development. Ministers of health and the environment provide oversight and regulate the sector, while municipalities maintain ownership of services provision. In general, deficiencies can be observed in sector management, as well as in medium- and long-term planning and programming. Municipalities typically lack management and economic capacity; notable omissions are seen in the legal framework; adequate control instruments to verify compliance and impose penalties are wanting; there are overlapping legislation—at times contradictory—and jurisdictional conflicts; and only a few countries have established specific laws dealing with solid waste.

Most countries do not have comprehensive solid waste management policies, and those that do often do not enforce or disseminate them. Few countries have comprehensive plans and strategic planning for the sector, and in many it is impossible to define a national lead agency for policy and plans. The few oversight responsibilities that are fulfilled are done so in a patchwork manner by the ministries of health and the environment. Municipalities set forth regulations for household, non-hazardous industrial, and hospital solid waste, and regulate rates with some executive control.

The Region's average cost for solid waste services is US$ 29 per ton, 70% of which corresponds to sweeping, collection, and transport. The rate, however, only covers 47% of service costs, and delinquent payments approach 50%. Sector-wide investment is limited compared to that which is made in electricity, water, and sanitation. In most countries, the service is supported by collection of a municipal fee, but the fee is not only for the cleaning service; rather, it is part of street lighting, property taxes, and other taxes.

It is estimated that only 22.6% of waste generated in the Region is deposited in a sanitary landfill; 23.7% ends up in controlled landfills, and 45.2% in open-air dumps or watercourses. Society's participation in solid waste management is limited and is only given effective expression when there is support from nongovernmental organizations.

The creation of microenterprises and cooperatives to manage solid waste is on the rise. These companies represent an economic municipal alternative, using low-cost technology and intensive labor, creating employment, and fostering community participation. Their participation in cleaning services is usually carried out with the support of nongovernmental organizations. Solid waste management cooperatives, although not numerous, provide services to the poorest segments of the population.

Basic Water and Sanitation in Critical and Emergency Situations in Latin America and the Caribbean

Natural disasters and their impact on existing systems constitute an "external" factor that represents a threat to water and sanitation services. Over the past decade, the Americas have been the second continent most affected by natural disasters (22). The effects of natural disasters of a catastrophic magnitude on all aspects of the economy and development have been obvious—particularly on water and sanitation systems—with economic losses of US$ 650 million during the 1994–2003 period alone. In the wake of Hurricane Mitch in Honduras, for example, socioeconomic conditions and infrastructure were set back 30 to 40 years (23). Moreover, since many of the Region's affected communities are geographically dispersed, in some cases the damages to small, sensitive systems never came to light.

Year after year, natural disasters strike many countries in the Region. During the last five years, natural disasters in the Americas have inflicted enormous loss of life, damage to water and sanitation infrastructure, and the subsequent difficulties of getting access to water suitable for human consumption, as well as enormous economic losses.

TABLE 8. Estimated damages[a] to drinking water and sanitation services, floods in Venezuela, December 1999.

Service	Damages		
	Total	Direct	Indirect
Drinking water	178.2	118.3	59.9
Sanitary sewerage system	38.3	38.3	0
Storm drainage	9.1	9.1	0
Greater expenditure/ lower earnings	17.3	0	17.3
Total	242.9	165.7	77.2

[a]In US$ millions.
Source: Economic Commission for Latin America and the Caribbean. The Socioeconomic Effects of the Floods and Landslides in Venezuela in 1999. Mexico City: ECLAC; 2000.

On 13–14 December 1999, torrential rains led to flooding and mudslides that affected 10 states in northern Venezuela, including the capital city of Caracas. National authorities estimated that more than 20,000 perished as a result. Water and sanitation services infrastructure suffered considerable damage. More than 200,000 people were affected, and more than 4,000 had to be given temporary lodging in La Guaira, Caracas, Maracay, and Valencia. A 2000 socioeconomic assessment conducted by the Economic Commission for Latin America and the Caribbean (ECLAC) estimated damages to water, sanitation, and run-off drainage systems to be approximately US$ 243 million (Table 8).

Earthquakes in El Salvador in January and February of 2001 caused great losses, and according to an ECLAC report on the disaster (24), reconstruction costs for water and sanitation systems infrastructure, both in urban and rural areas, totaled US$ 18.6 million and affected more than 200 water and sanitation systems. Close to US$ 400,000 alone was spent on water distribution using tanker trucks as part of the emergency relief efforts. According to data from the National Aqueduct and Sewerage System Administration of El Salvador, over a period of 138 days 98,700 m^3 of water was distributed, at a cost equivalent to US$ 4 per m^3.

On 23 June 2001, an earthquake struck the southern coast of Peru, mainly affecting the cities of Arequipa, Moquegua, Ilo, Tacna, Ica, and Cusco.

In July 2001, an intense drought occurred in El Salvador, Guatemala, Honduras, Nicaragua, and, to a lesser extent, Costa Rica. Data from ECLAC (25) indicate that the drinking water systems in Central America that used surface water sources were affected. The metropolitan area of Tegucigalpa, Honduras, was the hardest hit, and the company that provides water in this city incurred more expenses and earned less income during the entire year. ECLAC estimated that in addition to the foregoing, damages wrought by the drought reached approximately US$ 3.5 million.

In November 2001, Hurricane Michelle struck the Caribbean coasts of Nicaragua and Honduras, and the island nations of

Jamaica, the Bahamas, and Cuba, with the latter suffering the greatest extent of damages.

In November 2002, the Reventador Volcano, located 95 km to the northeast of Quito, Ecuador, erupted and shot out a significant amount of ashes that mostly affected Quito and the central provinces (in addition to Pichincha, Imbabura, Cotopaxi, Orellana, and Sucumbíos). Many water distributions systems, particularly water treatment plants, were damaged.

In September 2004, Hurricane Ivan, the worst storm of the season, left behind a trail of destruction in the Caribbean. The Cayman Islands and Grenada bore the brunt of the hurricane, although Cuba, Haiti, Saint Vincent and the Grenadines, and Jamaica also suffered its consequences.

While world attention focused on the Indian Ocean tsunami that struck South and Southeast Asia in late December 2004, flooding in Guyana was the worst natural disaster in this country's recent history. In January 2005, torrential rains equivalent to almost 10 times the average rainfall unleashed intense flooding in the coastal area, Guyana's most densely populated region. More than 300,000 people—close to half of the country's population—were affected. Moderate flooding is not unknown in Guyana, but January's extreme prolonged flooding was the worst experienced in a generation. At the apex of the crisis, more than 192,000 people in the capital of Georgetown, the East Bank, and West Demerara were affected. Three weeks later, 92,000 people still had water in or around their homes. The greatest difficulties faced by the authorities were drinking water coverage, ensuring water quality, sanitation, and basic refuse management.

In August 2005, in the United States, Hurricane Katrina first made landfall in Florida and then continued along the Gulf Coast to the states of Mississippi, Louisiana, and Alabama, where this Category 5 hurricane unleashed its destruction. Katrina flooded the historic city of New Orleans and caused the deaths of more than 1,300 people, becoming the most destructive natural disaster in U.S. history. The Mississippi Emergency Management Agency and the Federal Emergency Management Agency together allocated over US$ 9.4 billion in disaster relief aid in Mississippi, of which US$ 1.6 million was used to repair water control devices, such as irrigation ditches and reservoirs, and more than US$ 1.3 billion was earmarked for waste and rubble collection, including almost US$ 222 million for coastal waste and US$ 790 million for waste on flooded land.

In July 2005, Hurricane Emily struck several Caribbean islands and the Mexican and U.S. coasts. According to data from the Secretary of Government's National Center for Disaster Prevention and ECLAC, in Mexico, more than 226,000 inhabitants (in 43 localities in 11 municipalities, in an area covering approximately 35,000 km^2) had restricted water and sanitation services due to damages to these systems.

In October 2005, rains from Hurricane Stan in Central America and Mexico caused flooding and landslides in towns along the Atlantic coasts of Mexico, Guatemala, Nicaragua, and El Salvador.

The National Aqueduct and Sewerage System Administration in El Salvador reported sanitary infrastructure damage estimated at US$ 11.5 million, with Guatemala suffering losses of US$ 4 million to its water and sanitation facilities. Tropical storms Alpha and Beta followed Stan at the end of October 2005, striking Haiti and the Dominican Republic, as the conclusion to one of the most active and destructive hurricane seasons ever known.

Table 9 summarizes the main natural disasters recorded in the Americas during the 2000–2005 period.

AIR POLLUTION

Air pollution and its effect on humans is a growing public health concern. A wide variety of pollutants are found in the air in the form of gases, dust, or particulate matter that come from human activities as disparate as transportation, power generation, industrial processes, food preparation, and home heating. A limited number of other sources of pollution are the result of natural environmental processes such as climatic changes (it should be noted, however, that some of these changes are linked to human endeavors, i.e., the greenhouse effect due to carbon emissions). Significant differences exist both in the magnitude and sources of pollution in outdoor and indoor environments where people live and carry out their activities. There are further differences in pollution according to where it occurs; for example, in rural areas exposure to carbon emissions is more closely linked to pollutants arising from biomass combustion inside the home, whereas in urban areas pollution is particularly serious outdoors and is related more to the use of fossil fuels in transportation, power generation, and industry.

In response to concern over environmental pollution, several countries have proposed and ratified international treaties, specifically the Kyoto Protocol to the United Nations Framework Convention on Climate Change (26), the Montreal Protocol on Substances that Deplete the Ozone Layer (27), and the United Nations Millennium Declaration, which established the Millennium Development Goals (28), whose targets include decreasing, in upcoming decades, gas emissions and other pollutants that harm the environment. The following sections will address various dimensions of outdoor air pollution and its effects on human health.

Air Quality in the Americas

Increasing use of fossil fuels is the greatest source of outdoor air pollution in many cities of the Region and the world. The main pollutants created during this process are particulate matter, nitrogen oxides, sulfur oxides, carbon monoxide, and ozone.

Burning fossil fuels and biomass (principally firewood) causes environmental degradation and is therefore a serious concern that is addressed in MDG targets, specifically MDG 7's Target 9, which addresses sustainable development principles and envi-

TABLE 9. Leading natural disasters, by country, Region of the Americas, 2000–2005.

Countries affected	2000	2001	2002	2003	2004	2005
Argentina	F (May)			F (Feb., Apr.)		
Aruba					H (Ivan, Sep.)	H (Emily, Jul.)
Bahamas	H (Debby, Aug.)	H (Michelle, Nov.)		TS (Odette, Dec.)	H (Frances, Aug.) TS (Jeanne, Sep.)	H (Wilma, Oct.)
Barbados	H (Keith, Sep.) TS (Joyce, Sep.)	TS (Jerry, Oct.) H (Iris, Oct.)	TS (Lily, Sep.)		H (Ivan, Sep.)	H (Emily, Jul.)
Belize		TS (Chantal, Aug.) TS (Jerry, Oct.) H (Iris, Oct.)		TS (Claudette, Jul.)		H (Emily, Jul.) H (Stan, Oct.) H (Wilma, Oct.) TS (Gamma, Nov.)
Bolivia	F (Apr.)	F (Jan.)	F (Feb.)	F (Jan.) L (Apr.)	F (Jan.) D (Nov.)	
Brazil	L (Aug.)	F (Dec.)		F (Jan.)		
Canada						
Chile	F (Jun.)		F (May)			E (Jun.)
Colombia	F (May)			F (Dec.)	F (May, Oct.) H (Ivan, Sep.) E (Nov.)	F (Feb.) H (Wilma, Oct.) V (Galeras, Nov.)
Costa Rica	H (Keith, Sep.) TS (Joyce, Sep.)		F (May) F (Dec.)	E (Dec.)	F (May, Nov.) E (Nov.)	F (Jan.) F (Sep.) H (Stan, Oct.) H (Beta, Oct.)
Cuba	H (Debby, Aug.)		TS (Isidore, Sep.) TS (Lily, Sep.)	TS (Claudette, Jul.)	H (Charley, Aug.) H (Ivan, Sep.)	H (Dennis, Jul.) H (Emily, Jul.) H (Rita, Sep.) H (Wilma, Oct.)
Dominican Republic	H (Debby, Aug.)	TS (Jerry, Oct.) H (Iris, Oct.)	TS (Lily, Sep.)	E (Sep.) F (Nov.) TS (Odette, Dec.)	F (May) H (Frances, Aug.) H (Ivan, Sep.) TS (Jeanne, Sep.)	
Ecuador		V (Tungurahua, Aug.) FL (Jun.)	F (Mar.) V (Nov.)	V (Tungurahua, Jul.)		
El Salvador	H (Keith, Sep.) TS (Joyce, Sep.)	D (Jul.) E (Jan., Feb.) TS (Jerry, Oct.) H (Iris, Oct.)	F (Sep.)			TS (Adrian, May) F (Jun.) V (Santa Ana, Sep.) F (Oct.) H (Stan, Oct.) H (Beta, Oct.)
Guatemala	F (Jun.)	E (Jan.) D (Jul.) TS (Jerry, Oct.) H (Iris, Oct.)	V (Feb.) L (Sep.) TS (Lily, Sep.)	L (Apr.)	D (Nov.)	L (Jun.) F (Jul.) H (Stan, Oct.) H (Beta, Oct.)
Guyana						F (Jan.) L (Jun.)
Haiti	H (Debby, Aug.)	E (Jan.) D (Jul.) TS (Chantal, Aug.) TS (Jerry, Oct.) H (Iris, Oct.) H (Michelle, Nov.)	F (May) TS (Lily, Sep.)	TS (Odette, Dec.) F (Dec.)	F (May) H (Ivan, Sep.) TS (Jeanne, Sep.)	H (Dennis, Jul.) H (Emily, Jul.) H (Stan, Oct.) H (Wilma, Oct.) TS (Alpha, Oct.)
Honduras	H (Keith, Sep.) TS (Joyce, Sep.)	D (Jul.) TS (Jerry, Oct.) H (Iris, Oct.)	F (Sep.)	F (Sep.)	D (Nov.)	H (Stan, Oct.) H (Wilma, Oct.) TS (Beta, Oct.) TS (Gamma, Nov.)

(continued)

231

TABLE 9. (Continued).

Countries affected	2000	2001	2002	2003	2004	2005
Jamaica	H (Keith, Sep.) TS (Joyce, Sep.)	TS (Chantal, Aug.) TS (Jerry, Oct.) H (Iris, Oct.) H (Michelle, Nov.)	F (May) TS (Lily, Sep.) TS (Isidore, Sep.)	TS (Claudette, Jul.) TS (Odette, Dec.)	H (Charley, Aug.) H (Ivan, Sep.)	H (Dennis, Jul.) H (Emily, Jul.) H (Wilma, Oct.)
Mexico	V (Popocatépetl, Dec.) H (Keith, Sep.) TS (Joyce, Sep.) E (Aug.)	TS (Chantal, Aug.) H (Juliette, Sep.) TS (Lorena, Oct.) TS (Jerry, Oct.) H (Iris, Oct.) H (Michelle, Nov.)	F (Aug.) TS (Isidore, Sep.) TS (Lily, Sep.) H (Kenna, Oct.)	E (Jan.) TS (Claudette, Jul.) H (Ignacio, Aug.) H (Marty, Sep.) F (Sep.) TS (Larry, Oct.) H (Olaf, Oct.)	F (Apr.) H (Ivan, Sep.)	H (Emily, Jul.) H (Rita, Sep.) H (Stan, Oct.) H (Wilma, Oct.) TS (Gamma, Nov.)
Nicaragua	H (Keith, Sep.) TS (Joyce, Sep.) E (Jul.)	D (Jul.) H (Michelle, Nov.)	F (Sep.)		L (Jul.)	H (Stan, Oct.) H (Wilma, Oct.) TS (Beta, Oct.)
Panama	H (Keith, Sep.) TS (Joyce, Sep.)		F (Dec.)	E (Aug., Dec.)	F (Sep., Oct.)	F (Jan.)
Paraguay			F (May) D (Oct.)			D (Chaco)
Peru		F (Mar.) E (Jun.)	F (Feb.)	F (Jan.)	F/D (Feb.)	E (Sep.)
Puerto Rico					H (Frances, Aug.) TS (Jeanne, Sep.)	
Trinidad and Tobago		TS (Chantal, Aug.)			H (Ivan, Sep.)	H (Emily, Jul.)
United States					H (Charley, Aug.) H (Frances, Aug.) H (Ivan, Sep.) TS (Jeanne, Sep.)	H (Dennis, Jul.) H (Emily, Jul.) H (Katrina, Aug.) H (Rita, Sep.) H (Wilma, Oct.)
Uruguay	D (Feb.)	F (Jun.)				F (Aug.)
Venezuela	H (Keith, Sep.) TS (Joyce, Sep.) F (Nov.)		F (Jul.)		H (Ivan, Sep.)	F (Feb.) H (Emily, Jul.)
Other Caribbean islands[a]	H (Debby, Aug.) H (Keith, Sep.) TS (Joyce, Sep.)	TS (Jerry, Oct.) H (Iris, Oct.) H (Michelle, Nov.)	TS (Lily, Sep.) TS (Isidore, Sep.)	TS (Claudette, Jul.) TS (Odette, Jul.)	H (Frances, Aug.) H (Charley, Aug.) H (Ivan, Sep.) TS (Jeanne, Sep.)	H (Emily, Jul.) H (Dennis, Jul.) H (Stan, Oct.) H (Wilma, Oct.) TS (Gamma, Nov.)

F: Flood	TS: Tropical Storm	E: Earthquake	H: Hurricane
V: Volcanic Eruption	L: Landslide	D: Drought	

[a]Includes Anguilla, Antigua and Barbuda, Bermuda, British Virgin Islands, Dominica, French Guiana (France), Grenada, Guadeloupe (France), Cayman Islands, Martinique (France), Montserrat, Netherlands Antilles, Saint Lucia, Saint Vincent and the Grenadines, Saint Kitts and Nevis, and Turks and Caicos Islands.

Source: Data from ReliefWeb (http://www.reliefweb.int/rw/dbc.nsf/doc100?OpenForm). ReliefWeb was launched in October 1996 and is managed by the United Nations Office for the Coordination of Humanitarian Affairs.

ronmental resources conservation, and includes indicators on the use of energy and biomass, and atmospheric emissions.

According to a recent report (*29*), between 1990 and 2001 the average level of energy use in Latin America and the Caribbean, measured by petroleum consumption in kilos per dollar of gross domestic product (GDP), increased slightly from 0.18 to 0.19. Large increases (>0.05) were seen in Bolivia, Brazil, Haiti, Jamaica, Panama, Trinidad and Tobago, and Venezuela, however, while in the rest of the countries for which data are available, the general trend was decreasing (Table 10). During this same pe-

TABLE 10. Energy consumption and carbon dioxide emissions, by country, Region of the Americas, 1990–2000.

Country	Consumption of energy/$ of GDP[a]		Metric tons of CO_2 per 1,000 population	
	1990	2000	1990	2000
Antigua and Barbuda	...	...	421	3
Argentina	0.17	0.2	2,100	3,300
Bahamas	...	...	66	66
Barbados	...	...	21	12
Belize	...	...	16	28
Bolivia	0.22	0.27	76	77
Brazil	0.15	0.2	8,500	6,200
Chile	0.2	0.2	662	470
Colombia	0.14	0.1	2,000	1,200
Costa Rica	0.12	0.1	267	145
Cuba	...	...	778	504
Dominica	...	...	1	1
Dominican Republic	0.17	0.18	274	486
Ecuador	0.36	0.22	604	207
El Salvador	0.15	0.16	423	117
Grenada	...	...	4	4
Guatemala	0.16	0.18	357	256
Guyana	...	...	19	20
Haiti	0.12	0.17	...	169
Honduras	0.23	0.21	115	122
Jamaica	0.36	0.5	424	49
Mexico	0.21	0.2	12,000	2,200
Nicaragua	...	...	87	35
Panama	0.15	0.2	252	180
Paraguay	0.17	0.18	240	116
Peru	0.13	0.1	801	189
Saint Kitts and Nevis	...	...	6	3
Saint Vincent and the Grenadines	...	...	2	7
Saint Lucia	...	...	11	3
Trinidad and Tobago	0.73	0.8	138	79
Uruguay	0.11	0.1	416	102
Venezuela	0.42	0.5	3,300	2,500

[a]Energy use (equivalent in kilograms of petroleum) per dollar of GDP.

Source: Economic Commission for Latin America and the Caribbean. The Millennium Development Goals: A Latin American and Caribbean Perspective, Santiago: ECLAC; 2005.

riod, carbon dioxide emissions (CO_2) in Latin America and the Caribbean fell on average from 5,868 metric tons (MT) per 1,000 individuals to 3.072, a situation that was seen, in differing degrees, in most nations. Countries such as Argentina, Brazil, Colombia, Mexico, and Venezuela had CO_2 levels that were almost 25 times greater than in the rest of the Region in 1990. Furthermore, this group of countries with the highest CO_2 levels in 1990

succeeded in decreasing those values to almost half (average 3,080 MT).

Short- and long-term exposure to pollutants has been associated with an increase in mortality and morbidity due to respiratory and cardiovascular diseases (29). It is estimated that 800,000 premature deaths occur annually worldwide from respiratory and cardiovascular causes, lung cancer, and respiratory infections (in children under age 5) that are specifically linked to exposure to particulate matter (30).

In 2005, PAHO conducted a systematic search and review of scientific evidence presented in the Americas regarding the effects on health of exposure to particulate matter and the significance of this phenomenon for the Region. As part of this initiative, data were also gathered on concentrations of particulate matter of 10 μm in diameter (PM_{10}) reported by different urban areas in the Region (Table 11). The situation regarding outdoor air pollution varies a great deal. For example, in Arequipa, Peru, elevated concentrations of PM_{10} (up to 111 μg/m³) have been reported; in contrast, in other cities, annual concentrations are rather low, such as in Belo Horizonte, Brazil, (13 μg/m³) and San Juan, Puerto Rico, (32 μg/m³). In general terms, annual concentrations of PM_{10} in urban areas surpass national standards, as well as those established in the global air quality guidelines recommended by WHO (29, 31), although between 2000 and 2004 there was a decreasing trend in 7 out of 11 countries that had more than three years of recordings during this period (31).

Global air quality guidelines are based on the epidemiological and toxicological results of effects on health and represent a threshold level (i.e., the level under which no adverse effects would be seen). To the extent that the concentrations reported exceed those limits, it can be inferred that a significant number of people in the Region are exposed to concentrations that harm their health.

It is important to point out that there are notable variations in the availability of data on PM_{10} in the Region. In some cities, air quality monitoring is a longstanding practice; in other cities, the annual average concentration for the entire period was not available or was not recorded at all. The situation is similar for other pollutants that result from burning fossil fuels, and, in fact, data available for these are even more limited.

Air pollution is a major problem for urban areas because it affects the entire population. Due to its significance for public health, good air quality indicators are essential, and this is achieved through reliable monitoring systems. Adequate monitoring provides the foundation for developing air quality profiles with which to identify the extent of human exposure, for conducting epidemiological studies on the impact from such exposure, and for guiding selection, implementation, and assessment of prevention and control measures.

Another source of pollution, in addition to fossil fuel use, is the burning of biomass, whose impact on air quality is not well known. In 21 Latin American and Caribbean countries for which

TABLE 11. Average annual concentration of PM$_{10}$ (µg/m^3), selected cities of Latin America and the Caribbean, 2000–2004.

City/Country	Annual standard (µg/m^3)	Average annual concentration of PM$_{10}$ (µg/m^3)				
		2000	2001	2002	2003	2004
Arequipa, Peru	50	111	91	102	100	90
Belo Horizonte, Brazil	50	13	21	26	. . .	. . .
Bogotá, Colombia	65	58	64	66	66	66
Cochabamba, Bolivia	. . .	. . .	. . .	98	104	64
Fortaleza, Brazil	50	84	74	81	. . .	. . .
Guatemala City, Guatemala	. . .	. . .	54	. . .	. . .	. . .
Havana, Cuba	. . .	. . .	75	60	54	
La Paz, Bolivia	. . .	. . .	. . .	. . .	. . .	49
Medellín, Colombia	65	. . .	. . .	87	93	. . .
Mexico City, Mexico	50	71	60	65	64	54
Quito, Ecuador	50	. . .	. . .	. . .	. . .	54
Rio de Janeiro, Brazil	50	. . .	39	40	53	. . .
San Salvador, El Salvador	50	. . .	60	. . .	. . .	. . .
San Juan, Puerto Rico	50	32	31	31	32	30
Santiago, Chile	. . .	77	72	70	74	68
São Paulo, Brazil	50	52	49	51	48	41

Source: Pan American Health Organization. An Assessment of Health Effects of Ambient Air Pollution in Latin America and the Caribbean. Santiago: PAHO; 2005.

data are available, it is estimated that the per capita biomass consumption fell from 0.7 to 0.6 between 1990 and 2001. In Chile, El Salvador, Guatemala, Guyana, Honduras, Nicaragua, Panama, and Paraguay, however, this consumption continues to be very high and is between two and five times greater than the Region's average (Table 12).

Clearing farmland and eliminating agricultural waste by burning is a deeply rooted practice. In Brazil, for example, a total of 226,252 forest fire outbreaks were reported in 2005. This problem can extend beyond rural areas, since substances emitted by fires can travel great distances and affect air quality in urban areas, even in bordering countries.

The Effects of Air Pollution on Human Health

International epidemiological literature has shown that short- and long-term exposure to airborne pollutants in urban areas is associated with the appearance of a wide range of cardiovascular and respiratory conditions (Table 13). Furthermore, maternal exposure to such pollutants during pregnancy may be harmful to fetal development (*32*).

A review of literature on the effects of air pollution on health in the Americas (*29*) covering the 1994–2004 period identified 85 studies published in scientific journals. Most of these papers focused on urban populations in just a few Latin American countries: Brazil, Chile, Cuba, Mexico, Peru, and Venezuela. More than half of the articles reviewed were temporal series studies, which are designed to allow for estimating the impact of temporary (usually daily) variations of air pollutants on mortality and mor-

bidity using statistical models in which the daily number of deaths is related to daily concentrations. This design enables the effects of short-term exposure to be assessed.

The outcomes of short-term studies in the Region were similar to those reported in international literature. Temporary variations in particulate matter have been associated with an increase in daily mortality due to cardiovascular and respiratory causes. It has been further associated with an increase in hospital admissions from respiratory causes.

As part of the review of testing conducted, a quantitative analysis was carried out to calculate summary measures of the effects on mortality from exposure to PM$_{10}$, based on the results of temporal series studies. Such measures provide a more precise estimate of the exposure-response function, which can be used in formulating public policies to calculate health costs due to air pollution and benefits associated with reducing particulate matter concentrations. The measures estimated for Latin America were compared with those calculated for other regions of the world. In this meta-analysis, it was observed that the quantitative summary estimates for mortality in all age groups and in persons over 65 were similar in magnitude to figures from other parts of the world (Table 14).

In general, evidence from Latin America suggests that exposure to particulate matter is associated with an increase in mortality and morbidity. It should be noted that the summary estimates are based on studies conducted in three Latin American cities (Mexico City, Mexico; São Paulo, Brazil; and Santiago, Chile), and therefore the data are not necessarily representative of the Region of the Americas as a whole. Summary quantitative es-

TABLE 12. Per capita biomass[a] consumption, selected Latin American and Caribbean countries, 1990–2001.

Country	1990 level	2001 level	Difference
Bolivia	0.09	0.02	−77.8
Brazil	0.05	0.04	−20.0
Chile	0.14	0.18	28.6
Colombia	0.10	0.04	−60.0
Costa Rica	0.16	0.01	−93.8
Dominican Republic	0.08	0.03	−62.5
Ecuador	0.05	0.03	−40.0
El Salvador	0.17	0.16	−5.9
Grenada	0.04	0.05	25.0
Guatemala	0.30	0.27	−10.0
Guyana	0.28	0.29	3.6
Haiti	0.11	0.11	0.0
Honduras	0.25	0.16	−36.0
Jamaica	0.03	0.04	33.3
Mexico	0.07	0.06	−14.3
Nicaragua	0.22	0.22	0.0
Panama	0.13	0.13	0.0
Paraguay	0.27	0.18	−33.3
Peru	0.11	0.07	−36.4
Suriname	0.08	0.08	0.0
Uruguay	0.10	0.09	−10.0

[a]Includes firewood, sugar cane products, and other raw materials.

Source: Economic Commission for Latin America and the Caribbean. The Millennium Development Goals: A Latin American and the Caribbean Perspective. Santiago: ECLAC; 2005.

TABLE 13. Health effects attributed to short- and long-term air pollution[a] exposures.

Short-term effects
- Daily mortality
- Respiratory and cardiovascular hospital admissions
- Respiratory and cardiovascular emergency room visits
- Respiratory and cardiovascular primary care visits
- Use of respiratory and cardiovascular medications
- Days of restricted activity
- Work and school absenteeism
- Acute symptoms (wheezing, coughing, phlegm production, respiratory infections)
- Physiological changes (lung function)

Long-term effects
- Respiratory and cardiovascular disease mortality
- Chronic respiratory disease incidence and prevalence (asthma, chronic obstructive pulmonary disease)
- Chronic changes in physiological function
- Lung cancer
- Chronic cardiovascular disease
- Intrauterine growth restriction (intrauterine growth retardation, term low birthweight, small for gestational age)

[a]Includes particulate matter, nitrogen oxides, sulfur oxides, carbon monoxide, and ozone.

Source: Gouveia N, Maisonet M. Health Effects of Air Pollution. In: World Health Organization. WHO Air Quality Guidelines: Global Update 2005. Geneva: WHO; 2006.

timates were only calculated for some effects on health for some age groups and for some pollutants. Significant data are lacking in the Region on the effects of particulate matter exposure on child morbidity and mortality and adult morbidity.

In light of this situation, PAHO has responded by acknowledging the lack of data and information gathered and analyzed systematically on aspects such as exposure to pollutants and its potential effects and is stimulating and bolstering environmental monitoring processes in the Region's countries. At the same time, PAHO, together with professionals and groups of experts in the field from various centers of technical expertise in the Americas and other regions, is preparing technical guides on measuring environmental exposure and its effects, such as the air quality guidelines recently published. To strengthen the processes for attaining information and knowledge on this issue, PAHO has developed information, bibliographies, technical guides, methodologies, and training activities that are available electronically through its Virtual Library of Sustainable Development and Environmental Health.

TABLE 14. Quantitative summary estimates of percentage changes in mortality from all causes associated with a 10 μg/m^3 increase of PM$_{10}$, selected regions of the world.

	All causes, all ages	
Region	Percentage change (CI)	Reference
Asia	0.49 (0.23; 0.76)	HEI, 2004
Europe	0.60 (0.40; 0.80)	Katsouyanni, 2001
Latin America	0.61 (0.16; 1.07)	PAHO, 2005
United States	0.21 (0.09; 0.33)	Dominici, 2003
Worldwide	0.65 (0.51; 0.76)	Stieb, 2002
	All causes, over 65 years of age	
Europe	0.70 (0.50; 1.00)	Katsouyanni, 2001
Latin America	0.86 (0.49; 1.24)	PAHO, 2005
Worldwide	0.86 (0.61; 1.11)	Stieb, 2002

Source: Pan American Health Organization. An Assessment of Health Effects of Ambient Air Pollution in Latin America and the Caribbean. Santiago: PAHO; 2005.

CHEMICAL CONTAMINANTS

In the environmental health field, preventing or mitigating exposure to chemical contaminants is one of the priorities of government action. The globalization of contaminants and their presence in almost all phases of productive processes—from the extraction of raw materials to product processing, consumption, and finally, waste—place the entire population permanently at risk, particularly the most vulnerable groups: children, pregnant women, exposed workers, older adults, and the illiterate or barely educated, who have limited or no access to basic information about the toxicity of these substances.

Chemical waste has become a serious environmental problem that requires special attention. In Brazil, for example, in 2004, 1,964,380 people were identified as having been exposed to chemical products at 703 sites with contaminated soil. The Government made provisions for the following risk assessments to be conducted in areas exposed to contaminating waste: organochlorides (Cidade dos Meninos, State of Rio de Janeiro); lead (Santo Amaro da Purificação, State of Bahía); solvents (Campinas, State of São Paulo); and volatile organic compounds (Barão de Mauá, State of São Paulo) (33, 34).

In North America, the Commission for Environmental Cooperation (CEC)—created by Canada, Mexico, and the United States as part of the North America Free Trade Agreement (NAFTA)—used data available up to 2004 to identify children as the group that suffered the greatest exposure to dangerous chemical substances and recommended giving priority to preventive actions (35). Despite efforts being made in several countries and subregions of the continent, data available on chemical substances and their effects on the environment and health (acute intoxications and, fundamentally, chronic intoxications) do not reflect the magnitude of the problem. Of the different kinds of chemical substances increasingly used in the Region, metals and pesticides have required particular attention from health authorities due to problems arising in the last five years.

The CEC cites a study on metals that shows a drop in the average lead concentration in blood taken from children under 5 years old in the United States from 15 µg/dL in 1976–1980 to 1.7 µg/dL in 2001–2002. This decrease is linked to the elimination of lead sources in gasoline and paint, and to epidemiological surveillance. In Mexico, studies conducted from 1992 to 2005 on children in rural and urban areas indicated high lead concentrations, in some cases exceeding by more than five times the level of 10 µg/dL (35).

In the Amazon subregion, which encompasses Bolivia, Brazil, Colombia, Ecuador, Guyana, Peru, Suriname, and Venezuela, contamination from mercury used in gold production threatens the population's health. Brazil produces an average of 200 tons/year, and is thus responsible for emitting mercury into the atmosphere, soil, and rivers.

Studies have indicated the possibility of "natural" exposure to mercury in the Brazilian Amazon area. Average concentrations of this metal found in the hair of inhabitants living in communities in the State of Pará that are not directly exposed to anthropogenic mercury sources were high, at levels ranging from 3.98 to 8.58 µg/g. These values were higher than those found in individuals not exposed to mercury in some countries in the Northern Hemisphere, where the average mercury in hair does not reach 3 µg/g (36).

Pesticides also pose a serious public health problem in South America and the Caribbean. Several countries report on the amounts of pesticides utilized and cases of acute poisonings, as indicated in Table 15. Over the last 40 years, approximately 85,000

TABLE 15. Extent of pesticide use and reported cases of acute poisonings, selected countries of the Americas, 2000–2005.

Country	Pesticide use (kg)	No. of poisoning cases
Argentina	46,347,000 (2001)	3,881 (2001)
Barbados	295,000 (2002)	2 (2002)
Bolivia	6,700,000 (2000)	2,208 (2000)
Brazil[a]	131,970,000 (2001)	4,273 (2001)
Colombia	77,000,000 (2000)	2,763 (2005)
Chile	24,197,000 (2000)	804 (2005)
Ecuador	36,118,222 (2004)	1,991 (2004)
Saint Vincent and the Grenadines	546,000 (2002)	29 (2002)
Saint Lucia	44,000 (2002)	3 (2002)
Uruguay	7,600,000 (2000)	439 (2002)

[a]Fourth largest consumer in the world.
Source: Ministries of Health and Agriculture.

tons of DDT were sprayed in Mesoamerica (Mexico and the seven countries of the Central American isthmus) to control agricultural pests and mosquitoes that are malaria vectors. DDT is an extremely stable toxic compound that accumulates in living organisms, persists in soil for decades, and is transported by the water cycle to areas far removed from where it was originally utilized, thus contributing to environmental pollution all over the world. Central America is predominantly covered by agricultural and forest land where a constant increase in pesticide use has been observed. In 2001, imports of 46 million kg of active ingredients were recorded, which constitutes 1.5 times more per person than the worldwide average, according to WHO estimates. The utilization of chemical pesticides as the principal strategy for controlling pests has significant social costs, as it produces both acute and chronic harmful effects on human health and inflicts damage on the environment, animals, and food.

Interventions

In order to address problems that pesticide use has brought about in Mesoamerica, national governments and PAHO, through its Sustainable Development and Environmental Health Area, have implemented various subregional initiatives, two of which are described in the following paragraphs.

The Occupational and Environmental Aspects of Exposure to Pesticides in the Central American Isthmus project, better known as PLAGSALUD, was carried out between 1994 and 2003 with financial support from the Danish International Development Agency with the objective of reducing the prevalence of health problems linked to pesticides and supporting the implementation of sustainable agricultural alternatives. The project scored a number of important achievements, a few of which are described below.

Health surveillance. All countries involved were successful in establishing acute pesticide poisoning surveillance and incorporating it into their national epidemiological surveillance systems, thereby allowing needed prevention and control actions to be better targeted (*37*). As a result, reported poisonings initially increased. After various project interventions between 1999 and 2002, however, the number of acute poisoning cases reported dropped from 7,227 to 6,010, and the number of deaths fell from 867 to 712. The poisoning rate per 100,000 population decreased from 20.3 to 15.8; the mortality rate fell from 2.4 to 1.8; and the poisoning rate for agricultural workers went from 91.7 to 67.7 per 100,000 population. Indicators obtained from the surveillance systems, and the tools these provided, made local interventions to reduce health and environmental risk factors possible. This information also swayed decision-makers in the health, labor, education, agricultural, and environmental fields to promote and support adequate case treatment, develop prevention and control measures, and improve existing legislation regarding pesticides, not only at a municipal and national level, but also throughout the Central American subregion (*38*).

Intersectoral and interinstitutional coordination. One of the most effective and practical results of PLAGSALUD was the creation across Central America of more than 300 intersectoral local commissions on pesticides made up of representatives of the health, labor, education, environment, and agricultural sectors; city halls; nongovernmental organizations; workers' associations; and civil society. These commissions were the most vivid expression of the work done locally in Central America to reduce the negative effects of pesticides, raise community awareness, and promote the use of alternatives to agrochemicals.

Legislation. Guidelines developed for improving pesticide legislation over the course of the project facilitated many achievements. For example, in all seven countries, legislation governing pesticide restrictions and prohibitions was gathered and analyzed. Such legislation was also widely disseminated to relevant sectors to foster and consolidate institutionalized civil society participation in all stages of decision-making.

In addition, Agreement No. 9 regarding the prohibition of 107 pesticides and the restricted use of 12 others was approved at the XVI Special Meeting of the Health Sector of Central America and the Dominican Republic (RESSCAD) held in 2000. This forum brings the issue of health into the subregion's social development process, and its principal aim is to foster the sharing of experiences, and, above all, to obtain a commitment from participating governments to jointly address common environmental public health problems in a coordinated fashion in the spirit of the Central American integration framework.

Education. PLAGSALUD prepared and published educational materials designed for the general public, schoolchildren, workers, health professionals, and agricultural experts on a variety of topics, including acute pesticide poisoning diagnosis, treatment and prevention; health surveillance of pesticides; alternatives to pesti-

"We must be able to determine more precisely the essential limits of environmental quality so that we can set realistic standards that will not interrupt development on the one hand or compromise health on the other."

Abraham Horwitz, 1973

cide use (integrated pest management and organic agriculture); pesticide legislation; epidemiological status of acute pesticide poisonings; and research outcomes. This material continues to be used today, not only in Central America, but also in other Latin American countries. The creation of school-based organic vegetable gardens in several countries, an initiative supported by PLAGSALUD, deserves special mention. During the school year, students actively participated in tending vegetable gardens located near their schools, where they learned about the viability of growing agricultural products free of chemical pesticides and how this strategy could help them take better care of the environment.

Research. Professionals were trained in research methodology, both locally and nationally in all countries, which then made it possible to conduct studies on priority issues related to pesticides, generate data needed to carry out an adequate assessment of the situation, and propose appropriate interventions. Of note among this body of research are studies focusing on pesticide-related knowledge, attitudes, and practices; the underreporting of acute pesticide poisoning incidents (conducted in Belize, Costa Rica, El Salvador, Guatemala, Honduras, Nicaragua, and Panama); monitoring bodies of water (Honduras and Belize); determining levels of organochloride and organophosphorous pesticides in six water treatment plans in San Salvador, El Salvador; raising awareness among health services personnel regarding acute pesticide poisoning case management; pesticide exposure in women working in the flower-growing industry; assessing the level of awareness regarding pesticide use, management, and legislation among workers at agrochemical points of sale (Guatemala); and gender roles in social behavior regarding pesticide use in banana cooperatives (Panama).

A second noteworthy initiative undertaken by the Mesoamerican countries in conjunction with PAHO's Sustainable Development and Environmental Health Area is the Regional Program of Action and Demonstration of Sustainable Alternatives to DDT for Malaria Vector Control in Mexico and Central America, which is a four-year program (2004–2008) supported by the UNEP, the Global Environment Facility (GEF), and the CEC, and known as the DDT/UNEP/GEF/PAHO Program.

Malaria is a transboundary public health problem with multisectoral implications that affects approximately 89 million people in Mesoamerica, the majority of whom live in indigenous communities. Population growth, the rapid expansion of agricultural lands, environmental degradation, and high rates of migration among the affected population groups facilitate the disease's spread across national borders. Given this situation, and bearing in mind the negative repercussions of intensive DDT and other persistent insecticide use for both human health and the environment, PAHO, together with the Governments of Belize, Costa Rica, El Salvador, Guatemala, Honduras, Mexico, Nicaragua, and Panama, are executing the DDT/UNEP/GEF/PAHO Program (39), whose principal objective is to prevent the reintroduction of DDT into the subregion and to show that alternative methods to DDT for controlling malaria are both cost-effective and sustainable within the framework of community participation. The Program's three components are described in the following paragraphs.

Demonstration projects and dissemination. This component utilizes the comprehensive malaria vector control model (without DDT use), in which principles of epidemiology are blended with those of the social sciences through the active participation of the health, education, environmental, and agricultural sectors. The projects are based on the WHO Roll Back Malaria Partnership model and the successful Mexican experience. The projects incorporate a combination of interventions that address vector control, early diagnosis, and timely case treatment, and emphasize physical control, with measures focused on environmental sanitation, clearing the home and yard of potential vector breeding sites, and whitewashing dwellings. They also include biological control using larvivorous fish, biological larvicides, and other environmentally friendly forms of control. An important dimension of the project is to strengthen the principles of social equity through greater interventions coverage in indigenous rural communities that have historically been excluded and provided little or no health care. More than 80% of the inhabitants of the areas selected for these projects are from indigenous communities with high rates of malaria transmission. To this end, resources have been allocated so that new vector control modalities may be adapted to the unique culture of each community and implemented with the active involvement of local organizations and leaders. Discussion forums, in which indigenous leaders, local technicians, representatives of municipal governments, and authorities from various governmental sectors participate, have bolstered the indigenous communities' acceptance of new malaria control alternatives that do not depend on persistent insecticide use. Experience obtained from these projects can be used as a model that can be replicated not only in other countries in the Americas, but also in other regions of the world. The bottom-up approach, rooted in the active participation of local communities, nongovernmental organizations, and government institutions, also contributes to ensure the sustainability of the models introduced under the Program.

Strengthening of national institutional capacity to control malaria without DDT. This component has been instrumental in boosting national capacity to assess the risk of malaria

transmission. Furthermore, laboratory infrastructure has improved and the population has gained more awareness about malaria.

Elimination of DDT stockpiles. Under this component, the Program, in compliance with the Basil Convention on the Control of Transboundary Movements of Hazardous Wastes and Their Disposal, the Rotterdam Convention on the Prior Informed Consent Procedure for Certain Hazardous Chemicals and Pesticides in International Trade, and the Stockholm Convention on Persistent Organic Pollutants (POPs) (40, 41, 42), will allow 136 tons of DDT and 64 tons of other POPs—toxaphene, chlordane, hexachlorobenzene, aldrin, dieldrin, and mirex—to be safely eliminated from the eight countries involved in the DDT/UNEP/GEF/PAHO Program by incineration. These POPs, which are inadequately stored, pose a significant risk of contamination.

Chemical Safety in Latin America and the Caribbean

Actions regarding chemical safety in Latin America and the Caribbean have followed the recommendation from Chapter 19 of the Rio Declaration on Environment and Development's Agenda 21 regarding ecologically sound chemical management. The Third Session of the Intergovernmental Forum on Chemical Safety was held in Salvador da Bahia, Brazil, in October 2000. In February 2006, the International Conference on Chemicals Management defined the Overarching Policy Strategy and the Global Plan of Action for international activities on this issue. In line with this work, headway has been made in the following areas:

- Several countries in the Region of the Americas (Argentina, Brazil and Venezuela, among others) now have national chemical safety profiles, an instrument that enables existing infrastructure and management capacities for these products to be evaluated.
- Seventeen countries have one or more poison control centers that provide treatment and information.
- Several toxicology and chemical security networks have been created, enhancing information exchange on chemicals, both regionally in Latin America and the Caribbean (RETOXLAC), as well as nationally: REDARTOX (Argentina), RENACIAT (Brazil), RITA (Chile), LINATOX (Cuba), RETOMEX (Mexico), and REPATOX (Panama).
- Eight PAHO/WHO Collaborating Centers in the Region have actively supported chemical risk management and assessment activities.
- The Virtual Library of Sustainable Development and Environmental Health has gathered data on chemical substances, thereby strengthening human resources capacity in assessment and risk management through self-learning courses available through the Library. These courses include risk communication; assessment, treatment, and prevention

of acute pesticide poisoning; methodologies for identifying health risks at contaminated sites; and chemical disaster prevention, preparedness, and response.

- Work has begun on harmonizing reporting requirements for the most hazardous pesticides in Central and South America in order to decrease or eliminate exposure to these toxins.
- Countries have national integrated chemical substance management plans, although the current trend is to design and execute subregional plans that bolster national capacities (e.g., the Central American Subregional Plan, under the aegis of RESSCAD, and the Andean Subregional Plan).
- Efforts are under way to apply the new global chemicals classification and labeling system.

FOOD SAFETY

Chemical and microbiological food contamination continues to significantly affect public health and indirectly impact tourism and international trade in food. Foodborne diseases (FBD) are a worldwide problem that has been exacerbated over the past several decades due to changes in the international arena, such as population growth, poverty, rapid urbanization in developing countries, and increasing international trade in food for human and animal consumption, in addition to the appearance of new foodborne disease-causing agents and mutant microorganisms with greater pathogenicity. FBD can have serious consequences not only on health, but also on individual, family, and national finances, and the most vulnerable groups include children, the aged, and immunodepressed individuals. Studies conducted during the last 30 years on acute diarrheal diseases—the principal symptom of FBD—have shown a decline in associated mortality rates, but morbidity rates have remained relatively stable. These infections remain one of the main causes of morbidity and mortality in children under age 5, with 1.5 billion cases of diarrhea in the world annually, resulting in 21% of deaths in children under age 5, which, according to estimates, accounts for 1.5–2.5 million deaths every year (43).

The incidence of illnesses caused by microorganisms that are principally foodborne, such as *Salmonella* spp. and *Campylobacter* spp., has risen considerably in many countries. Data on South America from the WHO program for epidemiological surveillance of *Salmonella* and other enteric microorganisms (44) indicate that from 2000 to 2004 there was a 43.5% rise in the number of *Salmonella* isolations, for a total of 15,737. During this period, the most prevalent serotypes were *S. enteritidis* (40%) and *S. typhimurium* (16%) (44). Moreover, new and serious hazards have emerged in the food chain, such as infections from enterohemorrhagic *Escherichia coli* and bovine spongiform encephalopathy.

Chemical contaminants remain an important cause of FBD, a striking example of which is the massive methanol poisoning

that occurred in Nicaragua in September 2006. The Nicaraguan Ministry of Health reported 788 poisoning cases, resulting in 44 deaths. Likewise, natural toxins, such as mycotoxins and marine toxins, as well as environmental toxins such as mercury and lead, have been implicated in FBD outbreaks.

Deficiencies in epidemiological surveillance coverage in general persist throughout the Region, particularly as regards the FBD component, as well as outbreak detection and research, reporting, and analysis, and geographical inequalities. From 1993 to 2002, PAHO's regional FBD system received reports of outbreaks in 22 countries in the Region: of the 4,093 outbreaks in which an etiological agent was identified, 21% were caused by marine toxins (838 of them from ciguatoxin) and 4.6% by unspecified chemical contaminants. More recently, in a WHO consultation of experts on the burden of FBD that took place in September 2006 (45) it was determined that arsenic, cadmium, fluoride, lead, and methylmercury are the chemical FBD-causing agents for which the greatest quantitative data are available.

It is important to emphasize the link between tourism and food safety. Tourism is one of the biggest growth industries in the Americas, where the number of visitors has had a cumulative increase of 5% over the past decade (1990–2000). In several nations, tourism accounts for up to 25% of GDP and is the country's main source of employment and income. According to data from the World Travel and Tourism Council, in the Caribbean the industry provided 2.4 million jobs and generated economic activity worth US$ 35.3 billion in 2000, which is a nearly tenfold increase when compared to the US$ 3.8 billion generated in 1980. Therefore, all factors impacting quality and competitiveness are extremely important. FBD outbreaks in tourist areas and hotels have led to travel and reservation cancellations, as well as a growing concern on the part of the tourism and public health sectors, government authorities, and medical insurers. Several countries have shown an increase in the number of reports of "traveler's diarrhea" from different bacterial and viral agents associated with contaminated food. It is reported that 20%–50% of travelers suffer at least one episode of diarrhea (46). The direct cost associated with such episodes is also significant. Jamaica, for example, reports that medical treatment for each traveler affected represents a loss for the national economy of US$ 116.50, which is the total estimated cost per case (47).

Food safety and agrifood trade are also closely linked. Fresh products, which include vegetables, fruit, meat, and seafood, make up approximately half of all agricultural and food exports of developing countries. In Latin America, agricultural exports from Central America, the Southern Cone, and the Andean subregion account for 48%, 34%, and 23%, respectively, of all exports. In Brazil, agribusiness accounts for 33.8% of GDP, 44% of exports, and 37% of employment. All of this trade is governed by the World Trade Organization's Agreement on the Application of Sanitary and Phytosanitary Measures, whose standards play a key role in ensuring food safety, which in turn facilitates the achievement of sustained economic growth.

Countries have invested significant effort in improving their food safety control systems, such as in Uruguay's project under the Uruguayan Food Security Agency, Ecuador's and Venezuela's development of integrated national food control systems, and Colombia's and Peru's application of epidemiological surveillance systems, which have a FBD component. Nevertheless, weaknesses may still be detected in the food control systems in force, as shown in a PAHO study (48) featuring the organization of member countries' food safety systems in terms of their institutional framework. Using the cluster analysis technique, the study defined five task frameworks: food laws and regulations; food control management; inspection services; food monitoring/epidemiological surveillance and laboratory services; and information, education, communication, and training. The analysis performed generated seven clusters that satisfied 87% of the whole variability studied. Although the data obtained do not accurately reflect the reality of the countries, due to the fact that the information obtained was insufficient, they do reflect the trends observed in food safety systems of the countries assessed.

The first cluster is made up of the three countries whose food safety systems are in the best condition, reaching in all the task frameworks defined, a level of development that ranges from 96% to 100%, with an overall average of 99%. Thus, this cluster's degree of development is nearly equivalent to the ideal level. In contrast, the other two clusters, made up of 19 countries, have food safety systems that are less developed, ranging from 25% to 60%, with an overall average of 44% and 48%, respectively. These figures illustrate that these countries do not meet even half of the conditions of the ideal system proposed in the study and at the same time indicate where potential modernization efforts should be focused. The four remaining clusters, encompassing 11 countries, have an overall average development level that ranges from 58% to 81% and could be described as having food safety systems that are at mid-level development. Their full development could be reached with a coordinated restructuring and modernization program.

Finally, the morbidity, mortality, and disability burden due to FBD is not well defined in the countries in the Region. PAHO, in conjunction with national public health authorities, has organized several Region-wide activities designed to help countries strengthen their disease surveillance systems and determine the morbidity burden due to acute gastroenteritis. The data obtained will enable an evaluation to be conducted of the acute gastroenteritis burden of foodborne origin associated with specific pathogens commonly transmitted by food. For 2004, the Foodborne Diseases Active Surveillance Network in the United States, better known as FoodNet, estimated that the rate of acute foodborne gastroenteritis was 0.72 cases per person-year, which would indicate the existence of 195 million episodes nationally (49).

The first protocol of disease burden studies carried out jointly by WHO, PAHO, the Public Health Agency of Canada, U.S. Centers for Disease Control and Prevention (CDC), and the Cuban Ministry of Health concluded during the first half of 2006. Preliminary data from three sentinel sites, selected because of their cultural, economic, cultural, geographic and climatological differences, found that for each case of infection from Shigella spp. reported to the surveillance system, there were 688, 639, and 570 individuals that requested medical attention in their community, respectively (50).

This preliminary study clearly underlines the need to determine the true FBD burden. Estimating FBD underreporting and adapting improved microbiological and epidemiological methodologies to detect and report on pathogenic agents nationally will boost epidemiological analysis capacity for developing active FBD surveillance systems based on the cases diagnosed.

WORKERS' HEALTH

Work-related illnesses, injuries, and deaths are determined not only by traditional and emerging occupational hazards, but also by social determinants (employment situation, income level, gender, ethnic group), access to occupational health services and programs, and work practices that affect health. The structural characteristics of the Region's countries (including demographic and economic dimensions, as well as the relative share of private-sector participation) have led to deepening inequities that affect working conditions and workers' health. An ECLAC study determined that 20%–40% of the employed population still did not earn sufficient income to purchase a basic basket of goods (51). It also found that only 30% of all formal-sector workers received some type of occupational health services (52), which generally was geared towards treatment and not prevention or promotion. The rate of fatal occupational accidents was 2.5 times greater in Latin America and the Caribbean than in Canada and the United States (53).

Since 1992, the rate of fatal occupational accidents among Hispanic construction workers in the United States has been markedly higher than for non-Hispanic construction workers. In 2001 (the most recent year for which data are available), the rate of fatal occupational injury among Hispanic construction workers was 19.5 per 100,000 full-time workers, or 62.5% greater than the 12.0 per 100,000 for non-Hispanic construction workers (54). At the same time, 44.0% of workers in Latin America earn wages that place them below the poverty line and 19.4% under the extreme poverty line (55). In Honduras and Nicaragua, it is estimated that 8%–12% of all children and youth under the age of 18 live and work in the street. It is anticipated that the number of children who work will continue to rise due to rapid urbanization, unequal income distribution, economic crises, natural disasters, and poverty (56). Such inequities have been exacerbated by macroeconomic and social policy changes related to globalization; government, health, and social security reforms; the so-called labor market flexibilization; and longer workdays (*57*).

Nonetheless, it must be acknowledged that the number of Latin American and Caribbean children and youth who work has dropped. In Latin America in 2000, approximately 17.4 million children aged 5–14 worked (16.1% of all children in the Region), while by 2004, this figure had fallen to 5.7 million children (5.1% of the Region's total number of children). The number of economically active children therefore decreased by more than two-thirds over that four-year period. The recent economic activity rate (5.1%) for children now approaches that of a heterogeneous group of nations, including developing countries, emerging economies, and several Middle Eastern and North African countries (*58*).

The slightly positive trends seen in the labor market in Latin America and the Caribbean in recent years are in part thanks to three successive years of economic growth exceeding 4%. The unemployment rate for the total population rose only slightly in 2006, but increased 1.8% during the past decade, mainly because of the increase in the proportion of female workers, which rose from 41.5% in 1996 to 47.0% in 2006. The rate of female participation in the labor market increased from 46.1% in 1995 to 52.4% in 2006 (*59*).

Social protection varies considerably from country to country (Table 16), and not enough reliable, comparable data are available, as shown in the assessment survey of the PAHO Regional Plan on Workers' Health (*60*).

According to the International Labor Organization (ILO), between 1992 and 2002 the Latin American informal economy grew from 42.8% to 46.5%. Generally, informal employment is associated with greater occupational hazards, an absence of legal protection, health benefits, and other forms of social protection, as well as unstable working conditions and few opportunities to overcome a level of economic subsistence. Women, children, and aged are the least protected of all occupational groups (*61*).

Workplace Hazards and the Occupational Morbidity and Mortality Burden

Close to half of the Region's population spends a third of their lifetime working. According to WHO, two-thirds of workers are exposed to unsafe and unhealthy working conditions, in which several categories of risk factors are pervasive (Table 17) (*62*).

In a 2005 WHO report on the impact of occupational hazards on the global burden of occupational disease, five predominant factors were assessed: carcinogens, airborne particles, noise, ergonomic stressors, and injury hazards. The report indicates that in 2000 these hazards led to 850,000 fatalities in the world—almost 40% of the 2.2 million total deaths estimated by the ILO (*63*)—in addition to the loss of 24 million healthy life years.

Despite the gravity of the situation, in Latin America and the Caribbean the dearth of data and the obstacles to gathering reli-

able information on occupational injuries and diseases are notable. This is due to the dearth of adequate surveillance systems to define damages and their risk factors, underdiagnosis, underreporting, and the need for adequately trained medical and public health professionals. It is estimated that only 5%–10% of all occupational diseases are reported in developing countries. In Argentina, Brazil, Chile, Colombia, and Nicaragua, however, there is growing political interest, which, coupled with subregional integration processes, has led to significant legislative changes and strengthened occupational surveillance systems.

Occupational Accidents

The earlier-mentioned 2005 WHO report estimates that occupational accidents represent 8% of all accidents in the world and cause 312,000 deaths and a loss of 10 million disability-adjusted life years (DALYs). The agricultural, construction, and mining industries present the greatest number of risks for workers, especially in developing countries. The PAHO Regional Plan on Workers' Health assessment survey revealed that in 2003, among the Latin American and Caribbean countries with the most reliable data systems, the percentage of workers who had suffered accidents totaled 8.8% in Chile (*64*), 8.8% in Argentina, 6.8% in Colombia, 5.0% in the United States, and 2.0% in Canada. Many other countries could not provide these figures or only had data from years previous to the 2000–2005 period.

As regards occupational accidents trends, the Mexican Social Security Institute (IMSS) indicates that during the decade of 1992–2002, the rate of occupational accidents for every 100 insured workers fell from 6.6 in 1992 to 3.5 in 2002 for men, and from 2.7 to 1.3 for women during that same period (*60*).

In Chile, a 2004 occupational survey (*65*) showed that the rate decreased from 10.4% in 1997 to 7.1% in 2004. At the same time, the rate of fatal accidents dropped from 12% in 2003 to 9% in 2004 (*53*). These figures contrast with data provided by the 2005 Occupational Health Equity Report, which indicate a slight reduction in the rate of accidents between 1990 and 2002 (from 11.5% to 9.0%), and by the Superintendent of Social Security, which reported a decrease in the rate of accidents from 9.1% in 2000 to 8.8% in 2003 (*64*).

In Colombia, a constant increase can be observed in the number and rate of occupational accidents between 1994 and 2003; however, in 2004 these figures began to drop, and towards the end of 2005, 327,235 presumed occupational accidents were reported, of which more than 75% were described as being job-related, with a rate of 5.2% (*66*).

Occupational Diseases

Occupational diseases over the last several decades are characterized by mixed risk profiles, with a prevalence of "old epidemics," such as occupational respiratory diseases, dermatosis, occupational hypoacusia, and poisonings, together with "new epidemics," such as musculoskeletal disorders, chronic cardiovascu-

TABLE 16. Coverage under workers' compensation systems, selected countries of the Americas, 2001–2004.

Country	Year	% of economically active population	% of population employed	% of wage-earners and salaried workers	Source
Cuba	2004	79.4	100	NA	INSAT. Estimates from the PAHO Regional Plan Assessment Survey
Canada	2004	68.0	100	NA	Estimates from the PAHO Regional Plan Assessment Survey
United States	2004	63.0	75.4	81.5	University of Texas. Estimates from the PAHO Regional Plan Assessment Survey
Chile	2004	61.9	68.3	96.1	Ministry of Health. Estimates from the PAHO Regional Plan Assessment Survey
Panama	2002	56.7	66.2	NA	MSST. Estimates from the PAHO Regional Plan Assessment Survey
Costa Rica	2001	52.4	72.6	72.6	FISO/IDB
	2004	50.9	71.5	71.5	CCSS
Argentina	2004	32.3	45.1	59.1	SRT. Estimates from the PAHO Regional Plan Assessment Survey
Mexico	2003	28.7	29.4	NA	IMSS. Report to the Federal Executive Branch 2003–2004, June 2004
Guatemala	2001	24.6	NA	NA	FISO/IDB 2002
Colombia	2004	23.4	27.0		SENA. Estimates from the PAHO Regional Plan Assessment Survey
El Salvador	2000	19.6	24.5	47.2	FISO/IDB 2002
Nicaragua	2001	16.5	18.5	NA	FISO/IDB 2002
	2004	16.2	18.5	NA	Estimates from the PAHO Regional Plan Assessment Survey
Peru	2004	9.5	12.0	90.0	MSST. Estimates from the PAHO Regional Plan Assessment Survey
Brazil	2001	NA	40.0	NS	ILO 2003 Labour Overview
Ecuador	NA	NA	NA	NA	NA
Dominican Republic	2002	NA	NA	(9.0)	Number of insured unknown (ILO 2004)
Paraguay	2001	NA	9.0	NA	ILO 2003 Labour Overview
Uruguay	NA	NA	NA	NA	NA
Venezuela	NA	NA	NA	NA	NA

NA: data not available.
INSAT: National Institute of Workers' Health.
ILO: International Labor Organization.
FISO/IDB: Ibero-American Occupational Health and Safety Foundation/Inter-American Development Bank.
CCSS: Costa Rican Social Security Fund.
SRT: Office of the Superintendent for Workers' Compensation.
IMSS: Mexican Social Security Institute.
SENA: National Training Service.
MSST (Panama): Ministry of Labor and Social Security.
MSST (Peru): Occupational Health and Safety Bureau.

lar diseases, occupational stress, psychological harassment, and other emerging diseases, such a multiple chemical hypersensitivity, workplace-related cancer, and the effects of nanotechnology.

Exposure to asbestos, silica, and hazardous chemicals at the workplace is responsible for 9% of all cancers of the lung, trachea, and bronchus, and 2% of all cases of leukemia in the world. It is estimated that occupational exposure to carcinogenic agents led

to 102,000 deaths and 1 million DALYs in the world in 2000. The fraction of deaths and DALYs attributable to pneumoconiosis (silica, asbestos, and coal) and mesothelioma is 100%. In Brazil, more than 2 million workers—concentrated in the construction, mining, metal working, and non-metallic mineral processing industries—are exposed to silicon during more than 30% of the working day. In Bolivia and Peru, the prevalences are similar, al-

TABLE 17. Profiles of occupational risk factors, by type, Region of the Americas.

Risk factors	Principal economic activities where found	Consequences (effects)	Current situation in the Americas
Physical: • Noise • Vibrations • Radiation (ionizing and non-ionizing) • Extreme temperatures • Electromagnetic fields	• Mining • Agriculture • Construction • Fishing • Forestry	Hearing disorders and, in particular, deafness, are one of the leading causes of occupational morbidity in various countries in the Region. According to WHO, 16% of hypoacusia cases are attributable to exposure in the workplace. Diseases stemming from exposure to the other physical risk factors also cause significant occupational morbidity and disability in the Region.	The diverse complexity of etiology, diagnosis, and evaluation of physical risk factors present an obstacle to the formulation of comprehensive intervention strategies. These factors affect up to 80% of the workforce in developing countries.
Ergonomic: • Lifting heavy loads • Monotonous and repetitive work • Fast pace of work	• Mining • Agriculture • Construction • Services sector	Musculoskeletal disorders are one of the leading causes of occupational morbidity. WHO has estimated that 37% of all cases globally of lumbar-region pain are attributable to work-related situations.	Musculoskeletal disorders, particularly those affecting upper extremities or the lumbar region, are currently the most common occupational diseases in the countries of the Region. Such disorders are a significant disability, especially among young workers.
Biological: • More than 200 kinds of viruses, bacteria, fungi, parasites, molds, pollen, and organic dust	• Services sector (health workers) • Agriculture	Biological phenomena cause airborne and blood-borne infectious diseases, such as tuberculosis, HIV infection, and hepatitis, and emerging infections such as severe acute respiratory syndrome (SARS) and avian influenza infection in humans.	Several Latin American and Caribbean countries have reported that health workers run 1.5 to 2 times greater a risk of being infected by the hepatitis B virus. Nevertheless, vaccination coverage against this disease stands as low as 39% in several countries.
Psychosocial: • Occupational stress—Psychological harassment • Overburdening • Little control	• Services sector (financial, banking, insurance, telecommuting) • Agriculture • Manufacturing	Occupational stress and psychological harassment in the workplace are the most common consequences of this kind of risk. Post-traumatic stress syndrome is also of importance, especially among health workers. Occupational stress is also associated with cardiovascular and digestive problems and diseases of the immune system, among others.	Psychosocial risks are reported to be the second-most common cause of work-related problems among U.S. workers, and they increasingly are the cause of disability, productivity decreases, and absenteeism in several other countries in the Region.
Chemical: • Handling chemicals • Fire and explosions • Disposal of hazardous wastes	• Agriculture • Chemical industry • Manufacturing • Pharmaceutical industry • Chemical production	Exposure to harmful chemicals in the workplace are responsible for such conditions as acute pesticide poisonings, asthma, dermatitis, allergies, injuries to the peripheral and central nervous system, hepatic injuries, reproductive problems, and various kinds of cancer.	Between 1,500 and 2,000 chemicals are used intensively in various economic activities in the Region. In 2002, the acute pesticide-poisoning rate in Central America was 15.8 per 100,000 inhabitants, with a total 712 fatalities that year.

Source: Pan American Health Organization, Area of Sustainable Development and Environmental Health.

though silicotuberculosis is also reported. In 2005, 3,500–4,000 workers in Peru without social security coverage suffered from silicosis.

According to WHO estimates, nonmalignant chronic lung diseases caused 360,000 deaths and close to 6.6 million DALYs (63). In the year 2000, 11% of asthma cases worldwide were considered to stem from occupational exposure. The WHO report also estimated 0.8 million DALYs lost from ergonomic stressors and 4.2 million from hearing losses. For health workers, the report determined that 40% of hepatitis B and C and 1%–12% of all cases of HIV/AIDS are due to needlestick injuries.

At the end of the 1990s, when the PAHO Regional Plan on Workers' Health was drawn up, it was estimated that in Latin America and the Caribbean only 1%–4% of the cases of occupational diseases were reported, and it was proposed that strategies for diagnosis and recognition of these illnesses in the Region be strengthened. The results, however, are not very encouraging. The survey of the PAHO Regional Plan, recent studies, and other sources show that Chile reported a significant increase in the number of cases between 2000 (4,481) and 2004 (9,200). Argentina reported 5,630 cases for 2003, with a rate of 10 per 10,000 workers. Colombia reported a rate of 2.43 cases per 10,000 workers in 2003, while in the United States for that same year the rate was 33.3 cases per 10,000 workers. The remaining countries did not have national data available, although the great majority of them do have an official list of occupational diseases. The differences between the rates in the United States and Latin America stem from underreporting in the latter.

In Mexico, for example, between 1992 and 2002, the IMSS recorded 5,212,372 claims for workmen's compensation, of which only 0.9% were categorized as occupational diseases. The most frequent were hearing disorders and traumatic deafness, respiratory infections from different kinds of chemical exposure (pneumoconiosis, anthracosilicosis, and chronic bronchitis), and contact dermatitis. There is significant underreporting, given that more than 50% of all workers are not insured by the IMSS and do not contribute to the social security system.

In Costa Rica, occupational illness records are included as part of the occupational accident statistics, which is why it is difficult to distinguish and analyze them. By 2004, poisoning and intoxications (430) were included, as well as dysphonias (398), effects from climatological exposure (224), suffocations (101), effects from electricity (81), harmful effects from radiation (33), lumbagos (5,693), and others (4,474). Nevertheless, it is difficult to correlate reported exposure and injuries, as it is impossible to draw conclusions regarding the occupational disease situation beyond the fact that there is a relatively high number of lumbagos, intoxications (type unknown), and dysphonias. In Argentina, the Superintendent of Occupational Hazards indicated that in 2003 work-related health conditions accounted for 1.4% of the reported accident cases and estimated the incidence of occupational diseases to be 1 per 1,000 workers. The most frequent condition is hypoacusia, which accounts for more than 50% of the cases (67).

In Chile, the Superintendent of Social Security indicated that in 2004, 44.3% of occupational diseases led to temporary disability, 0.8% to partial permanent disability, and 0.01% to total permanent disability (eight cases) and one death. It was not possible, however, to find diagnoses recorded as such in this source. The Mutual Accident Insurance Association reported 4,481 work-related health conditions in 2000, principally skin injuries, osteoarticular disorders, upper and lower respiratory diseases, poisonings, and hypoacusia (68), a figure that remained stable during the 2000–2001 period.

In Colombia, the number of occupational diseases reported was approximately 700 cases a year for the 1996–1999 period, and close to 900 cases a year for the 2000–2003 period, with an annual average rate of 2 cases per 10,000 workers. In the last two-year period, the figures increased significantly, doubling by 2005, with 1,909 reported cases (a rate of 3.74 per 10,000 workers) (69). Among these illnesses, musculoskeletal afflictions continue to be the most frequent and costly, accounting for 33.8% of the total, despite underreporting and diagnostic difficulties. These were followed, in order of frequency, by chronic respiratory conditions, with 23.8% of the total; dermatosis, with 18.4%; and occupational hypoacusia, with 14.5%.

A study of occupational health conditions that was conducted among more than 12 million workers in Belize, Costa Rica, El Salvador, Guatemala, Honduras, Nicaragua, and Panama also acknowledged reporting and underreporting problems regarding occupational diseases in these countries (70). It is striking that in three countries—Costa Rica, Nicaragua, and Panama—several chronic health problems were reported as being associated with occupational exposure to pesticides, including a high incidence of skin injuries and chronic neurotoxic effects among workers who previously suffered organophosphorous insecticide poisonings and among male and female vector control workers on banana plantations who had been exposed to DDT.

Occupational Mortality

According to ILO data, global occupational mortality, due to both occupational accidents and diseases, has been increasing. The ILO assigned 11% of global fatal occupational accidents to Latin America and estimated close to 140,000 work-related fatalities in that subregion in 2003. Absolute numbers reveal that cases in Latin America and the Caribbean consist mainly of occupational accidents and violence, genitourinary disorders, circulatory diseases, malignant neoplasms, and communicable diseases. Circulatory system diseases and malignant neoplasms are among the leading mortality causes, making up close to 55% of total cases, followed by accidents and violence, at 22%.

Only 46% of the countries surveyed provided mortality statistics on occupational accidents and only 30% on occupational diseases. The work-related accident mortality rate ranged between 32.8% in Nicaragua to 4.0% in the United States. In Central America, PLAGSALUD-supported surveillance systems reporting on cases of acute pesticide poisoning fatalities show a progressively upward trend in the rate, which rose from 0.30 per 100,000 inhabitants in 1992, to 2.44 per 100,000 in 1999, and then decreased to 1.87% in 2002 (60).

International Policies and Partnerships

During the 2001–2005 period, important progress was observed in the field of occupational health in the Region, as reflected at the IV Summit of the Americas, held in Mar del Plata, Argentina, in November 2005. At this gathering, Heads of State committed to promoting "integrated frameworks of public environmental, employment, health, and social security policies to protect the health and safety of all workers" and fostering "a culture of prevention and control of occupational hazards in the Hemisphere" (*71*). Their commitment was born of intense and effective work on occupational health programs and best practices, and was based on strategic, programmatic, and operational partnerships between the labor, private, and academic sectors of national governments, including the Network of PAHO/WHO Collaborating Centers, and nongovernmental organizations, including the Hispanic Forum Network in the United States, and numerous international, regional, and subregional institutions, including WHO, ILO, the International Commission on Occupational Health, the United Nations Development Program (UNDP), GEF, the UNESCO Regional Office for Education in Latin America and the Caribbean, the Organization of American States (OAS) and its Inter-American Committee on Education, the Inter-American Conference of Ministers of Labor (IACML), the Inter-American Development Bank (IDB), the Central American Integration System, the Southern Common Market (MERCOSUR), and the Andean Community of Nations (CAN).

The synergetic work produced by these partnerships has mainly been guided by the Healthy Workplace Initiative, the cross-cutting strategy of PAHO's Regional Plan on Workers' Health that is geared towards institutional strengthening in the countries of the Americas through human resources training, establishing data systems, supporting applied research, disseminating information, managing workers' health systems, and sharing information on best practices and successful programmatic strategies.

Some noteworthy examples of progress achieved include the execution in Central America of consolidated programs on best practices by the OAS/IACML and ILO. Such programs have used the PAHO/CERSSO (Regional Center for Occupational Safety and Health) toolkit to implement the Healthy Workplace Initiative in the maquiladora and flower-growing industries. The cost-benefit analysis with the toolkit highlighted the fact that investments in the prevention of occupational accidents and diseases in the maquiladoras—for example, those introduced in Guatemala and the Dominican Republic—would yield a return on investment of between 3 and 33 times (*72*).

Also to be noted is PAHO's commitment to promote the inter-sectoral and Region-wide Strategic Alliance of Health, Labor, Education, Environment, and Occupational Health and Safety Initiatives as a horizontal technical cooperation tool aimed at seeking and strengthening synergies between sectors with common goals.

Another important step forward is the work done jointly with the ILO to bolster data systems and reduce factors that contribute to underreporting. In conjunction with the IACML and ILO, two basic regional indicators—fatal and nonfatal accidents, and pesticide poisonings—will be prepared. They will be the first indicators entered in a newly created PAHO joint database. The proposed database will be based on reliable data systems established in Argentina, Brazil, Chile, Colombia, Jamaica, Mexico, and Nicaragua, with strengthened diagnosis and occupational disease reporting, and the creation of occupational health observatories required by law. In order to disseminate data, PAHO has sponsored and provided technical support, jointly with the ILO, to a virtual occupational safety and health network, which operates as a discussion forum and brings together participants from 40 Spanish and Portuguese-speaking nations.

Furthermore, the Americas Regional Plan to Eliminate Silicosis was implemented with the support of PAHO/WHO Collaborating Centers, the U.S. National Institute of Occupational Safety and Health, the National Institute of Public Health of Chile, the Jorge Duprat Figueiredo Foundation for Medicine and Workplace Safety (FUNDACENTRO) in Brazil, and WHO's Occupational Health Program.

CHILDREN'S ENVIRONMENTAL HEALTH

Over the last decade, the demographic and socioeconomic dynamic in the Region has been characterized by rapid population growth, displacement of persons from rural areas to urban centers, poverty, a proliferation of informal human settlements, and overpopulation in the outlying areas of large cities, in addition to widespread industrial, commercial, and agricultural development. All of the foregoing has contributed to unprecedented pollution of the air, soil, and water, and the emergence of many diseases that affect society's most vulnerable groups, particularly children.

In industrialized countries, children face new risks and threats stemming from urban pollution and chemical and radioactive waste, as well as from changes to the social fabric due to an increase in psychotropic substances abuse, violence, and injuries from accidents. In developing countries, traditional risks persist, and these threats are heightened by a variety of factors, such as disorderly demographic growth, poverty, limited access to drinking water and basic sanitation services, and inadequate housing, which exacerbate conditions of inequality and inequity. The interplay of all these factors continues to manifest itself in the spread of diarrheal diseases, respiratory infections, and vector-borne diseases, in addition to the risk of poisoning from improper use and/or inadequate elimination of pesticides. Furthermore, the transformation of the environment caused by climate change, deforestation, droughts, and flooding increases the incidence of emerging and reemerging diseases.

Children are at a higher risk than adults to environmental hazards because they are more easily exposed to environmental threats and their still-developing bodies are more vulnerable to certain types of exposures that are harmful to human health. Behaviors typical of children's early developmental stages, such as putting objects in their mouths; crawling on their hands, knees, and stomach; climbing up to dangerous places; and, in general, exploring their surroundings and practicing new skills, intensify their level of exposure. When children live, play, learn, and/or work in degraded environments, these behaviors increase their level of risk to accidents, injuries, and communicable diseases. Poor children are the most affected, as they generally live in unsafe and polluted surroundings, and if their bodies are compromised by lack of adequate nutrition, their weakened immune system is less likely to be able to fight off disease and infection. In addition, poor children are more apt to become part of the workforce at an early age, to support either themselves or their families, and typically perform dangerous activities that increase the risk of injury and/or disease.

Better data are needed to have a more accurate understanding of the environments in which children live and of the complex interaction of the various types of threats to good health found in these environments. The best way to express this knowledge is through the use of specific indicators that not only point to environmental threats and their possible impact on health, but also furnish data for decision-making and assessment of interventions.

Political Commitments

Four international declarations specifically address the issues of poverty reduction, of investments in the environment for the purpose of sustainable development, and of the need for a commitment to the health and well-being of children as an investment in the future. These are the United Nations Conference on Environment and Development (Earth Summit) (73), the United Nations Millennium Declaration (74), the Johannesburg Declaration on Sustainable Development (75), and the Declaration of Mar del Plata (76).

United Nations Conference on Environment and Development (Earth Summit)

In 1992, during the Earth Summit that took place in Rio de Janeiro, Brazil, the leaders of the world's nations adopted historic principles of sustainable development. They likewise approved Agenda 21, which established a platform for integrated action for achieving socioeconomic development and securing environmental protection. Article 40 of the Rio Declaration on Environment and Development's Agenda 21 urges governments to draw up effective indicators for decision-making aimed at attaining sustainable development and executing and evaluating development interventions that could impact the environment and/or human health. The first principle of the Rio Declaration provides that "human beings are at the center of concerns for sustainable development. They are entitled to a healthy and productive life in harmony with nature." This principle seeks to focus political interest on economic development activities that concomitantly help to alleviate health problems and improve the population's well-being.

United Nations Millennium Declaration

In September 2000, world leaders adopted the Millennium Declaration, in which they recognize their ". . . collective responsibility to uphold the principles of human dignity, equality, and equity at the global level." The Declaration also sets forth the duty of leaders to meet, in particular, the needs of "the children of the world, to whom the future belongs," and establishes the goals of eradicating extreme poverty and hunger (the topic of MDG 1), reducing child mortality (MDG 4), and improving maternal health (MDG 5). In the Declaration, Heads of State resolve that by 2015 ". . . children everywhere, boys and girls alike, will be able to complete a full course of primary schooling" and will have "equal access to all levels of education." The Declaration also promotes gender equality and empowerment of women (MDG 3) and calls for measures to be adopted for bettering the lives of inhabitants of poor neighborhoods and strategies to be formulated "for decent and productive work for youth." It reminds the world of the commitments assumed to protect the environment and ecosystems and highlights the need to bequeath to future generations a planet rich in natural resources. The 18 MDG targets, which are measurable and quantifiable, were designed for use in assessing and reporting on annual progress made toward achieving the eight MDGs.

Johannesburg Declaration on Sustainable Development

The World Summit on Sustainable Development, held in Johannesburg, South Africa, in 2002, provided an unprecedented opportunity to strengthen the role of health in sustainable development. The first principle of the Rio Declaration was reaffirmed at this Summit, and it was further emphasized that health is not only a resource, but also a product of sustainable development. Therefore, development cannot take root as long as poverty and disease continue to weaken individuals, and the population's health cannot be sustained without an adequate response from health systems within a healthy environment. Countries were urged to fight poverty as a means for endowing the population with health and sustainable development.

At the Johannesburg Summit, the Healthy Environments for Children Alliance was launched for the purpose of reaching the health- and environment-related MDGs. The Initiative's overriding goal is to galvanize global action to eliminate health threats and risks to which children are exposed in the environments where they live, play, and learn. A significant number of risk factors were considered in these three contexts, including an inadequate quantity and quality of water supply; inadequate hygiene and insufficient sanitation; diseases transmitted by vectors; air pollution (e.g., from the use of solid fuels, tobacco smoke in the home); unintentional injuries (accidents) inside and outside of the home; exposure to chemicals (e.g., pesticides, lead); and unhealthy behaviors. The Initiative calls for integrated and coordinated local action with the participation of the health, social protection, environmental, educational, industrial, agricultural, and energy sectors. The World Summit on Sustainable Development emphasized the need for information-sharing among sectors and for a more in-depth analysis of the effects of development on the environment and public health to take place, with special attention being accorded to society's most vulnerable groups. To facilitate this process, the Global Initiative on Children's Environmental Health Indicators was created under WHO's leadership.

Declaration of Mar del Plata

The Declaration, signed in November 2005, reiterates the commitment to direct efforts toward strengthening and consolidating partnerships among ministries of health and the environment and health and environment-related sectors in the Region of the Americas. It recognizes the importance of coordinating efforts among these sectors and promotes public policies on sustainable development that strive to reduce poverty and inequity and protect public health in the countries of the Americas. In the Cooperation Agenda in the Declaration's Annex, Summit participants focus their efforts on regional and subregional integrated management of water resources and solid waste management, sound management of chemicals, and children's environmental health.

With regard to this last point, the issues highlighted include strengthening training with respect to children's environmental health at every level of the health care system; strengthening programs of education and incentives for public participation, as part of a broad strategy for promoting children's environmental health; incorporating the theme of children's environmental health into formal educational programs; promoting the organization of fora on children's environmental health, as well as incorporating this issue into other fora; developing strategies for the implementation of initiatives on children's environmental health; promoting cohort studies on the effects of pollution on children's health; promoting measures aimed at the reduction of environmental risks related to zoonotic diseases; promoting the establishment and networking of pediatric environmental health specialty units; and strengthening capacities to recognize and manage poisonings in children derived from pesticides and other chemicals.

Progress in Children's Environmental Health

The main activities carried out by PAHO in cooperation with countries were:

- In 2003, as part of Health in the Americas Week, a regional workshop was held in Lima, Peru, on key scientific and political issues in environmental health. During this meeting the PAHO-designed Healthy Environments, Healthy Children Initiative was launched, and consensus recommendations were drafted for improving children's health and controlling environmental threats in the Region (*77*).
- National and international intersectoral groups were mobilized to prepare country profiles on the state of children's environmental health (2004). The 18 national profiles submitted yielded a wealth of information and provided the basis for drafting a regional summary of data and results.
- To promote children's environmental health initiatives, promotional multimedia packages for instruction, education,

and awareness were prepared and made available to the public in English, French, Portuguese, and Spanish (2004). Under this project, a variety of messages were developed for print, radio, and television media outlets and targeted toward children and other community groups, with the goal of raising public awareness in the Americas regarding the importance of having clean, healthy, and safe surroundings to protect children from environmental hazards. Two thousand kits, each with a video, DVD, and resource materials, were prepared and distributed (*78*).

- PAHO's Sustainable Development and Environmental Health Area collaborated with Argentina, the Dominican Republic, Ecuador, and Paraguay in the drafting of national action plans on children's environmental health, which included creating environmental pediatric units. This activity was guided by data and other input from the earlier-described national profiles on children's environmental health.
- PAHO led initiatives on children's environmental health indicators, or participated in them, in its capacity as member of the consultative group of the Commission for Environmental Cooperation created under NAFTA. In 2006, the Commission published a set of indicators regarding three environmental health dimensions: air quality, exposure to chemical substances, and water quality (*79*).
- In 2004, PAHO organized a meeting in Costa Rica with Latin American and Caribbean countries in which the first set of children's environmental health indicators for the Region were identified. A background document and report on the meeting were prepared as tools to be used by participants to gather the necessary data upon their return to their respective countries (*80, 81*).
- In 2004, a technical report was written, in cooperation with the Regional Institute for the Study of Toxic Substances, on the effects of POPs on human health (*82*).
- In June 2005, PAHO presented a children's health and environment regional action plan at the Second Meeting of the Health and Environment Ministers of the Americas held in Mar del Plata, Argentina.
- PAHO's Sustainable Development and Environmental Health Area produced a scientific document on air pollution, based on data and experience from the entire Region, which largely focused on exposure to particulate matter and its impact on children's health. This document showed that due to generalized air pollution and high population density in many of the Region's urban areas, a large number of individuals were being exposed to harmful substances. A broad array of economic repercussions for society was highlighted, from a greater need for medical attention to a decrease in productivity and quality of life. This research was inspired by the Declaration that came out of the Johannesburg World Summit on Sustainable Development in 2002 regarding the need to reduce, in particular, the prevalence of

respiratory diseases and other health consequences from environmental pollution (*83*).

FOOD AND NUTRITIONAL SECURITY

An essential aspect of human health is food security, understood as suitable nutritional management resulting from a sound balance between the food available and nutritional requirements. Unmet basic needs regarding food, water, air, and others are the results of food and nutritional insecurity (*84*).

This phenomenon in general can be observed indirectly, by the prevalence of its manifestations, which are delayed and almost always irreversible. Alterations in physical growth and mental development; abnormal changes in body weight, with deficiencies and excesses; acute and chronic morbidity; obstacles to school performance and adult economic productivity; and mortality in all age groups are some of the short- and medium-term outcomes of food and nutritional insecurity, whose most belated manifestation is human underdevelopment.

It should be highlighted that although statistics on food and nutritional insecurity's manifestations are useful for gaining an overall vision of the problem's magnitude, as well as its social and geographic distribution, they are insufficient for guiding decisions and public policies that require data on the basic conditions that bring about food insecurity.

The MDGs highlight the relevance of food and nutritional insecurity; and MDG 1, specifically, sets out to reduce hunger and reinforces the significance of food and nutrition as an underlying cause of other problems and deficits that afflict humanity. In particular, Target 2 of MDG 1 proposes halving, between 1990 and 2015, the proportion of people who suffer from hunger. Specifically, the indicators for Target 2 focus on a reducing the proportion of the population unable to met minimum calorie requirements to lead a healthy life (undernourishment) and decreasing the percentage of children under age 5 who are underweight for their age (undernutrition).

This section will present information on undernourishment and nutritional anthropometry, bearing in mind the double burden of nutritional deficiencies and excesses in the Region of the Americas.

Undernourishment

As regards the target of reducing by half the proportion of the Region's undernourished population, between the 1990–1992 period and the 2000–2002 period, the undernourished population decreased from 13% to 10% (equivalent to 6.6 million people) (Figure 17). In the analysis by subregion, only the Southern Cone countries and Brazil have experienced a drop in both the rate (from 10% to 7%) and in the absolute numbers, as can be seen in Table 18. In the Andean subregion, the relative figures for under-

FIGURE 17. Changes in percentage of undernourished population, by country or subregion, Latin America and the Caribbean, 1990–2002.

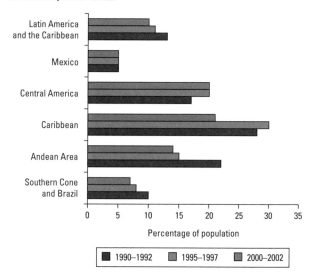

Source: Food and Agriculture Organization. The State of Food Insecurity in the World 2004. Rome: FAO; 2004.

nourished individuals fell during this period, but the absolute numbers increased slightly—by 200,000 to be precise—between the 1995–1997 and 2000–2002 periods. As Figure 17 shows, the Caribbean subregion as a whole experienced a 7% decrease over the entire 10-year period. During 1995–1997, however, there was an increase in both the proportion and the absolute number of undernourished persons, followed by a notable drop in both values. Mexico showed a constant rate of undernourished population throughout the period, and, therefore, the absolute number of undernourished individuals has grown in step with the population. Finally, Central America experienced a deterioration in each of the subperiods: in relative terms, the rate increased 18%, while in absolute terms, the rise was 48%, possibly as a result of the worsening situations in Guatemala and Panama.

TABLE 18. Undernourished population, by country or subregion, Latin America and the Caribbean, 1990–2002.

Subregion	Number (in millions) per period		
	1990–1992	1995–1997	2000–2002
Southern Cone and Brazil	21.4	18.6	17.4
Andean Area	20.0	15.2	15.4
Caribbean	7.8	8.9	6.7
Central America	5.0	6.5	7.4
Mexico	4.6	5.0	5.2

Source: Food and Agriculture Organization. The State of Food Insecurity in the World 2003 and 2004. Rome: FAO; 2003, 2004.

TABLE 19. Proportion of undernourished population, by category and country, Latin American and Caribbean countries, 2000–2002.

Very low <2.5%	Low 2.5%–4.0%		Medium 5%–19%	High 20%–34%	Very high ≥35%
Argentina	Chile Costa Rica Cuba Ecuador Uruguay	Brazil Colombia El Salvador Guyana Jamaica Mexico	Paraguay Peru Suriname Trinidad and Tobago Venezuela	Bolivia Dominican Republic Guatemala Honduras Nicaragua Panama	Haiti

Source: Food and Agriculture Organization. The State of Food Insecurity in the World 2004. Rome: FAO; 2004.

Using Region-wide data, the countries have been grouped in five categories by proportion of undernourished during the 2000–2002 period: from very low—<2.5%, to very high—≥35.0%. Table 19 and Figure 18 likewise illustrate disparities among the countries. In Figure 18, high levels of undernourishment are noted in Haiti, the Dominican Republic, Bolivia, Venezuela, Paraguay, Colombia, Peru, Trinidad and Tobago, Suriname, and countries of the Central American subregion, as compared to the Region-wide average.

With regard to food availability, most countries do not have enough data available on total caloric intake to allow dietary changes to be analyzed over time. They generally do have, however, data on the kinds of food consumed by their population, and this, in turn, sheds light on the dietary structure, showing the different proportions of energy that come from specific food groups. A study on trends in food consumption in Latin America and the Carib-

bean (*85*) indicates that harmful changes have occurred in diets, with a perceptible increase in the consumption of refined sugars; a reduction in the consumption of fruits, vegetables, and fiber; and an increase in the total intake of calories and fat, particularly saturated fats. There is clear evidence of a link between dietary changes that have taken place in the Region and the processes of globalization, modernization, and urbanization since 1980. Such changes are similar to those observed earlier in developed countries and constitute a higher dietary cost, which only middle and higher socioeconomic classes can afford. The gap, therefore, has widened between the groups that can habitually consume high-priced processed food and the poorest sectors that have maintained their traditional diets based on grains, vegetables, legumes, and tubers. Currently, however, even the poorest can purchase processed food high in fat and sugars, which has led to an increased incidence of overweight, obesity, and diabetes in the Region.

FIGURE 18. Prevalence of undernourishment in 24 Latin American and the Caribbean countries, 2000–2002.

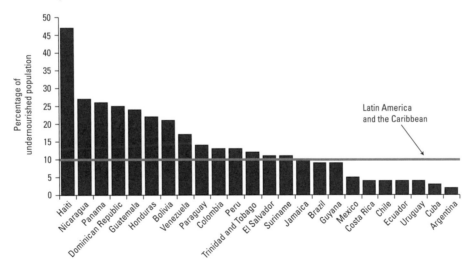

Source: Food and Agriculture Organization. The State of Food Insecurity in the World 2004. Rome: FAO; 2004.

Nutritional Anthropometry

All of Latin America and the Caribbean and its subregions experienced substantial improvements in the prevalence of underweight (low-weight-for-age) by age from 1980 to 2000. There was a 51% decrease in the entire Region, with the most marked drop occurring in the Caribbean (62%), followed by South America (56%). Data for Central America and Mexico reveal that the situation there also improved, but at a slower pace (44%). Figure 19 illustrates this indicator's situation during the 1996–2002 period among children under age 5 in selected countries. The average low-weight-for-age prevalence in Latin America and the Caribbean is estimated to be around 5%.

Of the 24 countries in Latin America and the Caribbean, only Guatemala remains among those with a high prevalence (20%–29%), according to the WHO classification (86). Based on this classification, Ecuador, El Salvador, Guyana, Haiti, and Honduras have rates that place them among the countries with mid-level prevalence (10%–19%), and the rest are grouped in the low category (< 10%).

The drop in the rate of low-height-for-age (stunting) in the Region between 1980 and 2000 was 44%, lower than the rate of reduction in low-weight-for-age (51%). In all subregions there were also improvements in the prevalences of low-height-for-age, and the pattern is identical to that described above regarding weight—the Caribbean countries have improved at a faster pace than the other countries, and Central America, although it shows progress, again has done so more slowly than the Andean and Southern Cone subregions. Figure 20 shows the disparities in the 1996–2002 prevalence of low-height-for-age in preschool-aged

children in Latin America and the Caribbean. The average rate of low-height-for-age in this region is estimated to be around 15%.

Of the 24 countries, only Guatemala has a very high prevalence of low-height-for-age (≥40%), according to the WHO classification. Bolivia, Ecuador, Haiti, Honduras, Nicaragua, and Peru are in the mid-level category (20%–29%), and the rest of the countries are in the low category (< 20%).

The Evolution of Overweight and Obesity in Latin America and the Caribbean

As has been suggested previously, many Latin American and Caribbean countries began their nutritional transition early and now have reached the stage of exhibiting noncommunicable chronic diseases associated with diet before other regions. The current situation in the Americas is one of contrasts, with countries such as Haiti and some areas of Central America still having pockets of hunger and poverty (87), while in other areas of the Region, the greatest burden of obesity has likewise moved toward the poor segments of the population. Brazil and Chile were the first to reach this stage, with studies conducted in both countries (88) indicating that the greatest burden of obesity has become concentrated in the poorest segments of the population. In the case of Chile, both sexes are affected, while in the case of Brazil, women are most affected. In Mexico, over only a short period of time, there has been a considerable increase in obesity rates (from 10.4% of the female population in 1987 to 24.4% in 1999), with a high prevalence of diabetes among adults (7%). The case of Cuba, however, exemplifies how changes of a macroeconomic

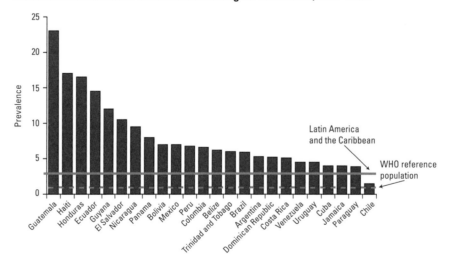

FIGURE 19. Prevalence of underweight-for-age in children under 5 years of age in 24 Latin American and Caribbean countries and at Region-wide level, 1996–2002.

Source: World Health Organization, Standing Committee on Nutrition. Fifth Report on the World Nutrition Situation: Nutrition for Improved Development Outcomes. Geneva: WHO; 2004.

FIGURE 20. Prevalence of stunting among children under 5 years of age in 24 Latin American and Caribbean countries and at the Regional level, 1996–2002.

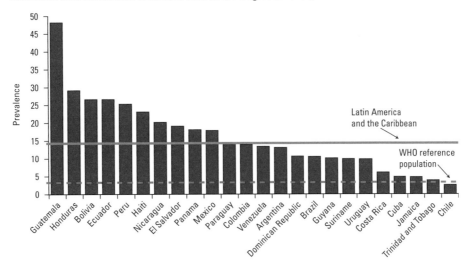

Source: World Health Organization, Standing Committee on Nutrition. Fifth Report on the World Nutrition Situation: Nutrition for Improved Development Outcomes. Geneva: WHO; 2004.

nature can have positive effects on caloric imbalances and obesity, as analysis suggests annual reductions of 0.64% in the prevalence of obesity in the female population between 1982 and 1998.

In comparison to the United State and Europe, where annual growth of the prevalence of overweight and obesity is 0.25, in Latin America and the Caribbean the corresponding growth rates are extremely high. Recent studies indicate an annual increase that ranges from 0.48 among Cuban females to 2.38 among Mexican females (*87*). Data available on overweight and obesity in the Americas highlight the need to make this dimension of malnutrition a priority, both due to the magnitude of the problem as well as its upward trend. During the 1992–2002 period, prevalences of overweight and obesity in children under 5 years of age in 11 countries were greater than the Latin American and Caribbean regional average, which is 4.4%. The specific rates are shown in Table 20.

Due to the special characteristics of the nutritional transition process in Latin America and the Caribbean, in the same household undernutrition in children and overweight in adults may be found to coexist. The foregoing demonstrates the nutritional deficiencies, excesses, and imbalances (lack of fortifying food, as well as macro- and micronutrients) that interact in the same social environment, a situation that places a double burden of morbidity on countries with high rates of social exclusion and obliges them to develop and apply simultaneously policies and programs aimed at preventing factors that give rise to both nutritional deficiencies and dietary excesses. The coexistence of overweight and obese mothers and chronically undernutritioned children in the

TABLE 20. Prevalence of overweight and obesity in children under 5 years of age, selected Latin American countries, 1992–2002.

Country	Prevalence (%)
Argentina	9.2
Dominican Republic	8.4
Chile	8.0
Bolivia	6.5
Peru	6.4
Uruguay	6.2
Costa Rica	6.2
Guatemala	5.4
Mexico	5.3
Cuba	5.2
Brazil	4.9
Regional average	4.4

Source: World Health Organization Global Database on Child Growth and Malnutrition. Available at: www.who.int/nutgrowthdb/en/.

same home can be seen in 16% of families, as revealed in surveys conducted in Guatemala and Honduras, such as the 2002 National Survey of Maternal and Child Health, carried out by the Ministry of Public Health and Social Assistance and the National Institute of Statistics of Guatemala, and the 2001 National Epidemiological and Family Health Survey, conducted under the auspices of the Honduran Association of Family Planning and Ministry of Health of Honduras.

251

TABLE 21. Classification of Latin American and Caribbean countries, according to the likelihood of reaching MDG child malnutrition reduction target.

	Extent of progress		
On course to reach target	Insufficient progress to reach target	Regressing	Data unavailable
Bolivia	El Salvador	Argentina	Belize
Chile	Guatemala	Costa Rica	Brazil
Colombia	Honduras	Panama	Dominica
Dominican Republic	Nicaragua		Ecuador
Guyana			Grenada
Haiti			Paraguay
Jamaica			Saint Kitts and Nevis
Mexico			Saint Lucia
Peru			Saint Vincent and
Venezuela			the Grenadines
			Suriname
			Trinidad and Tobago
			Uruguay

Source: World Bank. Repositioning Nutrition as Central to Development, a Strategy for Large-scale Action. Washington, D.C.: World Bank; 2006.

Towards a Regional Initiative

According to information gathered by the World Bank (*88*), of 17 countries in Latin America and the Caribbean that have data available from surveys or sequential studies to analyze trends, only 10 have a possibility of reaching the target of decreasing the percentage of children under age 5 who are underweight for their age (undernutrition) by 2015 (see Table 21).

According to an ECLAC publication (*89*), based on data from various United Nations specialized agencies, by the end of the 1990s, a reduction of approximately 55% had been achieved in undernutrition, according to the indicator for low-weight-for-age, higher than the 40% estimate originally anticipated for that period. Although the pace of progress in the Region suggests that the target will be reached by 2015, the prospects vary by country. According to the ECLAC publication, the goal has already been attained in the Dominican Republic, and in Bolivia, Mexico, Peru, and Venezuela it has been achieved by more than 75%. On the other hand, there are 17 countries whose achievement level is below 75%. Nine of these—Brazil, Chile, Colombia, El Salvador, Guatemala, Guyana, Haiti, Nicaragua, and Uruguay—show the minimum anticipated progress, or slightly above (i.e., progress of between 31% and 71%), and they will only be able to reach the target if policies and programs are maintained and no economic or environmental crises arise. Analysis of progress in Honduras, Jamaica, Panama, and Trinidad and Tobago seems to indicate that these countries are less likely to reach this target. Finally, the situation in Argentina, Costa Rica, Ecuador, and Paraguay shows a reversal.

In response to the persistence of the problems of malnutrition due to caloric, protein, and micronutrient deficiencies and the rapid appearance of new problems due to caloric excesses and other nutritional imbalances, the Governments of Latin America have signed declarations that call for implementation of collaborative efforts in the short, medium, and long term between nongovernmental organizations, public sector agencies, local governments, regional and international institutions, and civil society to address the issues of food and nutritional insecurity.

Based on these considerations, PAHO has drafted a Regional Strategy and Plan of Action on Nutrition in Health and Development aimed at responding jointly to health and nutrition issues in the Americas. The Strategy's objective is to contribute to the promotion of equity in health to fight disease and improve quality of life in the Region through adequate nutrition throughout the life cycle, especially among the poorest and most vulnerable groups, and by encouraging strategic and collaborative efforts among Member States and other partners to reach the MDGs. All of this points to a comprehensive evidence-based political nutrition agenda by 2015 that fosters and implements improvement regionally, subregionally, and nationally in the collective population's food security.

The proposed Strategy and its Action Plan, designed to garner participation at different levels to improve the Region's dietary situation, will focus on three dimensions that promote significant measurable and sustainable changes: food and nutrition in health and development; less-than-optimal nutrition and nutritional deficiencies; and the relationship between inadequate nutrition, physical inactivity, and noncommunicable diseases.

DISEASES AFFECTING FOOD SAFETY

The relationship between health and agriculture is of great importance for the well-being and quality of life of the peoples of the Americas. The sustainable production of food and achieving food and nutritional safety in the Region's countries are essential elements for eliminating hunger and reducing poverty. By enhancing food production, it is possible to increase the availability of animal protein, fruits, and vegetables, as well as increase family incomes and rural job opportunities, thereby improving overall living conditions and the population's health. The eradication of extreme poverty and hunger in Latin America and the Caribbean, in particular the elimination of chronic malnutrition in children under 5 years of age, constitute MDG commitments and are linked to the strategies for primary health care and local development (90).

Human health and animal health are closely interlinked. The emergence of infectious diseases such as HIV/AIDS over the last 20 years, and recent outbreaks of diseases such as bovine spongiform encephalopathy (BSE), variant Creutzfeldt-Jakob disease (vCJD), severe acute respiratory syndrome (SARS), and type A avian influenza (H5N1) have captured public attention, particularly given their ability to spread among different species, including humans. The globalization of trade in food, animals, and their derivative products, and the large number of people constantly traveling the world facilitate the rapid spread of infections (91). This not only causes direct economic losses to the livestock industry but also contributes to creating a global state of alert for public health risks. It is estimated that the increase in outbreaks of emerging and reemerging livestock diseases worldwide since the mid-1990s, including BSE, foot-and-mouth disease, avian influenza, and swine fever, has cost the world US$ 80 billion. Since 1968, PAHO has been driving the dialogue between the two sectors through its Inter-American Meetings, at the Ministerial Level, on Health and Agriculture (known as RIMSA, for its Spanish acronym) (92) as a mechanism to strengthen integrated actions on matters related to the interrelationship between human and animal health.

The following sections present the situation of the primary diseases that place animal production at risk and that, consequently, could affect food safety and cause major losses to the Region's national economies.

Foot-and-Mouth Disease

The 2001–2005 period witnessed major changes in the recording of foot-and-mouth disease in the Region. The year 2001 was characterized by an emergency situation in the Southern Cone, with 4,198 outbreaks of the type A virus in Argentina, Uruguay, and the State of Río Grande do Sul (Brazil). The situation was controlled with the firm intervention of these countries' animal health services, which focused on sacrificing infected animals and those in contact with them, controlling animal transit, strategic vaccinations, and seroepidemiological research. Simultaneously, the disease intensified in some regions and was reintroduced into others previously considered free of the disease both

with and without vaccination. Nevertheless, South America made progress in terms of zones and countries free of foot-and-mouth disease. Ecuador and Venezuela maintained their endemic status, with some epidemic situations between 2002 and 2004 (93–95). This situation of contrasts caused economic and social impacts in the productive sector, particularly due to the loss of international markets and the repercussions on labor relations and on businesses in the affected countries.

In 2002, an outbreak of the type O virus was recorded on a farm in the Department of Canindeyú, Paraguay, causing the country to lose its status as free of foot-and-mouth disease with vaccination. In 2003, the disease was recorded in the Gran Chaco region shared by Bolivia and Paraguay, and, after a year without outbreaks, in Argentina. Phylogenetic analysis conducted on samples of the O virus, isolated in the Southern Cone, demonstrated the existence of a pool of very similar viruses, according to biomolecular characterization studies, which has been perpetuated in the Region. PAHO's Pan American Foot-and-Mouth Disease Center (PANAFTOSA) led multinational technical cooperation missions to support the affected countries in identifying regional problems and proposing actions to mitigate the situation within the framework of a zone-based program with harmonized strategies to eradicate the disease.

In 2004, isolated outbreaks were recorded in Colombia, Brazil's Amazon region, and Peru, and control actions were taken (sacrifice of livestock, strategic vaccinations, and sanitary control of animals in transit). In all cases, seroepidemiological studies were conducted to demonstrate the absence of viral circulation. Colombia experienced an outbreak along its border with Venezuela, a country that suffered an epidemic, and subsequently, in early 2005, another outbreak appeared in the Department of Cundinamarca, in the country's central region, allegedly originating from a laboratory strain of the virus.

As a result of the 2001 emergencies, the Ministers of Health of the Southern Cone countries took the joint decision to establish a cycle of audits, to be coordinated by PANAFTOSA, of foot-and-mouth disease programs in the subregion with respect to regulatory structures and veterinary care services. Two cycles were executed: one in 2001 and another in 2002. Auditing is considered a strategic activity in the Hemispheric Program for the Eradication of Foot-and-Mouth Disease (PHEFA) for the 2005–2009 period (96).

PHEFA is the focal point for policies to eradicate foot-and-mouth disease in the Americas, and since 1988 this entity has prioritized the strengthening of national programs to eradicate the disease to eliminate the endemic situation in critical zones. Its strategies are based on a regional risk characterization, the development of efficient epidemiological oversight, and the strengthening of biosafety in handling the foot-and-mouth disease virus, both in production of the vaccine and in diagnostics.

To focus national and regional efforts on the goal of eradicating foot-and-mouth disease in the Americas by 2009, in March 2004,

"Economic progress in developing countries in recent years has brought about a dramatic increase in highway traffic. Despite the lack of reliable data, there are indications that, after communicable diseases, accidents are becoming the largest single cause of morbidity and mortality in many of the Region's developing countries."

Héctor Acuña, 1982

the Hemispheric Conference on the Eradication of Foot-and-Mouth Disease was held in Houston, Texas. The Inter-American Group for the Eradication of Foot-and-Mouth Disease, which was established at this gathering and is made up of public and private representatives from throughout the Americas, defined new guidelines to combat the disease in the Hemisphere.

In 2005, investments made in foot-and-mouth disease eradication programs were evaluated and it was noted that the direct expenditures of the countries and the private sector on national programs totaled approximately US$ 580 million in 2005 alone. Controlling the 2005 emergency in Brazil's central-western region cost approximately US$ 15 million in direct expenses alone. These amounts may be significant, but the country's foreign trade in meat products for 2004–2005 was approximately US$ 3 billion. The determining factors in the appearance of epidemic outbreaks of foot-and-mouth disease continue to be the weakening of national programs, especially in terms of the fragility of controls at international and regional borders, the low coverage of the epidemiological oversight systems, and the lack of harmonization of control and eradication actions, a responsibility of the national programs (*97*).

The effect of foot-and-mouth disease outbreaks on food safety may be evaluated at two points: the decline in production and productivity caused by the disease, and the direct and indirect losses due to the lack of competitiveness on the global market of the countries considered endemic. In addition, the lack of political will and of coordination between the public and private sectors, and the reluctance of the private sector to actively participate in national programs, could be reasons for the continued endemism in some countries, which in turn compromises overall progress in the Region toward achieving the disease's eradication.

Bovine Spongiform Encephalopathy

BSE, commonly known as "mad cow disease," is a foodborne, communicable, neurodegenerative, progressive, and fatal disease of the bovine nervous system, caused by an abnormal self-replicating protein known as a prion. The disease was first diagnosed in 1986 in the United Kingdom, where it spread epizootically and peaked in 1992–1993, with an average of 36,185 cases per year and an annual incidence of 6,445.08 per million bovines over 24

months old. The most widely accepted theory regarding the origin of the BSE epidemic is the recycling of proteins from ruminants infected with the disease. By May 2006, 189,854 cases had been reported in 25 countries, 97.11% of which occurred in the United Kingdom. Nevertheless, the epidemic curve is currently declining in this country, with only 225 cases being reported in 2005 (*98*). The public health significance of BSE arises from the appearance of human cases associated with a new variant of Creutzfeldt-Jakob disease (vCJD), a rare and fatal neurodegenerative disease related to the consumption of food products from cattle contaminated with BSE. Unlike traditional forms of CJD, vCJD affects younger patients (average age of 29, compared with 65 for CJD) and has a longer relative duration (averaging 14 months, compared with 4.5 months for CJD). This new human disease was first described in March 1996; since then, 129 cases have been reported in the United Kingdom, six in France, and one each in Canada, Ireland, Italy, and the United States. Of these cases, three in France and those in Canada and the United States are considered to be the result of exposure to the causal agent in the United Kingdom (*99*).

During 2000 and 2001, indigenous cases of BSE were detected in several European countries and in Japan. The 2003 detection of indigenous cases in Canada and the United States, countries previously considered free of this disease, continues to cause concern among public health authorities and consumers. According to available scientific and technical information, the Region of the Americas from Mexico southward is free of indigenous cases of BSE. In response to the recommendations made at regional meetings, PAHO has taken various actions to keep the Region free of BSE, thus avoiding the restrictions on global trade that have, in part, affected the availability of food products of animal origin. A risk self-evaluation guide has been drafted and training activities have been undertaken (*100*). Epidemiological oversight activities have also been undertaken and national professionals have been trained in immunohistochemical techniques for BSE diagnosis (*101*).

Avian Influenza

Global Situation

Avian influenza is a disease caused by type A strains of the influenza virus. It can naturally infect a wide variety of species, including humans, swine, horses, marine mammals, and birds. All known variants of the type A influenza virus have been isolated from birds, and only a few from mammals. Phylogenetic and ecological studies of the type A influenza virus show that wild aquatic birds are the natural reservoir and source of these viruses for the other species. Occasionally, devastating influenza epidemics have occurred in humans (most recently in 1918, 1957, and 1968). These have emerged from genetic modifications of the type A influenza virus from animals. There is also conclusive evidence of the risk of zoonotic infections from the type A influenza virus in animals (*102*).

Given that aquatic birds may be the source of all type A influenza viruses in other species, it is thought that the human pandemic strains emerged through one of three possible mechanisms: 1) a genetic rearrangement (occurring as a result of segmentation of the virus' genome) of type A influenza viruses from birds and humans infecting the same host; 2) a direct transfer of the entire virus from other species; or 3) reemergence of the virus that caused an epidemic long ago.

In the 20th century, the rapid emergence of antigenically different strains in human beings was recorded four times: in 1918 (H1N1), 1957 (H2N2), 1968 (H3N2), and 1977 (H1N1). In each case, they caused a pandemic. Between the pandemics, frequent epidemics have appeared as a result of a process called antigenic shift, in which two different strains of influenza combine to form a new subtype having a mixture of the surface antigens of the two original strains. Since 1996, the H7N7, H5N1, and H9N2 viruses have been transmitted from birds to humans but have apparently failed to spread massively in the human population (*103, 104*).

The influenza virus that infects birds can be divided into two groups differentiated on the basis of their pathogenic capacity. The most virulent viruses cause highly pathogenic avian influenza (HPAI), which can cause up to 100% mortality in the affected flocks. These viruses have been limited to the H5 and H7 subtypes, although not all of them cause HPAI. All the other subtypes cause a much milder disease, known as low pathogenic avian influenza (LPAI). Chickens and turkeys tend not to be natural hosts of the avian influenza viruses, but they do become infected when they come in contact with wild aquatic birds that are carriers (*105*).

Since 1996, transmission of the type A(H7N7), A(H5N1), and A(H9N2) viruses from birds to human beings has been detected, but there appears to have been no person-to-person transmission. In particular, the A(H5N1) virus has been causing an HPAI epizootic in domestic poultry and wild birds in various Asian countries since early 2003, with devastating consequences for poultry farming in the affected countries. More than 200 people have been infected, and of these, nearly one-half have died. Scientific reports warn of the potential appearance of a new influenza pandemic in humans, caused by H5N1. A(H5N1) outbreaks have also been reported in migratory birds in Asia, Europe, and Africa, some with an intercontinental migratory range; through June 2006, the epidemic had spread to 46 countries in Asia, Europe, and Africa (*98, 106, 107*).

The Importance of Poultry Production to Food Safety

Poultry production in the Americas is highly developed and represents a major economic activity due to its capacity to generate income and employment, in addition to providing high-quality, low-cost animal protein. According to FAO data (*106*), the Americas generate 46.9% of the 67 million tons of poultry produced and export 58.3% of the 7 million tons exported worldwide. Five countries in the Region produce 99% of the Region's exports (United States, Brazil, Canada, Argentina, and Chile), and 12 countries are responsible for 98% of the Hemisphere's production (United States, Brazil, Mexico, Canada, Argentina, Venezuela, Colombia, Peru, Chile, Ecuador, Guatemala, and Bolivia). Moreover, poultry meat and eggs are the most economical sources of animal protein and represent nearly 40% of the animal protein consumed per capita in the Region. There are also important activities highly dependent on poultry farming, such as grain production, trade, and the agricultural services and transport industry.

Industrial and semi-industrial poultry farming is a highly competitive economic activity in both domestic and export markets. In general, it has low profit margins per product unit, so companies require high levels of productive efficiency and low costs to be competitive, and they tend to be concentrated in order to leverage economies of scale. In this regard, health is one of the key factors for competitiveness because of the direct impact of disease on bioproduction indicators (an increase in costs and a decrease or loss of production), the consequences for the markets (both domestic and export) and consumption, and the impact on human health when infected poultry products enter a country. This is precisely the case with avian influenza, a disease with a great ability to spread and cause economic damage in addition to compromising human health.

The Regional Avian Influenza Situation

Avian influenza outbreaks of high and low pathogenicity have been recorded periodically in several countries in the Americas. In this Hemisphere, most of the known types of the influenza A virus have been found in wild aquatic birds.

Since 1959, cases of HPAI in domestic poultry have been reported in Canada, the United States, Mexico, and Chile. These outbreaks have caused direct losses to the affected countries of many tens of millions of dollars. It is important to note that the cases of HPAI have emerged from LPAI viruses. To date, all the HPAI outbreaks have been caused by H5 and H7 viruses.

In Canada and the United States, the presence of HPAI viruses has been reported in domestic poultry, primarily in commercial live bird establishments (for consumption or pets). Cases have also been recorded of HPAI caused by H5N2 in Mexico, Guatemala, and El Salvador, countries where oversight and control actions are undertaken with official systematic vaccination plans (*102*).

Risk of the Introduction and Spread of H5N1 Influenza in the Region

The rapid spread of the H5N1 virus in Asia since 2003 is due to the movement and legal and illegal trade of domestic birds and pets and to the movements of migratory birds. According to studies of avian migratory cycles, it is likely that the H5N1 virus will

255

arrive in the Region of the Americas through this mechanism, even before a potential pandemic is caused by the virus. The likely resulting epidemiological scenarios will depend on how it is introduced, the location and type of birds initially infected, and the detection capacity of the veterinary care systems (98).

The Region's domestic poultry production systems cover large areas with high concentrations of birds and are characterized by active population dynamics and a close epidemiological relationship among farms. These factors imply levels of risk of vulnerability and receptivity to the influenza virus sufficient for possible entry and establishment under conditions of endemism, inasmuch as the forms of control established are inadequate (106). A likely scenario after entry is that the infection would tend to take root (become endemic) in the poultry production systems with low biosecurity—that is, on small and medium-sized poultry farms, family poultry farms, and live bird establishments for consumption or pets. At this level, the impact would be greater, given that poultry farming generates direct food products for the rural family as well as economic income from the sale of the products (106).

The infection has also demonstrated a surprising level of aggressiveness, being capable of breaking through biosecurity mechanisms at poultry farms with the highest sanitary levels, and reaching the industrial poultry farming sector, affecting both meat and egg production. Given the level of integration and the number of birds in the sector, the potential for dissemination and the level of morbidity/mortality are quite high.

Based on this background, it can be estimated that the arrival of the infection in the Region could have a major impact on poultry farming, representing a true catastrophe in affected countries where it plays a major role in the national economy, with repercussions for the supply of low-cost animal protein for mass consumption to most of the population. The repercussions to the supply would be further aggravated by the impact of emergency control measures (flock destruction, quarantines) and trade restrictions, in addition to the impact on the environment caused by the need to dispose of thousands of tons of highly contaminated organic matter (106).

With respect to the risk the influenza virus poses to human health, as indicated earlier, transmission of the influenza virus between animals and humans has been confirmed, causing a wide range of disease (H7N7, H9N2, and H5N1). Occasionally, the influenza virus causes pandemics in humans when the following conditions are met: 1) the population lacks prior immunity against the pandemic virus; 2) the virus is transmitted from animals to humans; and 3) the virus acquires an efficient person-to-person transmission capacity. In the case of the H5N1 HPAI virus, it is considered to have acquired a high pandemic potential as it meets the first two conditions and has only to acquire the ability to be transmitted efficiently between persons to become a pandemic virus. It must be specified that the pre-pandemic conditions of the H5N1 HPAI virus have to date been met in the countries affected by it, primarily in Asia, where the HPAI epidemic coexists with a high exposure of persons by close contact with infected birds and the appearance of human cases (107, 108).

The Political and Technical Response

The emergence of avian influenza caused by highly pathogenic strains that can be transmitted from birds to humans represents a serious public health problem, given the risk of contagion of workers who are in close contact with the birds and the technicians responsible for oversight, diagnostics, and control of outbreaks, as well as the possible impact on food safety caused by losses in animal protein and trade restrictions. To respond to these problems, PAHO veterinary public health experts are providing guidance to countries on biosecurity measures to be incorporated to protect local populations, such as vaccination against seasonal influenza, the use of personal protection equipment, and the training of workers on standardized hygiene procedures. Likewise, coordination between the health, agriculture, and environmental sectors is fundamental. PAHO has promoted this coordination through RIMSA. At RIMSA 14, held in Mexico City in April 2005, the Ministers issued a resolution on the global risk of new and emerging zoonoses that provides guidance to countries regarding PAHO's technical cooperation and intersectoral actions (109).

Clearly, there is a broad scientific, technical, and political consensus that avian influenza, and particularly the global scenario for H5N1, represent a serious public health problem and pose a formidable challenge to prevention systems in public health (risk of zoonoses and pandemics) and animal health (economic impact on poultry production). The challenge posed by avian influenza for food safety is particularly significant because of the need to protect rural populations from the impact caused by losses of animal protein, decreased revenues, and the loss of jobs, all of which increase this group's vulnerability and poverty.

TOBACCO

Tobacco-related Morbidity and Mortality

Tobacco use continues to be one of the most significant risk factors for death and disease worldwide and in the Region of the Americas in particular. WHO's *World Health Report 2002* (110) estimated that, as a preventable cause of death, only high blood pressure outpaces tobacco use, which causes 5 million deaths annually worldwide, 900,000 of them in the Region of the Americas, according to 2000 figures. It also considered that tobacco use ranked fourth in the global burden of disease, with approximately 60 million DALYs (110).

Since the vast majority of cases of lung cancer are caused by smoking (including exposure to secondhand smoke), the specific mortality rates constitute a reasonable indication of the damage to health caused by tobacco use. Nevertheless, it is important to

TABLE 22. Mortality rates[a] from malignant neoplasms of the trachea, bronchus, and lung,[b] by country, Region of the Americas, 2000–2004.

Country	Year	Men	Women	Total
Antigua and Barbuda	2002	0.0	3.7	2.2
Argentina	2004	34.1	8.6	19.8
Bahamas	2000	12.8	6.8	9.7
Barbados	2001	8.0	1.2	4.1
Belize	2001	17.0	4.5	10.8
Brazil	2002	19.8	8.0	13.4
Canada	2003	43.0	25.6	33.3
Chile	2003	17.9	7.7	12.2
Colombia	2001	16.5	9.1	12.4
Costa Rica	2004	10.4	5.4	7.8
Cuba	2004	41.3	18.8	29.5
Dominica	2003	20.8	10.7	15.6
Dominican Republic	2004	13.8	8.4	11.1
Ecuador	2004	7.5	4.9	6.1
El Salvador	2003	7.4	6.3	6.7
Guatemala	2003	6.8	4.6	5.7
Guyana	2003	5.9	2.0	3.7
Haiti	2003	6.2	6.0	6.1
Mexico	2004	13.5	5.4	9.1
Nicaragua	2003	7.4	6.3	6.8
Panama	2003	16.4	8.1	12.1
Paraguay	2003	27.6	6.4	16.1
Peru	2000	14.2	8.3	11.0
Saint Lucia	2002	6.1	4.5	5.2
Saint Vincent and the Grenadines	2003	17.1	10.2	13.5
Suriname	2000	17.9	5.2	11.1
Trinidad and Tobago	2000	13.7	3.1	8.1
United States	2002	45.3	26.9	35.0
Uruguay	2001	52.9	6.8	26.9
Venezuela	2004	17.2	9.1	13.1

[a]Per 100,000 population; adjusted for age (all ages).
[b]Includes ICD-10 codes C33–C34.
Source: Pan American Health Organization, Health Analysis and Statistics Unit. Mortality and Population Information System.

note that the mortality rates for lung cancer reflect the guidelines for past tobacco use but not necessarily current smoking rates. Table 22 (*111*) shows the Region's mortality rates for malignant neoplasms of the trachea, bronchus, and lung.

Smoking is the number two modifiable risk factor for heart disease and the top modifiable risk factor for cancer. The INTERHEART study, conducted between 1998 and 2003 in 52 countries, determined that smoking approximately triples the risk of acute myocardial infarction in both males and females. Worldwide, smoking represented 36.4% of the population attributable risk (PAR) of acute myocardial infarction (44.0% in males and 15.8% in females) and 38.3% of the PAR in South America (*112*). According to other studies, smoking causes one-fifth (21%) of all deaths by cancer in the world: 29% in high-income countries and 18% in low and medium income countries (*113*).

Results published in 2005 and 2006 confirm prior findings that exposure to secondhand smoke increases the risk of disease in nonsmoking adults and children and also link this exposure to a greater risk of breast cancer in predominantly premenopausal nonsmoking young females (*114, 115*).

Tobacco Use and Exposure to Secondhand Smoke

Prevalence of Tobacco Consumption among Adults

There is no standardized system to monitor the prevalence of tobacco use among adults, thus allowing for comparisons between countries in the Americas. There are also few countries that have comparable data on smoking trends among adults, due to year-to-year methodological differences. These limitations regarding comparability should be considered when examining

TABLE 23. Smoking prevalence in the general population, by sex, selected countries, Region of the Americas, 2000–2005.

Country	Year of survey	Age group	Sex	Active smokers[a] (%)
Argentina	2005	18+	Men	35.1
			Women	24.9
			Total	29.7
Brazil (Rio de Janeiro)	2002–2004	15+	Men	19.8
			Women	15.9
			Total	17.5
Brazil (São Paulo)	2002–2004	15+	Men	23.1
			Women	17.5
			Total	19.9
Canada	2005	15+	Men	22
			Women	16
			Total	19
Chile	2003	17+	Men	48.3
			Women	36.8
			Total	42.4
Costa Rica	2000	12–70	Men	23.3
			Women	8.2
			Total	15.8
Mexico	2001	18–65	Men	42.3
			Women	15.1
			Total	27
Nicaragua	2001	15–49	Women	5.3
Peru	2005	12–64	Total	31.8
United States	2003	18+	Men	24.1
			Women	19.2
			Total	21.6

[a]Definition of "active smoker":
Argentina: has smoked in the last 30 days and at least 100 cigarettes in his/her entire life.
Brazil: "regular" smoker, no definition available.
Canada: includes daily and occasional smokers.
Chile: includes daily and occasional smokers.
Costa Rica: has smoked in the last month.
Mexico: no definition available.
Nicaragua: no definition available.
Peru: has smoked in the last 30 days.
United States: has smoked at least 100 cigarettes in his/her entire life and currently smokes every day or some days.
Source: Country survey data.

Table 23, which shows the most recent data available on smoking prevalence in the Americas between 2000 and 2005. As can be seen, the corresponding rates vary widely throughout the Region.

Prevalence of Smoking among Adolescents

The Global Youth Tobacco Survey presents comparable data on the prevalence of tobacco use among adolescents aged 13–15 (Figure 21). According to surveys conducted between 2000 and 2005, cigarette use (defined as the prevalence of having smoked cigarettes on one or more days during the previous month) was highest in Chile, with nearly 34% (figures for Santiago, 2003), and lowest in Antigua and Barbuda, with only 3.6% (national figures, 2004) (*116*). These values do not include the use of tobacco prod-

ucts other than cigarettes, although the use of these products may be significant in some countries.

Except in Chile, Argentina, and Uruguay, where the rates for girls are higher than those for boys (Chile: boys, 27.6%, girls, 39.2%; Argentina: boys, 17.2%, girls, 26.8%; Uruguay: boys, 22.2%, girls, 29.6%), the prevalence of smoking in the Region continues to be higher among boys. Available data on trends indicated that, in most countries, the prevalence of smoking among young people has remained relatively stable (Figure 22), although in some Caribbean countries such as Cuba, Suriname, Barbados, Bahamas, and Antigua and Barbuda, it seems to be on the decline, while in others, such as Chile and Grenada, an upward trend is observed.

FIGURE 21. Smoking prevalence among adolescents 13–15 years old, by sex, Latin America and the Caribbean, 2001–2005.

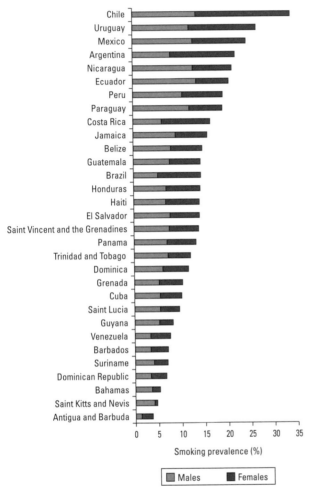

Smoking prevalence (%)

Males ■ Females

Source: World Health Organization, U.S. Centers for Disease Control and Prevention. Global Youth Tobacco Survey data.

FIGURE 22. Trends in smoking prevalence among adolescents 13–15 years old, selected countries of the Americas, 1999–2004.

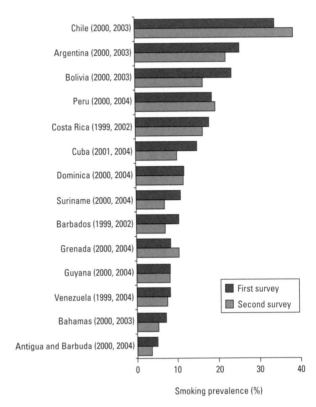

Smoking prevalence (%)

Note: The data represent national totals, except in the cases of the following countries, in which data were collected from a selected location (capital or another major city) and substituted: Argentina (Buenos Aires), Bolivia (La Paz), Chile (Metropolitan Santiago), Cuba (Havana), Peru (Lima), and Venezuela (Barinas).
Source: World Health Organization, U.S. Centers for Disease Control and Prevention. Global Youth Tobacco Survey data.

Per Capita Tobacco Consumption

Per capita consumption is estimated on the basis of tobacco production, import, and export data and can provide an idea of the trends in different countries over time (Figure 23). On the whole, per capita consumption is declining in the Region or is stable in almost all countries for which data are available, except Bolivia and Colombia.

Nevertheless, it is appropriate to note the following observations when using per capita consumption data: they are influenced by income levels and the price of the tobacco products with respect to income, and these factors can have a negative impact on otherwise successful antismoking efforts in a given country. In general, these data do not take into account the consumption of illegal imports (contraband or counterfeit), in such a way that, where this consumption is high, the data may not be an accurate

reflection of absolute consumption; the data included in Figure 23 represent three- or four-year averages. Year-to-year fluctuations can mask trends over longer terms (that could be the case, for example, in Brazil). It would be ideal to consider per capita consumption data together with prevalence data for a more complete picture of current tobacco use in the Region.

Exposure to Secondhand Smoke

The Global Youth Tobacco Survey determined that, in most countries, at least 30% of young people were exposed to tobacco smoke in the home at least once a week. Exposure was highest in Argentina (nearly 70%), Uruguay (65%), and Chile (56%). The lowest exposure rates were in El Salvador (15%), Saint Kitts and Nevis (17%), and Antigua and Barbuda (18%) (Figure 24) (*116*).

In an assessment of the concentration of nicotine in public places, airborne nicotine (which is a marker for exposure to environmental tobacco smoke) was found in 94% of the critical points

FIGURE 23. Cigarette consumption per capita (persons over 15 years old), selected countries of the Americas, 2000–2003 average compared to 1996–1999 average, percentage variation.[a]

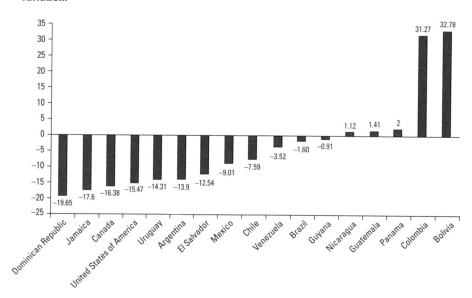

[a]Exceptions: Nicaragua and Panama compare 2001–2004 data with 1997–2000; Uruguay compares 2001–2004 data with 1998–2000.
Source: Calculations based on data from Guindon GE, Boisclair D. Cigarette consumption dataset 1970–2004. Prepared for the American Cancer Society, August 2005.

surveyed in seven Latin American countries (Argentina, Brazil, Chile, Costa Rica, Paraguay, Peru, and Uruguay) (*117*). In all the countries, the highest concentrations of nicotine were found in bars. They were also very high in many nonsmoking areas in bars and restaurants, indicating that the designation of separate seating areas for nonsmokers is an inefficient, and even self-defeating, strategy to control exposure to secondhand smoke.

Economic Considerations

In a 1993 study by the World Bank, it was calculated that the international tobacco market represents an annual global loss of US$ 200 billion in health care costs and lost productivity (*118*). In the United States, it is estimated that tobacco use was responsible for an average US$ 76 billion annually for the 1995–1999 period in direct medical costs for treatment of smoking-related diseases, and US$ 82 billion more during this same period in productivity losses due to deaths caused by tobacco (*119*). Moreover, the U.S.-based Society of Actuaries estimated the annual cost of exposure to environmental tobacco smoke at US$ 10 billion (US$ 5 billion in direct medical costs and US$ 5 billion in lost productivity) (*120*). In studies relating to Canada, the direct health cost from exposure to environmental smoke in newborns and children was calculated at nearly US$ 250 million in 1997, and the cost of fires attributable to tobacco use was US$ 81.5 million that same year (*121*).

In response to the concerns frequently expressed by governments, tobacco cultivation and production in the Region of the Americas represent a very small part of most countries' agricultural and manufacturing activities. Studies undertaken by PAHO in the Southern Cone countries confirmed that the percentage of land planted with tobacco was less than 1% in Argentina, Bolivia, Chile, and Uruguay. Even in Brazil, which is the world's largest exporter of tobacco leaf, tobacco employs less than 5% of the agricultural workforce (*120–124*). Employment in the tobacco industry represents just 0.003% of the industrial workforce in Uruguay, 0.02% in Brazil, 0.09% in Chile, and 0.46% in Bolivia. Tobacco manufacturing employs a higher proportion of the industrial workforce in Argentina (4.23%), but this percentage still represents a small minority of the industrial workforce (*122–126*).

In most countries, nearly 100% of the market share belongs to subsidiaries of British American Tobacco or Philip Morris International (*127*). This means that the earnings from the sale of tobacco products are transferred out of the countries and represent a net currency loss.

Status of Interventions

WHO Framework Convention on Tobacco Control

The most significant contribution to tobacco control in recent years has been the 2003 adoption of the WHO Framework Con-

FIGURE 24. Exposure of adolescents 13–15 years old to tobacco smoke at home, selected countries of the Americas, 2000–2005.

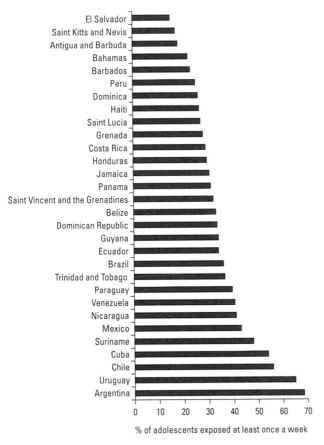

% of adolescents exposed at least once a week

Source: World Health Organization, U.S. Centers for Disease Control and Prevention. Global Youth Tobacco Survey data.

vention on Tobacco Control (FCTC) and its ratification by 142 Member States in December 2006 (*128*). The FCTC is legally binding, according to international law, in all signatory countries. It establishes specific regulations and obligations that cover a wide range of tobacco control policies and programs, including fiscal policy, legislation regulating tobacco use and its marketing, smoking cessation programs, control of the illegal trade, education and raising public awareness, and exchanging research and information.

As of December 2006, 21 PAHO Member States, together representing approximately half the population of the Americas, were signatories of the WHO FCTC. They are Antigua and Barbuda, Barbados, Belize, Bolivia, Brazil, Canada, Chile, Dominica, Ecuador, Guatemala, Guyana, Honduras, Jamaica, Mexico, Panama, Paraguay, Peru, Saint Lucia, Trinidad and Tobago, Uruguay, and Venezuela. Effective compliance with its provisions will have significant repercussions for tobacco use in the Region, and ultimately, for the morbidity and mortality caused by tobacco.

Smoke-free Environments

Smoke-free environments protect nonsmokers from the harmful effects of exposure to tobacco smoke. They also constitute, in terms of economic cost, one of the most effective measures for reducing tobacco use (*129*).

In March 2006, Uruguay became the first country in the Americas to impose an absolute ban on smoking in all indoor workplaces (including clubs, bars, and restaurants) and in all public establishments. Significant progress at various jurisdictional levels has also been made in Canada to prevent exposure to tobacco smoke (covering 74% of the population), the United States (45% of the total population), and Argentina (Santa Fe, Córdoba, and Tucumán, representing 21% of the entire country) (*130, 131*).

Public information campaigns have been undertaken to further support the creation of smoke-free environments in several countries, including Argentina, Barbados, Brazil, Costa Rica, Guatemala, Honduras, Peru, and Trinidad and Tobago. In other countries, however, progress toward comprehensive legislation to protect workers from exposure to environmental tobacco smoke has been much slower.

PAHO recently analyzed exposure to environmental tobacco smoke within the context of the rights protected by international legal instruments of the United Nations and the inter-American systems (*132*). These instruments and their enforcement mechanisms or agencies, such as the Inter-American Commission on Human Rights, offer clear directions to governments on how to protect workers and the general population from exposure to environmental tobacco smoke and open an appropriate legal channel for individuals to defend their right to healthy, smoke-free environments.

Taxes on Tobacco Products and Price-setting

The relationship between the prices of tobacco products and the population's income (accessibility of tobacco), as well as the relationship between these prices and those of other consumer products, are among the primary factors determining their purchase (*133*). Between 1990 and 2001, there were more countries in the Americas where the price of cigarettes fell with respect to income than those where it increased. The cost of 100 packs of cigarettes as a percentage of the average per capita GDP for the period 1999–2001 was highest in Ecuador (nearly 9%) and lowest in the United States (less than 2%) (*134*). Currently, no detailed analysis of the most recent changes in the accessibility (relative price) of tobacco is available, but this should be an important monitoring priority for understanding changes in per capita consumption.

Most countries do not pay due attention to the impact of the relative price (accessibility) on tobacco use, and fiscal policy has not been sufficiently utilized in the Region as a tool to reduce consumption. A result is that tobacco often becomes more—rather than less—economical (or accessible) over time. Nevertheless, some countries, including Mexico and Uruguay, have implemented moderate tax increases on tobacco use in recent years as a specific part of their antismoking efforts, or—as in the case of Jamaica—to finance medical costs. In 2006, Suriname significantly increased taxes on cigarettes, effectively doubling the sales price.

Health Risk Warnings on Tobacco Products

Conspicuous warnings on the risks to health printed on cigarette packs provide valuable information to smokers and motivate them to try to quit or reduce their consumption. Studies conducted in Brazil and Canada indicate that these warnings were very effective in communicating health risks and motivating smokers to try to quit and smoke outdoors, away from their families (135, 136).

Four countries in the Americas—Brazil, Canada, Uruguay, and Venezuela—currently require packs to carry printed warning images on them; Panama and several Caribbean countries also are considering the possibility of implementing this requirement.

Elimination of Tobacco Advertising and Promotion

Tobacco promotion has been correlated with an increase in consumption and the initiation of young people to smoking (137). Evidence exists that restrictions on promotion are effective only when they completely ban all or most forms of direct and indirect advertising (138). This is the case because when provisions restricting some form of tobacco advertising or its presentation in a given medium (e.g., radio, television) are approved, tobacco companies simply redirect their resources to types of promotion where the prohibition does not yet apply.

Although the FCTC requires countries to prohibit the promotion of tobacco within five years of the Convention's entry into force, in the Region of the Americas only Brazil (which allows promotion solely at points of sale), Canada (which allows some types of promotion), and Cuba impose restrictions on the promotion of tobacco use considered sufficiently broad to reduce consumption. Although in 2006 a law was approved in Chile banning many forms of tobacco advertising, its provisions fail to ban tobacco companies from advertising sponsorships and other forms of indirect advertising, and thus the law has not been effective. It is possible that the depiction of tobacco use in film has been the most important promotional vehicle in recent years. A great deal of research has confirmed that young nonsmokers exposed to such films are almost three times more likely to start smoking than those who are not exposed. The showing of tobacco use in films also increases young people's willingness to smoke (139). Public health agencies, including WHO, have provided their support to various principles that would reduce the impact of depicting tobacco use in films (140); to date, no major United States motion picture studio has agreed to apply these principles.

Tobacco Industry Activities

The Region's tobacco industry is an oligopoly controlled by the transnational corporations of British American Tobacco and Philip Morris International. PAHO and other agencies have documented the tobacco industry's strategies to counter effective tobacco control policies, using the tobacco companies' own allegedly probatory documents (127). One of the industry's most popular campaigns in the Region is the program called "Living Together in Harmony," which promotes smokers and nonsmokers sharing spaces as a tactic to neutralize laws requiring the establishment of smoke-free environments. This program was recently relaunched in Mexico (141), where there is growing community pressure to enforce laws that ban smoking. Another customary strategy is to use school smoking prevention programs aimed at young people. In fact, several governments in the Americas, through their health or education ministries, have contacted tobacco companies to have them cosponsor these programs, which have proven to be ineffective. British American Tobacco reports that it has sponsored health promotion programs for young people in Venezuela (142), and Philip Morris International has launched its "Yo tengo P.O.D.E.R." (I have POWER) program in schools in Uruguay. More recent initiatives by tobacco companies consist of voluntarily placing more conspicuous health warning messages on cigarette packs (143), to stay ahead of governments imposing stronger warnings.

The reactions of the tobacco companies reveal which control measures they perceive as most threatening to their sales and thus reinforce independent verifications to evaluate the efficacy of these measures on the reduction of tobacco use.

Tobacco in the Courtroom

In August 2006, in a civil lawsuit brought by the U.S. Department of Justice (United States v. Philip Morris et al.), the Federal Court for the District of Columbia found that several tobacco companies were guilty of illegal activities under the so-called RICO (Racketeer Influenced and Corrupt Organizations) statute, which pursues corrupt and criminal organizations, and ordered various measures including prohibiting the use of misleading terms such as "mild" and "low tar." The tobacco companies appealed, and the Federal Court of Appeals suspended the judgment and the above-mentioned prohibition, indicating that enforcement of the measures ordered by the lower court will not be required until the courts have ruled on all pending appeals (144).

Many legal class actions on behalf of a group of victims, individual claims, suits to recover medical expenses, and other legal actions remain pending in the United States and Canada. Nevertheless, British American Tobacco reports that the only other countries in the Region with more than five suits pending against the company are Argentina and Brazil (145).

Challenges and Priorities for the Future

The tobacco industry continues to be the principal obstacle to reducing the morbidity and mortality caused by tobacco in the

Americas. Second is the inability of public health systems in many countries to make prevention of tobacco use a high priority, rather than focusing on ineffective strategies in terms of cost, such as individual programs to quit smoking and school education programs (which do not work). Although some short-term studies monitoring school programs have reported a lower prevalence of tobacco use among young people, the evaluation of long-term efficacy provides convincing indications that they are not effective (146). Perhaps they can improve students' knowledge of the risks of smoking, but over the long term they do not reduce smoking in young people. The logical appeal of these programs, combined with their lack of efficacy in actually reducing smoking, explains why the tobacco industry has been supporting them for so long. Nevertheless, the situation is changing: the entry into force of the WHO FCTC has mobilized governments and nongovernmental organizations to strengthen actions to reduce tobacco use, placing greater emphasis on measures that have proven their cost-effectiveness and have a greater impact on the population.

A central achievement of the FCTC is the recognition by governments of the need to collaborate globally to ensure the exchange of success stories and the support of wealthy countries for the application of the FCTC in developing countries. The pending challenge rests on ensuring that the spirit of the FCTC is translated into action, providing more resources to the countries that need them most.

ALCOHOL

Worldwide, alcohol consumption has become one of the most significant risks to health. According to the *World Health Report 2002* (147), 4.0% of the burden of disease should be attributed to alcohol, equivalent to 58.3 million lost DALYs, and 1.8 million deaths, or 3.2% of all deaths in the world. Alcohol is the leading risk to health in developing countries with low mortality, where it is the cause of 6.2% of lost DALYs, and the number three risk in developed countries, where it represents 9.2% of lost DALYs. In the Region of the Americas, it is the leading risk factor among the 27 different factors evaluated for the burden of disease (148), as shown in Table 24.

The burden of disease caused by alcohol consumption in the Region is significant and exceeds global figures: 4.8% of deaths and 9.7% of DALYs in 2000 (compared with 3.2% and 4.0% worldwide, respectively) are attributable to alcohol consumption, and most occur in the Central and South American countries (149). It is estimated to have caused at least 279,000 deaths that year, a number proportionally higher than European and global averages (148). Intentional and unintentional injuries represented nearly 60% of all alcohol-related deaths and nearly 40% of the morbidity due to the same cause. Most of the burden of disease affects males (83.3%); 77.4% of morbidity affects the population aged 15–44, indicating that it primarily affects young peo-

TABLE 24. Primary risk factors for the burden of disease and percentage of total DALYs, Region of the Americas, 2000.

Amr-D[a]		Amr-B[a]		Amr-A[a]	
High mortality	%	Low mortality	%	Very low mortality	%
Alcohol	11.4	Alcohol	11.4	Tobacco	13.3
Low birthweight	5.3	Overweight	4.2	Alcohol	7.8
Unprotected sex	4.8	High blood pressure	4.0	Overweight	7.5
Lack of sanitation	4.3	Tobacco	3.7	High blood pressure	6.0
Overweight	2.4	High cholesterol	2.3	Low cholesterol	5.3
High blood pressure	2.2	Unprotected sex	2.1	Low intake of fruits and vegetables	2.9
Iron deficiency	1.9	Lead exposure	2.1	Physical inactivity	2.7
Smoke in the home (use of fuel)	1.9	Low intake of fruits and vegetables	1.8	Unprotected sex	2.6
High cholesterol	1.1	Lack of sanitation	1.6	Unprotected sex	1.1
Low intake of fruits and vegetables	0.8	Physical inactivity	1.4	Iron deficiency	1.0

[a]To facilitate cause-of-death and burden-of-disease analyses, the 192 Member States of WHO have been divided into five mortality strata on the basis of their levels of mortality in children under 5 years of age and in males ages 15–59. The Amr-D classification refers to developing countries in the Region of the Americas with high child mortality and high adult mortality, Amr-B to developing countries in the Region with low child mortality and low adult mortality, and Amr-A to developed countries in the Region of the Americas with very low child mortality and low adult mortality. Table 5 in this chapter lists the Region's countries by their corresponding A, B, and D mortality strata.

Source: Pan American Health Organization, Sustainable Development and Environmental Health Area, based on data from Rehm J, Room R, Monteiro M, Gmel G, Graham K, Rehn N et al. Alcohol use. In: Ezzati M, Lopez AD, Rodgers A, Murray CJL, eds. Comparative qualification of health risks: global and regional burden of disease due to selected risk factors (Vol 1). Geneva: WHO; 2004, pp. 959–1108.

TABLE 25. Comparison of mortality attributable to alcohol, by absolute number and percentage, Region of the Americas and worldwide, 2002.

	Region of the Americas		Worldwide	
	No. of deaths	Percentage of total attributable to alcohol	No. of deaths	Percentage of total deaths attributable to alcohol
Perinatal and maternal morbidity	203	0.1	3,057	0.2
Cancer	37,006	14.0	377,968	21.2
Neuropsychiatric morbidity	27,492	10.4	113,603	6.4
Cardiovascular diseases	−3,249[a]	−1.2[a]	196,646	11.0
Other noncommunicable diseases	46,657	17.6	237,985	13.3
Unintentional injuries	88,409	33.4	585,553	32.8
Intentional injuries	68,180	25.8	269,155	15.1
Total alcohol-related deaths	264,697	100.0	1,783,567	100.0
Percentage of deaths attributable to alcohol with respect to all deaths	4.4		3.1	

[a]The negative figures correspond to the number of lives saved by reduced alcohol consumption and its beneficial effects on cardiovascular diseases.

Source: Pan American Health Organization, Sustainable Development and Environmental Health Area, based on data from Rehm J, Room R, Monteiro M, Gmel G, Graham K, Rehm N et al. Alcohol use. In: Ezzati M, Lopez AD, Rodgers A, Murray CJL, eds. Comparative qualification of health risks: global and regional burden of disease due to selected risk factors (Vol 1). Geneva: WHO; 2004, pp. 959–1108.

ple and young adults during their most productive years. Table 25 summarizes alcohol-related mortality results for 2002, comparing the Region of the Americas with global figures, yielding very similar burden-of-disease results to those from 2000.

Alcohol Consumption, Health, and Social Problems

Alcohol consumption is widespread in most countries in the Americas, despite the fact that it is not free of risks. It is essentially an intoxicating drug that causes dependency and is primarily consumed for its psychoactive effects that alter perception and behavior. Alcohol addiction (usually called alcoholism) is a behavioral disorder characterized by dependence, involving deficient personal control of its consumption, growing tolerance to its effects, withdrawal, a desire to drink, and constant consumption, in addition to the numerous health and social problems that afflict drinkers.

Despite large subregional variations in per capita alcohol consumption, the average in the Americas, weighted by population, is 8.9 liters, well above the global average of 5.8 liters (*148*) (Table 26). Figure 25 shows alcohol consumption trends, by type of beverage, in Central and South America over the last 40 years. These trends reflect only recorded alcohol consumption and do not include home or clandestine production of alcoholic beverages, which are considered significant in the Region. The figures show that beer consumption is undergoing sustained growth, while wine consumption has fallen or stabilized. The consumption of distilled spirits has also increased over the years.

Several nations in the Region are major producers of alcoholic beverages, and the taxes on their sale represent a significant source of revenue for the respective national economies. Nevertheless, in countries such as the United States and Canada, where

earnings from alcohol are enormous, analysis of the costs of alcohol consumption indicates that they far exceed the revenues they generate. In the United States, the estimated economic cost of alcohol consumption in 1992 was US$ 148 billion, including more than US$ 19 billion spent on health care, but in 1998 it grew 25% to US$ 184.6 billion (*150*)—that is, approximately US$ 638 per capita. In Canada, the economic costs of alcohol consumption represent 2.7% of the GDP, equivalent to US$ 18.4 billion in 1992 (*151*). There are no similar studies available for the Region's developing countries.

It is estimated that in many of these latter countries, the consumption of alcohol produced or distilled illegally in the home, or smuggled as contraband, is on par with the consumption of commercially produced alcoholic beverages. This represents a challenge, both from an information perspective, since this consumption is difficult to record, and also from a public health perspective, since noncommercial alcohol production and its quality are not subject to any control. It is estimated that in most Latin American countries, 11%–55% of total alcohol consumption goes unrecorded (*152*).

Several interrelated factors combine to cause the harmful effects of alcohol. Alcohol consumption is characterized and measured by three important elements: the amount of alcohol consumed in one year, the amount consumed on a single occasion, and the context and circumstances under which it is consumed (*153*). In the Region, occasional excessive alcohol consumption is quite common. This represents a harmful pattern of consumption that damages health and translates into problems related to intentional and unintentional injuries, including homicides, traffic accidents, violence, drowning, falls, burns, poisoning, and suicides. At the same time, a significant proportion of people who have alcohol-related disorders, particularly dependence, over time present

TABLE 26. Alcohol consumption characteristics, by country, Region of the Americas, 2000.

Country	Per capita consumption[a]	Unrecorded consumption[b]	Drinking patterns[c]	Abstainers (%) Men	Abstainers (%) Women	Per capita consumption per drinker[d]
Argentina	16.3	1.0	2	7	21	19.0
Barbados	7.4	−0.5	2	29	70	14.8
Belize	6.4	2.0	4	24	44	9.7
Bolivia	5.7	3.0	3	24	45	8.7
Brazil	8.6	3.0	3	13	31	11.1
Canada	9.4	1.0	2	17	28	12.1
Chile	8.3	1.0	3	31	47	13.6
Colombia	8.3	2.0	3	31	47	13.6
Costa Rica	6.7	2.0	3	45	70	15.9
Cuba	5.7	2.0	2	29	70	11.4
Dominican Republic	5.7	1.0	2	12	35	7.5
Ecuador	5.5	3.7	3	41	67	12.0
El Salvador	4.6	2.0	4	9	38	6.0
Guatemala	3.7	2.0	4	49	84	11.2
Guyana	12.1	2.0	3	20	40	17.3
Haiti	5.4	0.0	2	58	62	13.5
Honduras	4.2	2.0	4	9	38	5.5
Jamaica	4.3	1.0	2	29	70	8.6
Mexico	8.2	4.0	4	36	65	16.7
Nicaragua	3.7	1.0	4	9	38	4.9
Paraguay	9.6	1.5	3	9	33	12.2
Peru	5.4	1.0	3	17	24	6.8
Suriname	6.0	0.0	3	30	55	10.5
Trinidad and Tobago	2.4	0.0	2	29	70	4.8
United States	9.5	1.0	2	28	43	14.8
Uruguay	9.5	2.0	3	25	43	14.4
Venezuela	9.6	2.0	3	30	55	16.8

[a]Liters of pure alcohol, including unrecorded consumption.

[b]Liters of pure alcohol.

[c]Hazardous drinking score, where 1 = least detrimental and 4 = most detrimental.

[d]Per capita consumption per drinker, in liters of pure alcohol, including unrecorded consumption.

Source: Rehm J, Monteiro M. Alcohol consumption and burden of disease in the Americas: implications for alcohol policy. Rev Panam Salud Pública 2005; 18(4/5): 241–248.

chronic health problems that ultimately translate into many years of life lost due to disability. All of this represents more than 50% of the total burden of disease related to alcohol. It is estimated that in Latin America and the Caribbean, more than 30 million people could be diagnosed with alcohol-related disorders, and more than 75% of this group have not received any medical care (*154*).

The widespread consumption of alcoholic beverages is associated with another wide range of consequences both for health and for society, including injuries related to sports and leisure activities, reduction of work productivity, various types of cancer, chronic liver disease, heart disease, and diseases of the central and peripheral nervous system. Alcohol-related problems also extend to other people, as occurs in domestic violence, child abuse, violent behavior, and the injuries or deaths of passengers in automobiles or of pedestrians caused by drivers under the influence of alcohol.

Drinking to the point of inebriation is a significant cause of alcohol-related injuries, causing the highest percentage of DALYs lost in all Latin American and Caribbean countries; it is also highly associated with unintentional injuries, negative social consequences, and a drop in industrial productivity. These negative consequences tend to have a particular impact on young people. While per capita alcohol consumption has decreased or stabilized in Canada and the United States, binge drinking, especially among young people, is on the rise in many of the Region's countries, including Mexico, Brazil, Peru, Bolivia, Uruguay, and Chile (*152*). In developing countries, young drinkers are adopting the consumption habits of their counterparts in developed countries (*155*). Young people run a higher risk than other age groups of being involved in accidents while driving under the influence of alcohol as well as engaging in violent behavior and having alcohol-related family problems.

FIGURE 25. Alcohol consumption among persons over age 15, by year and type of beverage, Central and South American countries, 1961–2003.

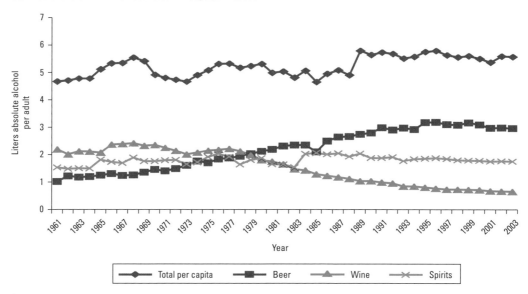

Source: Rehm J, Monteiro M. Alcohol consumption and burden of disease in the Americas: implications for alcohol policy. *Rev Panam Salud Pública* 2005; 18(4/5): 241–248.

Alcohol consumption is also associated with other high-risk behaviors, such as unprotected sexual relations or the use of other psychoactive substances. For this reason, alcohol use presents a high level of comorbidity with disorders caused by the use of other problem-causing substances, such as nicotine and illegal drugs. Recent studies also suggest an association between disorders caused by alcohol and HIV/AIDS and other sexually transmitted infections.

Finally, many of the social problems related to alcohol cannot be calculated precisely, but their repercussions are considered to have a very high cost for society in terms of neglect, suffering, destruction of the family environment, loss of family income (in addition to that caused by the loss of work productivity), psychological trauma in children of alcoholic parents, the long-term consequences of domestic violence, disruptions in community life, and academic failure, among others.

The Cultural Significance of Alcohol and Its Consumption in Indigenous Communities

In ancient civilizations throughout most of the Region of the Americas, alcoholic beverages were already known and consumed before contact with Europeans during the early 16th century. During their thousands of years of history, alcoholic beverages have been primarily produced locally, on a domestic scale or in small communities, using raw materials of local origin and traditional techniques passed from one generation to the next. These beverages, produced by the fermentation of grains, fruits,

or other organic substances, contained at most a low percentage of ethanol. They included wine, beer, hard cider, fermented yeast, and a variety of other beverages with ethyl alcohol content produced in specific geographical areas.

Beer, hard cider, *chicha* (a beverage made with fermented maize, traditionally consumed in Peru), and fermented yeast could not be preserved for long periods of time and means of transportation were limited, so what was produced locally was consumed relatively quickly. For the most part, these beverages were not sold in public marketplaces, but rather were consumed in the home, presented as symbols of generosity or hospitality, or shared in community festivals and religious celebrations and within the local trade circuits, to mark the end of the agricultural harvest or the completion of other types of collective undertakings. Alcohol production presupposes the existence of an agricultural surplus above the minimum necessary for subsistence. For this reason, and also given its potential to intoxicate, in many societies alcoholic beverages were considered special products: their consumption tended to be restricted to specific social classes of the population and certain political observances and religious ceremonies (*156*).

Later on during the 16th century, when distillation was discovered and spread on a commercial scale, the availability of alcoholic beverages increased substantially, and they could be accessed at any time of year, regardless of the season. Distilled beverages became a major part of colonial trade (*157*): rum flowed from the Caribbean to North America, and less expensive varieties of industrial alcohol, called commercial distilled spirits,

---

BOX 1. Brazilian City Reduces Alcohol-related Social Problems through Effective Legislation

The mayor of Diadema, an industrial city of nearly 400,000 inhabitants in the greater São Paulo area, submitted a bill in 2002 to require the city's 4,800 bars and restaurants to suspend sales of alcoholic beverages between the hours of 11 p.m. and 6 a.m. Since passage of this law, the number of homicides has dropped 47.4%; traffic accidents, 30%; violence against women, 55%; and the number of alcohol-related hospital admissions, 80%. Contrary to popular belief, after approval of the law, business activity intensified, investments increased, and job creation was stimulated. At least 120 additional municipalities have followed Diadema's example, and a similar law was recently passed in the State of Pernambuco. The Brazilian Federal Government is now offering additional financing for public order maintenance to municipalities that limit alcohol consumption and actively address urban violence issues (*162*).

---

were brought from Europe. Many of these beverages were distilled in the Region, including *aguardiente*, *cachaça* (a distilled beverage made from sugarcane, traditionally consumed in Brazil), *pulque*, and *pisco*.

Measures were frequently adopted to restrict and control the availability of alcohol: in tribal or rural societies, the consumption of alcoholic beverages tended to be limited to specific cultural celebrations and specific social hierarchies, as earlier noted. During colonization, alcohol was also used as a means of exploitation, so that the consumption of fermented beverages lost most of its cultural significance.

Over the intervening centuries, acculturation and close contact with nonindigenous and urban populations have led to widespread consumption of alcoholic beverages by indigenous groups, as well as serious social and health problems related to alcohol abuse and further aggravated by poverty. In 2002, Seale et al. (*158*) reported very high rates of alcohol use in an indigenous community in Venezuela—86.5% of males and 7.5% of females indicated that they drank excessively—while group discussions on this issue revealed that "traditional patterns of festive drinking of corn liquor had gradually been replaced by consumption of commercial beer and rum at more frequent intervals and with more negative social consequences."

In the indigenous communities of Bolivia, Brazil, Mexico, Nicaragua, and Panama, it has been reported that the consumption of alcohol was a long-established tradition, even before colonization (*159*), above all for therapeutic, medicinal, or ritual purposes, or together with food in certain celebrations. However, after colonization, the traditional beverages consumed by indigenous populations were gradually replaced by distilled beverages. Over time, alcohol consumption has increased and spread in indigenous communities, particularly among young males, who often drink until inebriated. The greater accessibility and availability of alcohol, as well as the lack of health, education, and other public services to address their basic needs, has combined with deficient

living and working conditions to produce high alcohol-related morbidity and mortality in these native communities (*160*).

In conclusion, cultural and social issues associated with alcohol have transcended its importance beyond the realm of being merely a commercial commodity (*161*), and although many people associate its consumption with pleasure and socializing, its use involves serious risks to personal health and social relationships (*152*). To address the risk posed to public health by the harmful effects of alcohol consumption, the development and implementation of coordinated, comprehensive, and effective strategies are required.

The Path Forward

Socioeconomic development tends to be associated with higher levels of alcohol consumption and the damages it causes, to the extent that people with higher disposable incomes will spend more on alcoholic beverages and drink excessively as accessibility and availability of alcoholic beverages increase (*161*). For those who live in poverty, the expenses represented by alcohol consumption can bankrupt the family's economy and greatly compromise opportunities for its members to obtain an adequate education, housing, nutrition, health care, and access to other goods and services (*160*). The advertising of alcohol and the low awareness level of the negative consequences of excessive drinking, combined with the absence of effective policies restricting the availability of alcoholic beverages and the lack of health services, leave those who abuse alcohol without the means to have their health needs addressed or choose healthier alternatives.

The information available is limited, but there is sufficient evidence that action must be taken both nationally and regionally. Prevention of the harmful effects related to alcohol, therefore, must be a public health priority in the Americas, and effective policies exist, as proven in countries in the Region and around the world (Box 1).

267

Effective policies to reduce alcohol-related mortality and disability also aim to reduce all forms of alcohol consumption through taxes and price controls and to limit alcohol's availability (e.g., times and points of sale, sales to minors). Policies can also focus on reducing specific types of cases, including legislation to prevent operating vehicles under the influence of alcohol, short interventions for young drinkers, and implementation of training programs to promote responsible alcoholic beverage service in public venues. Controlling the sale of alcoholic beverages to young people would support these policies and would help change the social norms related to alcohol consumption and abuse.

The following interventions are crucial for addressing the availability of and demand for alcoholic beverages, appropriate responses for treating the harmful social and health effects caused by alcohol abuse, and the need to create mechanisms to facilitate and consolidate efforts aimed at reducing its negative effects. These strategies are based on the latest data proving the efficacy of a wide range of policies against alcohol abuse, sponsored by WHO and published by Oxford University Press (*161*), and on an analysis of the cost-effectiveness of the various interventions in reducing alcohol-related mortality and morbidity (*163*).

- Create a system of taxes on alcohol expressly aimed at reducing the damages caused by its consumption and based on the products' alcohol content in order to provide a practical tool for increasing the cost of beverages in direct relation to their potential to produce harmful effects.
- Establish legal and regulatory mechanisms for the production, importation, retail sale, availability, and consumption of alcoholic beverages, including a minimum age for the consumption and purchase of alcoholic beverages; restrictions related to times, days, and points of sale; a license concession system to regulate wholesale and retail sales of alcoholic beverages, providing mechanisms to sanction those who sell them for any action that promotes or encourages damage to health and the negative social consequences of alcohol abuse; importation permits; control of illegal sales; and quality standards for production of alcoholic beverages.
- Appropriately strengthen agencies responsible for enforcing the laws and regulations regarding alcohol consumption.
- Consider alcoholic beverages as goods subject to special treatment in international trade agreements in order to reinforce national and local capacity in public health matters and control of alcohol markets.
- Use marketing campaigns to better inform the general public regarding the dangers of inebriation, driving under the influence of alcohol, and excessive consumption during pregnancy, among other things.
- Entrust a governmental or independent agency with the responsibility of monitoring and enforcing regulations and prohibitions related to advertising and promoting alcoholic beverages in the print media and on radio, television, the In-

ternet, and public signage, as well as at cultural, youth, and sporting events, paying particular attention to messages targeted to young people.
- Develop integrated interventions for the early detection of drinking problems and how to effectively address them and disseminate these at all primary health care services.
- Develop treatment methods for the various types of alcohol-related problems and integrate these into the general health system, ensuring their accessibility to vulnerable populations.
- Discourage driving under the influence of alcohol by measuring blood alcohol concentration (BAC) and establishing a low ceiling (BAC from 0%–0.05%) for drivers, adopting zero tolerance policies for new drivers who drink, as well as random blood alcohol testing, sobriety checkpoints, and suspension of drivers' licenses by simple administrative order.
- Develop information systems to monitor alcohol consumption and related problems as a way to provide input for the implementation of policy changes and enable an evaluation of their effectiveness.
- Support and finance local organizations in defining community-level social action strategies to address alcohol-related problems.

VIOLENCE

Intentional and Unintentional Injuries

In the Region of the Americas, violence and unintentional injuries entail particularly high costs associated with mortality, morbidity, and injuries. Intentional injuries, or injuries related to violence, may be interpersonal (homicide), self-inflicted (suicide), or collective. Unintentional injuries include those caused by traffic accidents, drowning, falls, burns, and poisoning.

The WHO *World Report on Violence and Health*, in broad terms, defines violence as "the intentional use of physical force or power, threatened or actual, against oneself, another person, or against a group or community, that either results in or has a high likelihood of resulting in injury, death, psychological harm, maldevelopment or deprivation" (*164*). This includes physical, sexual, or psychological harm, as well as that caused by deprivation, and is applied to domestic violence, primarily against children, women, and the elderly; violence inflicted by and against young people; and the various forms of group violence carried out for political, economic, or social reasons. A complex interaction of individual, relational, social, cultural, and environmental factors makes the Region of the Americas one of the most violent in the world. The ecological model included in the *World Report* aims to identify risk factors, including the high level of cultural tolerance for violence, the weakness of court systems, and social inequalities. In the area of individual and family relations, a history of having been a victim or witness to violence, family violence, and peer pressure are well-known risk factors for future violent behavior.

According to official figures, in the last decade there were between 110,000 and 120,000 homicides and between 55,000 and 58,000 suicides in the Region (*165*). Various studies have shed light on the factors that contribute to creating a climate that incites violence. Specialized studies indicate that the risk of women becoming victims of violence increases when they have five or more children, a family history of violence, economic problems, a lack of work, lack of education, or live in marginal, unsafe neighborhoods in urban areas (*166*). With respect to youth violence, the factors that increase the risk of young people engaging in violent behavior include dropping out of primary school, a lack of job opportunities, having a dysfunctional family, and having been victim or witness to violence in the family environment (*167, 168*). Moreover, while most victims of homicide are males aged 15–44 (*169, 170*), victims of nonfatal violence are generally women, children, and the elderly. At the individual, family, community, and national levels, violence has become the norm, and since violence is to a large extent a learned behavior, the cycle continues from one generation to the next.

In general, public financial resources to combat violence tend to be used to fight crime. The costs related to violence represent more than 12% of the GDP annually, exceeding the percentage of investments in health and education (*171, 172*).

Homicides

Homicide is a crime that consists of killing another person. The WHO definition expands this concept, which is described in the *International Classification of Diseases and Related Health Problems, Tenth Revision* (ICD-10) as "injuries inflicted by another person with the intent to injure or kill, by any means" and excludes injuries due to legal intervention and operations of war (*173*). Although there are a significant number of unrecorded cases, according to the data considered, in the Americas, Colombia has the highest reported rate per 100,000 population in the last two decades. However, rates have fallen significantly in recent years, from 64 per 100,000 in 2001 to 50 per 100,000 in 2003 and, finally, to 38 per 100,000 in 2005. Most of the victims and perpetrators were males from urban areas, and many of the violent deaths were the result of the ongoing armed conflict (*170, 174*). The decrease in deaths is due primarily to two factors: first, the Government's initiative to advance negotiations aimed at demobilizing the paramilitary organizations, and thus reducing politically related homicides; and second, the implementation of sustainable urban programs that promote peaceful coexistence and mutual respect, especially in Bogotá and Medellín, where intensive programs have been undertaken to improve city culture, reduce crime and violence, and reestablish coexistence and the urban infrastructure (*175, 176*). This series of violence prevention programs and projects resulted in a marked decline in the homicide rates per 100,000 population, which went from 80 per 100,000 in 1995 to 21 per 100,000 in 2005 (*177*).

> " *Air, water, and soil pollution and the exposure to toxic substances are the principal environmental health risk factors associated with development.* "
>
> Carlyle Guerra de Macedo, 1988

The homicide rates in Brazil, which increased from 11.4 to 28.4 per 100,000 population between 1980 and 2002, are among the highest in the Region. In 2000, 28% of all homicides in the Americas took place in Brazil. Young and adult males are the most frequent victims. In general, in the most populous cities, the homicide rates tend to be higher than the rate for the entire country. Thus, for example, while in the 1980–2002 period the homicide rate per 100,000 population more than doubled in all of Brazil, in São Paulo it tripled (*178*).

In Puerto Rico, homicides constitute the 12th leading cause of death, but the fifth among males. Between 1999 and 2003 the homicide rate per 100,000 population was 47.7 for males and 3.5 for females. Urban areas are the most frequent venues, and firearms the most common means. Contributing factors include high population density and urbanization, illicit drug use, drug trafficking, political violence, and organized crime. Trends in the homicide rate vary among countries. While homicide rates in the 15–29-year-old age group have fallen in the United States from 21.6 to 13.4 per 100,000 population, in Puerto Rico they have surged from 49.8 in 1999 to 54.1 in 2003. The Puerto Rican Government and the Center for Hispanic Youth Violence Prevention are working to address this problem by improving law enforcement and implementing educational programs (*179*).

In Central America, El Salvador and Guatemala have homicide rates above 30 per 100,000 population (Figure 26). In recent years, these countries have implemented "firm hand" or "iron hand" policies aimed at controlling and reducing crime, more specifically that of the youth gangs known as *maras*. However, these policies have not achieved the expected effect, since between 2000 and 2005 the homicide rates in Guatemala increased from 20.0 to 27.0 per 100,000 population (*180*). El Salvador experienced a decrease from 62.5 to 54.9 by 2005 (*181*). Despite problems in data collection systems, Honduras reported a homicide rate of nearly 53 per 100,000 population for 2005.

In contrast, other Central American countries have lower homicide rates. Between 2001 and 2005, Costa Rica's rates ranged between 5.6 and 7.2 (*182*); in Belize they fell from 21.0 to 15.4 (*183*); in Panama they fluctuated between 10.3 and 11.9 (*184*); and in Nicaragua they increased from 7.3 to 9.5.

Over the last 30 years, in Jamaica, the homicide rate has undergone sustained growth, reaching 45 per 100,000 population in 2004 (*185*); most victims were males aged 15–44 and residents of urban areas, and firearms and sharp objects were the methods most commonly used. It is important to point out that the homi-

FIGURE 26. Homicide rates per 100,000 inhabitants, selected Central American countries, 1996–2005.

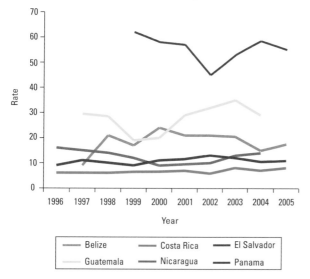

Source: Based on data from references 179–183 from this chapter.

cides were primarily related to fights or revenge rather than gang violence or assaults. In Jamaica, the cost of violence is enormous, with approximately US$ 10 million lost due to injuries related to violence and US$ 225 million lost due to all consequences of violence (*186*). In Venezuela, the homicide rate per 100,000 population increased from 19.4 in 1998 to 50.9 in 2003. Young males, particularly those living in the most vulnerable areas, are the most affected (*187*).

Youth Violence

Gang violence is currently one of the most visible forms of youth violence in the Region of the Americas. Between 20% and 50% of all violent crimes are attributed to gangs (*164, 181*), with gang-related homicide rates in El Salvador reaching nearly 50 per 100,000 population. Gangs generally display violent and criminal behavior, and their members are not concerned with concealing their identity or about the consequences of their actions (*188*).

In general, gang members are young, poor, and marginalized, from urban areas, outside the school system, have no work, and have experienced violence in the past (*169, 189, 190*). Migration to large cities, the lack of social options and of gun control, the inefficiency of security forces, corruption, and drug trafficking are factors that contribute to the growth and increased activity of youth gangs.

The increased violence of gangs seems to coincide with the end of the armed conflicts in Central America during the 1990s (*191, 192*). The epicenter of gang activity is El Salvador, Guatemala, and Honduras. However, the increased complexity of youth

gangs' organization, transnational and cross-border implications, migration, and the Region's deportation criteria make this an international issue. Police estimate that there are between 25,000 and 70,000 active gang members, whose sphere of influence extends beyond their urban zones to the most remote corners of Central America (*193*).

In response to the growing problem of youth violence, PAHO, with the support of the German Agency for Technical Cooperation, has executed the Promotion of Youth Development and Violence Prevention project in six Latin American countries: Argentina, Colombia, El Salvador, Honduras, Nicaragua, and Peru. This project proposed lines of action based on the following five governing principles: developing and executing interventions based on confirmed data and theoretical concepts, and evaluating them; stressing the promotion of health and well-being in the prevention of violence; leveraging human and material resources already existing in the respective countries and at the local level; using a gender-based perspective; and including the participation of young people and the entire community in the development of policies and programs. There is already significant documentation on the national and regional scale showing the progress of this initiative and the problems it is addressing (*194*).

Internal Population Displacement due to Violence

Colombia is the only country in the Region where massive internal population displacements are occurring (close to 2 million people over the last decade) as a result of the extended armed conflict that has affected the country for more than 40 years. The "displaced by violence" category was legally adopted by the Colombian Government in 1997 with Law 387, which defined a displaced person as "any person who has been forced to migrate within the national territory . . . because his or her life, physical integrity, security, or personal freedom has been violated or is directly threatened by domestic armed conflict, domestic disturbances and tension, widespread violence, massive violations of human rights, violations of international humanitarian law, or other circumstances" (*195*). The number of people displaced by violence reached its peak in 2004, when 424,863 persons were forced to abandon their homes (*196*). The PAHO/WHO Country Office in Colombia has created a "Health and Displacement" Web site (*197*), where it provides health situation information about the displaced population.

Information Systems on Violence and Injuries

The need for regional data on the magnitude of violence, its trends, and the effectiveness of prevention strategies is increasingly important, yet acquiring reliable information remains a challenge. As is the case with many reports on disease, data related to violence tend to be quite limited, contradictory, and, depending on the sector and the source, of relatively low quality.

Despite these deficiencies, existing data systems present several positive characteristics. For violence and injuries mortality data, there is general agreement to classify them by systematically applying the *International Classification of Diseases*. Several countries have become leaders in the field of data collection, with initiatives ranging from the use of a detailed, Internet-based notification results dissemination system, being monitored by El Salvador with the help of PAHO, to the use by police in Costa Rica of a satellite positioning system to locate the exact point where a traffic accident took place. Other countries, such as Brazil, have long had complex data collection systems providing information on traffic accident victims to a classification and distribution center. Finally, in many of the Region's countries, constructive dialogue and collective information systems have been established among the various agencies that collect data on injuries, including the local ministries of health and transportation and the police, to improve the quality and interpretation of the data included in them. It is encouraging that a growing number of countries recognize the need to have broad data systems, and political decision-makers should take these aspects into consideration when preparing new plans to address the issue of injuries.

Information Systems of Injuries from External Causes: Successful Initiatives

Surveillance Systems in Hospital Emergency Departments in Colombia, El Salvador, and Nicaragua

Since 2001, PAHO, together with the U.S. National Center for Injury Prevention and Control of the CDC, has been working with health authorities in Colombia, El Salvador, and Nicaragua to implement injury surveillance systems in hospital emergency departments. To do this, they are following WHO and CDC guidelines (*198*), based on the International Classification of Causes of Injury (*199*). The objective is to highlight the magnitude and impact of these injuries on health services. The information is used to promote the development of evidence-based injury prevention strategies. The surveillance system is being applied in 16 hospitals in Colombia, eight in El Salvador, and six in Nicaragua. Argentina, Brazil, Honduras, Jamaica, Peru, and Trinidad and Tobago also have hospital surveillance systems that apply similar methodologies and processes.

In hospital emergencies, a form is used to record the patient's medical history, and on it demographic data and other circumstances related to the event are collected daily, such as the intentionality, modus operandi, where the event took place, and what the victim was doing at the time. It contains three modules with variables for injuries related to 1) traffic accidents (information regarding the person(s) and vehicle involved), 2) interpersonal violence (relationship of the perpetrator to the victim), and 3) self-inflicted violence (triggering factors). Clinical information (location and seriousness of the injuries) and the assignment of the patient within the institution are also entered on the form. There is also space to record whether there are suspicions about alcohol or drug abuse. The flowchart presented in Figure 27 shows the steps taken in emergency rooms to gather and monitor patient data.

This system has determined that between 10% and 50% of all emergencies treated in national- and departmental-level hospitals are for injuries from external causes. It has also highlighted that injuries from external causes constitute a major public health problem and has raised awareness among the health authorities regarding the need to adopt public policies aimed at preventing them. In Nicaragua, in the summer, when large segments of the population travel to vacation in beach locales, the "Happy, Safe, and Healthy Summer" plan is implemented, and an intersectoral coordination committee made up of public and private entities and community organizations monitors injuries and supports preventive measures. The PAHO/WHO Country Office in El Salvador, in coordination with the Ministry of Public Health and Social Welfare, has created a computerized information program on injuries from external causes that is linked to a Web-based morbidity-mortality system into which the country's hospitals input information daily.

Observatories on Mortality Caused by External Injuries

Based on a model developed in 1993 in Cali, Colombia, where an intersectoral committee consisting of representatives of institutions that routinely recorded data on mortality caused by injuries from external causes met to share, unify, analyze, and disseminate relevant information about each victim of homicide, suicide, a traffic accident, or other unintentional causes, a series of violence observatories have been established, currently the responsibility of Instituto CISALVA (*200*) of Universidad del Valle, a PAHO/WHO Collaboration Center. The observatory operating in Pasto, Colombia, also records data on domestic violence from various sources as well as hospital surveillance. The Colombian model is also being implemented in various municipalities in El Salvador, Panama, and Nicaragua.

ROAD SAFETY

Since 1896, when the world's first fatality caused by a motor vehicle was reported, there is no doubt that human mobility has undergone a major transformation. While technological advances have improved the population's living conditions by cutting travel times and distances, they have also greatly increased the number and types of risks to human life, often resulting in injuries and death.

Among unintentional injuries, those caused by motor vehicles are at the top of the list. Globally, according to the *World Report on Road Traffic Injury Prevention* by WHO and the World Bank, "in 2002, nearly 1.2 million people died worldwide as a result of road traffic injuries, which represents an average of 3,242 persons

FIGURE 27. Flowchart for the hospital emergency injury surveillance system.

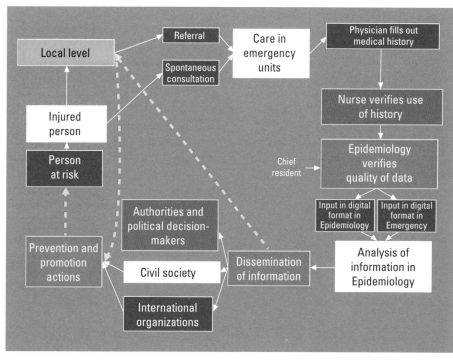

Source: Pan American Health Organization, Area of Sustainable Development and Environmental Health.

dying each day around the world from road traffic injuries" (*201*). In the Americas, approximately 130,000 individuals die each year, more than 1.2 million are injured, and hundreds of thousands are disabled as a result of collisions, crashes, or road accidents (*202*).

In 2002, the Region recorded 2,055,000 traffic-related injuries, with an average mortality rate of 16 per 100,000 population, ranging from 6.8 per 100,000 in Bolivia to 24.0 per 100,000 in Guatemala (*203*) (Table 27). Although most are avoidable, the lack of permanent, consistent policies compatible with the situation of each country further aggravates the problem. The existence of road infrastructure and vehicles in poor condition; inadequate knowledge and inappropriate conduct by drivers; alcohol abuse and other pervasive, risky social norms and behaviors; and lack of efficient emergency medical services are contributing factors.

Each road traffic injury generates short-, medium-, and long-term repercussions. The costs to society, families, and the health sector are considerable. Reports from some Latin American countries show the tremendous costs linked to roadway crashes.

At the family level, the aftereffects are oftentimes more acute. Injuries or death can bring about the total loss of a family's means of economic support, in addition to emotional pain. In Mexico, the loss of parents to accidents is the second leading cause of children being orphaned (*204*). Injuries caused by transit also constitute a source of stress on the legal system, a manifestation of the deterioration of public safety.

Who Has Accidents?

Users of public roads. Injuries caused by motor vehicles affect four categories of users of public roadways: pedestrians, occupants of motor vehicles (drivers and passengers), bicyclists, and motorcyclists. There are marked regional and national differences in the distribution of injuries (Figure 28). Low income countries in Latin America have a particularly complex mix of public roadway users; pedestrians and high-technology motor vehicles share the road with old and poorly maintained vehicles, in addition to bicycles, motorcycles, pushcarts, and vehicles drawn by animals. Roadway design is focused more on the needs of the motor vehicle traffic flow than on those of nonmotorized users. There are no legal regulations or social norms that facilitate sharing the streets and roads. This results in pedestrians, bicyclists, and motorcyclists becoming the most frequent victims of traffic accidents in developing countries.

Country data on the distribution of deaths by type of roadway user show the vulnerability of pedestrians in Latin America and the Caribbean, while the problem in Canada and the United States revolves largely around vehicle occupants.

Gender. In accordance with global trends, road collisions have a disproportionate impact on males throughout the Americas: in the last decade, between 75% and 80% of deaths were among

TABLE 27. Mortality caused by traffic accidents, selected countries, Region of the Americas, 2000–2006.

Country	Rate (per 100,000 population)	Year
Argentina	9.5	2002
Belize	26.7	2006
Bolivia	6.8	2003
Brazil	19.9	2004
Canada	9.0	2003
Chile	9.9	2002
Colombia	11.8	2005
Costa Rica	14.2	2004
Cuba	10.6	2003
Ecuador	15.6	2000
El Salvador	16.9	2005
Guatemala	24.0	2005
Jamaica	14.8	2003
Mexico	15.0	2001
Nicaragua	9.1	2005
Panama	13.2	2006
Peru	10.5	2003
Trinidad and Tobago	14.9	2003
United States of America	14.6	2000
Venezuela	22.7	2002

Sources: Argentina, Ministerio de Salud, Dirección de Estadísticas e Información de Salud. (Argentina)

Taller de Sistemas de Vigilancia de Lesiones de Causa Externa con énfasis en el Tránsito. El Salvador, 30–31 January 2007. (Belize, El Salvador, Guatemala, Panama)

Seminario Internacional sobre Seguridad Vial, Organización Panamericana de la Salud, Brasilia, 28–30 June 2004. (Bolivia, Brazil, Colombia, Costa Rica, Cuba, Jamaica, Mexico, Nicaragua, Peru)

Canada, Statistics Canada. Age-standardized mortality rates by selected causes, by sex. Available from: http://www40.statcan.ca/l01/cst01/health30a.htm. Accessed on 27 February 2007. (Canada)

Chile, Comisión Nacional de Seguridad de Tránsito; Instituto Nacional de Estadística (INE). (Chile)

Ecuador, Instituto Nacional de Estadística y Censos. 2001. (Ecuador)

Trinidad and Tobago, Ministry of Planning and Development, Central Statistical Office. Available from: http://www.cso.gov.tt/statistics/psvs/default.asp. Accessed on 11 June 2004. (Trinidad and Tobago)

Maynard M. Death rate on highways rises, and motorcycles are blamed. The New York Times. 23 August 2006. (United States)

FIGURE 28. Traffic accident mortality, by type of road user,[a] selected countries, Region of the Americas, 2000–2003.

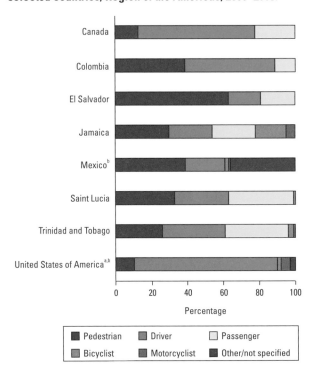

[a]Roadway user categories are not homogeneous for all countries.
[b]The data from Mexico and the United States do not differentiate between drivers and passengers; therefore, the portion of the bars for these two countries representing drivers corresponds to the total number of drivers and passengers deceased.
Sources: Canada, 2002: Canadian Motor Vehicle Traffic Collision Statistics, 2002, http://www.tc.gc.ca/roadsafety/tp/tp3322/2002/page3.htm.
Colombia, 2002: National Institute of Legal Medicine.
El Salvador, 2003: National policy registry.
Jamaica, 2003: Ministry of Health and Jamaica Constabulary Force.
Mexico, 2000: Consejo Nacional de Prevención de Accidentes.
Saint Lucia, 2001: Traffic Department, Royal Saint Lucia Police Force.
Trinidad and Tobago, 2003: Carr BA. Spotlight on motor vehicle injury and deaths in Trinidad and Tobago (1998–2003). PAHO; 2004.
United States, 2002: National Highway Traffic Safety Administration.

males, and between 20% and 25% were among women. Injuries caused by traffic accidents were the eighth leading cause of death among males and the 14th among females, and the roadway mortality rate was 23.9 per 100,000 population for males, three times higher than the rate for females of 7.7 per 100,000 population. Furthermore, in 2002, these injuries were the sixth leading cause of DALYs lost among males (3,109,083) and the 14th among females (1,141,861) (*201*).

Age distribution. In the distribution of deaths caused by road traffic in the Americas by age group in 2002, adults aged 15–29 represented 32% of the burden of mortality caused by road traf-

fic accidents, followed by adults aged 30–44, with 25%. In Argentina, adults aged 15–24 had the highest proportion (one in five) of traffic-related deaths during the 1993–2002 period (*205*). In Colombia, the higher rates of traffic-related deaths corresponded to adults aged 60 and older. Among females, those 60 and older were also the most affected (23% of total deaths), followed by females aged 25–34 (15%) (*206*). In Venezuela, adults aged 20–44 represented more than 50% of all traffic-related deaths between 1993 and 2002. The proportion of deaths among children aged 0–14 in Venezuela fell slightly, from 13% in 1993 to 10% in 2003; at the same time, the proportion of deaths among adults aged 45–59 increased (*207*).

In Cuba, more than half the traffic-related deaths between 1993 and 2002 were adults aged 19–44 (*208*). In Trinidad and Tobago, traffic accidents were the second leading cause of death among adults aged 15–34 in 1999 (*209*). In Costa Rica, the proportion of traffic-related deaths for adults aged 60 and older has fallen since the early 1990s from 22% of all deaths in 1993 to 15% in 2002 (after experiencing a slight upturn in 1999 and 2000) (*210*). This trend in the Americas is consistent with global trends. Despite the fact that the population aged 15–59 are the most economically productive, and, consequently, their death or disability has major repercussions on each country's economic and social costs, the highest mortality rates in the Region in 2002 were for the population over age 60: for males, 35.2 per 100,000 population, and for females, 14.4 per 100,000 (*211*).

Strategies for Improving Road Safety

Traffic-planning strategies to address this problem have followed the traditional methods used in developed countries already familiar with this serious phenomenon. The persistence of deficient road safety conditions, however, highlights the inadequacy of the prevailing available strategies.

New ideas and interventions are required to make road traffic more equitable and safe. To find the most appropriate solutions, rather than considering the primary factors in isolation (the public road user, roadway, and vehicles), it is essential to consider the broad physical, political, institutional, technical, and law enforcement context as a whole as well as its influence on road safety.

In developing countries, in terms of road safety, the entire road traffic context is dangerous for all forms of transportation but primarily for pedestrians, bicyclists, and motorcyclists, and this fact has a profound influence on the nature and number of traffic accidents. The political context also affects road traffic safety, since the decision-making process and the policies adopted tend to favor motor vehicles. The institutional context, characterized by its placing of responsibility for roadway policy in the hands of the regional authority and not municipal administrators, has represented an obstacle for local investment and the adoption of solutions more closely linked to local problems and needs. The technical context also plays an important role. Transportation and road traffic planners belong to agencies with a strict technical tradition and often neglect broader social approaches to problems; they are not required to prioritize safety and cannot be held legally responsible for the safety consequences of the plans they develop.

Another problem for improving traffic planning is the lack of reliable data relating to accidents and their victims, from various sectors, such as transportation, police, and health care. The conditions under which laws and regulations are or are not enforced also contribute to maintaining high rates of accidents and traffic-related deaths. Traffic laws and regulations are applied, above all, with an emphasis on optimizing traffic flow, but this can in no way imply negligence in their strict enforcement and in the effective punishment of offenders (*212*).

Intervention and Prevention

PAHO's work to prevent injuries caused by traffic accidents is based on the primary recommendations of the earlier-mentioned WHO report (*201*) as well as those arising from international conferences and consultations. In summary, these recommendations are to identify a governing body; evaluate the problem, the policies, and the institutional environment; prepare a national strategy and plan of action; allocate human and financial resources to address the problem; take specific actions and support the development of national capacity and international cooperation; define objectives; improve legislation and insurance coverage for the most vulnerable; and effectively ensure that public spaces (e.g., streets and roads) respond to the population's needs and ensure care for the victims. In October 2005, the United Nations General Assembly approved a resolution establishing the organization, between 23 and 29 April 2007, of activities around the world aimed at demonstrating the need to develop and apply plans aimed at reducing road traffic injuries.

Immediate professional care of road traffic victims saves lives. In Venezuela, the Interministerial Commission for Road Traffic Care, Prevention, and Education; the Ministry of Health and Social Development; and the Venezuelan Society of Public Health coordinate the Program to Prevent Accidents and Other Violent Acts, one objective of which is to improve the care for victims (*207*). In Mexico, the National Accident Prevention Council has developed a prehospital care model, with an Emergency Medical Management Center serving as the base for organizing, standardizing, categorizing, providing, and evaluating quality, equitable emergency medical care (*213*). Peru has organized emergency care networks and is making progress on the recording and epidemiological surveillance system that provides valuable data to improve care and prevention strategies (*214*).

Thus, there is a body of knowledge on successful experiences, as well as others that have failed, that must be considered when defining policies to address these problems. It is clear that successful experiences can be replicated if the context and situation in which they will be implemented are taken into account. Road safety is one component of public safety, and its objective is to protect all people, including tourists. Consequently, road safety issues concern both government officials and the general population. People feel safe not only when their life, well-being, property, and dignity are not threatened by acts of crime and violence, but also when they can enjoy public spaces without the risk of road traffic injuries.

HEALTH PROMOTION

Recognition of the need to address the social determinants of health, the renewal of the primary care strategy, and new currents in thought on public health have revolutionized the debate on social processes and their effects on health and facilitated the emergence of an approach that promotes health through public policy formulation (*215*).

The Ottawa Charter for Health Promotion (Canada, 1986) (*216*), by reinforcing the principles adopted in 1978 at the International Conference on Primary Health Care in Alma-Ata (Kazakhstan) and the theories on the determining social factors for health, had a positive influence on health policies and programs (*217*). PAHO's concept of health promotion is based on the Ottawa Charter, which is defined as "the process of enabling people to increase control over, and to improve, their health." Therefore, health promotion actions must be oriented toward the various areas of daily life and must be supported by public policies that influence social conditions and lifestyles, which, in turn, take shape as healthy behaviors. The conceptual framework of health promotion is based on the principles established in the Ottawa Charter and further developed by subsequent international and regional summits, such as the Adelaide Recommendations on Healthy Public Policy (Australia, 1988), the Sundsvall Statement on Supportive Environments for Health (Sweden, 1991), the Bogotá Declaration on Health Promotion and Equity (Colombia, 1992), the Caribbean Charter for Health Promotion (Trinidad and Tobago, 1993), the Jakarta Declaration on Leading Health Promotion into the Twenty-first Century (Indonesia, 1997), the Mexico Ministerial Statement for the Promotion of Health: From Ideas to Action (2000), the Health Promotion Forum in the Americas (Chile, 2002), and the Bangkok Charter for Health Promotion in a Globalized World (Thailand, 2005).

The health promotion strategy has been placed on the agenda of the PAHO Governing Bodies by Resolution CD37.R14 (PAHO 1994) and the Regional Plan of Action for Health Promotion in the Americas CE113/15 (PAHO 1994), as well as Resolution CD43.R11 and the accompanying document CD43/14 (PAHO 2001). The issue of health promotion has also been established within the subregional integration processes, through RESSCAD and the health ministers of Central America and the Dominican Republic, and REMSAA, its counterpart in the Andean subregion.

Diseases whose origins are more associated with people's behaviors and lifestyles are the leading causes of morbidity and mortality. Addictions, obesity, sedentary lifestyles, inadequate nutrition, and domestic violence are some of the risk factors whose effects are being felt with growing intensity. Few countries have adopted effective health policies and measures to modify these risky behaviors, despite numerous health education programs and various social communications campaigns undertaken in many nations. The scant positive results are due in part to the persistence of approaches based on programs operating in vertical and linear health services focused on a single factor and having little community participation. The medicalized model continues to have a disproportionate influence, based on an approach focused on the disease and on the individual risk factors which fails to consider the influence of the social conditions and determinants of health. Health interventions must consider the increased complexity of today's problems and strengthen intersectoral work.

The health promotion movement faces a complex context in the Region of the Americas. On the one hand is the conceptual development of a new approach to public health, and on the other is a context of social development in countries with profound inequalities. The integration of health promotion was initially based on experiences and proposals that arise in developed countries faced with a reality of poverty and inequalities. This contradiction with the reality of the systems became even more profound during the 1990s in countries undergoing structural changes in their health services. Nevertheless, the new social perspective on health has influenced academic thought and some health policies and programs with various methods and levels of depth.

The Bogotá Declaration (1992) (*218*) highlighted the aspects of equity and violence and was aimed at a proposal of intersectoral health management with the leadership of the health sector. Since that time, countries such as Argentina, Brazil, Costa Rica, Chile, Cuba, Mexico, and Peru have developed more integrated care models and adopted a more preventive approach in public health interventions (*219*). The health situation in the Caribbean laid the groundwork for the Caribbean Charter (1993), which underscores the importance of the strategy of chronic diseases prevention and maintenance of healthy lifestyles. The core issue addressed in the Mexico Ministerial Statement (2000) encourages governments to take active leadership with vision, ensuring the commitment of the public and private sectors and civil society in the development of public policies and plans for activities that benefit health, all with the objective of undertaking public health interventions that strengthen the potential for people's health with an ecological approach and applying the principles of equity, justice, democracy, the creation of conditions for full social participation, and intersectoral cooperation (*220*). The Mexico Ministerial Statement established a commitment to place health promotion on international political and development agendas, a commitment reaffirmed in the Bangkok Charter and in various WHO and PAHO resolutions.

In fulfillment of the Mexico Statement and the 2001 PAHO Resolution CD43.R11, a progress report was drafted on health promotion in the Region of the Americas. The preliminary version of this analysis was presented at the Health Promotion Forum in the Americas, held in Santiago, Chile, in 2002. Subsequently, a survey was conducted to assess the institutional capacity for health promotion development, organized into parts I and II, in which 28 and 27 countries in the Region participated, respectively. The results of these surveys were presented at the 6th Global Conference on Health Promotion, held in Bangkok, Thailand, in 2005. In part I, the survey proposes eight key fields or areas for monitoring national capacity in health promotion: 1) policies and plans; 2) core competencies and capacities; 3) cooperation mechanisms within the government; 4) services (pro-

FIGURE 29. Profile of institutional capacity for health promotion development in the Region of the Americas, 2005.

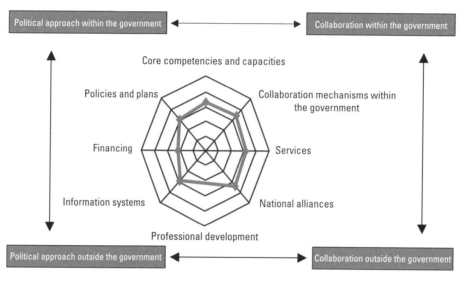

Source: Institutional capacity map for health promotion development. Part I of survey; *N* = 28 countries.

gram execution); 5) alliances between the government, the private sector, and nongovernmental organizations; 6) professional development; 7) information systems; and 8) financing for health promotion. In general terms, the results of this preliminary analysis are heterogeneous and show that some countries have weaknesses related to policies and plans, professional development, information systems, and financing. Figure 29 shows the general profile of the institutional capacity for health promotion in the Region. The analysis of the data and results of part II permitted a more detailed mapping of national capacity in health promotion in critical areas, including plans of action, public policies, reorientation of health services, civic participation, and advocacy networks.

The results of part II of the survey indicated that in about 45% of the countries, health promotion holds a relevant position in national public policy and that fewer than half the countries have a political or legal framework that supports health promotion (Figure 30).

This analysis also shows that the countries in the Region have used different approaches for the development and application of healthy public policies and that the approaches respond to different social, political, and economic circumstances. For example, Brazil has adopted the participatory budget model and has taken actions to adapt and implement public health policy demonstration areas at the municipal level, with the support of the municipal and state health boards. Argentina has stimulated a profound debate on the impact of the economy on health determinants, which has strengthened its social policies and furthered tobacco control policies and the training of health care personnel in health

promotion competencies. Chile has implemented the health promotion policy known as Vida Chile, with an intersectoral approach aimed at improving health determinants. Brazil, Canada, Paraguay, and Uruguay have developed specific policies to address the health risks posed by tobacco, alcohol, and the lack of road safety. Barbados has established social participation mechanisms for the establishment of policies through public consultations at the national and community levels. The United States has encouraged civic participation through the establishment of its Healthy People 2010 public policy. In Trinidad and Tobago, acts and national policies were approved to promote health with broad-based community involvement.

The creation of environments that favor health has gained enormous momentum over the past decade. In 95% of the countries surveyed, some initiative is under way to create healthy environments, and in 70% of the countries there are strategic plans at the municipal level. The initiative is based on both the political commitment of mayors and other local authorities and on the active participation of citizens to define their collective needs and establish local plans to address them (*221*). Nevertheless, although most healthy cities and municipalities have intersectoral plans and full community participation, the monitoring, development, and evaluation of evidence regarding these issues continue to represent a major challenge. Only 35% of the countries reported that the initiatives to create healthy environments have been evaluated (*222*).

The establishment of networks and alliances has been a key factor in the dissemination and exchange of experiences between municipalities and countries. In 75% of the countries surveyed,

FIGURE 30. Distribution of thematic areas of health promotion, Region of the Americas.

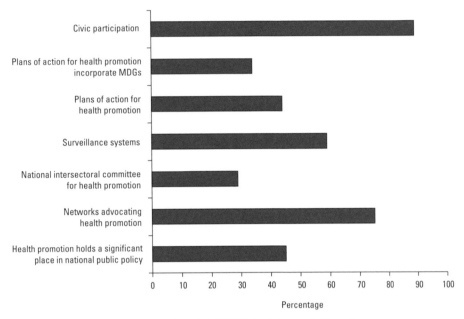

Source: Institutional capacity map and comparative analysis 2002–2005. Part II of survey; *N* = 27 countries.

there are health promotion advocacy networks (Figure 30). Networks promoting the creation of healthy cities and municipalities are one example of best practices, since through intersectoral work they have improved health conditions in many urban areas. While the regional network has been difficult to sustain, national networks in Argentina, Chile, Costa Rica, Cuba, Mexico, Paraguay, and Peru have proven their sustainability over time. The Safe and Healthy Sister Cities initiative implemented along the U.S.-Mexico border area is an example of cooperation to resolve problems requiring a bilateral approach. This network of cities, formed out of the building of alliances between local governments with the social participation of stakeholders from a variety of sectors, has had great success. The action plans are structured based on binational agreements and are planned and evaluated by the community.

Complementing and enhancing the healthy cities and municipalities concept are the health-promoting schools and healthy housing strategies, which similarly have been the fruit of the work of networks and alliances and effective community participation.

The health-promoting schools (HPS) strategy promotes the development of knowledge, abilities, and skills in the school environment aimed at minimizing risky behaviors and supporting the adoption of healthy lifestyles. Based on the results of a survey conducted in 2001 in 19 countries in the Region, 53% of the participating countries reported having adopted this strategy. Among them, Canada, Chile, Colombia, El Salvador, and Mexico are implementing the initiative nationally. Based on the information obtained in the survey, the Plan of Action 2003–2012 for the Health-Promoting Schools Regional Initiative was developed and

adopted by HPS networks at their third annual meeting in Quito, Ecuador, in 2002 (*223*). The countries participating in this initiative are now moving forward to develop procedural guides for HPS certification and accreditation.

The healthy housing initiative has helped to promote and protect the health of the Region's most vulnerable populations from environmental hazards in the home and has contributed to the integrated local development of communities. It is estimated that the housing deficit in Latin America and the Caribbean is approximately 23 to 28 million units. This precarious housing situation affects the population's health, particularly the poorest and most vulnerable segments, such as children, the disabled, and the elderly, who spend much of their time at home. The Inter-American Healthy Housing Network (VIVSALUD), made up of 12 countries, disseminates, together with the United Nations Human Settlement Program and ECLAC, guidelines for national and local authorities on the primary components of the healthy housing strategy. Regional implementation of the community program started in Colombia called "Toward healthy housing: Long live my home!" has been promoted, and for this, more than 300 professionals and technicians have been trained in bioclimatic architecture, sustainable construction, vector elimination, and healthy housing. The Canada Mortgage and Housing Corporation promotes the concept of healthy housing and publishes guides and pamphlets on housing-related health issues.

Analysis of the map of institutional capacities for health promotion (Figure 30) also shows that nearly 90% of the countries surveyed reported having mechanisms and opportunities for ac-

"Accelerated urban growth, industrial expansion, and agricultural development in Latin American and Caribbean countries in recent years have triggered a sharp rise in environmental contamination in the Region, which has, in turn, resulted in heightened environmental hazards to human health."

George A.O. Alleyne, 1994

tive civic participation. The most common forms of civic participation are public consultations and forums. Social and community participation represents a fundamental strategy for health promotion, and it is achieved by building networks in which representatives of multiple sectors and nongovernmental organizations participate.

Moreover, 90% of the countries have some policy to reorient health services beyond preventing and treating disease. For example, in Nicaragua and Costa Rica, as well as in Mexico City, Mexico, and Bogotá, Colombia, integrated care models are being incorporated into health and social development plans. Mexico has an operational model and is establishing an integrated health promotion service throughout the country. The principle of comprehensive care is guiding health reform in Brazil and is the focus of the family health strategy. Programa Puente, in Chile, and the recently started Programa Juntos, in Peru, integrate primary health care services with other social services targeting the family. FOROSALUD, a broad federation of civil society organizations in Peru, and the Congresses for Health and Life in Ecuador, are actively demanding the reorientation of health services with an intersectoral and integrated vision. Argentina has also redirected its services, particularly through its social and community health programs. But these processes still face multiple challenges, from a lack of adequate resources to a profound operational fragmentation of services in many uncoordinated, parallel, duplicate, and overlapping subnetworks, in a context in which the institutional and organizational segmentation of the Region's health systems is on the rise.

Building intersectoral consensus is fundamental for health promotion. Of the countries that participated in the surveys on institutional capacity for health promotion, approximately 30% have an intersectoral council or committee at the national level (Figure 30). The experiences of Argentina, Brazil, Chile, Canada, Costa Rica, Cuba, Mexico, Peru, and the United States, among others, offer examples of committees, consortia, and other forms of collaboration and alliances between social organizations and government agencies to implement public policies and other strategic actions for health promotion (*224, 225*). Despite the progress made, intersectoral collaboration still faces significant challenges in many countries, due in part to public administration segmentation (lack of communication between sectors) and

coordination with their provincial or departmental jurisdictions, the verticality of many programs, and professional training, which tends not to favor the interdisciplinary approach.

The results of the analysis of the institutional capacities show that, in 60% of the Region's countries, there is a system of surveillance related to health risk factors (Figure 30). For example, in Canada, Chile, Colombia, Ecuador, Guatemala, the United States, and Venezuela, work is being done to establish a surveillance system for social and epidemiological indicators of the social determinants of health as well as the social and behavioral risk factors.

In addition to strengthening surveillance, the Global Program on Health Promotion Effectiveness, a joint initiative of PAHO/WHO, the International Union for Health Promotion and Education, and the CDC, has given a significant boost to strengthening the capacity to evaluate health promotion initiatives and has facilitated the dissemination of best practices in health promotion. Argentina, Brazil, Cuba, Mexico, and Peru have adopted methodologies and developed initiatives to evaluate health promotion.

PAHO has collaborated with various countries in developing public policies through strengthening technical working groups and the exchange of information between them through the networks of institutions involved in healthy settings—municipalities, schools, housing, the network of health promotion collaboration centers, and centers of excellence, such as the Inter-American Consortium of Universities—to strengthen the training and development of professionals in this field. The development of methodological guides for the strategic planning and evaluation of health promotion interventions and activities has been a point of collaboration between countries, as has the evaluation of institutional capacities for health promotion undertaken in 2002 and 2005. PAHO is also working jointly with other organizations to execute health promotion initiatives. In this regard, UNICEF, FAO, and the World Food Program have collaborated on the dissemination and strengthening of the HPS initiative. The United Nations Educational, Scientific, and Cultural Organization (UNESCO), together with PAHO, through an established agreement, has contributed to the training of instructors to improve health education and the teaching of life skills in schools in the Region's countries. UNDP has contributed to strengthening community action and has supported local development. Likewise, UNEP contributed to improving basic sanitation and environmental health. Alliances have also been forged with the CDC, the European Union, the Canadian International Development Agency, the U.S. Agency for International Development, the Kellogg Foundation, and other organizations to strengthen health promotion in the Region.

In the two decades since the approval of the Ottawa Charter, considerable progress has been made in assessing health promotion as an essential public health function and strategy. Nevertheless, putting the issue of health promotion on the agenda of the health sector itself and in development plans remains a challenge. Some countries are making major efforts to develop national health promotion plans, agreed on in the Mexico Ministerial Statement. In Chile, the national action plan for health promotion, coordinated by the Consejo Intersectorial Vida Chile, is a good example. Many provinces in Canada have health promotion plans, with very creative, comprehensive programs and resources. Other countries, such as Peru, have established national health promotion policies as a strategic framework for developing a wide range of health promotion activities.

Since the holding of the 4th International Conference on Health Promotion in Jakarta, Indonesia, in 1997 (226), efforts to forge intersectoral alliances to increase the efficacy of health promotion initiatives have multiplied, especially with respect to the adoption of intersectoral approaches that involve the government as a whole, given their impact on economic and social policies. In the spirit of commitments made at the 5th Global Conference on Health Promotion held in Mexico City, Mexico, in 2000, PAHO has promoted numerous initiatives to evaluate the effectiveness of health promotion and the impact of public policies on health. Continuing to strengthen evidence of the efficacy and cost-effectiveness of health promotion and determining the most appropriate combination of strategic actions are urgent needs. The visibility of public opinion as a tool to change living conditions and lifestyles has been strengthened, and social participation has been stimulated to implement education and communication initiatives aimed at promoting the adoption of healthy behaviors (227). Collaboration has also been undertaken on the reorientation of health services to incorporate health promotion concepts and strategies and on strengthening leadership in the health sector regarding this area.

The progress of health promotion in the Region highlights the importance of all the initiatives that have grown out of the Ottawa Charter as well as the diversity of results, depending on the context of each country. Nevertheless, there are limits and problems that must be examined in depth to establish strategies and mechanisms to ensure the continued consolidation and sustainability of health promotion in the Region. Health promotion faces various challenges. On the one hand, the broader concept of health promotion must be disseminated as a public health strategy that addresses the gamut of social determinants of health. Based on this understanding, it is essential for governments to exercise their leadership and ensure the commitment of all sectors to work on the social determinants of health and develop public policies that promote solidarity and increase the well-being of the population. On the other hand, strengthening the health sector's role in the development of health promotion is key, given its ability to enlist support and its capacity to coordinate with other sectors to carry out health promotion actions, thus reducing social inequities and improving the quality of life.

States' commitment to the MDGs represents an excellent opportunity to invest additional needed resources in health promotion activities. Going back to the surveys on institutional capacity for health promotion, in 45% of the participating countries there is a plan of action to promote health that is being applied nationwide. Of these countries, 35% report having a health promotion action plan that incorporates the MDGs (Figure 30).

While it is true that multiple initiatives have been undertaken and resolutions adopted to address the social determinants of health (poverty, education, nutrition, and basic services) in the Region, it is also true that the social, economic, cultural, environmental, and political conditions, as well as inequities, continue to represent a major challenge for all countries. The recent establishment of the global Commission on Social Determinants of Health represents a unique opportunity to fight inequity and design and implement public policies in line with the Ottawa Charter and the documents that have followed it through the Bangkok Conference in 2005.

HEALTHY SPACES

In recent years, there has been a significant increase in interventions addressing the determinants of health. Nevertheless, social and economic inequities continue to erode the health conditions of many population groups. The establishment of healthy settings is an effective health promotion strategy to protect and improve the health and quality of life of the Region's population. Municipal and local governments can address the factors determining poverty and inequity, and their influence on health, by creating healthy, sustainable public policies; implementing healthy settings; forging alliances between the public and private sectors; strengthening support networks; mobilizing the media; and adopting an active role in promoting health.

The Region's rapid urbanization in recent decades poses a major challenge for health promotion. Various factors act on today's urban settings and affect the health and quality of life of their inhabitants. Among others, the chaotic growth of cities, disorganized industrial development, and high rates of rural-to-urban migration contribute to the formation of marginal areas as well as the proliferation of makeshift housing, increased poverty, environmental contamination, and increasing rates of disease and violence.

Data provided by the United Nations for monitoring MDG Target 11 ("by 2020, to have achieved a significant improvement in the lives of at least 100 million slum dwellers") show concern about trends in the lack of housing security in the Region's urban areas. While the percentage of the Region's urban population living in makeshift settlements fell from 35% in 1990 to 32% in 2001, the number of inhabitants increased from 111 million to 127 million (228). In other words, although the proportion of the total population living in makeshift urban settlements fell, this did not reduce the total number of people living in them. There are also great disparities among countries. In Belize, Bolivia, Guatemala, Haiti, Nicaragua, and Peru, more than one-half of the

---

BOX 2. Agreements and Strategies for a Healthy Community

PAHO/WHO believes that a community begins to be healthy when its political leaders, local organizations, and citizens commit and organize to continuously and progressively improve the conditions of health and well-being of all their inhabitants; when a social contract is established between the local authorities, community organizations, and public and private sector institutions; and when local planning is used as a basic tool, including social participation in management, evaluation, and decision-making.

The healthy municipalities and communities strategy is a process that reflects the commitment undertaken by the local government to prioritize health promotion through:

— the establishment of healthy public policies;
— the creation of settings that support and benefit health;
— the strengthening of community action;
— the development of personal skills in health issues; and
— the reorientation of health care services toward health promotion.

---

urban population lives in makeshift settlements, while in Antigua and Barbuda, Aruba, the Bahamas, Barbados, Bermuda, Chile, Cuba, Grenada, Guyana, the Netherlands Antilles, Puerto Rico, Saint Kitts and Nevis, Saint Vincent and the Grenadines, Suriname, and Uruguay, less than 10% of the urban population lives in such conditions (228).

The creation of healthy municipalities and communities is a strategy that contributes to improving the social, economic, and environmental factors that influence the quality of life, health, and human development of the Region's urban populations. To create healthy municipalities, various cities and communities have agreed to push health promotion actions, to utilize a community and multisectoral approach, and to prioritize public health in the development of municipal plans and policies (Box 2). Since the 1980s, this initiative has been an effective strategy for participatory health promotion at the local level. As its benefits have become visible, the healthy municipalities and cities movement in the Region has grown significantly (Table 28). Countries such as Argentina,

Brazil, Canada, Chile, Costa Rica, Cuba, El Salvador, Mexico, Paraguay, Peru, and the United States have established national networks (in addition to integrating many of them into the Healthy Municipalities, Cities, and Communities Network of the Americas) and are contributing to the strategy's consolidation in the Region by including healthy spaces initiatives in their work programs. Within the framework of the healthy municipalities and cities strategy, PANAFTOSA initiated a special line of technical cooperation for local development beginning in 2000. The focus of this technical cooperation, called productive municipalities, includes primarily national zoonoses programs, since many of the actions on this issue are decentralized and fall on municipal agencies.

Examples in the Americas of Healthy Municipalities and Communities

In Argentina, the National Healthy Municipalities and Communities Network has undergone sustained growth since 2002,

TABLE 28. Growth of the healthy municipalities and communities (HMC) movement in selected countries of the Americas, 2000–2005.

Country	Total municipalities in the country	Healthy municipalities				National or regional HMC network
		2000	%	2005	%	
Argentina	2,171	4	0.2	182	7.4	Yes
Costa Rica	81	40	49.4	56	70.0	Yes
Cuba	169	79	46.8	98	58.0	Yes
Mexico	2,438	1,000	41.0	1,875	77.0	Yes
Paraguay	600	10	1.7	35	6.0	Yes
Peru	1,800	30	1.7	574	32.0	Yes
Uruguay	19	0	0	10	52.0	No

Source: Pan American Health Organization, Sustainable Development and Environmental Health Area, country reports.

favoring the development of local promotion and prevention projects, the implementation of healthy public policies, and the strengthening of community participation. The Argentine network is made up of 216 municipalities (of a total of 2,171). One of the focuses of its actions has been to raise the awareness of local governments regarding the importance of integrating all civil society stakeholders, as well as different areas of the government, into healthy municipalities and communities projects. The Argentine network has major political support, as expressed at the National Healthy Municipalities and Communities Conference held in August 2006 with the presence of the country's Vice President, several federal cabinet ministers, 24 provincial health ministers, more than 200 mayors from around the nation, PAHO representatives, and members of the Argentine Federation of Municipalities. At the Conference, the Statement entitled "Toward a National Plan for Healthy Living" was signed, whereby the signatories committed to promote the implementation of public policies that emphasize the social determinants of health and strengthen disease prevention and health promotion actions at the local level. The issues most commonly addressed in the healthy municipalities framework in Argentina are physical activity, healthy nutrition, smoke-free environments, solid waste management, and addiction prevention (229).

In Bolivia, the Productive and Healthy Communities strategy, launched in 2004, has contributed to economic development in small communities, and thus to reducing internal migration and poverty. Farmers in the Chacaltaya community increased sales of their agricultural and livestock products (mainly vegetables) and thereby generated more revenue for the community. Community members were also trained in economic management and the cost-effectiveness of solar heating. In 2004, PAHO/WHO and the Chacaltaya community signed a series of letter agreements to perform ecotourism, agricultural, and livestock activities. The objectives achieved include establishing a community pharmacy, constructing solar heating greenhouses for the community's own use and sale, installing solar-powered hot-water showers, establishing health services for the local school, constructing a small plant to produce llama jerky (fresh meat, dried in the sun, in areas built for this purpose), and farming trout for their own consumption and for sale in the capital city of La Paz. Community members were also trained in economic and financial analysis, as well as in marketing in La Paz supermarkets, so as to obtain fair prices to contribute to the community's sustainability. As a result of this activity, the municipality of La Paz and the communities won a competitive bid with the IDB to build a hotel and tourism enclave at an estimated value of US$ 100,000 that is expected to be operational in late 2007. Currently, the Ministry of Rural Development, Agriculture, and the Environment and other national and international institutions are implementing this model in other highly vulnerable areas of the country.

In Brazil, the states of Ceará, Goiânia, Mato Grosso do Sul, Paraná, Pernambuco, Rio de Janeiro, Rio Grande do Sul, Rio Grande do Norte, São Paulo, and Tocantins are participating in the healthy municipalities and communities initiative. Brazil does not have a national healthy municipalities and communities network, but does have several regional networks. The Network of Potentially Healthy Municipalities in the region of Campinas started with six municipalities and now has 30, representing 2 million inhabitants. The Brazilian healthy municipalities and communities strategy is being implemented jointly with various social agendas that share the same values and principles, such as Programa 21, the environmental primary care program, the participatory budget, and the productive municipalities movement. The major challenge is to coordinate the efforts around networks that consider social inclusion, participation, solidarity, equity, sustainability, and intersectoral cooperation. In Rio de Janeiro's Vila Paciencia district, between 2002 and 2004, 25 projects were implemented, including such activities as health fairs, children's recreation, training in nutrition, and mobilization for cleaning up the community, directly benefiting more than 1,000 people. In Curitiba, Paraná, as of 2005, the healthy environments initiative had mobilized 143 local institutions to develop and implement health promotion activities (230).

Canada was one of the first countries in the Americas to apply the healthy municipalities and communities strategy. The Ontario Healthy Communities Coalition was established in 1992, with the mission of working with Ontario's diverse communities to strengthen their social, environmental, and economic well-being (231). The Québec Network of Healthy Cities and Towns was established in 1988 and now includes 140 member municipalities, representing more than 50% of Québec's population (232).

Costa Rica's healthy, ecological cantons initiative has benefited from great popular support. The country's national network, founded in 1996, includes 56 municipalities (70% of the national total). An annual contest that is held to select the best healthy, ecological canton initiatives and the subsequent publication of results and information on the initiatives have served to stimulate growing interest and strengthen the national network.

The first healthy municipality in Latin America was officially declared in Cuba in 1989, within the framework of the Global Project of Cienfuegos. In 2006, the 14 provinces and the special municipality of the Isle of Youth were incorporated into the movement. The Cuban National Network of Municipalities for Health, established in 1994 with 14 municipalities, now includes 98, representing 58% of the country's total of 169. This country is promoting the Productive Municipality Atlas initiative to expand analytical and management capacities in municipal contexts by using the Geographic Information System in Epidemiology developed by PAHO health analysis and information systems experts. The initiative's primary achievements include developing local case-treatment capacity, consensus-building for health promotion actions, strengthening intersectoral strategic alliances, and exchanging experiences.

The experience of the United States began in 1988, with the California Healthy Cities and Communities project, covering more than 70 communities. This initiative's achievements include establishing community gardens for 140 families; implementing a road safety program for bicyclists and pedestrians, resulting in an increase in helmet use from 26% to 53% in one year; and a clean-up campaign, obtaining a 45% reduction in community garbage (233). Since 1991, Indiana University's center for the establishment of healthy cities has laid the foundation for promoting healthy municipalities and communities programs, research, and resources in the country (234). Members of the Indiana Healthy Cities network work on constructing nature trails, drafting anti-tobacco ordinances, improving health services coverage, and reducing violence.

The Mexican Network of Municipalities for Health was established in 1993 with 13 municipalities. Since then, it has managed to consolidate the 31 state networks grouped into regional networks. It currently includes more than 1,800 municipalities out of a total of 2,438 (77%). Most of the network's municipalities are also part of the National Healthy Communities Program. The network has held 13 annual national meetings in which mayors, the health sector, and other sectors have exchanged knowledge and best practices and national and international experts have presented novel methods and successful experiences for modifying determinants of health at the municipal level. The involvement of various sectors in municipal health promotion projects and the participation of municipalities in a contest to obtain federal resources for the program resulted in the financing of 1,059 municipal health projects between 2002 and 2006. The projects' focuses include healthy communities, zoonosis control, care and improvement of the environment, prevention and control of vector-borne diseases, solid waste management, drivers' education, addiction prevention, health education, healthy markets, child and adolescent health, adult and older adult health, reproductive health, basic sanitation, HIV/AIDS, tuberculosis, proper water use and consumption, and oral health. The Healthy Municipalities Network and Program constitute effective strategies for promoting public policies and intersectoral actions aimed at a greater commitment to health by the population and various levels of the government through political activities, programs, services, research, and training.

In Paraguay in 2002, 24 municipalities established the Healthy Municipalities Network; currently it includes 35 municipalities (15% of the country's 230 municipalities) that jointly undertake activities aimed at creating healthy and productive settings. In 2002, a novel collaborative experience called Healthy Borders was implemented between two municipalities in Paraguay and one in Argentina (Nanawa, Falcón, and Clorinda) to provide drinking water to all three municipalities. Another success story is the Emboscada project, which combines improvements in health protection for workers through the Healthy Quarries project with proposals for alternatives to the only source of employment (worm farming and family garden projects) and improvements in waste management, school settings, and child and maternal health care. In 2004 an agreement was signed between the Ministry of Public Health and Social Welfare, the Ministry of Education and Culture, and the Government of Misiones for the joint implementation of health-promoting schools initiatives and healthy municipalities and communities in all the province's municipalities. Today, 22 schools are receiving assistance to obtain their HPS accreditation. In 2005, the municipalities in the network performed a wide range of activities aimed at creating healthy and productive environmental settings, including waste removal in exchange for milk or baskets of goods, separation of contaminated waters, and tree planting and ecological garden projects.

In Peru, communities, together with local government, the public sector, and nongovernmental organizations, have been actively working on the healthy municipalities and communities strategy since 1996. The Ministry of Health's General Directorate of Health Promotion is investing in provincial and local training to carry out healthy settings initiatives. The National Network of Healthy Municipalities and Communities includes 574 municipalities and 10 regional networks (Arequipa, Ayacucho, Huancavelica, Andahuaylas, Callao, Lambayeque, La Libertad, Cusco, Cajamarca, and Loreto) (235). The Ministry of Health is implementing the Healthy Municipalities and Communities Program, which includes 757 municipalities (41% of the nation's total). These municipalities are carrying out activities related to maternal health, child nutrition, education, gender, road safety, smoke-free environments, physical activity, immunizations, and dengue prevention, among others. Various health public policy workshops have been held on specific issues of municipal interest, resulting in various publications. The Ministry of Health has organized several regional workshops and meetings to raise the awareness of mayors and disseminate experiences. Concrete results and achievements of the healthy municipalities initiatives include:

- the sectoral political will that led to the establishment of a General Directorate of Health Promotion in the Ministry of Health, with related resources, interventions, and policies, to promote the healthy municipalities and communities strategy;
- the strengthening and growth of the Peruvian Network of Healthy Municipalities and Communities;
- a strategic alliance between the Peruvian Network of Healthy Municipalities and Communities, PAHO, the Ministry of Health, and the AMARES (Support for Health Sector Modernization) project to drive the healthy municipalities process in the country;
- the incorporation of the healthy municipalities and communities initiative into established local development plans and the municipalities' participatory budget; and
- the approval of municipal ordinances and resolutions favoring the creation of healthy municipalities and communities.

In Trinidad and Tobago, the healthy municipalities and communities movement began in 2002, with the development of a multisectoral team proposal called the Healthy Spaces Initiative. Promotion workshops were held for each regional health authority to design initiatives to support the healthy communities. Through this initiative, some rural communities began to work on issues of food safety, sanitation, youth capacity-building, and improvement of health services, among others. In the Plum Mitan community, specific results obtained include the construction of water tanks while a technical study was conducted to determine a permanent source, access to health services by providing transportation to the health center in another town, training in fish farming and personal care, and basic computer literacy. It also increased women's involvement in the community's decision-making processes. The community's quality of life has improved with sustainable interventions supported by governmental and technical cooperation agencies, but the most important outcome is that the community has learned and is mobilizing resources for its own improvement.

With the support of local governments, the Ministry of Health has incorporated the initiative into its institutional framework, thus promoting the development of competencies to strengthen planning, monitoring, and evaluation of health promotion activities at the regional health authority and local levels, and the establishment of collaboration with civil society. Forums have also been established for community participation, and the community council is involved in national forums and conducts local development interventions. The initiative has allowed the experience to be shared with nongovernmental organizations, community organizations, government agencies, and private entities inside and outside the Caribbean subregion.

In Uruguay, the Ministries of Public Health, and of Livestock, Agriculture, and Fisheries, in collaboration with municipal administrations, other national organizations, and PAHO/WHO, launched the productive and healthy communities project, which combines assistance with the creation of jobs and other microenterprise activities rooted in community initiatives. It is important to note that the Uruguayan municipalities and departments cover a territory that includes both large urban areas (cities) and small population centers (towns and villages). In 10 municipalities (of a total of 19), there are one or more communities participating in this project. The activities undertaken include the coordination and enhancement of the production of rural traditional cheese makers, the creation of spaces to market local agricultural and livestock production, productive development and ecocultural tourism, and the implementation of food safety programs. The concrete achievements of the productive and healthy communities initiative include training and information on the various aspects of the strategy for 646 people; the consolidation and strengthening of 52 microenterprise projects; and the carrying out of 73 health program activities.

Healthy Housing Initiatives

Housing conditions have been recognized for some time as one of the primary factors determining human health. Healthy housing alludes to a residential space that promotes the health of its dwellers. This space includes the house (the physical shelter

where the people reside), the home (the group of people living under the same roof), the setting (the physical and psychosocial environment immediately outside the house), and the community (the group of people identified as neighbors by the residents). Healthy housing poses no risk factors, or makes them controllable or preventable, and includes agents that promote health and well-being (236).

Although the housing deficit in Latin America and the Caribbean is difficult to calculate because of the lack of standardized methodologies and information to measure it, it is estimated to range between 23 and 28 million units, while the qualitative deficit is approximately 26 million units.

The proportion of homes with access to secure tenure (that is, the right of all individuals and the group to the effective protection of the State against eviction from the land or residence) improved in relative terms regionally between 1990 and 2000 and represents approximately 80% of owners and tenants. Nevertheless, in countries such as Colombia, Costa Rica, Guatemala, Mexico, Nicaragua, and Paraguay, a reduction in the percentage of homes with secure tenure has been observed. Durability of construction materials improved in 70%–76% of housing between 1990 and 2000, which in absolute terms means an improvement for more than 17 million housing units in the 15 Latin American and Caribbean countries considered. In some cases, however, such as those of Ecuador and Paraguay, the situation has worsened. The lack of housing security in the Region could affect the health of millions of people, particularly the poorest and most vulnerable, such as children under age 5, those suffering from chronic diseases such as HIV/AIDS, the disabled, and older adults (228). Since 1995, the healthy housing strategy has contributed to strengthening activities that promote and protect the health of these populations and contribute to integrated local community development. The strategy includes strong political commitment, solid technical and intercultural expertise, ongoing intersectoral collaboration, the adoption of a multidisciplinary approach, and a high level of community participation. For these reasons, an effective mechanism for implementing the strategy is the establishment of national, intersectoral, and multidisciplinary healthy housing networks associated with VIVSALUD. In 2005, the VIVSALUD network developed its plan of activities for the next two years with the following lines of action (236): evaluation of the impact of health policies, plans, programs, and projects with a focus on equity; strengthening surveillance systems for risk factors and protective factors for health; research on the relationship between housing and health; the implementation of evaluation-action-participation projects; capacity-building and development; and institutional development of the network.

HEALTH-PROMOTING SCHOOLS

Health promotion and primary health care are fundamental strategies for addressing the social determinants of health and

"Millions of families in the world exist—or struggle to survive—in wretched, overcrowded, and unsafe slums, shacks, tents, ghettoes, and settlements. They are exposed to harsh weather. Rats and insects bring diseases to their homes. Poor ventilation, little light, and the need for constant repair aggravate the tragedy. These conditions are especially oppressive for children—their bodies, their growth and development, and their dreams. They live with no clean water, decent sanitation, or basic services that many in the world enjoy daily and take for granted. Yet they are our fellow human beings, a precious human capital, and we have the mission to reduce the environmental hazards they face in order to improve their health."

Mirta Roses, 2007

therefore promote the achievement of the MDGs under a commitment to equity. The school is conceived as an engine of health and community development, and therefore any approach to health at the various levels, from early to vocational education, strengthens the school-based approach to respond to the various challenges in its life cycle, while also strengthening the links between the health and education sectors.

PAHO's Health-Promoting Schools Initiative has been working at the preschool, primary, and secondary levels of education and has confirmed the need to work on health promotion interventions focused on the family-schools-health center triangle. The incorporation of HPS into early education involves greater collaboration between the first level of health care and early education centers. This approach opens the possibility of working with mothers from the first months of pregnancy, supporting the processes of early stimulation that will result in better conditions for the intellectual development of children. Recent studies in neuroscience (237) confirm the need to develop educational and health programs that, together with adequate nutrition, prioritize care to boys and girls in vulnerable situations to provide more equitable conditions. Starting with early education, the health-promoting school constitutes a privileged educational space for working with the mother and her child to modify behavior patterns leading to greater stimuli for learning and to ensure that healthier settings are established. Health education from an early level also has an impact on reducing infant morbidity and mortality.

The Health-Promoting Schools Regional Initiative (238) in the Americas, which grew out of multiple international consultations, was officially launched by PAHO in 1995. The purpose of the Initiative is to train future generations to have the knowledge, abilities, and skills necessary to promote and care for their own, their families', and their communities' health as well as to create and maintain healthy environments for study, work, and coexis-

tence. Through this Initiative, PAHO/WHO is supporting Member States in the development and execution of health promotion activities, consensus-building, and forging alliances between the health, education, and other sectors, and through associations of parents, students, and other pertinent organizations. The Initiative is focused on three main components: 1) an integrated approach to health education including the teaching of life skills; 2) the creation and maintenance of healthy physical and psychosocial environments; and 3) providing health services and healthy foods choices, psychological guidance, and opportunities for physical activity and the development of active lifestyles.

The first component provides students with the knowledge they need to recognize, adopt, develop, and cultivate the skills necessary to achieve and maintain an optimum level of well-being and quality of life. These skills are built on personal, family, and community values and by considering the individual, social, and cultural needs and characteristics of the students. Thus, this component strengthens self-esteem and the capacity to acquire and maintain hygienic habits and healthy lifestyles. The information facilitates the development of knowledge, skills, and abilities aimed at establishing and maintaining healthy behaviors through participatory interventions, including group discussions and community work projects.

Life-skills education and the acquisition of psychosocial competencies promote the adoption and maintenance of behaviors, attitudes, and habits that allow students to respond to life's demands and challenges, including creative, thinking, and communication skills. Students learn to value personal relationships, effectively utilize the resources of their immediate community, and adopt and maintain healthy behaviors. HPS promotes a sense of responsibility and enhances the ability to resolve often-problematic situations through dialogue and negotiation, as factors that prevent violence and tools for peaceful coexistence. This, in turn, facilitates integrated human development and a sense of civic responsibility.

The second component develops the capacity to create and maintain schools and school-related facilities in proper conditions of cleanliness and security, including basic sanitation facilities, the water supply, and the various physical spaces used as well as a psychosocial environment free of physical, verbal, and psychological aggression, or any other form of violence. This component devotes special attention to the emotional climate of the school and to the social interactions that affect the well-being and productivity of students and school staff as well as to the ongoing training of the faculty and the implementation of health promotion strategies aimed at family members within the framework of parents' associations and community organizations.

The third component facilitates the strengthening of the relationship between teams in the health, education, and other pertinent sectors and their capacity to complement and strengthen each other. Through this component, health problems can be detected and prevented, including risk factors and harmful habits.

BOX 3. What Do Health-promoting Schools Do?

- *They implement policies* that support individual and collective dignity and well-being and offer multiple growth and development opportunities for children and adolescents in a context of learning and strengthening the school community, with the participation of faculty, students, and their families.
- *They define strategies that promote and support learning and health,* using all available means and resources to do so and involving personnel in the health and education sectors and community leaders in the performance of planned school activities (e.g., comprehensive education for health and life-skills training, strengthening of protective factors, reduction of risk behaviors, facilitating access to school health services and nutrition and physical education programs).
- *They involve all members of the school and community,* including teachers, parents, leaders, and nongovernmental organizations, in decision-making and the implementation of interventions to promote learning, healthy lifestyles, and community health projects.
- *They have a working plan* to improve the physical and psychosocial environment in the school and its surrounding area (including rules and regulations for environments that are free of smoke, drugs, and any form of violence and that ensure access to clean drinking water, healthy foods, and sanitary facilities), and try to set an example by creating healthy school environments and activities that extend beyond the school itself.
- *They implement actions* to evaluate and improve the health of students, teachers and other school personnel, families, and community members in general and work with local leaders to ensure access to health and referral, social work, nutrition, and other services as well as spaces for physical and other recreational activities.
- *They provide adequate, effective training* and educational materials to teachers and students.
- *They have a local education and health committee* in which parents' associations, nongovernmental organizations, and other community organizations actively participate.

Access to health services and healthy food also facilitates the early detection of nutritional deficiencies or diseases.

The principal functions and tasks of health-promoting schools are summarized in Box 3.

Progress of the Initiative

The Health-Promoting Schools Regional Initiative is in full development in the countries of Latin America and the Caribbean, as noted by 90% of the participants in the first regional survey on HPS carried out in 2001 (*239*), the results of which appear in Table 29.

The survey confirms that most of the Region's countries have school health promotion initiatives, ranging from the use of educational space to increase vaccination coverage or the identification of vision problems to comprehensive health promotion activities at three levels: classroom, school, and school-community relations. However, most of these programs are the responsibility of the respective ministries of health, who use the educational spaces to oversee student health with school doctors or nurses. The coverage of such experiences is quite heterogeneous among the countries, but for the most part they focus on urban and public institutions versus schools in rural and marginal urban areas where the social determinants of health are more accentuated.

PAHO Member States are currently defining criteria and procedures for HPS accreditation and certification, as well as standards and minimum requirements for accreditation and certification by ministries of health and education, HPS monitoring activities, information requirements, and the frequency with which the accreditation and certification processes should take place. These activities are being undertaken within the context of the Health-Promoting Schools Regional Initiative and with the participation of school directors, faculty, and administrative staff; other organizations in the educational community; students; and parents.

The role of joint national health and education commissions is significant, given their capacity to promote the mobilization of all necessary participants and material resources. Technical collaboration for implementation of this strategy consists of disseminating the knowledge and the methodology and promoting the exchange of experiences between countries. For this purpose, regional and subregional meetings have been held in which the establishment and extension of Latin American and Caribbean Networks of Health-Promoting Schools have been supported.

The creation and strengthening of these networks have provided a forum for the exchange of ideas, resources, and experiences between countries, in order to feed the motivation and enthusiasm of participating teachers, students, and parents as well

TABLE 29. Results of first regional survey of health-promoting schools (HPS) in Latin America and the Caribbean, 2001.

Level of dissemination of HPS approach	Ninety-four percent of the countries are developing the HPS Initiative. The proportion of HPS with respect to all schools is very heterogeneous country-to-country, depending on the level of the strategy's implementation.
	In 90% of the cases, the strategy is applied in public elementary schools in urban areas; in 60% of the cases, it is executed in preschools, and also in 60% of the cases, in secondary schools.
National health promotion policies and plans for the school population	Ninety-four percent of the countries have a broad legislative and political framework regarding school health.
	Eighty-two percent of the countries have specific policies or legislation on HPS. Most policies pertinent to this initiative emerged beginning in 1997, and in 82% of the cases, between 1999 and 2001, coinciding with the official launch of the PAHO/WHO regional initiative in 1995.
Multisectoral coordination mechanisms to support health promotion in the schools	Sixty-five percent of countries have formed joint national commissions on health and education, and when cases of other forms of collaborative work are taken into account, this figure reaches 75%.
Health education	All countries have incorporated health education into their school curriculum programs. The most commonly used method consists of including it as a cross-cutting objective. The prevailing trend of incorporating it as a cross-cutting objective coincides with and is related to educational (curriculum) reform processes.
Formation of and participation in national and international HPS networks	Forty-seven percent of the countries have some sort of participation in the Latin American Network of Health-Promoting Schools (LANHPS). In most cases, this participation consists of attending network meetings.
	Twenty-nine percent of countries have formed national HPS networks. In 2004, almost all Latin American countries participated in the fourth LANHPS meeting.
Financing of school health programs and activities	Thirty percent of the countries have a budget allocated to school health.

Source: Ippolito-Shepherd J. Las escuelas promotoras de la salud en América Latina. Resultados de la Primera Encuesta Regional. Serie Promoción de la Salud No. 3. Washington, D.C.: OPS; 2005.

as advocates of health promotion in schools. The Latin American and Caribbean Networks of Health-Promoting Schools were created from multiple regional consultations over the past decade.

The first meeting of the Latin American Network of Health-Promoting Schools (LANHPS) was held in 1996 in San José, Costa Rica, with an initial membership of 10 countries, and the first meeting of the Caribbean Network of Health-Promoting Schools (CNHPS) was held in 2001 in Bridgetown, Barbados, with an initial membership of 14 countries. The second LANHPS

gathering took place in 1998 in Mexico City, and the third in Quito, Ecuador, in 2002. This provided the opportunity to share experiences and strengthen the joint national commissions of the participating countries.

The fourth LANHPS meeting took place in San Juan, Puerto Rico, in 2004 (*240*) and included official health and education delegates from Argentina, Brazil, Chile, Costa Rica, Cuba, the Dominican Republic, El Salvador, Guatemala, Haiti, Honduras, Mexico, Nicaragua, Panama, Paraguay, Peru, Puerto Rico, and

BOX 4. Successes of the Health-promoting Schools Initiative in Various Countries of the Americas

Argentina. The HPS program was established in the province of Salta in 1998 by the Interministerial Health and Education Team, whose work is aimed at decentralization through the training of interdisciplinary teams and the strengthening of networks with intersectoral collaboration between government ministries. A project is currently under way that will add 100 schools and health services in the province to the 52 that already exist.

Bolivia. A program focusing on reproductive health with a gender perspective, prevention of HIV/AIDS and other sexually transmitted infections, avoidance of teen pregnancy, and prevention of sexual abuse of children and gender violence was implemented nationally in 14 municipalities, benefiting 177 schools and 57,691 students and involving 1,407 teachers.

Brazil. In response to the need to develop health education interventions and activities in the school environment, to define intra- and intersectoral strategies for implementing health actions for basic public education, and to engage social stakeholders in these processes, in 2005 the Intersectoral Chamber of Education for Health in the School was created with the joint participation of the Ministries of Health and Education. The institutionalization of health promotion in schools as a public policy strengthens the possibilities for integrating the issue into Brazil's National Health Policy. Successful examples include the following:

— In Rio de Janeiro, diagnostic studies, identification of key stakeholders, production of educational materials, and partnerships with universities and nongovernmental organizations are stimulating decentralized and intersectoral activities that facilitate greater access by the school community to health services.

— In the municipality of Embu, São Paulo, in 2002, the HPS strategy was implemented as an intersectoral project in partnership with the Federal University of São Paulo. The education-for-health activities have three priority themes: the environment, sexuality, and promoting peace.

— In the State of Tocantins, the school is a formal educational setting, but it is also an institutional, social, and political environment affected by culture. These aspects are important for the support and sustainability of health promotion strategies. In this context, the interdependence between management, training, and the teaching-learning process is highlighted for intersectoral collaboration and the results and impacts obtained. The HPS strategy in Tocantins considers these dimensions indivisible focal structures.

Chile. Since 1997, the HPS strategy has been developed jointly between the education and health sectors. Since 1999, the work has been strengthened by the incorporation of the institutions responsible for kindergarten-level education. In 2004, institutions linked to the environment and drug prevention joined the efforts under way. That year, effective intersectoral work took place in more than 3,000 schools across the country (nearly 30% of the national total) at the preschool, elementary, and secondary levels. In 2001, an accreditation process began and by 2004, 2,554 institutions had been granted HPS status.

Colombia. The Healthy Schools for Peace Program is a strategy that strives to integrate activities of the health and education sectors with the community to promote healthy lifestyles in the school setting. The program's first phase is to raise community awareness, followed by a diagnostic phase to define the specific health promotion and prevention activities to be implemented. The program incorporates a three-pronged rights-based approach: the right of a child to freedom from violence, the right to health care, and the right to healthy coexistence.

Cuba. In Cuba, the objective of the *Seminternado de Primaria-Agustín Farabundo Martí* initiative is motivation and stimulation to enhance the quality of life of the educational community. "My happy, healthy house" diplomas are presented to students whose families do not engage in the harmful habits of smoking and alcohol use; "Learning to grow" diplomas are awarded for reflective, creative achievements; and "Nature is my friend" diplomas are given for proper caring for plants, animals, and water and promoting their appropriate use in human nutrition.

(continued)

BOX 4. (*continued*).

El Salvador. The Healthy School Program focuses on the provision of school meals as a tool to satisfy students' immediate nutritional needs, increase their concentration and learning capacity, and thus maximize their education opportunities while in the classroom. In addition, 300 schools have planted school gardens to increase students' knowledge of healthy, wholesome food choices and improve their nutritional status.

Mexico. In Mazatlán, Sinaloa, the Intersectoral Healthy Education Program aims to strengthen self-health care among 778 students and raise their awareness about environmental protection. The school community, health personnel, and municipal authorities jointly developed a program that focuses on health education, prevention and detection of health problems, and healthy environments.

Peru. In the national capital of Lima, the HPS strategy builds leadership qualities in students by encouraging their participation in activities based on their own personal interests and motivations. The Clean Hands, Happy Faces project promotes personal hygiene and sanitation practices to improve student health; in 2004, a government agreement was signed calling for the project's educational materials and methodology to be disseminated nationwide to 2,000 additional schools. In Belén, Department of Loreto, health promotion activities focus on the maintenance of clean schoolyards and classrooms and on the incorporation of education modules (hygiene, nutrition, dengue and malaria prevention) into the school curricula.

Venezuela. In Aragua, in order for a educational center to be HPS-certified, it must meet such specific criteria as having a minimum of two trained health-promoting teachers among its faculty, implementing a health promotion plan based on the results of health diagnostics conducted in the school, ensuring that the school cafeteria offers healthy food choices, having an operational oral health program, designing and carrying out integrated community health projects, and maintaining a school emergency safety system. In Miranda, play activities are used to train new readers and future blood donors. Through the composition of stories and the painting of group murals, students learn about the importance and usefulness of blood donation in a creative and stimulating environment.

Venezuela as well as participants from Aruba, Australia, Canada, Colombia, Ecuador, Italy, Spain, the United States, and Trinidad and Tobago. The event also included the active involvement of representatives of Comprehensive Primary Health Care Programs; of the Industrial University of Santander, Colombia (PROINAPSA), a PAHO/ WHO Collaborating Center; as well as nongovernmental organizations and representatives of the private sector, academic institutions, and international organizations, for a total of 115 participants from 26 countries. Seven working committees were created that discussed seven key issues for strengthening HPS: 1) the organization, structure, and management of LANHPS; 2) human resources training for health promotion in the schools; 3) research, evaluation, and surveillance of protective and risk factors; 4) development of materials and educational tools for health promotion and education for a healthy life in the school setting; 5) HPS accreditation and certification; 6) strategic alliances and horizontal cooperation mechanisms between countries to strengthen health promotion in the schools; and 7) curriculum reform for the inclusion of health promotion and education for a healthy life in the schools. The meeting also facilitated the technical validation of the document *Dadores de vida: Guía Metodológica para Educadores* (Givers of Life: A Methodological Guide for Educators). After the fourth meeting of LANHPS, the

Puerto Rican Network of Health-Promoting Schools was established in Puerto Rico.

In its Plan of Action 2003–2012, PAHO highlights the importance of promoting the Latin American and Caribbean networks to strengthen and expand HPS throughout the Americas. Its primary objectives are to disseminate the HPS concept; to mobilize political will and multisectoral and multidisciplinary work, particularly in the health and education sectors; to create forums in which schools can share their experiences, thus ensuring enrichment from processes that are under way; to develop training programs for health and education personnel; to promote the preparation of educational material with novel approaches and the use of participatory methodologies; to disseminate evaluation methodologies and good practices; to promote the use of electronic media between network participants; and to strengthen institutional capacity to implement school health programs with a comprehensive approach incorporating gender equality principles. Box 4 describes the variety of HPS activities being undertaken in the Region.

Regionally, the HPS Initiative has allowed technical collaboration and the development of specific activities (*223*). The success of the training and committee work is evident in the ongoing commitment demonstrated by the seven committees and their members, who are currently finalizing proposals for a series of Regional Guides to be presented at the Fifth Meeting of LANHPS. Other noteworthy activities include:

- The promotion and strengthening of school health programs with an integrated approach, disseminating the HPS concept among the Region's countries, through regional and subregional meetings, the distribution of informational and promotional material, and participation in pertinent national and international forums.
- Technical collaboration with member countries to consolidate intersectoral coordination mechanisms; to analyze and update public policies; to strengthen institutional capacity; to support dissemination and inclusion of the life-skills approach; to develop, disseminate, and promote the use of instruments for rapid diagnosis and analysis; and to create strategic alliances.

HPS provides the opportunity to improve the health of children and adolescents, who represent the countries' most valuable human resource. Ensuring the physical and mental growth and development of the school-age population is essential for securing sustainable improvements in the population's quality of life and a social responsibility assumed by all governments committed to achieving the Millennium Development Goals.

References

1. Prüss-Üstün A, Corvalán C. Preventing disease through health environments. Towards an estimate of the environmental burden of disease. Geneva: WHO; 2006.
2. Zimmerman R. Social equity and environmental risk. Risk Anal 1993;13(6): 649–66.
3. Organización Panamericana de la Salud/Programa de las Naciones Unidas para el Medio Ambiente; Fundación Oswaldo Cruz. Proyecto GEO Salud. En búsqueda de herramientas y soluciones integrales a los problemas de medio ambiente y salud en América Latina y el Caribe. Mexico City: OPS; PNUMA; FIOCRUZ; 2005.
4. Firpo de Souza M. Public health and environmental justice in Brazil: joint perspectives (Presented at the International Colloquium on Environmental Justice, Work, and Citizenship). September 2001, Universidade Federal Fluminense, Niterói, Brazil.
5. Roque JA Environmental equity: reducing risk for all communities. Environ 1993;35(5): 25–28.
6. Pan American Health Organization. Water for Life. Equity and Quality of Services. International Decade for Action: 2005–2015. Available at: http://www.bvsde.paho.org/bvsadiaa/DIAA/docs/materiales/folletoeng2005.pdf.
7. Ramírez GL. La visión de políticas sobre el derecho humano al agua potable en el Perú. Preliminary document. 2004.
8. World Water Council. Fourth World Water Forum. Mexico City, March 2006. Available at: http://www.worldwaterforum4.org.mx/home/home.asp.
9. Nicaragua, Ministerio de Salud. Informe final de la evaluación rápida de la calidad del agua en Nicaragua. Managua: Ministerio de Salud; 2005.
10. Pan American Health Organization. Report on the Regional Evaluation of Municipal Solid Waste Management Services in Latin America. Washington, DC: PAHO; 2005.
11. World Health Organization; United Nations Children's Fund. Mid-term Evaluation of the Joint Monitoring Program on Water Supply and Sanitation. WHO/UNICEF; 2006.
12. Pan American Health Organization. Health, Drinking Water, and Sanitation in Sustainable Human Development. Washington, DC: PAHO; 2001. (Document cd43/10). Available at: http://www.paho.org/English/GOV/CD/cd43_10-e.pdf.
13. United Nations Human Settlements Program. The Challenge of Slums: Global Report on Human Settlements. UN-HABITAT; 2003. Available at: http://hq.unhabitat.org/mediacentre/documents/whd/GRHSB6.pdf.
14. Pan American Health Organization, Virtual Library of Sustainable Development and Environmental Health. BVSDE: Assessment 2000. Drinking Water and Sanitation: sector information. Available at: http://www.cepis.org.pe/sde/ops-sde/eva2000.html.
15. Meeting of the Ministers of Health of the Americas. Ottawa Declaration on Tobacco and Sustainable Development. Ottawa, Canada; 2002.
16. Meeting of the Ministers of Health of the Americas. Declaration of Mar del Plata. Mar del Plata, Argentina, 2005.
17. Costa Moreira J, Oliveira da Silva AL, Meyer A, de Esparza MLC. Improving environmental and health laboratories in Latin America and the Caribbean countries: diagnosis of the analytical capabilities and identification of the most important problems. CEPIS/PAHO; CDC; 2003.
18. International Atomic Energy Agency; Pan American Center for Sanitary Engineering and Environmental Sciences; Pan American Health Organization. Interlaboratory test comparison for environmental analytical laboratories of Latin America and the Caribbean (ARCAL RLA 8031 and RLA 2021 projects). IAEA; PAHO; CEPIS; 2004. Available at: http://www.iaea.org/programmes/aqcs/int1054/download/arcal_pt.pdf.
19. Jouravlev AS. El abastecimiento de agua y saneamiento en las ciudades de Iberoamérica. III Congreso Ibérico sobre Gestión y Planificación del Agua. La directiva marco del agua: realidades y futuros. CEPAL; 2002.
20. Joint Group of Experts on the Scientific Aspects of Marine Environmental Protection. A sea of troubles [research report]. GESAMP; 2001.
21. World Health Organization. Guidelines for safe recreational water environments. Vol. 1. Coastal and fresh waters. Vol. 2.

Swimming pools and similar recreational-water environments. Geneva: WHO; 2003.

22. Pan American Health Organization. Inter-American Water Day 2004: Water and Disasters [brochure]. Available at: http://www.bvsde.paho.org/bvsadiaa/diaa04/diaa2004/folleto.pdf.

23. Organización Panamericana de la Salud. Crónicas de desastres: huracanes George y Mitch. Washington, DC: OPS; 1999.

24. Comisión Económica para América Latina y el Caribe. El terremoto del 13 de enero de 2001 en El Salvador. Impacto socioeconómico y ambiental. Mexico City: CEPAL; 2001.

25. Comisión Económica para América Latina y el Caribe. El impacto socioeconómico y ambiental de la sequía de 2001 en Centroamérica. Mexico City: CEPAL; 2002.

26. United Nations. Kyoto Protocol to the United Nations Framework Convention on Climate Change. New York: UN; 1998. Available at: http://unfccc.int/resource/docs/convkp/kpeng.pdf. Accessed January 2007.

27. United Nations Environment Program. Montreal Protocol on Substances that Deplete the Ozone Layer. Geneva: UNEP; 2000.

28. Economic Commission for Latin America and the Caribbean. Millennium Development Goals: A Latin American and Caribbean Perspective. Santiago: ECLAC; 2005.

29. Pan American Health Organization. An Assessment of Health Effects of Ambient Air Pollution in Latin America and the Caribbean. Washington, DC: PAHO; 2005.

30. Cohen AJ, Anderson HR, Ostro B, Pandey KD, Krzyzanowski M, Kuenzli N, et al. Mortality impacts of urban air pollution. In: Ezzati M, López AD, Rodgers A, Murray CJL (eds.). Comparative quantification of health risks: global and regional burden of disease attributable to selected major risk factors. Vol. 2. Geneva: WHO; 2004. pp. 1353–1433.

31. World Health Organization. WHO Air Quality Guidelines Global Update 2005. Report on a working group meeting, Bonn, Germany, 18–20 October 2005. Copenhagen: WHO; 2006.

32. Maisonet M, Correa A, Misra D, Jaakkola J. A review of the literature on the effects of ambient air pollution on fetal growth. Environ Res. 2004;95:106–15.

33. Câmara VM, Tambellini AT. Considerações sobre o uso da Epidemiología em saúde ambiental. Rev Bras Epidemiol. 2003;6(2):95–104.

34. Brazil, Ministério da Saúde, Coordenação Geral de Vigilância em Saúde Ambiental, Secretaria de Vigilância em Saúde. Avanços e perspectivas da vigilância em saúde ambiental no Brasil. Brasilia: CGVAM/SVS; 2006. Unpublished.

35. Commission for Environmental Cooperation. Children's Health and the Environment in North America: A First Report on Available Indicators and Measures. Montreal: CEC; 2006.

36. Santos ECO, Cámara VM, Jesús IM, et al. A contribution to the establishment of references values for total mercury levels in hair and fish in Amazonia. Environ Res. 2002; 90(1):6–11.

37. Pan American Health Organization. Sanitary Surveillance of Pesticides: experience of PLAGSALUD in Central America. Washington, DC: PAHO; 2004.

38. Pan American Health Organization. Epidemiol Bul. 2001; 22 (4). Available at: http://www.paho.org/spanish/sha/EB_V22n4.pdf.

39. Pan American Health Organization; United Nations Environment Program; Global Environmental Facility. Regional Program of Action and Demonstration of Sustainable Alternatives to DDT for Malaria Vector Control in Mexico and Central America. Washington, DC: PAHO; 2002.

40. United Nations Environment Program. Minimizing hazardous wastes: a simplified guide to the Basel Convention. Geneva: UNEP; 2002.

41. United Nations Environment Program; Food and Agriculture Organization of the United Nations. Rotterdam Convention on the Prior Informed Consent (PIC) Procedure for Certain Hazardous Chemicals and Pesticides in International Trade. Geneva: UNEP; 2005.

42. United Nations Environment Program. Stockholm Convention on Persistent Organic Pollutants (POPs). Geneva: UNEP; 2002.

43. Kosek M, Bern C, Guerrant RL. The magnitude of the global problem of diarrheal disease from studies published 1992–2000. Bull World Health Organ 2003;81(3):197–204.

44. Binsztein N, Fernández A, Caffer MI, Agudelo CI, Arias MI, Ugarte C, et al. WHO Global Salm-Surv (WHO GSS) in the South American Region: five years (2000–2004) of Salmonella surveillance. International Conference on Emerging Infectious Diseases, Atlanta, Georgia, 21 March 2006.

45. World Health Organization. WHO Consultation to Develop a Strategy to Estimate the Global Burden of Foodborne Diseases. Geneva, 25–27 September 2006. Available at: http://www.who.int/foodsafety/publications/foodborne_disease/burden_sept06/en/.

46. Diemert DJ. Prevention and self-treatment of traveler's diarrhea. Clin Microbiol Rev. 2006;19:583–94.

47. Torres R, Skillicorn P. Montezuma's revenge: how sanitation concerns may injure Mexico's tourist industry. Cornell Hotel and Restaurant Administration Quarterly. 2004;45(2): 132–44.

48. Pan American Institute for Food Protection and Zoonoses. Assessment of the Food Safety Systems in the America Region. INPAZ/PAHO; 2004. Available at: http://www.panalimentos.org/evaluacion/evaluacion.sia.ingles/index.html.

49. Flint JA, Van Duynhoven YT, Angulo FJ, DeLong SM, Braun P, Kirk M, et al. Estimating the burden of acute gastroenteritis, foodborne disease, and pathogens commonly transmitted by food: an international review. Clin Infec Dis. 2005;41:698–704.

50. Aguiar Prieto PH, Castro Domínguez A, Pérez E, Coutin Marie G, Triana Rodríguez T, et al. Carga de la shigelosis en tres sitios centinelas de Cuba. 2005. Available at: http://www.sld.cu/galerias/pdf/sitios/vigilancia/rtv0405.pdf.

51. Economic Commission for Latin America and the Caribbean. Social Panorama of Latin America. Santiago de Chile: ECLAC; 2006.

52. Castro G. Los riesgos del trabajo en América Latina. International Social Security Review. 2005;58(2–3):125–39.

53. International Labor Organization, Policy Integration Department, Bureau of Statistics. LABORSTA: online statistics. Geneva: ILO; 2006.

54. Dong C, Platner J. Occupational fatalities of Hispanic construction workers from 1992 to 2000. Am J Ind Med. 2003; 45(1):45–54.

55. International Labor Organization. Labor Overview 2005. Geneva: ILO; 2005.

56. World Bank. Regional activities: Latin America and the Caribbean [Web site]. World Bank; 2006.

57. Bullinger HJ. The changing world of work: prospects and challenges for health and safety. Magazine of the European Agency for Safety and Health at Work. 2000;2:8–13.

58. International Labor Organization. The End of Child Labor: Within Reach. Geneva: ILO; 2006.

59. International Labor Organization. Global employment trends brief. Geneva: ILO; 2007.

60. Fundación Iberoamericana de Seguridad y Salud Ocupacional; Inter-American Development Bank. Survey on the Regional Workers' Health Plan. FISO/IDB; 2002.

61. International Labor Organization. Labor Overview 2005: Latin America and the Caribbean (First Semester Advance Report). Geneva: ILO; 2005.

62. Eijkemans G. WHO occupational health fact sheet. Geneva: WHO; 2007.

63. Fingerhut M, Nelson DI, Driscoll T, Concha-Barrientos M, Steenland K, Punnett L, et al. The contribution of occupational risks to the global burden of disease: summary and next steps. Med Lav. 2006;97(2):313–21.

64. Chile, Ministerio de Salud. Equidad en salud ocupacional, la salud de los trabajadores de Chile [PowerPoint presentation by the Minister of Health]. 2005.

65. Chile, Dirección de Trabajo, Departamento de Estudios. Encuesta Laboral 2004. Relaciones de trabajo y empleo en Chile. Resultados de la Cuarta Encuesta Laboral. Santiago de Chile; 2005.

66. Colombia, Ministerio de la Protección Social. Estadísticas del sistema general de riesgos profesionales; 2005. Available at: http://www.minproteccionsocial.gov.co/MseContent/images/news/DocNewsNo658301.pdf.

67. Argentina, Superintendencia de Riesgos del Trabajo. Anuario estadístico 2003. Accidentes de trabajo y enfermedades profesionales. Buenos Aires: SRT; 2004. Available at: http://www.srt.gov.ar/nvaweb/data/data2003.htm.

68. Heiremans E. Las mutualidades de empleadores en Chile. In: Federación de Aseguradores Colombianos. Memorias del Primer Encuentro Internacional de Riesgos Profesionales. Bogotá: FASECOLDA; June 2001.

69. Colombia, Ministerio de la Protección Social. Estadísticas del sistema general de riesgos profesionales; 2005. Available at: http://www.minproteccionsocial.gov.co/MseContent/images/news/DocNewsNo658301.pdf.

70. Wesseling C, Aragón A, Morgado H, Elgstrand K, Hogstedt C, Partanen T. Occupational health in Central America. Int J Occup Environ Health. 2002;8:125–36.

71. IV Summit of the Americas. Declaration of Mar del Plata. Mar del Plata, Argentina, November 2005.

72. Amador-Rodezno R. An overview to CERSSO's self evaluation of the cost-benefit on the investment in occupational safety and health in the textile factories: a step by step methodology. Pan American Health Organization; Regional Center for Occupational Safety and Health; 2005.

73. United Nations. Report on the United Nations Conference on Environment and Development. Earth Summit. Rio de Janeiro, June 1992.

74. United Nations. Resolution adopted by the General Assembly. 55/2. United Nations Millennium Declaration. New York: UN; 2000. Available at: http://www.un.org/millennium/declaration/ares552e.htm.

75. World Health Organization. Johannesburg Declaration on Sustainable Development. Johannesburg: WHO; 2002.

76. Meeting of the Ministers of Health of the Americas, Mar del Plata, Argentina, 16–17 June 2005.

77. Pan American Health Organization. Report on the Workshop on Environmental Threats to the Health of Children in the Americas. Lima: CEPIS; 2003.

78. Pan American Health Organization. Healthy environments: healthy children [toolkit for the classroom]. Washington, DC: PAHO; 2004.

79. Commission for Environmental Cooperation. Children's Health and the Environment in North America. A First Report on Available Indicators and Measures. Montreal: CEC; 2006.

80. Ruiz A, Henao S, Galvão L. Indicadores de salud ambiental: una herramienta para lograr la salud de los niños. Washington, DC: OPS; 2004.

81. Ruiz A. Taller sobre indicadores de salud ambiental para los niños de América Latina y el Caribe. Informe final. San José: OPS; 2004.

82. Partanen T, Wesselin C. Efectos sobre la salud humana de los contaminantes orgánicos persistentes: aldrín, dieldrín, endrín, clordano, DDT, toxafeno, mirex, heptacloro, hexaclorobenceno, los bifenilos policlorados, Dioxins-Para-Dibenzo policlorados y dibenzofuranos policlorados. Un examen. Costa Rica; 2004.

83. Pan American Health Organization. An Assessment of Health Effects of Ambient Air Pollution in Latin America and the Caribbean. Washington, DC: PAHO; 2005.

84. Delgado HL, Palma P, Palmieri, M. La iniciativa de seguridad alimentaria nutricional en Centroamérica. Guatemala: INCAP/OPS; 1999.

85. Bermúdez O, Tucker L. Trends in dietary patterns of Latin American populations. Cad Saúde Pública. 2003;19 Sup. 1:S87–S99.

86. World Health Organization. Physical status: The use and interpretation of anthropometry. Report of a WHO Expert Committee. WHO Technical Report Series 854. Geneva: WHO; 1995.

87. Popkin BM. An overview on the nutrition transition and its health implications: the Bellagio meeting. Public Health Nutrition. 2002;5(1A): 93–103.

88. World Bank. Repositioning Nutrition as Central to Development, A Strategy for Large-Scale Action. Washington, DC: International Bank for Reconstruction and Development/World Bank; 2006.

89. Economic Commission for Latin America and the Caribbean. The Millennium Development Goals: A Latin American and Caribbean Perspective, 2005. Santiago de Chile: ECLAC; 2005.

90. Roses M. Integración entre salud y agricultura para el bienestar y la calidad de vida. Available at: http://mirtaroses.paho.org/index.php?language=es-es en 13/0906.

91. Gibbs EPJ. Emerging zoonotic epidemics in the interconnected global community. Veterinary Record. 2005;157: 673–79.

92. Pan American Health Organization. 13th Inter-American Meeting, at the Ministerial Level, on Health and Agriculture (RIMSA 13). Final report. Washington, DC: OPS; 2003. Available at: http://bvs.panaftosa.org.br/textoc/rimsa13-fr-2003ing.pdf.

93. Organización Panamericana de la Salud. Informe de situación de los países presentado por el Centro Panamericano de Fiebre Aftosa a la COSALFA XXVIII. OPS; 2002.

94. Pan American Health Organization, Pan American Foot-and-Mouth Disease Center. South American Commission for the Fight against Foot-and-Mouth Disease (COSALFA) XXIX. Final Report. Rio de Janeiro: PANAFTOSA; 2003.

95. Pan American Health Organization, Pan American Foot-and-Mouth Disease Center. South American Commission for the Fight against Foot-and-Mouth Disease (COSALFA) XXX. Final Report. Rio de Janeiro: PANAFTOSA; 2004.

96. Pan American Health Organization, Pan American Foot-and-Mouth Disease Center. Action Plan Hemispheric Program for Eradication of Foot-and-Mouth Disease (PHEFA), 2005–2009. Washington, DC: PAHO; 2004.

97. Organización Panamericana de la Salud. Informe de situación de los países a la COSALFA XXXIII. Centro Panamericano de Fiebre Aftosa. OPS; 2006.

98. World Organization for Animal Health. Geographical distribution of countries that reported BSE confirmed cases since 1989. Paris: OIE; 2006. Available at: http://www.oie.int/eng/info/en_esb.htm.

99. World Health Organization. Variant Creutzfeldt-Jakob disease. WHO; 2006. Available at: http://www.who.int/zoonoses/diseases/variantcjd/en/.

100. Organización Panamericana de la Salud, Centro Panamericano de Fiebre Aftosa. Listado de verificación de los sistemas de prevención y vigilancia de las encefalopatías espongiformes bovinas. PANAFTOSA/OPS; 2003. Available at: http://www.panaftosa.org.br/inst/DOWNLOAD/evaluacion_EEB.pdf.

101. Organización Panamericana de la Salud, Centro Panamericano de Fiebre Aftosa. Los recursos de diagnóstico para EEB identificados por PANAFTOSA. OPS; 2006. Available at: http://www.panaftosa.org.br.

102. Organización Panamericana de la Salud, Centro Panamericano de Fiebre Aftosa. Situación actual y perspectivas de acción en relación a influenza aviar (IA) en América. Documento de trabajo. Conferencia Hemisférica de Vigilancia y Prevención de la Influenza Aviar. Brasilia: OPS; 2005.

103. Webster R. Influenza: an emerging disease. Emerg Infect Dis. 1998;4(3):437–41.

104. Horimoto T, Kawaoka Y. Pandemic threat posed by avian influenza A viruses. Clin Microbiol Rev. 2001 Jan:129–49.

105. Swayne DE, Suárez DL. Highly pathogenic avian influenza. Rev Sci Tech Off Int Epiz. 2000;19(2): 463–82.

106. Food and Agriculture Organization of the United Nations. Livestock statistics. Rome: FAO; 2006. Available at: http://faostat.fao.org/site/568/default.aspx.

107. World Health Organization. Cumulative number of confirmed human cases of avian influenza A/(H5N1) reported to WHO. September 2006. Available at: http://www.who.int/csr/disease/avian_influenza/country/cases_table_2006_09_30/en/index.html.

108. World Health Organization. Avian influenza: assessing the pandemic threat. January 2005. Available at: http://www.who. int/entity/csr/disease/influenza/H5N1-9reduit.pdf.

109. Pan American Health Organization. Report on the 14th Inter-American Meeting, at the Ministerial Level, on Health and Agriculture (RIMSA 14). Washington, DC: PAHO; 2005. Available at: http://www.ops-oms.org/English/GOV/CD/cd46-14-e.pdf.

110. World Health Organization. The World Health Report 2002. Reducing Risks, Promoting Healthy Life. Geneva: WHO; 2002.

111. Pan American Health Organization. Health Statistics from the Americas. Washington, DC: PAHO; 2006.

112. Teo KK, Ounpuu S, Hawken S, Pandey MR, Valentin V, Hunt D, et al. Tobacco use and risk of myocardial infarction in 52 countries in the INTERHEART study: a case-control study. Lancet. 2006 Aug 19;368(9536):647–58.

113. Danaei G, Vander Hoorn S, López AD, Murray CJ, Ezzati M. Comparative risk assessment collaborating group (cancers). Causes of cancer in the world: comparative risk assessment of nine behavioural and environmental risk factors. Lancet. 2005 Nov 19;366(9499):1784–93.

114. United States, California Environmental Protection Agency, Office of Environmental Health Hazard Assessment. Health effects of exposure to environmental tobacco smoke: final report. Sacramento: OEHHA; 2005. Available at: http://www.oehha.ca.gov/air/environmental_tobacco/2005etsfinal.html. Accessed 31 October 2006.

115. United States, Department of Health and Human Services, Centers for Disease Control and Prevention. The health consequences of involuntary exposure to tobacco smoke: a report of the Surgeon General. Atlanta: HHS; CDC; 2006.

116. United States, Department of Health and Human Services, Centers for Disease Control and Prevention; World Health Organization. Global Youth Tobacco Survey (GYTS). Available at: http://www.cdc.gov/tobacco/global/surveys.htm #gyts.

117. Navas-Acien A, Peruga A, Breysse P, Zavaleta A, Blanco-Marquizo A, Pitarque R, et al. Secondhand tobacco smoke in public places in Latin America, 2002–2003. JAMA. 2004; June 9;291(22):2741–45.

118. Barnum H. The economic burden of the global trade in tobacco. Tob Control. 1994;3:358–61.

119. United States, Department of Health and Human Services, Centers for Disease Control and Prevention. Annual smoking-attributable mortality, years of potential life lost, and economic costs, United States, 1995–1999. Morb Mortal Wkly Rep. 2002 Apr 12;51(14):300–3.

120. Behan D, Eriksen M, Lin Y. Economic effects of environmental tobacco smoke [report]. Schaumburg, Illinois: Society of Actuaries 2005. Available at: http://www.soa.org/ccm/cms-service/stream/asset/?asset_id=13389116&g11n.

121. Adams EK, Melvon C, Merritt R, Worrall B. The costs of environmental tobacco smoke (ETS): an international review. Background Paper for the International Consultation on Environmental Tobacco Smoke (ETS) and Child Health, 11–14 January 1999. Geneva: WHO; 1999.

122. Gonzáles-Rozada M. Economía del control del tabaco en los países del Mercosur y Estados Asociados: Argentina: 1996–2004. Washington, DC: OPS; 2006.

123. Alcaraz VO. Economía del control del tabaco en los países del Mercosur y Estados Asociados: Bolivia. Washington, DC: OPS; 2006.

124. Iglesias R. Economía del control del tabaco en los países del Mercosur y Estados Asociados: Brasil. Washington, DC: OPS; 2006.

125. Debrott Sánchez D. Economía del control del tabaco en los países del Mercosur y Estados Asociados: Chile. Washington, DC: OPS; 2006.

126. Ramos A. Economía del control del tabaco en los países del Mercosur y Estados Asociados: Uruguay. Washington, DC: OPS; 2006.

127. Pan American Health Organization. Profits over people. Tobacco industry activities to market cigarettes and undermine public health in Latin America and the Caribbean. Washington, DC: PAHO; 2002.

128. World Health Organization. WHO Framework Convention on Tobacco Control. Geneva: WHO; 2003.

129. World Health Organization. Policy recommendations on protection from exposure to second-hand tobacco smoke. Geneva: WHO; 2007.

130. Canada, Physicians for a Smoke-free Canada. Fact-sheet. Background on protection from second-hand smoke in Canada [Web page]. Ottawa: Physicians for a Smoke-free Canada; 2006. Available at: http://www.smoke-free.ca/fact-sheets/pdf/Q&A-smokefreecommunities.pdf.

131. United States, American Nonsmokers' Rights Foundation. Smokefree air on the increase—More than 50% of U.S. population to be protected by smokefree air laws [Press release]. Berkeley: Americans for Nonsmokers' Rights; 2006. Available at: http://www.no-smoke.org/pdf/smokefreeair-increase.pdf.

132. Pan American Health Organization. Exposure to Second-hand Tobacco Smoke in the Americas: A Human Rights Perspective. Washington, DC: PAHO; 2006.

133. World Bank. Curbing the Epidemic: Governments and the Economics of Tobacco Control. Washington, DC: World Bank; 1999.

134. Blecher EH, van Walbeek CP. An international analysis of cigarette affordability. Tob Control. 2004; 13:339–46.

135. Brazil, Instituto Datafolha. Encuesta de opinión pública realizada el abril de 2002 [data from the Instituto Nacional del Cáncer and the Ministerio de Salud of Brazil].

136. Hammond D, Fong GT, McDonald PW, Cameron R, Brown KS. Impact of the graphic Canadian warning labels on adult smoking behaviour. Tob Control. 2003;12: 391–95.

137. Hammond R. Tobacco advertising and promotion: The need for a coordinated global response. Background paper for the WHO international conference on global tobacco control law: towards a WHO Framework Convention on Tobacco Control. World Health Organization; 2000.

138. Saffer H. Tobacco advertising and promotion. In: Jha P, Chaloupka F, eds. Tobacco control in developing countries. Washington, DC: World Bank; WHO; 2000.

139. Dalton M, Sargent J, Beach M, Titus-Ernstoff L, Gibson J, Ahrens M, et al. Effect of viewing smoking in movies on adolescent smoking initiation: a cohort study. Lancet. 2003; 362(9380):281–5.

140. United States, Smoke Free Movies. [Web page]. Available at: http://www.smokefreemovies.ucsf.edu/index.html. Accessed in December 2006.

141. Mexico, British American Tobacco. Acomodando a ambos, "fumadores" y "no fumadores" [Web page]. Monterrey: British American Tobacco Mexico; 2006. Available at: http://www.batmexico.com.mx/oneweb/sites/BAT_5NNAR K.nsf/vwPagesWebLive/DO5PKSKK?opendocument&SID =&DTC=&TMP=1. Accessed December 2006.

142. British American Tobacco. Social Report 2005 [Web page]. British American Tobacco; 2005. Available at: http://www. bat.com/OneWeb/sites/uk__3mnfen.nsf/vwPagesWeb Live/C1256E3C003D3339C12571690056085D?opendocu- ment&DTC=&SID. Accessed in December 2006.

143. Argentina, Nobleza Piccardo. Leyendas de advertencia [Web page]. Available at: http://www.noblezapiccardo.com/ OneWeb/sites/NOB_58LMXM.nsf/vwPagesWebLive/DO6H GQHP?opendocument&SID=&DTC=&TMP=1. Accessed in December 2006.

144. United States, Department of Justice. National Campaign for Tobacco-Free Kids. Special report: Justice Department Civil Lawsuit. Available at: http://www.tobaccofreekids. org/reports/doj/. Accessed 6 December 2006.

145. British American Tobacco. Annual Review and Summary Financial Statement 2005. Available at: http://www.bat.com/ OneWeb/sites/uk__3mnfen.nsf/vwPagesWebLive/DO52AK 34?opendocument&SID=&DTC=&TMP=1. Accessed 6 De- cember 2006.

146. Wiehe SE, Garrison MM, Christakis DA, Ebel BE, Rivara FP. A systematic review of school-based smoking prevention trials with long-term follow-up. J Adol Health. 2005;36: 162–69.

147. World Health Organization. The World Health Report 2002. Reducing Risks, Promoting Healthy Life. Geneva: WHO; 2002.

148. Rehm J, Monteiro M. Alcohol consumption and burden of disease in the Americas: implications for alcohol policy. Rev Panam Salud Pública. 2005;18(4/5):241–48.

149. Rehm J, Room R, Monteiro M, Gmel G, Graham K, Rehn N, et al. Alcohol use. In: Ezzati M, Lopez AD, Rodgers A, Mur- ray CJL, eds. Comparative quantification of health risks: global and regional burden of disease due to selected risk factors (Vol. 1). Geneva: WHO; 2004. pp. 959–1108.

150. Harwood H. Updating estimates of the economic costs of alcohol abuse in the United States: estimates, update meth- ods, and data report. Prepared by the Lewin Group for the National Institute on Alcohol Abuse and Alcoholism, 2000.

151. Single E, Robson L, Xie X, Rehm J. The economic costs of alcohol, tobacco and illicit drugs in Canada. Addiction. 1992;93(7):99–100.

152. World Health Organization, Department of Mental Health and Substance Abuse. Global Status Report on Alcohol 2004. Geneva: WHO; 2004.

153. Rehm J, Room R, Graham K, Monteiro M, Gmel G, Tempos C. The relationship of average volume of alcohol consump- tion and patterns of drinking to burden of disease: an overview. Addiction. 2003;98:1209–15.

154. Kohn R, Levav I, Caldas de Almeida JM, Vicente B, Andrade L, Caraveo-Anduaga JJ, Saxena S, Saraceno B. Los trastornos mentales en América Latina y el Caribe: asunto prioritario para la salud pública. Rev Panam Salud Pública. 2005; 18(4/5):229–40.

155. World Health Organization. Global Status Report: Alcohol and Young People. Geneva: WHO; 2001.

156. Mandelbaum D. Alcohol and culture. In: Marshall M (ed.). Beliefs, behaviors and alcoholic beverages. Ann Arbor: Uni- versity of Michigan Press; 1979. pp. 14–30.

157. Pan L. Alcohol in colonial Africa. Vol. 22. Helsinki: Finnish Foundation for Alcohol Studies; 1975.

158. Seale P, Shellenberger S, Rodríguez C, Seale JD, Alvarado M. Alcohol use and cultural change in an indigenous popula- tion: a case study from Venezuela. Alcohol and Alcoholism. 2002;37(6):603–8.

159. Organización Panamericana de la Salud. Alcohol y salud de los pueblos indígenas El Alto, Capital Aymara. La Paz: OPS; 2006.

160. Room R, Jernigan D, Carlini-Marlatt B, Gureje O, Makela K, Marshall M, et al. Alcohol in developing societies: a public health approach. Vol. 46. Finnish Foundation for Alcohol Studies/WHO; 2002.

161. Babor T, Caetano P, Casswell S, Edwards G, et al. Alcohol: no ordinary commodity. Research and Public Policy. Oxford: Oxford University Press; 2003.

162. Duailibi S, Ponicki W, Grube J, Pinsky I, Laranjeira R, Raw M. Does restricting opening hours reduce alcohol related vi- olence? Am J Public Health. 2006. (In press).

163. Chisholm D, Rehm J, Van Ommeren M, Monteiro M. Reduc- ing the global burden of hazardous alcohol use: a compara- tive cost effectiveness analysis. J Stud Alcohol. 2004;65: 782–93.

164. Pan American Health Organization. World Report on Vio- lence and Health. Washington, DC: PAHO; 2003. (Scientific and technical publication No. 588).

165. Pan American Health Organization. Health Situation in the Americas. Basic Indicators. Washington, D.C.: PAHO; 1996–2005.

166. Ellsberg M, Peña R, Herrera A, Liljestrand J, Winkvist A. Candies in hell: women's experiences of violence in Nicaragua. Soc Sci Med. 2000;51(11):1595–1610.

167. El Salvador, Equipo de Reflexión Investigación y Comuni- cación; Instituto de Encuestas y Sondeos de Opinión; Insti- tuto de Investigaciones Económicas y Sociales; Instituto Universitario de Opinión Publica. Maras y pandillas en Cen- troamérica. Pandillas y capital social. Vol. II. San Salvador: UCA Editores; 2004.

168. Santacruz M, Concha-Eastman A, Cruz JM. Barrio adentro. La solidaridad violenta de las pandillas. San Salvador:

OPS/OMS; Universidad Centro América J.S. Cañas; Instituto Universitario de Opinión Pública; 2001.

169. Peres MFT. Violência por armas do fogo no Brasil—Relatorio Nacional, São Paulo, Brasil. Universidade de São Paulo, Núcleo de Estudos da Violência; 2004.

170. Colombia, Instituto Nacional de Medicina Legal y Ciencias Forenses. Forensis, Datos para la vida. Bogota; 2001–2005. Available at: http://www.medicinalegal.gov.co/.

171. Londoño, JL, Gaviria A, Guerrero R (eds.). Asalto al desarrollo. Violencia en América Latina. Washington, DC: Banco Interamericano de Desarrollo, Red de Centros de Investigación; 2000.

172. Programa de las Naciones Unidas para el Desarrollo. Cuánto le cuesta la violencia a El Salvador. San Salvador: PNUD; 2005.

173. Pan American Health Organization; World Health Organization. International Classification of Diseases and Related Health Problems (ICD-10). Vol. I. Washington, DC: PAHO/WHO; 2003.

174. Garfield R, Llanten Morales CP. The public health context of violence in Colombia. Rev Panam Salud Pública. 2004;16(4): 266–71.

175. Concha-Eastman A. Ten years of a successful violence reduction program in Bogota, Colombia. In: McVeigh C, Hughes K, Lushey C, Bellis MA (eds.). Preventing violence: from global perspective to national action. Liverpool: Center for Public Health, John Moores University; 2005. pp. 13–18.

176. Guerrero R, Concha-Eastman A. An epidemiological approach for the prevention of urban violence: the case of Cali, Colombia. Journal of Health and Population in Developing Countries. 2001;4(1). Available at: www.jhpdc.unc.edu.

177. Colombia, Sistema Unificado de Información sobre Violencia y Delincuencia de Bogotá. Available at: http://www.suivd.gov.co.

178. United States, Department of Health and Human Services, Centers for Disease Control and Prevention. Homicide trends and characteristics, Brazil, 1980–2002. Morb Mortal Wkly Rep. 2004 Mar 5;53(8):169–71.

179. United States, Department of Health and Human Services, Centers for Disease Control and Prevention. Homicides among children and young adults, Puerto Rico, 1999–2003. Morb Mortal Wkly Rep. 2006 Apr 7;55(13):361–64.

180. Guatemala, Instituto Nacional de Estadísticas. 2000–2005.

181. El Salvador, Mesa Técnica, Policía Nacional, Fiscalía General de la República, Instituto de Medicina Forense. [Data from 2005]. Fiscalía General de la República. [Data from 1999–2004].

182. Costa Rica, Instituto Nacional de Estadística y Censos. 1996–2005. Available at: http://www.inec.go.cr/.

183. Belize, Ministry of Health. Homicide rates. 2001–2005.

184. Organización Panamericana de la Salud/Organización Mundial de la Salud. Informe de la jornada de trabajo sobre indicadores de seguridad humana. Panama, August 2006.

185. Ward E. Application of an injury surveillance system for targeting interventions or violence prevention. In: McVeigh C, Hughes K, Lushey C, Bellis MA (eds.). Preventing violence: from global perspective to national action. Liverpool: Center for Public Health, John Moores Univesity; 2005. pp. 53–58.

186. Lemard G, Hemenway D. Violence in Jamaica: an analysis of homicides 1998–2002. Inj Prev. 2006 Feb;12(1):15–18.

187. Briceño-León R. Violencia interpersonal y percepción ciudadana de la situación de seguridad en Venezuela. Unpublished; 2006.

188. Cruz JM (ed.). Maras y pandillas en Centroamérica. Vol. IV. Las respuestas de la sociedad civil organizada. San Salvador: UCA Editores; 2006.

189. Honduras, Asociación Cristiana de Jóvenes; Save the Children. Las maras en Honduras. Investigación sobre pandillas y violencia juvenil, consulta nacional. Plan Nacional de Atención. Ley especial. Tegucigalpa: Frinsa Impresos; 2002.

190. Castro M, Carranza M. Las maras en Honduras. In: Maras y pandillas en Centroamérica. Vol. I. Managua: UCA Publicaciones; 2001.

191. Smutt M, Miranda JL. El fenómeno de la violencia en El Salvador. San Salvador: PNUD; 1998.

192. Cruz JM, Portillo PN. Solidaridad y violencia en las pandillas del gran San Salvador. Más allá de la vida loca. San Salvador: UCA Editores; 1998.

193. United States, United States Agency for International Development, Bureau for Latin American and Caribbean Affairs, Office of Regional Sustainable Development. Central America and Mexico Gang Assessment. April 2006.

194. Organización Panamericana de la Salud. Fomento del Desarrollo Juvenil y Prevención de la Violencia. OPS/GTZ; 2006. Available at: http://www.paho.org/CDMEDIA/FCHGTZ/principal.htm.

195. Colombia, Organización Panamericana de la Salud. Salud y desplazamiento. ¿Quiénes son los desplazados por la violencia?

196. Colombia, Sistema Único de Registro. Registro único de población desplazada. 2005. Available at: http://www.accionsocial.gov.co/SUR/Registro_SUR_Acumulado.xls.

197. Organización Panamericana de la Salud. Available at: http://www.disaster-info.net/desplazados/. Accessed 27 February 2007.

198. World Health Organization. Holder Y, Peden M, Krug E, Lund J, Gururaj G, Kobusingye O (eds.) Injury Surveillance Guidelines. Geneva: WHO; 2001. Available at: http://www.who.int/violence_injury_prevention/en/.

199. World Health Organization. International Classification of External Causes of Injury. Available at: http://www.iceci.org.

200. Colombia, Universidad del Valle, Instituto de Promoción de Coexistencia y Prevención de Violencia. Available at: http://www.cisalva.univalle.edu.co/.

201. Pan American Health Organization. World Report on Road Traffic Injury Prevention. Washington, DC: PAHO; 2004.

202. Acero-Velásquez H, Concha-Eastman A. Road safety: a public policy problem in the Americas. Washington, DC: PAHO; 2004.

203. World Health Organization. Injury severe enough to need medical attention. Available at: http://www.who.int/health info/statistics/gbdwhoregionincidence2002.xls.

204. Hijar M, Vásquez-Vela E, Arreola-Risa C. Pedestrian traffic injuries in Mexico: a country update. Injury Control and Safety Promotion. 2003;10:37–43.

205. Argentina, Ministerio de Salud de la Nación, Dirección de Estadísticas e Información de Salud. 2002.

206. García González M. Muertes en accidentes de tránsito. Forensis 2002: datos para la vida. Bogotá: Centro de Referencia Nacional sobre Violencia; 2003.

207. Venezuela, Comisión Interministerial para la Atención, Prevención y Educación Vial. Coordinación programa prevención de accidentes y otros hechos violentos. (Presented at the Seminario Internacional sobre Seguridad Vial, Pan American Health Organization, Brasilia, 28–30 June 2004.)

208. Cuba, Ministerio de Transporte, Comisión Nacional de Vialidad y Tránsito; Ministerio de Salud Pública; Policía Nacional Revolucionaria; Instituto Medicina Legal. Perfil nacional sobre seguridad vial, 2004. (Presented at the Seminario Internacional sobre Seguridad Vial, Pan American Health Organization, Brasilia, 28–30 June 2004.)

209. Trinidad and Tobago, Ministry of Planning and Development, Central Statistical Office. Available at: http://www.cso.gov.tt/statistics/psvs/default.asp. Accessed 11 June 2004.

210. Costa Rica, Ministerio de Salud. Perfil nacional sobre seguridad vial, 2004.

211. World Health Organization. Global Burden of Disease Project, 2002. Version 1.

212. Vasconcelos EA. Strategies to improve traffic safety in Latin America. (Presented at the World Bank Taller de Consulta en América Latina: Revisión de la Estrategias para Transporte Urbano, Santiago, Chile, 6–9 November 2000.)

213. Mexico, Consejo Nacional para la Prevención de Accidentes. Modelo de Atención Prehospitalaria.

214. Peru, Policía Nacional; Ministerio del Interior; Instituto de Medicina Legal; Ministerio de Salud. Perfil nacional sobre seguridad vial, 2004.

215. Pan American Health Organization. 47th Directing Council. Health Promotion: Achievements and Lessons Learned from Ottawa to Bangkok. CD47/16. Washington, DC: PAHO; 2006.

216. World Health Organization. Ottawa Charter for Health Promotion. First International Conference on Health Promotion, Ottawa, Canada, 17–21 November 1986.

217. World Health Organization. Adelaide Recommendations on Healthy Public Policy. Second International Conference on Health Promotion, Adelaide, Australia, 5–9 April 1988.

218. Pan American Health Organization, World Health Organization; Colombia, Ministerio de Salud. Declaration of the International Conference on Health Promotion. Bogota: PAHO/WHO; 1992.

219. Pan American Health Organization. Health Promotion: An Anthology. Washington DC: OPS; 1996. (Scientific publication No. 557).

220. Mexico Ministerial Statement for the Promotion of Health. Fifth Global Conference on Health Promotion. Mexico City, Mexico, 5 June 2000.

221. Sundsvall Statement on Supportive Environments for Health. Third International Conference on Health Promotion, Sundsvall, Sweden, 9–15 June 1991.

222. Organización Panamericana de la Salud/Organización Mundial de la Salud. Guía de evaluación participativa para municipios y comunidades saludables. OPS/OMS; 2003. Available at: http://www.bvsde.ops-oms.org/bvsdemu/fulltext/guiaeval/guiaeval.html.

223. Pan American Health Organization. Health Promoting Schools: Strengthening of the Regional Initiative. Washington, DC: PAHO; 2003.

224. Chile, Ministerio de Salud. Presentación de la experiencia de Chile. Santiago de Chile; January 2006.

225. United States, Department of Health and Human Services. Healthy People 2010. Washington, DC: Department of Health and Human Services; 2000. Available at: http://www.health.gov/healthypeople.

226. Jakarta Declaration on Leading Health Promotion into the 21st Century. 4th International Conference on Health Promotion, Jakarta, Indonesia; 21–25 July 1997.

227. Cerqueira MT, Conti C, De La Torre A. La promoción de la salud y el enfoque de espacios saludables en las Américas. In: FAO. Food, Nutrition and Agriculture. 2003;33:36–44.

228. Economic Commission for Latin America and the Caribbean. The Millennium Development Goals: a Latin American and Caribbean Perspective, 2005. Santiago de Chile: ECLAC; 2005.

229. Argentina, Red Argentina de Municipios y Comunidades Saludable. 2006. Available at: http://municipios.msal.gov.ar/.

230. Akerman M, Mendes R (eds.). Participating evaluation of healthy cities, communities and environments: the Brazilian trajectory—memory, thoughts and experiences. São Paulo; Midia alternativa; 2006.

231. Canada, Ontario Healthy Communities Coalition. 2006. Available at: http://www.healthycommunities.on.ca/.

232. Canada, Réseau québécois de villes et villages en santé. 2006. Available at: http://www.rqvvs.qc.ca/anglais/ reseau/intro.htm.

233. United States, Center for Civic Partnerships. 2006. Available at: http://www.civicpartnerships.org.

234. United States, Indiana University, WHO Collaborating Center for Healthy Cities. 2006. Available at: http://www.iupui.edu/~citynet/citynet.htm.

235. Peru, Red de Municipios y Ciudades Saludables. 2006. Available at: www.miraflores.gob.pe/redmunicipiosaludables.

236. Organización Panamericana de la Salud. Vivienda saludable: reto del milenio en los asentamientos precarios de América Latina y el Caribe. Guía para las autoridades nacionales y locales; 2005.

237. Zuluaga J. Neurodesarrollo y estimulación. Bogotá: Editorial Médica Panamericana SA; 2001.

238. Ippolito-Shepherd J, Cerqueira MT, Ortega D. Iniciativa Regional Escuelas Promotoras de la Salud en las Américas. IUHPE Promotion and Education 2005;XII(3–4):220–29.

239. Ippolito-Shepherd J. Las escuelas promotoras de la salud en América Latina. Resultados de la Primera Encuesta Regional. Serie Promoción de la Salud Nº 3. Washington, DC: OPS; 2005.

240. Organización Panamericana de la Salud/Organización Mundial de la Salud. Memoria de la Cuarta Reunión de la Red Latinoamericana de Escuelas Promotoras de la Salud y Asamblea Constitutiva de la Red Puertorriqueña de Escuelas Promotoras de la Salud, San Juan, Puerto Rico, 11–16 de julio de 2004. Serie Promoción de la Salud Nº 11. Washington, DC: OPS/OMS; 2006.

Chapter 4
PUBLIC POLICIES AND HEALTH SYSTEMS AND SERVICES

Health is a critical contributor to the success of social policies that enable the attainment of national goals of social and economic development. Attaining those goals depends on effective health policies. Notwithstanding, addressing health policy issues that shape the health system poses problems, because social needs are multidimensional, adverse effects can be cumulative, resources are finite, and, frequently, solutions lie outside the health sector. Consequently, introducing changes to enhance the role of the health system as a core social institution that is also able to create wide-ranging opportunities in the design and delivery of goods and services requires a systemic approach to public policies and policymaking. Public policy can be understood as a set of authoritative decisions produced by any branch and at any level of government and framed in a set of normative guidelines. Public policies communicate goals, means, strategies, and rules for decisionmaking in public administration and legislation. Laws, rules, regulations, operational and judicial interpretations and decisions, statutes, treaties, and executive orders are examples of such policies. Although there are no universally agreed definitions of public policies, they reflect a government's responses to conditions or circumstances that generate or will generate needs for a considerable number of people. Ideally, those responses coincide with the public interest. Furthermore, governments use public policies for political, moral, ethical, and economic reasons, or when the market fails to be efficient. A government also has the option of not responding—that is, public policy is "what government does and what government chooses to ignore" (*1*). Conversely, public policymaking is a central function of government and an essentially political process. As such, it involves relationships of power, influence, conflict, and cooperation where values, interests, and motivations shape the final design and implementation. Indeed, politics actually define who gets what, when, and how in society (*2*).

Health policies are important because they directly or indirectly affect all aspects of daily life, actions, behaviors, and decisions. They can prohibit behavior that is perceived as risky, promote behavior considered beneficial, protect the rights and well-being of targeted populations, encourage certain activities, and provide direct benefits to citizens in need. Regulatory policies can set professional accreditations; establish price controls on goods and services; define quality, safety, and efficacy standards in health services; and address social regulation issues, such as social security, occupational safety, immunization, food and drugs, and environmental pollution.

The Region of the Americas offers a broad array of subregional, national, and local health system experiences and evinces countless common trends, achievements, and challenges. For example, health system trends include the changing role of government in health care from sole provider to regulator and/or coordinator, the asymmetrical expansion of private health insurance, the privatization of social security institutions (affecting pensions and other forms of social security) and health services, and the expansion of public/private partnerships. Yet, along with the ascendancy of the market, civil society has increased its participation in policy development across the Region through partnerships, associations, organized groups, or representatives to advance issues of interest.

An important lesson learned from the legacies of previous health sector reforms, particularly decentralization and devolution, is that these transformations did not always result in greater and better access, equity, services, accountability, or even local participation. The incomplete achievement of those goals was, in some instances, associated with local conditions that were ignored. In the context of globalization, this is an increasingly significant factor due to the tensions between global and local interests, where the contours of "community" become more diffused, yet more heterogeneous (*3*). Recent experiences increasingly show that successful interventions value local knowledge and capacity, are tailored to heterogeneous conditions and populations, and learn lessons from the exchange, adaptation, and adoption of other successful interventions.

Policy innovation in health and health care is a challenging undertaking, mostly because systemic transformations in an era of global change that defy prevalent values and practices require significant resource commitments and often pose political risks. A case in point is that, despite escalating demands posed by demographic and epidemiological trends, competing needs, and resource limitations, the governments of the Americas, individually or collectively, continue to be committed to achieving high-performing systems that are capable of ensuring equitable access to services and social security, broadening coverage, and strengthening safety nets. However, it has been impossible to solve persistent problems in the production, acquisition, and regulation of pharmaceuticals, vaccines, and medical technologies, despite improvements in the legal and normative frameworks of the health system, including aspects related to stewardship, regulation, financing, insurance, quality, and harmonization.

The renewal of primary health care represents a substantial contribution to those goals, and the process rekindles longstanding commitments and represents a way forward to better public health. Systems based on primary care will further ongoing efforts to provide comprehensive care centered on promotion, prevention, and rehabilitation, jointly with patients, their families, and communities. The critical role of human resources for health figures prominently on the regional agenda, and unless these resources are competent, equitably distributed, and fairly compensated, health system goals will be unattainable.

The central role of health policies, health systems, and health services is to meet needs, mitigate risks, and protect populations from harm, disease, and disability; yet, potentially, they can also have a role in increasing disparities and exclusion. Although a more-detailed analysis is warranted, some factors enabling one or the other role include flawed initial structural conditions, weak governance, or even the delayed realization of benefits. Additionally, the limited ability of an increasingly devalued public sector, including health, to formulate policy has hampered the application of available knowledge, the presentation of convincing advocacy, and the implementation of policy. Too-slow execution and organizational and managerial misalignments may have jeopardized the desired goals of quality and safety in health services, including the effectiveness of drugs, medical technologies, and clinical services, which depend on the delivery of quality health services.

In effect, unwieldy conditions—pluralistic societies, uncertain conditions, unstable institutional landscapes, and a fragmented organizational base—can thwart the best intentions. Indeed, there are no universal policy prescriptions, and even a good decision does not guarantee a good solution. Moreover, the quality of health policies and the viability of equity-enhancing health system changes are constrained by history, culture, politics, economics, and the social foundations of the contexts where they are applied. Almost all aspects of economic and social policy influence health conditions and consequently health disparities. A closer alignment of health policies with equity-oriented social development policies that also consider issues of effectiveness and accountability is encouraging. Nevertheless, the coherence between social and economic policy and the subordination of social and health policy to decisions in other policy domains are still unresolved in most countries. Safeguarding the principle of universal access and achieving meaningful health gains will require not only changing current views on health policies, health systems, and services, but also challenging new forms of governance between the state and society—issues that transcend the health sector.

ORGANIZATION, COVERAGE, AND PERFORMANCE OF NATIONAL HEALTH AND SOCIAL WELFARE SYSTEMS

Values, Principles, and Purposes of Health Systems

A health system is understood to comprise the set of institutions responsible for interventions in society that are mainly responsible for health (4). These health interventions or actions embrace care for individuals and their environment for the purpose of promoting, protecting, or restoring health, or compensating for permanent disabilities, regardless of whether health agents are public, governmental, nongovernmental, or private (5). Health systems are a reflection of core social values that are also expressed in the legal and institutional frameworks that form the setting in which health policies are formulated.

Some of the values, principles, and purposes that most countries of the Region establish for their health systems in their constitutions or laws are:

- *Values*: right to health, universality, solidarity, equity, dignity, sustainable development, democratic governance.
- *Principles*: efficiency, effectiveness, quality, social participation/control, comprehensiveness of care, interculturality, decentralization, and transparency.
- *Purposes*: protection of the health of individuals and improvement of the quality of life, reduction of inequalities and inequities, alignment of services with the population's requirements, provision of financial protection from the risks and consequences of falling ill, and meeting people's expectations while respecting their dignity and autonomy and guaranteeing their right to privacy.

Countries organize their health systems with a view to upholding national values and principles, achieving their purposes, and attaining their health objectives which, in turn, generates different ways of managing the system and regulating its operation, providing and allocating funds, and delivering health services. The definition of the health system, its different subsystems, the organizations that comprise them, and the relations between them are mentioned in constitutions, general health laws, or health codes in all the countries of the Region. These normative frameworks establish the relations between the public system and the different subsystems, including the private subsystem, and the subsystems for social security, education, and training of health human resources. Almost all the Region's constitutions recognize health as a human right, but history shows that governments and societies have obtained better results in drafting health legislation than in making the changes needed in their health and social welfare systems to assure that right.

Background

The specific characteristics of each health system depend on the history and political and socioeconomic conditions of each country, the influence that is exerted by different interest groups, and the interplay of political forces. The history of the creation and development of health systems in the Region is closely bound to the development of social security schemes in the context of paternalistic governments that formed in the West at the beginning of the 20th century and which reached their height during the period immediately following World War II. The institutional frameworks and structures of social welfare systems vary widely with regard to relations between the government, the market, society, and the family (6).

The modes of operation of paternalistic governments had a great influence on the development of health systems; however, their organizational models are idealistic and do not actually exist in a pure state in reality, and, consequently, none of them was fully applied by the countries. On the contrary, the incorporation of partial versions of the models gave rise to a number of very different institutions, with separate organizational arrangements for the management/regulation, financing/insurance, and provision of services.

In short, the Region's health systems were based on Western social security models, but unlike the models followed in most European countries, the Latin American and Caribbean subsystems were directed to specific population strata, grouped by social class, income, occupation, formal employment, ethnic origin, and urban or rural status, whose result was social segregation consisting of stratification in the exercise of the right to health. As a consequence, the traditional organizational structure of health systems in Latin America and the Caribbean consisted of unintegrated subsystems targeted to specific population groups, which led to greater segmentation and fragmentation and seriously affected performance.

Segmented systems present sharp differences in their guarantees of the rights of members, per capita expenditure levels, and the degree of access to services by different population groups, weak stewardship marked by insufficient regulatory frameworks and inadequate supervision, and high transaction costs. They are also regressive and underfinanced, with direct or out-of-pocket payments predominating, and can entail catastrophic risks for the financial security of families.

Service delivery networks were established for each subsystem, with limited integration and communications between their constituent units, both within the same subsystem and between the different subsystems and for different levels of complexity. Services were concentrated mainly in the wealthier urban areas and in the salaried population and this led to inefficient use

Segmentation and Fragmentation of Health Systems

Segmentation is the coexistence of subsystems with different modes of financing, membership, and delivery of health care services, each of them "specializing" in different population segments, depending on their employment, income level, ability to pay, and social status. This kind of institutional arrangement consolidates and deepens inequity in access to health care between different population groups. In organizational terms, segmentation is the coexistence of one or more public entities (depending on the degree of decentralization or deconcentration), social security programs (represented by one or more entities), different financers/insurers, and private suppliers of services (depending on the extent of market mechanisms and entrepreneurial management introduced during sector reforms in the 1980s and 1990s).

Fragmentation of the health services delivery system is the coexistence of various units or facilities that are not integrated into the health network. The presence of numerous health agents that operate separately does not allow for suitable standardization of the content, quality, or cost of care and leads to the establishment of service networks that have no coordination, coherence, or synergies, and that tend to ignore each other or compete with each other, which leads to increases in transaction costs and promotes inefficient allocation of resources in the system as a whole.

of sector resources that failed to protect the very poor, the informal sector, and, in many countries, indigenous groups, Afro-descendants, and rural and marginal-urban populations. The provision of health services in the Region has been marked by overlapping and unnecessary duplication of care networks and the lack of complementarity among services and continuity of care. This prevents individuals from receiving comprehensive care, stands in the way of establishing adequate quality standards, and fails to guarantee the same level of care for individuals covered by different systems. This operational fragmentation can be ascribed to several factors, including structural segmentation, problems with governance, the lack of integrated planning, interactions between the public and non-public sectors that are often inadequate, and the weakness of referral and counter-referral mechanisms (7, 8). In some countries, such as Brazil, Canada, Chile, Costa Rica, and Cuba, changes were made to break down the barriers that separate these different institutional realms; but in most countries of the Region barriers still exist and their health systems are highly segmented and fragmented, with the consequent population segregation.

Summary of Sector Reform in the Region in the 1980s and 1990s

It is impossible to analyze the changes in the field of health during the 1980s and 1990s without considering the general macroeconomic reforms that took place in most of the countries in the world in those decades. Also worth bearing in mind is the process of globalization which, by promoting extensive liberalization of international movements of capital and entrenching the processes of transnationalization of industry, played a key role in defining policies that had a great influence on the health

sector. Those processes have led as well to a broader discussion of the viability and future of social welfare systems around the world, in circumstances in which the widespread application of structural adjustment policies has led to sweeping changes in the labor market, coupled with the weakening of the social services provided by the State, the rise of the private sector as a major player in areas traditionally occupied by the public sector—such as the administration of social services and natural monopolies—and the reduction in governments' ability to lead and regulate, with the consequent deepening of segmentation and fragmentation associated with the appearance of new pension and insurance plans and new ways of delivering health services.

The public health protection schemes offered by institutions that reported to the ministries of health and social security were insufficient since they excluded millions of people from access to health goods and services (9–11), which also translated into high out-of-pocket expenditure that persists. Studies show that when personal spending accounts for a significant percentage of total expenditure on health, the ability to pay becomes the determining factor in the demand for personal care (4).

As part of the macroeconomic reforms in the 1980s and 1990s, the countries of the Region introduced a series of changes in their health systems, aimed fundamentally at improving effectiveness, guaranteeing financial sustainability, promoting decentralization, and assigning a larger role to the private sector. The results of these reform processes differ, and their legacy can be seen in how the systems are organized today. Some of the advantages and disadvantages are presented in Table 1.

In general, health reforms failed to consider the peculiarities of each country as they relate to geography, social and demographic structure, history and political culture, and the extent to which sector institutions were developed. They tended to adopt

TABLE 1. Main advantages and disadvantages of health sector reforms in the 1980s and 1990s in Latin America and the Caribbean.

Advantages	Disadvantages
The different functions performed by health systems were identified and in many countries they were separated. The private sector became more important in insurance and the provision of health care services.	The creation, promotion, and deregulation of the markets for insurance and the provision of health care services led to the proliferation of competing middlemen. This intensified the segmentation of the system, increased transaction costs, and weakened the stewardship function of the ministries of health.
The idea of fiscal discipline was introduced in the public health sector, with stress on financial sustainability. New sources of financing for health care were sought.	Public expenditure was cut drastically in most of the countries. The application of strict cost control led to losses in public health infrastructure and human resources which, in turn, led to the deterioration of health outcomes. The introduction of user quotas and other payment mechanisms at the point of care increased direct out-of-pocket expenditure.
Service management improved in many countries, in some cases through the establishment of management commitments. The use of efficiency criteria in the provision of health services was introduced.	The introduction of a quasi-market logic in the public health sector adversely affected public health functions. Promotion of competition among insurers and suppliers to attract clients with the ability to pay deepened segmentation. The incorporation of financial incentives for the provision of individual health services led to stressing curative actions over preventive ones.
Different mechanisms, procedures, and instruments were applied to extend coverage and reach bypassed groups. Many countries adopted the idea of creating "basic packages'"for the poor or for specific groups.	The introduction of basic packages for the poor deepened the segmentation of health systems. The creation of separate funds for the population with the ability to contribute and for those without that ability led to a loss of solidarity in the system and worsened inequity in access to health care and health outcomes. Coverage did not increase as expected, and in many cases the rise in demand for health services could not be met owing to the scant resources allocated to improving the supply of health care services.
In most countries, efforts were made to increase local participation in the administration of services through decentralization.	Incomplete decentralization undermined the stewardship capacity of the ministry of health and increased geographic inequity in the provision of health services.

Source: Based on the Country Health System Profiles (2000–2002) available at www.lachealthsys.org.

models promoted across-the-board by multilateral lending agencies, which stressed financial and managerial changes, deregulation of the labor market, privatization, and decentralization.

These reforms also paid little attention to the impact of the changes on health sector players and interest groups, particularly health care workers. They did not promote the requisite coordination and synergy between system functions, ignoring their complex interrelations, and failed to encourage the definition of national health objectives. As a result, although some of the reforms were intended to develop a regional agenda based on greater pluralism, efficiency, and quality in the delivery of health services, in practice, government leadership capacity was undermined, the overall operation of the health system was weakened, and health issues were relegated to the background.

Organization, Coverage, and Performance of Health Systems

The degree of integration and types of interactions in a health system are crucial for determining its capacity to respond to the demands of beneficiaries. Other key elements that will act as constraints on the good performance of the systems are: the absence or insufficiency of prepaid and shared risk systems, and the predominance of direct or out-of-pocket payments; and weak or embryonic mechanisms for stewardship/regulation that make it difficult to define the rules of the game for players (user-service provider, insurer, financer) and for governments to provide adequate oversight to ensure that the rules are followed. Broadly speaking, the closer the integration within a single system or between the different subsystems in a mixed system, the better the response capacity of the system as a whole, and the lower the operating costs (12).

Single systems are, by definition, integrated vertically (a single entity carries out all functions) and horizontally (a single entity covers the entire population), while mixed systems can have different degrees of integration or segmentation/fragmentation, either of system functions or of the different population groups covered, with each subsector maintaining its own system of financing.

From the standpoint of users, the demand for health goods and services is shaped by the organizational characteristics and structure of the health system. Segmentation of financing and insurance, population segregation, and fragmentation of the delivery systems mean that members of different plans, both private and public, and people with the ability to pay but who are not members of an insurance plan, many self-employed, small entrepreneurs, merchants, etc., turn to public establishments if they offer good-quality, highly complex services, or are the only service providers in a given geographic area.

A large percentage of the low-income population also uses private health services—particularly pharmaceutical services, traditional medicine, or low-complexity medical care—as an alternative, given the barriers to access, the restricted supply, and the lack of comprehensiveness of public services, and the fact that they are excluded from health insurance plans and therefore must pay out-of-pocket. In turn, owing to the limitations on benefit plans or administrative barriers to the use of services, middle- and high-income groups that contribute to social security also have recourse to parallel modes of financing by buying individual or collective private insurance—the phenomenon of dual coverage—or paying out-of-pocket, which creates distortions in social security financing and demand.

In this context, the performance of health systems can be analyzed on the basis of the organizational structure and coverage of the different subcomponents, as can be seen in Table 2.

Social Exclusion and Barriers to Access to the Health System

In tandem with institutional segmentation in health systems and population segregation, the operational fragmentation observed in the delivery of services is a major source of exclusion of groups and inequity in access to health services, owing to institutional/legal, economic, cultural, geographic, ethnic, gender, or age barriers. In Latin America and the Caribbean, an estimated 20–25% of the population (close to 200 million people) has no regular and timely access to the health system (13). Conservative figures indicate that in the United States, more than 46 million people lack adequate health care coverage.

Recognition of social exclusion in health care, defined as "the lack of access of certain groups or people to various goods, services and opportunities that improve or preserve health status

and that other individuals or groups in the society enjoy" (14), has constituted a major step forward in describing and understanding the phenomena that affect access to health care.[1]

The main causes of exclusion in health care vary from country to country but in general are related to poverty, rural location, informal sector employment, unemployment, and factors linked to the performance, structure, and organization of health systems (Table 3). Exclusion is essentially the denial of the right to satisfy health needs and demands to citizens who do not have enough money or who do not belong to the dominant social groups.

Changes in the Agenda for Social Welfare and Strengthening of Health Systems, 2001–2005

The discussion of what should be understood by social welfare and what is the institutional venue in which health policies should be formulated and implemented has grown in importance in recent years in Latin America and the Caribbean, in a regional scenario dominated by four elements: (1) the questioning of the sector reforms carried out in the 1980s and 1990s; (2) the absence of a social safety net capable of acting as the foundation for social development in a new context and replacing the system previously provided by governments, social security institutions, or both; (3) the commitment to attain the Millennium Development Goals (MDGs) by 2015; and (4) a growing concern over the problems of inequity, exclusion, and poverty that prevail in the countries of the Region.

In this context, new institutional arrangements have arisen to replace or complement the earlier models. Some of them represent radical changes in the way the government organizes itself to formulate and implement social policies and, within this overarching project, they incorporate health institutions and actions such as the Unified Health System in Brazil, the Ministry of Social Welfare in Colombia, the Social Security Health System in the Dominican Republic, the national health insurance systems in Aruba, Bahamas, and Trinidad and Tobago, and the Explicit Health Guarantees Program in Chile.

Other countries opted to establish limited plans for the financing and delivery of health goods and services intended to eliminate barriers to access and improve health outcomes for specific population groups. Thus were established the Universal Mother and Child Insurance Program (SUMI) in Bolivia, the Comprehensive Health Insurance Program (SIS) in Peru, voluntary public insurance (Seguro Popular de Salud) in Mexico, and the provincial mother and child health insurance plans in Argentina. The Law on Free Maternity and Child Care was passed in

---

[1] To help the countries characterize and measure health exclusion, PAHO/WHO, with support from the Swedish International Development Agency (SIDA), prepared and validated a methodological guide that has been applied in eight countries (Bolivia, Dominican Republic, Ecuador, El Salvador, Guatemala, Honduras, Paraguay, and Peru), in two of Mexico's states, and in five inter-municipal associations in Honduras.

TABLE 2. Health systems in the Americas: population coverage by subsystem, 2001–2006.[a]

Country	Year	Source[b]	Subsystem	Coverage by subsystem
Anguilla	2006		Public	. . . The Health Services Authority (decentralized agency of the Ministry of Health) is responsible for public health care.
			Private	. . . Private health care services are offered to the population with the ability to pay or through private health insurance.
Antigua and Barbuda	2006		Public	. . . The government finances public health care.
			Social Security	. . . All workers contribute to the public insurance plan and the medical benefits plan.
			Private	. . . Private health insurance.
Argentina	2001	Mesa-Lago C. Las reformas de salud en América Latina y el Caribe: su impacto en los principios de la seguridad social. CEPAL, 2005.	Public	37.4% of the population has access to the public health services system operated by the federal and provincial health ministries.
			Social Security	51.2% employee benefit plans (obras sociales).
			Private	7.9% prepaid medicine.
			Other	3.2% dual insurance coverage, mainly through private plans (voluntary membership in prepaid plans, mutuals, etc.).
Aruba	2006		Public	100% general health insurance.
			Private	The private supply has begun to grow without much regulation.
Bahamas	2005	Web site of the Ministry of Health of the Bahamas: http://www.bahamas.gov.bs/. Bahamian Report of the Blue Ribbon Commission on National Health Insurance, 2004.	Public	100% with access to primary care and other health services or technologies in the country, with public health functions and the provision of collective and individual care.
			Social Security	All public and private employees are required by law to contribute to the National Insurance Office. Parliament is currently debating a national health insurance system.
			Private	51% of the population buys private health insurance.
Barbados	2006		Public	100% access to national health services.
			Private	20%–25% health insurance offered to large organizations and credit cooperatives.
Belize	2006	Web site of the Ministry of Health of Belize: http://www.health.gov.bz/.	Public	100% access to Ministry of Health services. The national public health system guarantees individuals and the population universal access to health care through the public services network and programs. 30% buy services through the national health insurance (estimate June 2006).
			Private	Private medical services are growing in urban areas. Private health insurance is offered in Belize City.

TABLE 2. (continued)

Country	Year	Source[b]	Subsystem	Coverage by subsystem
Bermuda	2000	Bermuda Health Systems and Services Profile, 2005, http://www.gov.bm.	Social Security/ Private	95% insurance coverage (85% by the major medical package; 10% by basic health coverage). Health insurance plans for public employees, private insurance for private employees and the self-employed; insurance for employees of large companies. The National Health Insurance Commission offers a low-cost health insurance plan.
			No coverage	4% have no health insurance; 1% SD.
Bolivia	2003–2004	Instituto Nacional de Seguros de Salud (INASES), Protección en salud desagregada por prestador, Bolivia, 2003.	Public	30% access to the services of the Ministry of Public Health and Sports (theoretical coverage).
			Social Security	25% (National Health Fund [CNS] 20.8%; other health insurance funds 4.2%, including the Oil Industry Health Fund [CPS], University Social Security [SSU], the Private Banks Health Fund [CSPB], the Military Social Insurance Fund [COSSMIL], CSC, CSCO, SINEC, COTEL).
			Private	12% out-of-pocket payments for services and private medical insurance.
			No coverage	45% with no access to health services. 72.8% with no public or private medical insurance.
Brazil	2003–2006	Agência Nacional de Saúde Suplementar (ANS), Ministério da Saúde, Brasil, Caderno de Informação de Saúde Suplementar. Rio de Janeiro, 2006.	Public	80.4% covered exclusively by the Unified Health System (SUS) (basic coverage 98%; Family Health Program coverage 68.4%).
			Private	19.6% supplementary medical care (private company collective plans 14.4% and individual and family plans 5.2%); 3.8% supplementary dental plans. Private insurance beneficiaries maintain their full right to coverage under the SUS.
British Virgin Islands	2006	Web site of the Government of the British Virgin Islands: http://www.bvi.gov.vg/. Agreement to develop the medical insurance program of the British Virgin Islands, 2006.	Public	. . . The Public Health Department provides health care for youths under 15 years and the elderly.
			Social Security	. . . Compulsory membership for employers, employees, and the self-employed.
			Private	50% of local medical consultations are private sector. People not covered by the Public Health Department or by social security must pay for services, although they are heavily subsidized.
Canada	2006	Web site of the Ministry of Health of Canada: http://www.hc-sc.gc.ca/index_e.html. Dewa CS, Hoch JS, Steele L. Prescription drug benefits and Canada's uninsured. J Law Psychiatry. 2005 Sep–Oct; 28(5):496–513; Health Affairs 25(3): 878–879; 2006.	Public	100% Medicare (composed of 13 provincial or territorial health plans) covers necessary hospitalization, medical care, surgery, dental, and some chronic care services, except for prescriptions.
			Private	65% of the population has private health insurance for services not covered by Medicare (50% for dental services and 30% for drugs).

TABLE 2. (continued)

Country	Year	Source[b]	Subsystem	Coverage by subsystem
Cayman Islands	2006		Public	. . .
			Social Security	24% CINICON, government social insurance provider.
			Private	59%
			No coverage	17%
Chile	2003		Public	100% services guaranteed under the Universal Access with Explicit Guarantees (AUGE) plan (public or private provision).
			Social Security	68.3% National Health Fund (FONASA) (legal coverage).
			Private	17.6% health insurance institutions (ISAPREs).
			Other	3% armed forces.
			No coverage	12.8% with no known public or private medical insurance (are often covered by other private mechanisms).
Colombia	2004	Cardona JF, Hernández A, Yepes, F. La seguridad social en Colombia. Rev Gerenc Polit Salud. 2005; 4(9)81–99.	Public	29% "vinculados" (population not members of a social security regime but with access to limited services and benefits paid for with national, regional, and municipal resources); theoretical coverage under the basic care plan (collective public health).
			Social Security	67.1% (32.8% contributive regime; 34.3% privately insured, health promoters [EPS], subsidized and partially subsidized regime; public insurers, subsidized regime administrators [ARS]). (The contributive and subsidized social security regimes and the different partially subsidized plans have different programs of services and benefits.)
			Other	3.9% special regimes (armed forces, police, oil industry workers).
Costa Rica	2003	Mesa-Lago C. Op. cit.	Public	100% collective public health.
			Social Security	86.8% Costa Rican Social Security Fund (CCSS) (75% employees, pensioners, and dependent family members; 11.8% indigents paid for by the government).
		Conferencia Interamericana de Seguridad Social (CISS). Reformas de los esquemas de la seguridad social; e Informe sobre la seguridad social en América, 2004.	Other	Workplace risk insurance covers 71% of the economically active population.
			Private	30% of the population (regardless of whether they belong to the CCSS) use private services either directly or through delegation by the CCSS at least once a year.
			Partial coverage	12.1% to 14.7% emergency service coverage by the compulsory automobile insurance (SOA).
Cuba	2006		Public	100% National Health System.

TABLE 2. (continued)

Country	Year	Source[b]	Subsystem	Coverage by subsystem
Dominican Republic	2001	OPS. Exclusión social en salud en países de América Latina y el Caribe, 2004.	Public	60.0% access to Ministry of Health/Secretary of State for Public Health and Social Welfare (SESPAS) services (estimated theoretical coverage). SESPAS has the goal of covering 76% of the population.
			Social Security	7.0% Dominican Social Security Administration (IDSS).
			Private	12.0% private health services paid for by companies and personal insurance.
			Other	5.0% (3% armed forces and police; 2% privately obtained insurance).
			No coverage	16.0% with no access to health services. 76.4% with no public or private health insurance.
Ecuador	2006	Palacio A. Programa de aseguramiento universal de salud, Ecuador, 2006. Mesa-Lago C. Op. cit. OPS. Exclusión en salud en países de América Latina y el Caribe, 2004.	Public	28% access to Ministry of Public Health services (theoretical coverage).
			Social Security	21% Ecuadoran Social Security Administration (IESS); 11% (9% general insurance, 2% pensioners); Rural Social Insurance 7%; armed forces and police 3% (Armed Forces Social Security Administration [ISSFA], Police Social Security Administration [SSPOL]).
			Private	26% (nonprofit 6% [Benevolent Board, NGOs, and municipal organizations]; for profit 20% [private health insurance 3%; out-of-pocket for private services 17%]).
			No coverage	27% with no access to health services. 76% with no public or private medical insurance.
El Salvador	2006	Conferencia Interamericana de Seguridad Social (CISS). Op. cit., 2005. Mesa-Lago C. Op. cit. Encuesta de la Dirección General de Estadística y Censos (DIGESTYC), 2002. OPS. Exclusión social en salud en El Salvador, 2004, http://www.lachealthsys.org.	Public	40.0% access to Ministry of Public Health and Social Welfare services (theoretical coverage). The ministry's goal is to cover 81% of the population.
			Social Security	15.8% Salvadoran Social Security Administration (ISSS).
			Other	4.6% (military health plan 3%, and teachers' plan 1.6%).
			Private	1.5% to 5.0% private medical insurance and out-of-pocket payment for health services.
			No coverage	41.7% with no access to health services. 78.0% with no public or private medical insurance.
Grenada	2006	National Strategic Plan for Health, 2006–2010. Web site of the Ministry of Health.	Social Security	. . . Health care is offered by public health services.
			Private	. . . Some people have individual or group private insurance.
Guadeloupe, French Guiana, and Martinique	2006		Social Security	100% universal health insurance plans, based on compulsory wage deductions and public subsidies. 25% to 33% have supplementary coverage.
			Private	Private and public health services private care under the universal insurance plan.

TABLE 2. (continued)

Country	Year	Source[b]	Subsystem	Coverage by subsystem
Guatemala	2005	Mesa-Lago C. Op. cit. OPS. Exclusión en salud en países de América Latina y el Caribe, 2004.	Public	27.0% Ministry of Health exclusively with a basic care package (theoretical coverage). The ministry's goal is to cover 60% of the population with the basic package.
			Social Security	18.3% Guatemalan Social Security Administration.
			Private	30.0% mainly through NGOs and other institutions that offer a basic care package. 10.0% out-of-pocket. 0.2% private insurance coverage.
			No coverage	12.8% to 27.4% with no access to health services. 82.2% with no public or private medical insurance.
Guyana	2006		Public	. . .
			Social Security	. . . There is no national health insurance system. The National Health Plan administers a social insurance program that is compulsory for employees and self-employed workers from 16 to 60 years of age.
Haiti	2004	Haiti, Ministère de la santé publique et de la population. OPS/OMS, Analyse du secteur de la santé, 2004.	Public	21% access to Ministry of Public Health and Population services.
			Social Security	1% public employees medical insurance.
			Private	37% (for profit, including out-of-pocket expenditure on basic private services 19%; nonprofit, NGOs, religious missions, and international missions 18%).
			Other	70% of the population goes to traditional healers first.
			No coverage	40% with no access to health services. 99% with no public or private medical insurance.
Honduras	2004–2006	OPS. Exclusión social en salud en países de América Latina y el Caribe, 2004. Ministerio de Salud de Honduras. Plan Nacional de Salud, 2001–2006.	Public	60% with access to Ministry of Health services (theoretical coverage).
			Social Security	18% Honduran Social Security Administration.
			Private	5% private health insurance.
			No coverage	30.1% with no access to health services. 77% with no public or private medical insurance.
Jamaica	2005	Web site of the Ministry of Health of Jamaica: http://www.moh.gov.jm/. Jamaican Survey of Living Conditions, 2001.	Public	95% of hospital care and 50% of ambulatory care are covered by public institutions.
			Social Security	13.9% of the population had health insurance in 2001.
			Private	50% of ambulatory and diagnostic services and most pharmaceutical services.

TABLE 2. (continued)

Country	Year	Source[b]	Subsystem	Coverage by subsystem
Mexico	2002–2006	Web site of the Secretaría de Salud de Mexico: http://www.salud.gob.mx/. Mesa-Lago, C. Op. cit. Frenk J, et al. Health system reform in Mexico 1: Comprehensive reform to improve health system performance in Mexico. Lancet 2006; 368:1524–1534.	Public	41.8% federal and state health departments (theoretical coverage, corresponds to the uninsured population, informal sector workers, the rural population, and the unemployed). 14.8% Seguro Popular (estimated on the basis of 5.1 million member families in November 2006).
			Social Security	58.2% Mexican Social Security Administration (IMSS): 45.3% (IMSS 34.3%; IMSS Oportunidades 11%); Public Employees Social Security and Services Administration (ISSSTE); 7% (Public Employees Social Security and Services Administration), PEMEX (Petróleos Mexicanos), armed forces, navy department and other insurance for government employees 5.9%.). Some of the insured are covered by more than one insurance plan.
			Private	2.8% private health insurance (5%-23% of IMSS affiliates also have private insurance).
			No coverage	1% with no access to health services.
Montserrat	2006	Web site of the Ministry of Education, Health, Community Services and Labour http://www.mehcs.gov.ms.	Public	100% primary and secondary level services. Ministry of Health, Department of Health, and Department of Community Health.
Netherlands Antilles	2006		Social Security	100% public health insurance (PPK "pro-paupere kaart") for the poor or people with preexisting conditions; public insurance for blue collar workers; insurance fund for retired public sector employees; and private plans.
Nicaragua	2004	Mesa-Lago C. Op. cit.	Public	60.0% access to Ministry of Health services (estimated theoretical coverage).
			Social Security	7.7% Nicaraguan Social Security Administration (INSS) (members and families, spouses and children under 12).
			Private	4.0% out-of-pocket payments.
			Other	0.4% armed forces and government.
			No coverage	27.9% with no access to health services.
Panama	2004	Conferencia Interamericana de Seguridad Social (CISS). Op. cit., 2004. Gobierno de Panamá, Plan de Desarrollo Social, 2000–2004.	Public	35.4% Ministry of Health (theoretical coverage). Corresponds to the uninsured population of the Social Security Fund (CSS) which by law must be covered by the Ministry of Health.
			Social Security	64.6% Social Security Fund.
			No coverage	20.0% without access to health services.
Paraguay	2005	Mesa-Lago, C. Op. cit. OPS. Exclusión social en salud en países de América Latina y el Caribe, 2003.	Public	35% to 42% access to Ministry of Health services (estimated theoretical coverage).
			Social Security	18.4% Social Welfare Administration (IPS) or some other kind (individual, work, family, military, police, or foreign).
			Private	7.0% out-of-pocket payment.
			No coverage	38.6% with no access to health services. 81.1% with no public or private health insurance.

TABLE 2. (continued)

Country	Year	Source[b]	Subsystem	Coverage by subsystem
Peru	2006	Perú, Ministerio de Salud. Seguro Integral de Salud, 2006.	Public	27.8% Ministry of Health comprehensive insurance plan.
			Social Security	28.1% (EsSalud 25.1%; health service providers (EPS), armed forces and police 3%).
			Private	10.0% private (2% out-of-pocket and 8% traditional medicine).
			No coverage	42.1% with no public or private health insurance.
Puerto Rico	2003		Public	40.0% Medicaid.
			Social Security	26.0% (Medicare 14%; public employees 12%).
			Private	37.0% private health insurance.
			No coverage	7.1% with no public or private health insurance.
Saint Kitts and Nevis	2006		Public	100% Ministry of Health. Services not available on the island are financed through public subsidies.
Saint Lucia	2000, 2002	Ministry of Health, Human Services, Family Affairs and Gender Relations. Proposals for Health Sector Reform 2000.	Public	Ministry of Health.
			Social Security	. . . National Insurance Plan and private health insurance for individuals and groups. A national health plan (universal health care) for secondary and tertiary care through a public-private mix is in the process of being introduced.
Saint Vincent and the Grenadines	2006		Public	. . . Ministry of Health.
			Social Security	. . . National Health Insurance Plan.
Suriname	2005		Public	54% (30% Ministry of Health; 24% Ministry of Social Affairs).
			Social Security	27% State Medical Insurance Fund (SZF) (21% Medical Mission; 6% with government subsidies).
			Private	13% private insurance (10% employer insurance plans; 3% private medical insurance).
			Other	1%
			Uninsured	5%
Trinidad and Tobago	2006		Public	. . .
			Social Security	The government's goal is to implement national health insurance in 2007.
			Private	Private employers offer health insurance.
Turks and Caicos Islands	2005		Public	80% Ministry of Health (theoretical coverage).
			Social Security	The government is considering the creation of a national health insurance authority to administer a national universal health insurance plan.
			Private	20% of the population has private medical insurance.

TABLE 2. (continued)

Country	Year	Source[b]	Subsystem	Coverage by subsystem
United States	2005	Web site of the Kaiser Family Foundation, 2006, http://www.kff.org.	Public	20.6% Medicaid.
			Social Security	16.1% Medicare.
			Private	45.5% private health insurance, usually offered by the employer.
			No coverage	17.8% have no public or private medical insurance or government-subsidized insurance.
Uruguay	2006		Public	45.3% Ministry of Health and the State Health Services Administration (ASSE).
			Social Security	45.0% mutuals.
			Other	7.6% (5.3% armed forces plan; 2.3% police forces plan).
			Private	1.8% private full-coverage insurance.
Venezuela	2000 2005 2006	Mesa-Lago C. Op. cit. OPS. Barrio adentro: derecho a la salud e inclusión social en Venezuela, 2006.	Public	65.6% Ministry of Public Health (estimated theoretical coverage of the population not insured by the Venezuelan Social Insurance Administration [IVSS]). Misión Barrio Adentro provides primary care for 73% of the population.
			Social Security	34.4% IVSS.
			Private	30.0% (estimated, can be a mix of public and private).

[a]Methodological notes: This table is not intended to provide an exhaustive or exclusive classification/topology, but to synthesize the most recent information available for each country. When data for a given subsystem are not available, the corresponding line was omitted to shorten the table. In some cases the percentages may add up to more than 100% owing to duplication of insurance in some groups that belong to more than one protection plan or to less than 100% owing to lack of information.

[b]When a specific source is not given, the information is taken from materials prepared during 2006 by the PAHO/WHO Country Offices for the publication *Health in the Americas*, 2007 edition. If another source is mentioned, it is additional.

TABLE 3. Social exclusion in health care: incidence and main causes, selected countries of the Americas.

Country	Social exclusion (%)			Main causes of social exclusion
	Incidence	Barriers to access	Insufficient supply	
Bolivia	77	60	40	Poverty/mother's lack of education/ethnic origin
Ecuador	51	41	59	Insufficient health infrastructure
El Salvador	53	54	46	Lack of transportation to health centers
Honduras	56	45	55	Insufficient health infrastructure/insufficient supply of services
Paraguay	62	53	47	Ethic origin: being monolingual in Guaraní/lack of other public services (electricity, sanitation)
Peru	40	54	46	Poverty/living in rural areas/ethnic origin

Source: Pan American Health Organization; Swedish Agency for International Development. Exclusion in Health in Latin America and the Caribbean, 2003.

Ecuador, and the social welfare program known as the Barrio Adentro was started up in Venezuela. Health coverage was extended to rural populations in Guatemala, El Salvador, and Honduras, and a family protection policy was introduced in Nicaragua. The appearance of these new institutional arrange-

ments or plans to extend social health protection is a sign that the importance of this issue is being recognized and a new approach is being sought to guide changes in health systems.

The central place occupied by the fight against poverty, social exclusion, and inequity on the political agenda of the countries and international agencies in their attempts to attain the MDGs led to a growing consensus in the first five years of the 21st century on a new approach to making changes in health systems, centered on the concept of social protection of health as a universal human right that is no longer contingent on employment or other individual or group characteristics and is guided by a renewed strategy for primary health care. The high priority attached to health in the MDGs underlines that health is not just the result of greater development, but rather lies at the very heart of development itself.

In 2002, the countries of the Americas, meeting at the 26th Pan American Sanitary Conference, approved Resolution CSP 26.R19, which expresses a commitment to provide all their citizens with access to health goods and services under equal conditions of opportunity, quality, and dignity, combating inequities in the use of those goods and services and in health outcomes by extending the social protection of health, understood as "the guarantee that society gives through the public powers to enable an individual or group of individuals to satisfy their health needs and demands, without the ability to pay acting as a restriction."

At the Special Summit of the Americas in 2003, the governments of the Region approved the Nuevo León Declaration, which outlines three objectives: economic growth with equity to reduce poverty, social development, and democratic governance. Social protection of health was considered essential for national progress and the countries undertook to adopt broader strategies for disease prevention, health care, and promotion, with particular stress on the most vulnerable sectors of society. In 2005, the 58th World Health Assembly approved Resolution WHA58.33 (15), which urges the member states to strengthen their health systems and gear their policies toward universal coverage and sustainable financing.

Accordingly, the main challenge facing the Latin American and Caribbean countries in the new millennium is to "guarantee universal social protection of health for all citizens by eliminating or reducing avoidable inequalities in coverage, access, and use of services as much as possible, and assuring that every person receives care based on their needs and contributes to system financing according to their possibilities" (16). Some countries have already taken up the task, reorienting their health systems toward social protection, based on the principles of primary health care, so they can contribute to building more equitable and inclusive societies, better attuned to the new needs of the population of the Region. Examples include the definition of national health objectives aligned with the population's health requirements, particularly those of the most disadvantaged groups; the implementation of mechanisms to integrate the operations of the social security and ministry of health systems, reducing fragmentation in the delivery of services and improving geographic equity; the introduction of a single comprehensive plan that guarantees health care for the entire population regardless of the type of insurance, the type of provider, or the user's ability to

contribute, in order to reduce segmentation in insurance and improve equity; the use of tools to analyze equity and exclusion in health care and to include economic, social, ethnic, cultural, and gender elements in the definition of health plans and policies; the creation of primary care services directed to families; the analysis of the performance of public health functions as a key to formulating health policies; the enhancement of the stewardship and leadership function of national health authorities by creating institutional conditions for sector and intersectoral steering and planning in the development of health actions; the startup of mechanisms to regulate and supervise the actions of the different players who participate in producing health care; the incorporation of health as a central element in social dialogue to define a country's productive platform; and the insertion of health policies into the broader institutional framework of the social welfare system, alongside income, labor, employment, housing, and education. These examples of the search for mechanisms to eliminate population segregation and institutional segmentation, reduce operational fragmentation, and combat exclusion in health care inform the direction that the public health agenda will take in the coming years.

NATIONAL HEALTH EXPENDITURE AND FINANCING OF NATIONAL HEALTH CARE SYSTEMS AND SERVICES

National Health Expenditure in the Americas and Other Regions, 2004: Public Spending Rises with Countries' Level of Economic Development

In 2004, worldwide health care expenditure was estimated as 8.7% of the global economy (US$ 4,500 billion).[2] In the same year, world per capita income was estimated as US$ 8,284 and per capita health expenditure as US$ 742. Table 4 compares national health expenditure in the Americas and different parts of the world in 2004. As the table shows, health expenditure is relatively high in high-income countries. Those countries, including Canada and the United States, accounted for 15% of the population and 71% of global health care expenditure. Average per capita spending on health in this group of countries is estimated at US$ 3,226. When the low- and middle-income countries of the world are grouped together, including the countries of Latin America and the Caribbean, they accounted for 85% of the population in 2004 but only 29% of global health care expenditure. Average per capita health expenditure in low- and middle-income countries is estimated to be US$ 248.

Within the Americas Region, the figures reported in Table 4 illustrate the stark differences in expenditure on health. Canada

---

[2] Unless otherwise specified, the figures are in US dollars of the year 2000, adjusted by purchasing power parity (US$ PPP 2000), as reported in the World Development Indicators Database of the World Bank (July 2006).

TABLE 4. National expenditure on health care in the Americas and other regions, 2004.

Region	Per capita income, US$ PPP 2000	National expenditure on health as a percentage of GDP	National expenditure on health per capita in current US$	National expenditure on health per capita, US$ PPP 2000	Public/private ratio	Expenditure on public health as a percentage of GDP
Americas	18,149	12.7	2,166	2,310	47/53	6.0
Canada	28,732	10.3	2,669	2,875	71/29	7.3
United States	36,465	13.1	5,711	4,791	45/55	7.2
Latin America and the Caribbean	7,419	6.8	222	501	48/52	3.3
High-income countries[a]	28,683	11.2	3,449	3,226	60/40	6.7
European Union	25,953	9.6	2,552	2,488	74/26	7.1
Other high-income countries	24,490	8.2	1,997	1,997	64/36	5.2
Low- and middle-income countries[b]	4,474	5.5	79	248	48/52	2.6
Eastern Europe and Central Asia	7,896	6.5	194	514	68/32	4.5
Middle East and North Africa	5,453	5.6	92	308	48/52	2.7
South Asia	2,679	4.4	24	119	26/74	1.1
East Asia and the Pacific	4,920	5.0	64	247	38/62	1.9
Sub-Saharan Africa	1,820	6.1	36	111	40/60	2.4
All regions and countries	8,284	8.7	588	742	58/42	5.1

[a]Includes Canada and the United States.
[b]Includes Latin America and the Caribbean.

Source: Prepared by the Health Policies and Systems Development Unit, Health Systems Strengthening Area, Pan American Health Organization; data on development indicators from the World Bank and PAHO's database on national health expenditure.

and the United States account for 39% of the population and 86% of total health care expenditure, while Latin America and the Caribbean account for 61% of the population but just 14% of expenditure. Average per capita national health expenditure in the countries of Latin America and the Caribbean is estimated to be US$ 501. The figure for Canada (US$ 2,875) is almost six times higher than the average for Latin America and the Caribbean. Average per capita spending on health in the United States (US$ 4,791) is even higher than Canada's, and is more than nine times greater than the average for Latin America and the Caribbean.

The Region of the Americas accounted for a relatively large share (44%) of global health care expenditure. The share of national health expenditure (NHE) as a percentage of gross domestic product (NHE/GDP) is estimated to be about 12.7%. This figure is higher than for the European Union countries (9.6%) and significantly higher than for the Latin American and Caribbean region taken alone (6.8%). Spending on health is one of many factors that define the preventive and curative levels of care achieved and national health expenditure can be a good indicator of inequalities in access to services, not only between regions but within them and between income groups in the same country.

The analysis of the public/private mix of national health expenditure helps to understand the degree of efficiency of the government and of the market that controls health resources. Resources channeled through public institutions are vulnerable to government failure due to misallocation, underutilization, or low

productivity of public resources. Resources transferred between consumers and providers through the purchase and sale of health goods and services, including the purchase of health insurance, are subject to market failures. Public policy discussion of issues related to efficiency should be based on the relative weight of the public and private sectors in expenditure—the public/private mix of national health expenditure (Table 4).

As Table 4 shows, there are variations in the composition of the public/private mix of national health expenditure in different regions of the world.[3] The ratio of public/private national health expenditure varies from 74/26 in the European Union where countries have universal health care systems to 26/74 in the low-income countries of South Asia. In the Americas, the mix varies from a public/private ratio of 71/29 in Canada, which has remained rather stable over the last decade, to about 45/55 in the United States and around 48/52 in Latin America and the Caribbean. Among the developed countries, the United States appears to be the most market-oriented national health care system. There is no clear pattern in the relationship between the public/private mix of national health expenditure and the level of income per capita. However, the share of public health expenditure

---

[3]Public health expenditure usually includes disbursements by central and local governments and mandatory social health insurance schemes. Private expenditure includes out-of-pocket spending by households and the payments made by various institutional sectors of the economy through health insurance and prepaid health plans.

as a percentage of GDP provides a better indicator of the role of government in the provision of health goods and services,[4] and is positively correlated with a country's level of economic development. For example, public health expenditure represents around 7.1% of GDP in high-income countries of the European Union, around 7.3% of GDP in Canada, and 7.2% of GDP in the United States, while the figure is about 3.3% for countries of Latin America and the Caribbean.

National Health Expenditure and the Public/Private Mix of National Health Care Systems in the Americas 2004–2005: Cross-Country Comparisons[5]

The total amount of national resources spent on health care expressed as a percentage of the national economy varies significantly in the countries of the Americas. The wide differences suggest that although per capita income may have some role in explaining the share of GDP devoted to national health, other factors may be playing a more important role in determining the level and composition of national health expenditure. Whether countries spend relatively more or less of their GDP on health is more influenced by policy decisions and reflective of the way in which national health systems are organized and financed.

Depending on the structure of national health care systems, the Region exhibits large variations in the public/private mix of national health expenditure. Table 5 summarizes this information by presenting GDP per capita, total national health expenditure as a percentage of GDP, per capita national health expenditure, and the relative weight of public and private expenditure as a percentage of overall national health expenditure.

As mentioned, there is no clear pattern in the relationship between the public/private mix of national health expenditure and the levels of per capita income in countries. There may be a slight

association between these factors, but at all income levels there are significant variations in the composition of the mix. The public/private composition of national health expenditure ranges from 93/7 in Antigua and Barbuda, where there is national health insurance, to 27/73 in Guatemala. In Table 6, national health care systems have been classified by type of health system and by level of income. The national health care systems of the countries of the Americas are classified either as predominantly public systems (with public expenditure exceeding 66% of total national health expenditure), mixed systems (with public expenditure ranging from 50% to 66%), and predominantly private market-oriented systems (with public expenditure amounting to less than 50%).

The more fundamental issue may be that the provision of public health services tends to be weaker in poorer countries, particularly in those that lack a predominantly public health system. The mild association between a larger share of private expenditure and the country's per capita income mentioned earlier is probably due to weak public health services in countries such as Bolivia, Ecuador, Guatemala, Haiti, Honduras, Jamaica, Nicaragua, and Paraguay. In general, where extensive coverage of the population exists under public health care systems or social insurance systems, private spending tends to account for a smaller share.

Changes in the Composition of National Health Expenditure: Trends in Total Expenditure and the Growing Role of Private Insurance and Pre-paid Health Plans

The dynamics and nature of national health expenditure have changed over time in Latin America and the Caribbean. Recent trends include one period from 1980 to about 1995, and a second very different period from 1996 to 2005. During the 1980s, national health expenditure in the Americas as a percentage of GDP rose steadily, and this occurred amidst general economic stagnation affecting most Latin American and Caribbean countries. The regional economy grew slowly during the 1980s, at a rate of 1.2% per year. Average per capita income declined from US$ 6,600 in 1980 to US$ 6,200 in 1990. During that period, national health expenditure grew faster than the economy, at around 1.4% a year. Per capita expenditure, in real terms, increased from US$ 380 to US$ 420. During the 1990s, most of the Latin American and Caribbean economies experienced a significant recovery in their rate of economic growth. National health expenditure grew at an even faster pace. The NHE/GDP ratio rose from 6.8 in 1990 to 7.1 in 1995. Per capita health expenditure reached around US$ 480. From the early 1980s to the mid-1990s, the share of national health expenditure as a percentage of GDP grew substantially, from around 5.9% in 1980 to around 6.8% in 1990 and reached about 7.1% in 1995.

Since the mid-1990s, the Region has experienced a period of accelerated economic growth. Expenditure on health care-related goods and services grew more slowly than the economy, and the

---

[4]The term "provision" is used as defined in the literature on public finance. It is not limited to the government's production of health care services; it includes regulatory and mandatory systems that ensure that an adequate amount of a particular type of good or service (health care services or health insurance) is available or used (consumed) by the population.

[5]Because of differences in concepts, classifications, and/or accounting procedures, the data presented in this section may differ from estimates reported in the country chapters and/or by other international organizations. Methods and data sources used in the estimates presented here are similar to the ones used in PAHO's Basic Health Indicators 2006, and can be consulted at: http://www.paho.org/english/dd/ais/BI-brochure-2006.pdf. The concepts, classifications, and accounting procedures used in the regular production of estimates of national health expenditure for the 48 countries and territories of the Americas are based on the guidelines of the United Nations System of National Accounts (SNA 1993), the Government Finance Statistics Manual of the International Monetary Fund (GFS 2001), the new international standards developed under the framework of the United Nations Statistical Commission, and the Statistical Conference of the Americas (SCA-ECLAC). Implementation of harmonized estimates of economic and financial indicators at the country level would assure that those indicators would be available for use in policymaking. National health accounts in the countries of the Americas include the development of economic and financial indicators related to health, health care services, and national health care systems.

TABLE 5. National health expenditure in the Americas: per capita, percentage of GDP, and public/private ratio, 2004.

Country	GDP per capita, US$ PPP 2000	National expenditure on health as a percentage of GDP	Per capita national expenditure on health, US$ PPP 2000	Public/private ratio
Anguilla	8,310	6.9	573	68/32
Antigua and Barbuda	11,567	9.4	1,084	93/7
Argentina	12,222	8.6	1,045	55/45
Aruba	21,515	14.2	3,064	89/11
Bahamas	15,955	6.1	969	52/48
Barbados	17,217	8.1	1,389	53/47
Belize	6,201	5.5	341	77/23
Bermuda	70,313	9.8	6,914	38/62
Bolivia	2,499	7.1	178	59/41
Brazil	7,531	7.0	530	49/51
British Virgin Islands[a]	36,947	1.8	681	...
Canada	28,732	10.3	2,959	71/29
Cayman Islands[a]	31,614	3.3	1,049	...
Chile	9,993	8.3	827	53/47
Colombia	6,669	6.0	402	57/43
Costa Rica	8,714	8.5	738	60/40
Cuba[a]	3,483	6.3	220	...
Dominica	5,186	6.5	335	68/32
Dominican Republic	6,846	4.7	320	29/71
Ecuador	3,642	4.6	166	48/52
El Salvador	4,633	6.2	287	39/61
French Guiana	7,774	...	...	...
Grenada	7,372	7.7	571	59/41
Guadeloupe	7,759	...	...	...
Guatemala	3,964	6.5	259	27/73
Guyana[a]	4,080	1.1	45	...
Haiti	1,714	5.7	98	47/53
Honduras	2,644	6.0	160	58/42
Jamaica	3,826	7.0	267	36/64
Martinique[a]	14,026	...	...	...
Mexico	9,010	5.5	497	44/56
Montserrat	3,072	7.2	220	85/15
Netherlands Antilles	15,481	12.9	1,997	91/9
Nicaragua	3,340	8.0	266	41/49
Panama	6,689	6.8	453	66/34
Paraguay	4,423	6.6	290	33/67
Peru	5,219	3.8	197	61/39
Puerto Rico[a]	23,987	3.5	828	...
Saint Kitts and Nevis	11,606	4.3	497	57/43
Saint Lucia	5,819	5.8	337	57/43
Saint Vincent and the Grenadines	5,880	4.5	267	86/14
Suriname[a]	6,188	3.8	237	...
Trinidad and Tobago	11,196	4.9	551	60/40
Turks and Caicos Islands	10,212	3.4	348	...
United States	36,465	13.1	4,791	45/55
US Virgin Islands[a]	13,938	3.0	416	...
Uruguay	8,658	9.0	781	71/29
Venezuela	5,554	6.3	348	56/44

[a]Public expenditure only.

Source: Pan American Health Organization, Health Systems Strengthening Area, Health Policies and Systems Development Unit.

TABLE 6. Classification of national health care systems in the Americas (type of system and income level), 2004.

Type of health system	Income level: Low *(Under US$ 4,000)*	Income level: Middle *(Over US$ 4,000; under US$ 11,000)*	Income level: High *(Over US$ 11,000)*
Predominantly public system		Anguilla	
		Belize	Antigua and Barbuda[a]
Public expenditure exceeds 66% of national health care costs	Cuba[a]	Dominica	Netherlands Antilles[b]
		Montserrat[a]	Aruba[b]
		Panama[b]	Canada[b]
		St. Vincent and the Grenadines	
		Uruguay[b]	
Mixed system[b]		Chile[b]	Argentina[b]
		Costa Rica[b]	Bahamas
Public expenditure exceeds 50% but is under 66% of national health care costs	Bolivia	Grenada	Barbados
			Saint Kitts and Nevis
			Trinidad and Tobago
	Honduras	Peru	
	Nicaragua	Saint Lucia	
		Venezuela	
Predominantly private, market-oriented systems	Ecuador	El Salvador	Bermuda
Public expenditure is less than 50% of national health care costs	Guatemala	Brazil	United States
	Haiti	Mexico	
	Jamaica	Paraguay	
		Dominican Republic	

[a]Can be classified as national health services systems.

[b]Countries with extensive social security or compulsory medical insurance systems that cover 50% or more of the population (see Table 7) can be classified as having national health insurance systems.

Source: Based on Table 5.

share of national health expenditure as a percentage of GDP declined to 6.8%. From 1990–2000 to 2004–2005, total spending on health care services grew by an average of 4% a year, slightly slower than the economy. The share of national health expenditure as a percentage of GDP declined from around 7.1% in the mid-1990s to about 6.8% in 2004–2005. During that time, the level of per capita expenditure on health remained practically constant (around US$ 500). Overall, the Latin American and Caribbean region spent about US$ 305 billion on health care in 2005. This figure is 50% higher than the level of US$ 190 billion in 1980, and 5% higher than in 2000 (around US$ 291 billion).

From 1980 until 2005, the composition of national health expenditure underwent significant changes. The economic and fiscal crisis of the 1980s severely curbed government spending capacity. In 1985, governments spent less on health care than in 1980. Public expenditure as a share of GDP declined from around 2.9% in 1980 to 2.6% in 1985. During the 1980s, private expenditure grew faster than public expenditure. The share of private expenditure as a percentage of GDP increased from 3.2% in 1980 to about 3.8% in 1990. Figure 1 shows the changes in the composition of national health expenditure for Latin America and the Caribbean for 1980–2005.

The recovery of economic growth during the 1990s had a positive impact on public health expenditure. (Public health expenditure includes central government, local government, and public insurance spending.) From 1990 to 1997, public health expenditure grew continuously, rising to 3.4% of GDP in 1995–1997. It declined slightly to 3.2% in 2000 and remained at that level for the next three years. There have been changes in the composition of public health expenditure: central government expenditure decreased during the 1980s, then increased with the economic recovery in the 1990s. Local government expenditures on health were low in the 1980s, grew in the 1990s and, after peaking in 1995, have been declining since 1998. Public health insurance program expenditures decreased slightly in the 1980s, before rising in 1990; they declined in the 1990s, but apparently improved again during 2004–2005.

Most of the increases in private spending on health care came from a significant rise in household out-of-pocket expenditure and rapid growth in private health insurance and pre-paid medical plans. Household out-of-pocket spending grew when government spending declined during the 1980s, peaking in 1990. Out-of-pocket spending has declined since then, consistent with the increase in spending on private health insurance. Private health

317

FIGURE 1. Changes in the composition of national health care expenditure over time, Latin America and the Caribbean, 1980–2005.

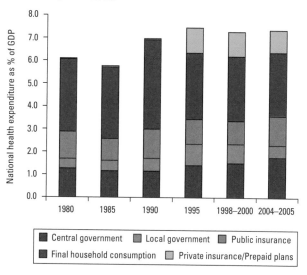

Source: Pan American Health Organization, Health Systems Strengthening Unit. Database on national health expenditure.

insurance and pre-paid health plans amounted to about 2% of total private spending in the early 1980s. With growth in the market for private health insurance and prepaid plans, private expenditure on these items rose steadily through the late 1980s and early 1990s, accounting for about 27% of total private spending in the mid-1990s. It has remained fairly constant since then at about 1.2% of GDP.

Public Health Care Systems: Expenditure and Coverage of Government and Social Health Insurance Plans

The organization and financing of national public health care systems in the Americas are reflected in expenditures on health goods and services by central and local governments (provincial, state, and departmental), either directly or indirectly through the health and maternity programs of social security institutions or mandatory (social) health insurance schemes (depending on the accounting practices of the countries, these expenditures may or may not be included as part of government finances). There are large differences in Latin America and the Caribbean in total public expenditure on health, in the magnitude of public resources spent through social security and other public insurance schemes, and in the coverage of public health insurance plans. Table 7 illustrates the wide differences between countries in public expenditure on health as a percentage of GDP, and the spending and coverage levels of health insurance systems during 2004–2005.

Total public health expenditure as a percentage of GDP in the Region ranges from a high of around 12.7% (Aruba) to a low of 1.1% (Guyana). Countries with the largest share of public expenditure as a percentage of GDP are those whose national health systems provide universal or near-universal coverage of services through national health insurance schemes. The central government is directly involved in the provision of health care services to all or most of the population in those countries. For example, Cuba and some English-speaking Caribbean countries have total public health expenditure of 6% of GDP or more; the Netherlands Antilles and Aruba have total public health expenditure of around 12% or more of GDP. Countries with public health insurance schemes covering more than two thirds of the total population, such as Chile, Costa Rica, and Panama, spend between 4.4% to 5.0% of GDP on this item. Canada is the only country in the Region providing universal coverage, with total public health expenditure of around 7.3% of GDP.

Other countries exhibit high levels of public expenditure on health but lower levels of coverage, such as Colombia and the United States. The relatively high share of public expenditure as a percentage of GDP in Colombia is associated with the introduction of a new compulsory public health insurance scheme in the early 1990s, which increased coverage from around 20% in the early 1990s to about 52% in 2004–2005. The United States spends about 7.2% of GDP on public health, with a coverage rate of just over 30% of the population. The main components of that expenditure are the social insurance systems targeted to the poor (Medicaid), to persons over 65 years old (Medicare), and to children (State Children's Health Insurance Program—SCHIP).

Public expenditure per capita varies considerably throughout the Region, ranging from US$ 45 in Haiti to over US$ 2,000 in Aruba, Bermuda, Canada, and the United States. In countries with public health insurance, there are significant differences in per capita expenditure per beneficiary, ranging from a high of about US$ 7,150 in the United States to a low of about US$ 136 in Bolivia. In general, health expenditure per beneficiary of public health insurance is more than twice as high as public health expenditure per capita.

Social security institutions have low population coverage in countries with predominantly private market-oriented systems. This is true in Ecuador (20.4%), Guatemala (17.8%), El Salvador (16.8%), and Paraguay (10.9%). A similar level of low coverage is observed in low-income countries with mixed health systems such as Honduras and Nicaragua.

Some countries in the Region have implemented publicly financed health programs targeted to vulnerable groups. Implementation of these programs has actually increased the level of overall public health spending. These programs have been financed through the creation of specific taxes to raise funds for improving maternal and child health. The programs have been implemented in an incremental manner. The box on page 320 presents a short summary of key information on how two of

TABLE 7. Public health expenditure and public health insurance coverage in the Americas, 2004–2005.

Country	Total population (millions)	Total public expenditure on public health as a percentage of GDP	Expenditure on social security and public health insurance including the total of the preceding column as a percentage of GDP	Coverage of social security and public health insurance plans as a percentage of the total population	Per capita public expenditure in US$ PPP 2000	Expenditure on health per public health insurance beneficiary in US$ PPP 2000
Anguilla	0.01	4.7			388.3	
Antigua and Barbuda	0.08	8.7			1,005.1	
Argentina[b]	38.37	4.7	2.5	49.6	574.4	609.1
Aruba[a]	0.10	12.7	12.7	100.0	2,732.4	2,732.4
Bahamas	0.32	3.1			502.5	
Barbados	0.27	4.3			739.0	
Belize	0.28	4.2			262.0	
Bermuda	0.06	3.7			2,624.9	
Bolivia	9.01	4.2	1.5	27.8	105.1	136.1
Brazil	183.91	3.4			259.5	
British Virgin Islands	0.02	1.8			680.6	
Canada	31.97	7.3	7.1	100.0	2,097.5	2,040.0
Cayman Islands	0.04	3.3			1,048.8	
Chile[b]	16.12	4.4	3.7	83.5	441.7	437.0
Colombia[b]	44.92	3.4	3.0	67.8	229.4	294.9
Costa Rica	4.25	5.0	4.5	87.8	440.0	449.0
Cuba	11.24	6.3			220.2	
Dominica	0.07	4.4			228.0	
Dominican Republic	8.77	1.4	0.5	0.0	94.1	
Ecuador	13.04	2.2	1.0	20.4	80.1	177.6
El Salvador	6.76	2.4	1.2	16.8	111.0	331.6
French Guiana	0.20					
Grenada	0.11	4.5			334.8	
Guadeloupe	0.45					
Guatemala	12.29	1.8	0.9	17.8	71.1	192.1
Guyana	0.75	1.1			45.3	
Haiti	8.41	2.7			46.3	
Honduras	7.05	3.5			93.4	
Jamaica	2.64	2.5			95.7	
Martinique	0.44					
Mexico	103.80	2.4	1.7	56.4	217.9	275.0
Montserrat	0.01	6.1			186.0	
Netherlands Antilles[a]	0.18	11.7	11.7	100.0	1,811.2	1,811.2
Nicaragua	5.38	3.3	1.9	10.7	108.8	
Panama	3.18	4.5	2.9	62.7	298.8	
Paraguay	6.02	2.2	1.0	10.9	95.7	
Peru	27.56	2.3	1.1	27.3	120.1	
Puerto Rico	3.89	3.5			827.8	
Saint Kitts and Nevis	0.05	2.5			285.1	
Saint Lucia	0.16	3.3			192.9	
Saint Vincent and the Grenadines	0.12	3.9			228.3	
Suriname	0.45	3.8			237.0	
Trinidad and Tobago	1.30	3.0			332.0	
Turks and Caicos Islands	0.02	3.4			348.5	
United States	293.66	7.2	5.9	30.1	2,633.0	7,149.8
US Virgin Islands	0.11	3.0			415.6	
Uruguay[b]	3.44	6.4	4.5	44.8	554.1	876.1
Venezuela	26.13	3.5	1.3	38.3	194.4	192.9

[a]Public health insurance accounts for more than 96% of total public expenditure.

[b]Includes the costs of public health insurance plans financed through compulsory contributions: Argentina (Obras Sociales); Chile (FONASA and ISAPRES); Colombia (Health Social Security Funds, contributive and subsidized); Uruguay (IAMCS).

Source: Pan American Health Organization, Health Systems Strengthening Area, Health Policies and Systems Development Unit, Washington DC, PAHO, August 2006.

Financing of Mother and Child Health Care Programs in Bolivia and Ecuador

In both Bolivia and Ecuador, universal publicly financed mother and child health insurance has been introduced through national laws and decrees. The Universal Mother and Child Insurance (SUMI) was established in Bolivia in January 2003 to replace the Basic Health Insurance (SBS) and the National Maternal and Child Insurance (SNMN). SUMI was established as a broad, universal, and free insurance plan for pregnant women, and it covers up to six months after delivery, in addition to covering care for children from birth to age 5. In 2005, Law 3.250 extended SUMI coverage to all women up to 60 years of age. The basic health services covered by SUMI rose in number from 92 to 546 and are provided by institutions in the public and social security network and by health centers operated by NGOs, churches, and other institutions.

SUMI is mainly financed with funds from the national treasury, municipal tax transfer payments (CTM), and the National Solidarity Fund (FSN). Between 1999 and 2005 financing for mother and child health insurance rose from US$ 8 million to US$ 24 million. The initial figure of US$ 8 million was doubled in 2002 with the inclusion of the CTM and FSN contributions, and it is estimated that the program has the capacity to disburse between 70% and 85% of total funding. After the SNMN was introduced in 1996, mother and child health coverage in Bolivia expanded to cover 55% of the population in 2005.

Estimated per capita expenditure on mother and child health rose from about US$ 11 in 1999 to US$ 25 in 2005 for each person assisted. That amount is not sufficient to cover services for the entire potential beneficiary population. Even with a sustained increase in service coverage and higher disbursement capacity by SUMI, financing will continue to be insufficient to cover all services for the entire potential beneficiary population.

In Ecuador, the Free Maternity and Child Care Law of 1994 was implemented for the first time in 2000 through the National Maternity and Child Insurance (SNMI). The law establishes that 3% of the special consumption tax (ICE) will be used to finance the insurance, complemented by contributions from the National Child Nutrition Fund (FONNIN) and international cooperation agencies that contribute funds to local governments. The latter finance activities in their respective jurisdictions (municipalities) and cover the costs of transportation in obstetrical and pediatric emergencies. The estimated budget for the Free Maternity and Child Care Law does not include funds from the Ministry of Health's general budget that the government authorizes each year to subsidize salaries, unit equipment, instruments, and maintenance of installations or establishments.

Financing for SNMI rose from approximately US$ 8 million to US$ 20 million between 1999 and 2005. This steady increase is due to the special tax allocated directly to the insurance. In 1999 it initially covered nine services which were gradually increased to 42 by 2003. Over the same period, the number of beneficiaries jumped from 793,000 to 3 million, while per capita expenditure per beneficiary increased from about US$ 6 to US$ 10. National estimates suggest that the average per capita package costs US$ 34, so that current financing does not cover all the programmed services. The sustainability of this insurance depends on the government's capacity to increase taxes for this purpose and on efficiency in the use of funds.

Source: Adapted from Gordillo A, 2006. Pan American Health Organization, Health Systems Strengthening Area, Health Policies and Systems Development Unit.

these programs are financed: the Universal Mother and Child Insurance Program in Bolivia and the Free Maternity and Child Care Program in Ecuador.

Private Expenditure on Health by Households

For most countries of the Region private spending on health care is an important component of general national health expenditures, even in countries with relatively high levels of government spending and countries where public health insurance coverage is relatively high or universal. However, in general, there seems to be an inverse ratio between the relative importance of public health care systems and the relative importance of private health expenditure.

Household expenditure on health services as a percentage of total household spending measures the health care costs borne by families, directly through out-of-pocket spending, or indirectly through household and company spending on pre-paid medical plans and private health insurance plans. It also measures the differential impact of increases in health care costs on household budgets.

The share of private household expenditure on health as a percentage of GDP is an indicator of the significance of private consumption of health goods and services compared to the total income and expenditure of an economy. The differences in the level of household spending on health care in per capita terms—adjusted for purchasing power parity—is an indicator of differences in actual access and utilization of health care services in different countries of the Region. Household spending on private health services represents a significant percentage of total consumer spending in most countries of the Region. The estimates of the relative importance of household spending on health care presented in Table 8 correspond to the weight of the cost of health goods and services in a country's official consumer price index (CPI).[6]

Table 8 shows the sharp differences in the relative importance of household spending on health goods and services as a percentage of the total household consumption. These differences range from 10% in Argentina and 8.5% in the United States, to less than 2% in Antigua and Barbuda, Aruba, and Saint Vincent and the Grenadines. In countries with relatively high levels of government expenditure and public health insurance coverage, such as Canada, Chile, and Costa Rica, household spending on health care represents between 5% and 6% of total household consumption. In low-income countries, such as Haiti, Honduras, and Peru, the share is low, at about 3% of total household consumption. This private household expenditure is over and above the value of the health care services received free of charge from governments or social security institutions. The differences in these shares illustrate the large differences in the potential impact of increases in health care costs on household budgets between countries. Similarly, the large differences in private household expenditure expressed as a percentage of GDP indicate the relative importance of public policies to manage the market failures that are typical of private health care markets.

Large regional differences in the level of household expenditure in per capita terms point to the wide inequalities in access to

and utilization of private health care services in the countries of the Americas. Table 8 summarizes different indicators for assessing the relative importance of private health expenditure, estimated on the basis of the weight of household expenditure on health goods and services.

Private health insurance and pre-paid health plans are becoming important mechanisms for financing private health costs. The rapid increase in resources spent on private health insurance and pre-paid health plans is the most important factor in recent trends in national health expenditure and has become a major factor shaping the health care markets of the countries. This trend poses a major public policy challenge. Regulations must be designed to ensure efficiency in the functioning of the health insurance and pre-paid health plan markets, and to address inequalities that exist in countries of the Americas in access to health care. The scale of the markets for private health insurance and pre-paid health plans seems to be determined by the size of the public health care system, the extent of population coverage, the services covered under public health insurance systems, and the presence (or absence) of policies regulating the functioning of those markets. The presence of multinational and large national corporations in different countries, rather than a country's income level, seems to be an important factor in explaining the relative importance of the markets for private health insurance and pre-paid health plans.

Shortfalls in coverage by public health care systems do not appear to be a sufficient reason for a private health insurance market to develop. In the case of Mexico (as in South Korea, Greece, and Turkey), private health insurance markets are relatively undeveloped, despite gaps in coverage of the public health care system. On the other hand, even in countries with near-universal public health insurance systems, such as Costa Rica, large firms will provide their employees with complementary private health insurance to reduce waiting times at public facilities and/or to provide access to "better quality care."

Because of the lack of regulation, many individuals with private health insurance rely on subsidized health care services at public hospitals to keep their insurance premiums low. Private health insurance may be used to cover a limited set of medical services. The most expensive and unusual medical procedures are not included in private insurance plans on the assumption that infrequent, costly procedures will be provided at subsidized public hospitals. This poses an additional problem in terms of the potential impact on the use and financing of public hospitals. It also creates an additional public policy challenge that needs to be addressed.

---

[6] A consumer price index (CPI) measures changes over time in the average prices of goods and services that a reference population acquires, uses, or pays for. A CPI is estimated as a series of summary measurements of the period-to-period proportional change in the prices of a fixed set of consumer goods and services of constant quantity and characteristics, acquired, used, or paid for by the reference population. Each summary measurement is constructed as a weighted average of a large number of elementary indices. Each of the elementary indices is estimated using a sample of prices for a defined set of goods and services obtained in, or by residents of, a specific region from a given set of outlets or other sources of consumption of goods and services. For a detailed description of the different names and components of the item "health and medical care" used in different countries see the footnotes and methodological notes to PAHO's Health Situation in the Americas: Basic Indicators 2006. PAHO/HDN/HA/06.01; Washington D.C.; September 2006.

Description of Household Expenditure on Health

Analyzing household expenditure on health is a way to measure the financial burden families face in seeking health care, and to understand the choices families make in allocating resources

TABLE 8. Private health care expenditure by households, Region of the Americas, by country, 2004.

Country	Health care expenditure by families as a percentage of total household spending	Health care expenditure by families as a percentage of GDP	Per capita health care expenditure by families in US$ PPP[a]
Anguilla	3.1	2.2	184.4
Antigua and Barbuda	2.8	0.7	79.4
Argentina	10.0	6.9	845.4
Aruba	2.9	1.5	331.1
Bahamas	4.4	2.9	466.5
Barbados	5.9	3.8	649.6
Belize	6.0	4.1	251.6
Bermuda	...	...	...
Bolivia	...	...	...
Brazil	5.9	3.6	270.2
British Virgin Islands	...	...	...
Canada	6.4	3.5	1,005.3
Cayman Islands	...	...	...
Chile	6.0	3.9	385.5
Colombia	4.0	2.6	172.2
Costa Rica	5.0	3.4	298.5
Cuba	...	...	...
Dominica	3.2	2.0	106.5
Dominican Republic	...	...	...
Ecuador	3.4	2.7	85.8
El Salvador	...	...	...
French Guiana	...	...	...
Grenada	...	...	...
Guadeloupe	...	...	...
Guatemala	5.5	4.7	187.7
Guyana	...	...	...
Haiti	3.2	3.2	55.2
Honduras	3.7	2.5	66.4
Jamaica	7.0	4.5	171.2
Martinique	...	...	...
Mexico	...	...	...
Montserrat	6.9	5.3	162.3
Nicaragua	5.1	4.7	157.2
Panama	...	...	...
Paraguay	...	...	...
Peru	2.9	2.0	106.4
Puerto Rico	...	...	...
Saint Kitts and Nevis	3.7	1.8	212.0
Saint Lucia	3.6	2.5	143.8
Saint Vincent and the Grenadines	1.0	0.6	38.4
Suriname	...	...	...
Trinidad and Tobago	3.6	2.0	219.3
Turks and Caicos Islands	...	...	...
United States	8.5	5.9	2,157.8
US Virgin Islands	...	...	...
Uruguay[b]	3.8	2.8	242.2
Venezuela	4.2	2.8	153.2

[a]United States dollars adjusted for purchasing power parity (PPP), year 2000.

[b]Excludes contributions and payments to public health insurance systems and the medical services of collective health institutions and mutuals.

Source: Pan American Health Organization, Health Analysis and Statistics Unit (HA), Health Situation in the Americas: Basic Indicators 2006. Washington, DC: PAHO; 2006.

TABLE 9. Distribution of household expenditure on health care (%) by quintile, selected countries of the Americas.

| Country | Year | Total | Approximate income or expenditure by quintile | | | | |
			1	2	3	4	5
Argentina	1996–1997	8.6	9.2	8.6	7.8	8.2	9.0
Brazil	1995–1996	6.5	8.3	6.5	6.9	7.1	6.3
Dominican Republic	1996	6.3	29.1	14.7	9.4	7.7	3.5
Guatemala	1998–1999	7.3	3.9	5.9	7.0	8.3	7.8
Jamaica	1998	2.6	2.4	2.5	2.5	2.6	2.7
Mexico	1996	2.9	3.7	3.3	3.3	2.9	2.8
Paraguay	1996	10.7	14.0	13.8	10.9	10.1	8.8
Peru	1997	4.4	4.3	4.8	4.7	4.0	4.5
Uruguay	1994–1995	13.0	11.0	14.0	15.0	13.0	11.0

Source: Pan American Health Organization, Health Systems Strengthening Area, Health Policies and Systems Development Unit. August 2006

to purchase health goods and services. The analysis may also provide some limited insight into other issues, such as health sector equity and access to health services. A number of factors play a role in whether or not households have access to and make use of health care services, such as family income, time constraints, the cost of services and transportation, the availability and quality of services, cultural preferences, and an awareness of the need to seek treatment. Families have their own priorities that influence the decision about when and where to seek care. Furthermore, health services are not a homogeneous product and often the price of comparable services can vary considerably from private to public sector providers (where services may not cost anything), thus rendering expenditure data even less useful. Nevertheless, the relative share and composition of spending on health in a household's budget and comparisons across income groups can provide important information on family choices, and often reflects the availability of public resources and services.

Table 9 provides data on the percentage of household resources allocated to health across income groups for nine countries of the Region. The share of total household expenditure that is devoted to health tends to be relatively stable across income groups within a country, usually differing by only a few percentage points. In absolute terms, however, wealthier income groups spend far more than the poor do on health goods and services. A rough average for the Region suggests that the richest 20% of the population spends up to 12 times more than the poorest 20%. For the nine countries included in Table 9, a weighted average was constructed for household spending on health. Using these data, households on average allocated 6% of their expenditure to purchase health goods and services: however, the poorest quintile spends 7.3% on health care, and the richest quintile spends 5.9%. In six countries in Table 9, the poorest quintile spends a larger share of its resources on health than the richest quintile. In some countries, such as the Dominican Republic and Paraguay, the poor spend considerably more on health care than the rich. In the Dominican

Republic, health care expenditures comprise 29.1% of spending for the poorest quintile, but only 3.5% for the richest; in Paraguay, health care expenditures comprise 14% of spending for the poorest quintile, and just 8.8% for the richest. In other countries, health expenditures are roughly equal in the poorest and richest quintiles. Guatemala is the only country where the richest quintile spends more on health care than the poorest quintile.

Private expenditure on health as a share of total household spending tends to decrease as income increases. Two factors seem to be the driving force in this trend. The first is the relatively recent impact of private insurance on household health care spending. The increasing degree of private insurance coverage in the upper income groups, with premiums paid largely by employers, reduces out-of-pocket spending in those income quintiles. The second factor relates to the gaps in public health system coverage. The poorest income quintiles have limited access to formal health insurance programs, because they are primarily composed of agricultural and informal laborers who are not covered by them. The poorest income quintile may also have more limited access to public health facilities, given that they tend to be located in or near urban areas, which may not be easily accessible for people living in rural areas. With governments allocating the majority of resources to secondary and tertiary facilities in predominantly urban areas, public subsidies may disproportionately favor the cities and the upper-income quintiles rather than reducing the burden on the lowest-income groups in rural areas.

Distributive Impact of Government Health Expenditure

There appears to be considerable variability in the effectiveness of health expenditure as a distributive tool. The analysis of government health expenditure suggests there are large differences in the distributive impact of government expenditure on health by income groups, both across countries and within coun-

TABLE 10. Distribution of the benefits of government expenditure on health in selected countries of Latin America and the Caribbean, by quintile.

Country	Q1	Q2	Q3	Q4	Q5
Argentina[a]	31.0	18.0	26.0	18.0	7.0
Argentina, 1991[b,c]	38.7	16.6	25.5	14.8	4.5
Bolivia, 1990[c]	15.2	14.7	24.4	24.4	21.3
Brazil, 1994[c,d]	31.5	26.5	19.5	14.2	7.5
Colombia, 1970[a]	21.4	26.9	19.0	25.9	6.8
Colombia, 1974[a]	28.0	22.0	20.1	17.7	12.2
Colombia, 1993[a]	27.4	25.6	18.7	15.9	12.5
Colombia, 1997[c]	17.5	19.7	22.2	20.7	19.7
Costa Rica, 1986[c]	27.7	23.6	24.1	13.9	10.7
Chile[a]	31.0	25.0	22.0	14.0	8.0
Chile, 1996[c]	30.9	23.2	22.2	16.5	7.2
Ecuador, 1995[a]	12.5	15.0	19.4	22.5	30.5
Ecuador, 1994[c]	18.8	41.9	16.0	16.3	7.0
Guatemala, 1998–1999[a]	12.8	12.7	16.9	26.3	31.3
Jamaica, 1993[a]	25.3	23.9	19.4	16.2	15.2
Peru, 1997[a]	20.1	20.7	21.0	20.7	17.5
Uruguay, 1993[c]	34.9	19.9	22.1	13.2	10.0
Average[c, e]	26.9	23.3	22.0	16.7	11.1

[a]Estimates reported by Suárez-Berenguela R, 2001, page 142.

[b] Household distribution by income less social security contributions, income tax, and government subsidies.

[c] ECLAC estimates (ECLAC 2000; ECLAC 2001). Per capita income quintiles, includes public expenditure on health care and nutrition.

[d] The data are for the city of São Paulo only.

[e] Average for the countries included in the ECLAC study, only.

Sources: Suárez-Berenguela R. Health systems inequalities in Latin America and the Caribbean. In: Invertir en salud. Beneficios sociales y económicos. (Publicación Científica y Técnica No. 582). OPS; 2001.

Economic Commission for Latin America and the Caribbean. Equity, Development and Citizenship. Final Version. Santiago, Chile: ECLAC; 2000.

Economic Commission for Latin America and the Caribbean. Social Panorama of Latin America 2000–2001. Santiago, Chile: ECLAC; 2001.

tries. Paradoxically, there seems to be an inverse relationship between a country's level of income and the distributive impact of government expenditure on health. The distributive impact of government expenditure was found to be progressive in countries with relatively higher income levels (Argentina, Chile, Costa Rica, and Uruguay) and regressive in countries with lower levels (Bolivia, Ecuador, and Guatemala). The distributive impact of health expenditure was found to be neutral in the case of Peru. Table 10 examines the distribution of the benefits of government expenditure on health by socioeconomic quintiles for Latin America and the Caribbean.

Colombia is the only country where it was possible to observe trends in government expenditures on health over time, from 1970 to 1997, due to the availability of a series of data sets. A shift can be observed from a progressive to a regressive distribution. The poorest 20% of the population received more than 21% of government health expenditure in 1970 and around 28% in 1974. In 1997, the poorest 20% received just 17.5%. The wealthiest 20% of the population benefited the most from these changes in dis-

tributive impact: it received almost 7% of government health expenditure in 1970; but in 1997 it received almost 20%.

Public spending on health has a significant redistributive impact favoring the poor in countries where expenditure represented 2.5% or more of GDP (Argentina, Colombia, Chile, and Jamaica). Public spending favoring the rich was observed in countries where government expenditure on health represented around 1% of GDP or less (Ecuador and Guatemala). In most countries, financing of the (public) system was regressive, based on indirect taxes. Changing the financing of the health systems from an indirect tax-based system to a direct tax-based system reduces regressivity.

Specific policies may contribute to improving the distributive impact of government expenditure on health. For example, only the case of Brazil was considered progressive where in 1997–1998, an earmarked tax on financial transactions and direct taxes on net company profits were the main sources of revenue of the Ministry of Health. Redirecting public expenditure to policies aimed at heightening individuals' perceptions of their own health status and health risks may be an effective way to narrow the gap between actual and self-assessed health status, to make people aware of their health service needs, and to increase the demand for those services.

Public expenditure and fiscal revenues are the main tools that a government can use to achieve more equitable financing and access to health care services. Higher levels of taxation are required to finance government activities, similar to schemes used by governments in the now developed countries. However, most of these fiscal instruments are not fully utilized in developing countries, including those in Latin America and the Caribbean. Low-income countries in the region face a vicious cycle of weak governments and lack of funds to set up institutions strong enough to enforce tax codes and fiscal policies and to ensure the sustainability of social programs.

Public policy choices influence the levels of public expenditure on health and social programs. Wide differences in the distributive impact of government spending on health care services and public health programs suggest that in most countries of the Region, there is ample room for making better use of government financing and expenditure tools with a view to achieving more equitable financing for health care services and access to them. Data presented in this section suggest that governments of countries in Latin America and the Caribbean, particularly those in low-income countries, have the potential to use existing fiscal tools more effectively to address health and equity issues.

In conclusion, governments have considerable room to maneuver to enhance the distributive impact of public expenditure on health. They can increase health resources, reduce regressivity in health financing, and redirect public expenditure to interventions that lead to greater utilization of health care services by the poor.[7] Results from a number of studies, including those conducted by the project Equity in Latin America and the Caribbean/Investment in Health, Equity, and Poverty on the distributive impact of government expenditure on health, suggest that the relative size of that expenditure makes a difference in terms of equity in financing for health services as a percentage of GDP.

HEALTH LEGISLATION

Legislation provides health policies with the support required to move from the political sphere into the legal framework. With regard to health systems and services, legislation establishes a platform of guarantees with counterpart obligations, defines the roles to be played by national and international public, private, and social institutions and their functions and interactions, and establishes the model that will put into effect national health ob-

---

[7]For more information on the distributive impact of public expenditure on health, see Investments in Health: Social and Economic Returns. PAHO Scientific and Technical Publication No. 582 (available in PDF format).

"We are making every effort to obtain original articles penned by the highest authorities in the Americas on topics of interest related to matters of public health."

Hugh Cumming, 1927

jectives, all of which is accessible through the judicial system. In the last five years, several of the countries of the Region continued revising their legal frameworks with a view to providing a legal footing for policies aimed at restructuring health services and systems. This included redefinition of the responsibilities of the health ministries/departments and the design of plans to extend coverage, including the regulation of private sector participation, quality assurance and control mechanisms, participation by civil society, and consolidation of individual health rights.

Legal Framework for Health System Stewardship and Regulatory Functions

The legislation that restructures health systems reformulates the functions of the ministries and departments, stressing their stewardship and regulatory roles. In 2002 Supreme Decree No. 26.875 was approved in Bolivia, which redefines the national health system and establishes organizational and functional responsibilities based on management levels. Under this arrangement, the Ministry of Health and Social Insurance (today the Ministry of Health and Sports) is responsible for the national leadership and regulatory function. Technical management is the responsibility of the Departmental Health Service (SEDES) and the municipalities, through the Local Health Directorates (DILOS), which are the highest local authority. In Chile, under Law No. 19.937 of 2004, the Ministry of Health is made responsible for leadership and regulation in the field of health, including the formulation, evaluation, and updating of the Universal Access with Explicit Guarantees (AUGE) system. In Colombia, Law No. 790 of 2002 merged the Ministry of Labor and Social Security and the Ministry of Health into the Ministry of Social Welfare to implement the social safety net established in Law No. 789 of the same year, one of whose objectives is to provide timely access to good quality basic health services. Also, Decree No. 205 of 2003 defined the functions of the Ministry of Social Welfare, which is the lead agency in the system.

Ecuador promulgated the National Health System Institutional Law and its Enabling Regulations (Decree No. 3.611 of 2003) to make exercise of the right to health effective by guaranteeing equitable and universal access to comprehensive health services. Under these norms, the national system is decentralized, deconcentrated, and participative in its activities and its functions include coordination, service provision, insurance, and financing. The function of system coordination is the responsibility of the

Ministry of Health at all levels. Nicaragua enacted the General Health Act (Law No. 423 of 2002) and its Enabling Regulations (Decree No. 001 of 2003) which regulate the different health activities and define the Ministry's sphere of competence and responsibilities, which include regulation of the benefit regime that it establishes and its status as the lead agency in the sector.

In Peru, the Ministry of Health Act (Law No. 27.657 of 2002) establishes that it is the agency that leads, regulates, and promotes the national health system to achieve the full development of individuals. Subsequently, Law No. 27.813 of the same year established the National Coordinated Decentralized Health System (SNCDS) to provide comprehensive health care for the population and progress toward universal social security, and also conferred the status of lead agency on the Ministry of Health. In the Dominican Republic, the General Health Act (Law No. 42 of 2001) regulates all the actions that permit the government to make effective the right to health protection recognized in the constitution. This act organizes the national health system, which is headed by the Secretary of State for Public Health and Social Welfare (SESPAS). In Venezuela, Decree No. 3.753 of 2005 partly reforms the organization and operation of the central public administration. As a result, the Ministry of Health and Social Development became the Ministry of Health, with responsibilities for the preparation, formulation, regulation, and monitoring of comprehensive policies for the health of the population.

In the English-speaking Caribbean, legislation was passed to create regulatory systems under the supervision of authorities, commissions, and committees, with the goal of making the administration of hospitals and other health care institutions more effective and efficient. The British Virgin Islands Health Service Authority Act of 2004 makes that authority responsible for administering the Peebles Hospital and community health services. The act establishes a council appointed by the Minister of Health, whose functions include the design of policies based on the territory's health requirements and the development and implementation of a quality assurance program subject to the Ministry's policies.

In Guyana, the Regional Authorities Act and the Ministry of Health Act were passed in 2005. The first creates regional authorities to deliver and administer services and programs in specific zones and makes the Ministry responsible for applying the law and establishing parameters to enable the authorities in question to carry out their functions. The Ministry of Health Act defines that institution's functions, which include control of health services and their development in a comprehensive, balanced, consistent, and equitable manner. The 2002 Institution-Based Health Services Act of Saint Kitts and Nevis establishes a directorate to manage and administer institutional health services (17). In Canada, an Order in Council of 2004 created the Public Health Agency of Canada with the mandate of fostering communications with the provinces, providing leadership in health surveillance, and initiating community action programs (18).

Regulation of Financing, Insurance, and Private Sector Involvement in Health Care

In Argentina, a package of essential benefits was approved and guaranteed by health insurance agents under the Mandatory Emergency Medical Program (PMOE), which was to remain in effect until 31 December 2002. The period was extended to 2003. Law No. 25.929 of 2004 expands the mandatory benefits that all Obras Sociales (employee benefit plans) and pre-paid medical institutions are required to provide, including pregnancy, labor, delivery, and post-partum care, which are fully incorporated into the Mandatory Medical Program (PMO) as part of a regime of rights for parents and newborns. In 2005, Decree No. 317 issued by the country's president approved Obras Sociales' system of regional contracting, which will be implemented gradually in the country's different regions and whose purpose is to avoid middlemen in contracts between the Obras Sociales groups belonging to the system and service providers. This decree establishes general guidelines to assure medical coverage for the beneficiaries of Obras Sociales.

In 2001, Belize amended the Social Security Act to establish a national health plan that covers the provision of the public and private health services determined in the act. Bolivia promulgated the Universal Mother and Child Insurance (SUMI) in 2002 to provide free care for pregnant women (from conception to six months after delivery) and children up to age 5, which is universal, comprehensive, and free of charge, at all levels of public care. SUMI is financed jointly by the national government, municipal taxes, and a special account called *Diálogo 2000*. Local Health Directorates (DILOS) have been established as the highest local health care authority.

In Canada, two recent decisions by the Supreme Court will have an impact on the Medicare system. One is related to the debate over what services are "medically necessary" or "medically required" as defined in the Canada Health Act; and the other opens the door to removing the ability of the provincial governments to prohibit private insurance for services covered with public funds. Nonetheless, the provinces are making efforts to strengthen Medicare. In British Columbia the Medicare Protection Act was amended to prohibit extra charges for services diagnosed as medically necessary, in order to address situations created by private for-profit clinics. Ontario passed legislation that supports its Medicare commitments and re-introduced an additional mandatory health care contribution (the health care premium tax) (18).

In Chile, Law No. 19.996 establishes the General Health Guarantees Regime, which is a regulatory instrument that forms part of the Health Services Regime referred to in Law No. 18.469, whose Article 4 regulates the exercise of the constitutional right to health protection and establishes the 1985 health benefits regime. The General Health Guarantees Regime includes explicit guarantees related to access, quality, financial protection, and timeliness, which must be mandatorily assured by the National Health Fund (FONASA) and the Health Insurance Institutions (ISAPREs).

Under the new structure, the Office of the Superintendent of Health takes on a relevant role. It is a decentralized agency with legal status and its own assets that reports to the country's president through the Ministry of Health. The Office of the Superintendent, which acts through the Health Insurance Institutions Administration and the Health Care Providers Administration, is responsible among other things for overseeing and controlling the ISAPREs and overseeing compliance with obligations, including those relating to the Health Guarantee Regime. It also oversees and controls the National Health Fund and supervises all public and private health care providers with respect to accreditation and certification and compliance with accreditation standards.

In Colombia, Legislative Act No. 01 of 2001 amends some of the articles of the 1991 Constitution and creates the general participation system for departments, districts, and municipalities, also establishing criteria for the distribution of resources, with emphasis on equity. As a consequence, Law No. 715 of 2001 was promulgated, which defines the responsibilities of the national and subnational entities in the health sector and the system for the distribution of financial resources. In Ecuador, the National Health System Institutional Law establishes a comprehensive health care plan guaranteed by the government as a strategy for accessible public health protection with compulsory coverage for the entire population, through the public and private network of suppliers, whose structure is based on a multicultural approach. This plan defines the care model, which stresses primary care, health promotion, and interrelations with traditional and alternative medicine, or both, and includes mechanisms for deconcentrated, decentralized, and participative management. The plan is intended to achieve universal coverage through three coordinated regimes—the contributing, the non-contributing, and the voluntary—incorporating public, private, and mixed health service providers.

In El Salvador, Legislative Decree No. 775 of 2005 promulgated the Law on the Basic Comprehensive Health System and Decree No. 1.024 of 2002 established provisions relating to health and social welfare guarantees. Health is defined as a public good and the country's constitution makes the provision of public health services mandatory. The decree prohibits privatization, concession, or the purchase of services or any other modality intended to transfer to private institutions the provision of public health services or the social security services delivered by the Salvadoran Social Security Administration.

In 2002, the United States passed the Health Care Safety Net Amendments, which created the Healthy Community Access Program that provides health care for persons with no health insurance (or insufficient insurance) through joint actions by suppliers, organizations, and local governments. The program was to conclude in fiscal year 2006. The Medicare Prescription Drug Improvement and Modernization Act (MMA) of 2003 modifies the Medicare + Choice option by including a component to cover prescription drugs, called Medicare Advantage. The reform affects access to

medicines, while transferring part of Medicare responsibilities to private plans and to the beneficiaries themselves. Under the Deficit Reduction Act of 2005, the federal government required proof of citizenship to accede to Medicaid benefits and the State Children's Health Insurance Program (SCHIP). Several states, including Massachusetts and Maine (Dirigo Health Initiative), have passed legislation involving extensive reforms of their health systems. The Massachusetts Plan provides universal health coverage, making it compulsory to participate, while the Dirigo Plan, although it has the same goal, does not make it mandatory to join (19).

In 2002, Grenada passed the Private Hospitals and Nursing Homes Act, which regulates those institutions through the Private Hospitals Committee. In Jamaica, the 2003 National Health Fund Act implements the national health insurance plan, known as the National Health Fund, as a contributing plan intended to improve the quality of life of the population. The plan includes the provision of certain health benefits for all the country's residents, without distinction by age, gender, or income (17).

In 2003, Mexico reformed its General Health Act to establish the social health protection system, which is financed jointly by the federal government, the states and the Federal District, and beneficiaries. A Department of Health resolution of the same year published the operating rules and management and evaluation indicators for the Health for All or Seguro Popular de Salud Program, which is a voluntary public insurance plan to implement the system. The main targets of the Seguro Popular are families and individuals who are not enrolled in social security institutions and who do not have any other health insurance. Also, a 2001 Department of Health resolution establishes a National Committee for the action program "Arranque Parejo en la Vida" (Fair-Start Program), whose objective is to contribute to health care for women during pregnancy, delivery, and the puerperium, and adequate health care of children from birth to 2 years of age, through close monitoring and evaluation of the actions introduced under the program.

Peru passed Law No. 27.812 in 2002, which establishes the sources of financing for the Comprehensive Health Insurance (SIS) to make it sustainable over time and enable it to comply with its objectives, and Decree 9-2002-SA of 2002 regulates its organization and functions. One of the sources of financing for the SIS is transfers from the Permanent Solidarity Fund created by Law No. 27.656 of 2002, whose sole intent is to promote access for the excluded population to good quality services. As a complement, Decree No. 3-2002-SA of 2002 established regulations governing the services delivered by the SIS in order to incorporate the services grouped into the mother and infant, child, and youth components as priorities. The Dominican Republic promulgated Law No. 87 of 2001, which creates the Dominican Social Security System, structured into three regimes—contributing, subsidized, and subsidized contributing—with the goal of achieving universality. Members are guaranteed free choice between the National Health Insurance, as a public insurer, and the Health

Risk Administrators, which can be public, private, or mixed. Also in the Dominican Republic, the regulations governing Family Health Insurance and the Basic Health Plan were established in Resolution No. 48-13 of 2002, which are intended to govern the provision of family health insurance benefits, conditions, limitations, and exclusions throughout the country.

In Uruguay, Decree No. 133 of 2005 created the Consultative Council for Implementation of the Integrated Health System within the Ministry of Public Health, whose main objective is health policy. In Venezuela the Social Security System Institutional Law was promulgated in December 2002 to make the right to social security effective. The regimes it establishes include the Health Benefits Regime, which will be the responsibility of the Ministry of Health and Social Development and will be managed through the National Public Health System, through policies, structures, and actions targeted to universality, equity, promotion of health and the quality of life, and comprehensive services.

Regulation of the Quality of Care

A number of countries have issued regulations governing the quality of care. In Argentina, Resolution No. 482 of 2002 approves regulations on the organization and functioning of the social services area in the establishments that form part of the National Medical Care Quality Assurance Program. In Decree No. 140 of 2004, Chile approved the Health Services Organization Regulations that introduce audits to assure the quality of services. In Costa Rica, Decree No. 30.571 of 2002 approves general regulations on the authorization and functioning of health facilities and Law No. 8.415 of 2004 adds a paragraph to Article 30, Chapter IX, of Law No. 7.593 on the Public Services Regulatory Authority to include failure to observe quality standards and principles in the delivery of public services among actions that are subject to sanction. In Resolution No. 06 of 2005, Honduras issued the Regulations on the Control of Products, Services, and Establishments of Health Interest.

In Mexico, a 2002 decision by the General Health Council laid the groundwork for a National Medical Care Establishment Certification Program, and in 2003, the council issued Internal Regulations governing the Health Services Facilities Certification Committee, which is intended to support the council in coordinating and developing the national certification program. The General Health Act of Nicaragua establishes the System for Health Sector Quality Assurance and its regulations introduce audits of the quality of medical care.

In Dominica, the 2002 Hospitals and Health Establishments Act regulates the licensing of those facilities and others that the government operates and maintains. In Saint Kitts and Nevis, the 2002 Institutional Health Services Administration Act establishes an executive management committee, whose functions include coordinating oversight of activities related to service quality with the Ministry of Health. In 2004, an act established the Accreditation Council of Trinidad and Tobago. The council, appointed by

the president, has the mandate of providing guidance and advice regarding the accreditation and recognition of post-secondary and tertiary education institutions, including those offering health education, and of promoting quality standards. The 2003 Public Hospitals Authority (Medical Staff) By-laws of the Bahamas establish a series of committees whose function is to guarantee the quality of services and ensure that medical staff comply with the policies, guidelines, and regulations (17).

Channels for Participation by Civil Society

In regard to civil society participation, the Management Model and Local Health Directorates (DILOS) Law and the Universal Mother and Child Insurance Law of Bolivia establish that management will include participation by the public to comply with national health policy and implement local directorates. Chile's Law No. 19.937 establishes users consultative councils to advise local health directors on policies and the definition and evaluation of institutional plans. In Law No. 715, Colombia establishes the need to promote mechanisms on all levels for adequate participation by society in the full exercise of citizen rights and duties in the field of health and social security. Ecuador's National Health System Institutional Law includes the promotion of participation and control by society and the observance of user rights among the functions of the National Health Councils and the Canton Health Councils. The Dominican Republic's General Health Law creates grass-roots organizations, neighborhood associations, and organizations of users and patients as consultative bodies of the National Health Council. Venezuela issued Decree No. 2.745 of 2003, which creates the Presidential Committee for the Implementation and Institutional Coordination of the Comprehensive Program for Primary Health Care, known as Barrio Adentro, as a new management model based on the principles of interdependence, coordination, accountability, cooperation, and active and predominant participation by the organized community. For its part, the Social Security System Institutional Law establishes that on account of their public relevance, community organizations have the right and duty to participate in decision-making for planning, execution, and control of specific policies in public health institutions.

Enhancing Health Rights

The general health laws of Nicaragua and the Dominican Republic contain chapters referring to the rights and duties of public and private sector users and the rights, duties, and responsibilities of the population in relation to health, respectively. In Bolivia, the Professional Practice Act of 2005 (Law No. 3.131) establishes the rights and duties of patients and medical professionals, medical audits, and management of the quality of health care services. The regulations to that act, issued in Supreme Decree No. 28.562, also of 2005, include the obligation to publicize those rights and duties and require medical professionals to know the native language used at the place where they practice. The regulations also refer to standards and protocols for managing the quality of services.

In Canada, the federal government reformed the Labor Code to allow up to eight weeks of compassionate leave with pay for persons caring for relatives with terminal illnesses. Most of the provinces have reformed their labor codes along the same lines. The Personal Information and Electronic Documents Protection Act has been in force since 2002 and includes the protection of health information (18). In Costa Rica, Law No. 8.239 of 2002 on the rights and duties of users of all public and private health services creates the office of the Auditor General of Health Services as a deconcentrated agency of the Ministry of Health with the mandate of promoting continuous improvement in health services. In Panama, Law No. 68 of 2003 regulates the rights of patients, healthy individuals, and professionals at public and private health facilities with regard to information and free and informed decisions for clinical and therapeutic purposes. In Mexico, the Resolution of the Department of Health publishing the regulations for the management and evaluation of the Health for All Program (Seguro Popular de Salud) includes a list of the rights and duties of members.

In the United States, the federal government has not acted to regulate the health management organizations, but in 2005 nine states (Arkansas, North Carolina, Colorado, Connecticut, Indiana, New Hampshire, Rhode Island, Texas, and West Virginia) issued detailed patients' bills of rights for the members of those organizations (19).

HUMAN RESOURCES

The Importance of Health Human Resources and Their Development

The main challenge in the field of health human resources is to achieve recognition of their importance in the countries of the Region as a whole, and there has been a promising change in that regard. After two decades in which health imbalances sharpened and health human resources were viewed more as a cost that needed to be reduced than as an investment, since 2004 these resources have gradually been recognized as core components for the development of health.

Many national and international initiatives underline their relevance and urge that efforts be concentrated in this field. In 2006, WHO dedicated World Health Day to recognizing the work of health professionals under the motto "Working Together for Health" and defined this area as a priority for its 2006–2015 work plans. The adoption of the Millennium Development Goals—in which improvement in different health indicators plays a central role—has underlined the importance of having sufficient qualified human resources to make faster progress. Different studies on the possibilities of attaining the MDGs have recognized that success hinges largely on health human resources. Institutions such as Harvard University, private foundations such as the

Rockefeller Foundation, Atlantic Philanthropies, and the Bill and Melinda Gates Foundation, and cooperation agencies such as the Swedish Agency for International Development (SIDA) joined WHO in designing the Joint Learning Initiative (JLI) which decries the lack of investment, efforts, and financing in this field and declares that the goal of attaining the health-related MDGs will not be met without the active participation of the health workforce (20).

In recent years, statistics have been compiled on the impact of human resources availability on the health situation, and it has been demonstrated that the number and quality of health workers is directly related to the degree of coverage of immunizations, the scope of primary care, and the survival of infants, children, and mothers. An econometric study conducted in 2004 in 117 countries by the JLI concluded that the density of health care personnel has a significant impact on maternal, infant, and under-5 child mortality and that this correlation exists independently of any income improvement policies, poverty reduction programs, or increases in education for girls that may have existed (21).

In past decades, the issue of human health resource development in the Americas did not have a high profile, which is apparent from the fact that between 1980 and 2001, PAHO's Governing Bodies did not approve any resolution in that regard. More recently, however, the Region has not been left untouched by the global movement that has come to realize the importance of health personnel, as is clear from the growing concern of governments and the place occupied by the issue on the agendas of their meetings and in their commitments (22, 23). At the same time, the close relationship between the availability of health workers and the health status of the population is beginning to be recognized. When countries are grouped by the availability of human resources (low, medium, and high) it is apparent that mortality from certain causes declines as the number of human resources increases (Table 11).

An evaluation of the impact of the Family Health Program in Brazil in the period 1990–2002 indicates that the infant mortality rate dropped in those 12 years from 49.7 to 28.9 per 1,000 live births, as the program's coverage rose to 36%. The analyses suggest that, after controlling for the other health determinants, an increase of 10% in the coverage of the program was associated

TABLE 11. Selected mortality rates and coverage of deliveries in groups of countries by the availability of health human resources.

Human resources per 10,000 population	Maternal mortality rate per 100,000 live births	Infant mortality rate per 1,000 live births	Mortality rate in children under 5 years per 1,000 live births	Deliveries (attended by qualified personnel)
< 25	148	31	43	74%
25 to 50	65	22	25	95%
> 50	9	7	8	99%

Source: Pan American Health Organization. Basic Indicators. PAHO 2005.

with a drop of 4.5% in infant mortality (*24*), a figure that is similar to the one obtained in a study conducted for the JLI, which found that an increase of 10% in health human resources leads to a drop of between 2% and 5% in maternal, infant, and under-5 child mortality.

In this context, in 2005 the Seventh Regional Meeting of the Observatories of Human Resources in Health was held in Toronto, Canada, attended by 28 countries and many cooperation agencies. During the event, the Toronto Call to Action was drafted which was intended "to mobilize institutional actors, both national and international, of the health sector and other relevant sectors and civil society, to collectively strengthen the human resources in health through both policies and interventions, in order to achieve the Millennium Development Goals and according to the national health priorities to provide access to quality health services for all the peoples of the Americas by the year 2015" (*25*). Five key challenges were identified at the meeting:

1. Define long-range policies and plans to better adapt the workforce so it will be prepared to meet expected changes in the health systems and to better develop the institutional capacity for defining those policies and revising them periodically.
2. Place the right people in the right places to achieve an equitable distribution of health workers in the different regions so that they match the specific health needs of the population.
3. Regulate the displacements of health workers to ensure access to health care for all the population.
4. Create ties between health workers and health organizations that result in a commitment to the institutional mission to guarantee quality health services for the entire population.
5. Develop mechanisms for cooperation between training institutions (universities and schools) and health services institutions so that the education of health workers can be adapted to a universal and equitable model for providing quality care to meet the health needs of the population.

A survey conducted in 28 countries of the Region in 2005 (*26*) asked about the status of the five challenges in each of them and found that more progress was necessary. The following sections review the situation in the Region with respect to those challenges, in both their qualitative and quantitative aspects.

Long-Range Policies and Plans to Better Adapt the Workforce to Health Requirements and Develop the Institutional Capacity to Put Them into Practice

Human Resource Planning Processes and Their Characteristics

The production and use of information on human resources varies from country to country. In the period under considera-

tion, the availability and use of information for decisionmaking has improved in many countries in the Region, but it is also true that limitations in both these aspects persist in many others. In the survey mentioned earlier, 75% of the 28 countries admitted that they did not have sufficient information about health workers, their occupations, and skills. Some countries make great efforts to know the number of physicians and nurses they have and in general they obtain information from preexisting databanks (population censuses, records of professional colleges, etc.) but there are few which, like Brazil, obtain original information intended to respond to specific problems.

Notwithstanding, information on health human resources has been improving in many countries. In the Dominican Republic, Guatemala, and Costa Rica, information systems are being organized on the health workforce, while others, such as Bahamas, Canada, Colombia, Cuba, Jamaica, Mexico, Suriname, and Trinidad and Tobago, have relatively stronger information systems on health human resources.

Institutionalization of National Management of Human Resource Development

The institutional complexity of the field of human resources has led to the creation of collective bodies for discussion, negotiation, and coordinated decisionmaking in a growing number of countries. Many others have also promoted institutionalization of the capacity to lead the national development of health human resources. Some, such as Brazil, Chile, Cuba, Peru, and Honduras, have human resource directorates or similar bodies, whose functions include guidance and support for sector development of health human resources. Others have bolstered the capacity of their health ministries or departments to lead national processes to develop those resources. For example, Guatemala established a unit in charge of human resource development in the Ministry of Public Health and Social Welfare (MSPAS); in Brazil, the Department of Health Employment and Education Management carries out functions involving information, planning, investigation, regulation, and advisory services on human resources. Peru, with the creation of the Human Resources Development Administration, and Chile, with its Human Resources Management Division, have strengthened the administrative units responsible for sector development of health human resources.

Notwithstanding, of the 28 countries consulted in 2005 about the capacity of the directorates or agencies of the ministries or departments of health responsible for compiling information, planning, and proposing human resource policies, 23 responded that there are major weaknesses in this field (*26*).

Regulation of Professional Practice by Health Human Resources

The regulation of professional practice differs from country to country, but in general the subject is gaining in importance. In most countries, this responsibility lies with the professional colleges, while the health authorities remain relatively in the background. In Costa Rica, only the colleges of physicians, dentists, and pharmacists have a professional recertification system. In the Dominican Republic, regulations have recently been drafted on professional certification and recertification. Other countries are implementing periodic recertification processes. In the Bahamas, for example, the Health Professions Council requires that professional licenses be renewed annually. In Bolivia, a professional recertification process has been developed based on accreditation of the certificates obtained. The Nursing Council of Jamaica has established a biannual registration system. In Mexico, the medical specialty councils certify and recertify professionals in their respective specialties. In Canada, the authorities in each province and territory define most of the regulatory mechanisms. And in Peru, professional recertification has only been implemented for the medical profession and efforts are being made to establish similar mechanisms for the colleges of nursing, midwifery, and dentistry.

Subregional efforts in the field of regulating professional practice include initiatives to establish agreements for reciprocal recognition of diplomas for teaching purposes and for the pursuit of postgraduate studies in the universities of the MERCOSUR member countries.

Placing the Right People in the Right Places to Achieve an Equitable Distribution of Health Personnel

Availability of Health Personnel

The Region has 1,872,000 physicians and 3,580,000 nurses, for an average of 22 and 42 per 10,000 population respectively. Recently (2000–2004) these rates have increased at an annual pace of 0.15 for physicians and 0.20 for nurses.

Positive growth of health human resources is being maintained but the increase is tending to be smaller. In the period 1980–1992, annual average growth in the number of health professionals throughout the Region was 5.8% for physicians and 8.2% for nurses, with the figures falling in 1992–2000 to 3.7% and 2.7%, respectively. In the period 2000–2004, the trend became more marked, with annual average growth of 1% in the number of physicians and of 0.8% for nurses. These values also indicate that the drop in the number of nurses is considerably larger than for physicians.

Many countries in the Region do not have the necessary personnel to achieve minimum levels of health services coverage.[8] In contrast, another group of countries has five times more personnel available. The average density of health professionals per person in the groups of countries with low, medium, and high in-

dexes is 18.4, 27.7, and 122.6 (human resources per 10,000 population), respectively.[9] It should be noted that as long as the rate for health professionals in the group of countries with low indexes (18.4) is below the minimum parameter proposed by WHO (25 professionals per 10,000 population), the goal of having 80% of childbirths attended by professionals will not be attained.

The 15 countries with the lowest health personnel density contain 19% of the Region's population and have 10% of the physicians and 3% of the nurses, while the 11 countries with the highest density have 40% of the population and 52% of the physicians and 90% of the nurses. When the situation of these groups of countries in the year 2000 is compared with 2004, the concentration of health personnel can be seen to rise. In the former year, the countries with the most health personnel had 73% of the Region's physicians and nurses, while they now have 77%.

The total density of health personnel (physicians plus nurses per 10,000 population) in the countries with higher density was 122.6, which represents a moderate increase since 2000 (120.1). The group with medium density has a health personnel rate of 27.7 (similar to the rate in 2000). In the countries with lowest density, the availability of human resources increased in the period 2000–2004 from 13.3 to 18.4 per 10,000 population, while infant mortality fell from 34.0 to 31.4 and mortality among children under 5 fell from 51.6 to 42.6 deaths per 1,000 live births.

The health personnel rate of several of the countries in the group with lowest availability is significantly below the minimum density required to achieve basic coverage: Haiti (3.6), Paraguay (9.1), Bolivia (10.8), Guyana (11.2), Honduras (11.9), and Guatemala (13.3). To achieve the minimum rate, the countries in question will require 124,000 physicians and nurses— with Haiti needing 18,000, Guatemala 14,500, Bolivia 12,000, Paraguay 9,500, and Honduras 8,500.

In the period 2000–2004 significant increases were reported in health personnel in some countries: Bolivia increased its rate by 120%, Nicaragua by 88%, Paraguay by 44%, Costa Rica by 25%, and Colombia by 24%; but in other countries the rates fell: Saint Vincent and the Grenadines by 18%, Belize by 15%, and Guatemala by 13%.

Particular mention should be made of Cuba, which provides training for health human resources, particularly physicians, and accepts students from other countries. To date, 8,222 students from 24 countries, 20 of which belong to the Region, are enrolled in the Latin American School of Medicine (ELAM) in Havana. In 2005, ELAM graduated the first generation, composed of 1,372 physicians from the Region. Also, the Santiago de Cuba School is

---

[8]To calculate the number of physicians and nurses for a given population, WHO and the JLI have proposed using a measurement known as "health human resources density" which consists of the sum of these two categories for all the countries per 10,000 population. The measurement thus obtained is imperfect because it does not consider any of the other health workers, but it is the only viable measurement for making global comparisons.

[9]To analyze the availability of health personnel, the countries were grouped according to the density of human resources, into three categories: (1) countries with a rate exceeding 50 per 10,000; (2) countries with a rate between 25 and 50; and (3) countries with a rate under 25, in accordance with WHO's World Health Report 2006, which indicates that a density of 25 professionals per 10,000 population is needed to assure a minimum level of coverage (defined as 80% of childbirths attended by trained health personnel).

currently training 726 students from three countries, including Haiti, a country that has 128 recent graduates.

With regard to the MDGs, it is interesting to note that if the rate of growth in human resources in the period 2000–2004 does not pick up, some countries will not achieve the requisite goal of 25 health professionals per 10,000 population by 2015. Paraguay will need 32 years, Bolivia 15, Colombia 11, and Ecuador 9, and in all cases, that period extends beyond 2015. The situation of countries with negative human resources growth, such as Belize and Guatemala, is even more serious (it was not possible to determine the growth rate in some countries, for instance Guyana, Haiti, and Honduras, owing to the lack of information).

The lack of trained human resources is a problem that extends beyond the complex and lengthy process of training health professionals, and the countries with the largest health personnel needs have great difficulty in creating and financing positions that can attract and keep those professionals in the places where they are needed most.

Health Personnel Composition

The Region as a whole has 21.8 physicians per 10,000 population, which is an increase of just 0.6 over 2000. Cuba is the leading country in the Region with regard to the availability of physicians per person at approximately 60 per 10,000, a figure that rank it second in the world for this indicator. The rates of physicians per person in Uruguay and Argentina are also among the highest in the Region (over 30 per 10,000 population). At the other extreme, Haiti and Guyana have rates of 2.5 and 2.6 physicians per 10,000 population.

Trends in the rates for physicians per capita varied enormously throughout the Region, from a reduction of 11% in Guatemala, to an increase of 165% in Nicaragua and 130% in Bolivia. The rate of nurses per capita for the Region as a whole is 41.7 per 10,000, which is almost double the rate for physicians; however, growth is tending to slow rapidly. Trends in the rate for nurses per capita differed from country to country. In Costa Rica the rate rose by 178%, and in Bolivia by 100%, while it fell in Nicaragua by 58%, in Belize by 24%, and in Guatemala by 12%.

The rate of nurses per capita was high in the United States (97.2 per 10,000 population), in Bermuda (89.6 per 10,000), and in Canada (73.4 per 10,000); with nurses outnumbering physicians in a ratio of 3 to 1 in the United States, Canada, and some of the English-speaking Caribbean countries. Physicians outnumber nurses in a ratio of 5 to 1 in the MERCOSUR countries. The concentration of nursing personnel in the Region is clear when we consider that in 2004, 83% of nurses worked in the United States or Canada.

Data from population surveys and censuses conducted in 13 countries of the Region (Belize, Bolivia, Costa Rica, Chile, Dominican Republic, Ecuador, El Salvador, Honduras, Mexico, Nicaragua, Panama, Trinidad and Tobago, and Venezuela), which have a total of 2.4 million health workers, indicate that the percentage of women lies between 65% and 70%. Different docu-

ments stress that the numerical importance of women in the health sector reveals gender inequities, since senior positions are mainly held by men, in both public and private institutions.

Public Budgets for Human Resources

Expenditures for salaries and other outlays related to health personnel are one of the largest items in the Region's health budgets. Budget constraints and lack of financial leeway, given that the budgets of the public health institutions are financed by the ministries of the economy, affect many countries. The 2005 consultation showed that in 64% of the countries, the budget of public health institutions is not sufficient to cover the population's main needs. Health budgets make it impossible to plan adequately for demographic and epidemiological needs, with the required numbers and types of personnel. Furthermore, 75% of the countries consulted in 2005 estimate that the planning and preparation of the budgets for public health institutions is inadequate and does not allow them to have sufficient workers in the more remote and poorer areas (*26*).

Health institutions and authorities have relatively weak capacity to negotiate budget allocations. Part of these difficulties stem from the existing limitations on obtaining and processing reliable information that links spending on services to outcomes in terms of the population's health. There are some exceptions: Canada, where each jurisdiction has the power to adjust health personnel in function of needs; Cuba, where the budget is tailored to requirements; Brazil, where the Family Health Program transfers specific resources to relocate professionals in primary care services; and Chile, where recent legislative reforms have led to greater flexibility in the staffing of health services.

Displacement of Health Workers

Distribution of Health Personnel

The shortage of health workers in some countries is aggravated by the tendency of professionals to live in urban areas, which restricts the already limited access to services by the rural population. Only nine of the 28 countries of the Region reported being satisfied with the information available on the distribution of health personnel in relation to the population. At the same time, 82% of the countries acknowledged weaknesses in the adoption of policies and implementation of plans to mobilize and attract health workers to the regions where they are most badly needed (*26*).

There are marked differences in the urban-rural distribution of health human resources. Generally speaking, there are 1.5 to 4 times more physicians available in urban zones than the national average and 8 to 10 times more than in rural zones (Table 12).

In most of the countries for which information is available on the concentration of health personnel, the proportion of physicians and nurses available in the areas with highest and lowest concentrations is less than 10 to 1, while in other countries (Ar-

TABLE 12. Rates of physicians and nurses per 10,000 inhabitants in provinces and departments of high and low distribution in selected countries of the Americas, 2000–2005.

	Year	Physicians			Nurses		
		High	Low	Ratio	High	Low	Ratio
Argentina	2000	105.0	10.4	10/1	7.2	0.3	24/1
Bolivia	2001	5.3	1.3	4/1	4.6	0.8	6/1
Colombia	2000	14.7	6.0	2/1	4.3	1.9	2/1
Ecuador	2001	24.4	5.7	4/1	9.2	1.5	6/1
Guatemala	2004	30.5	4.5	7/1	n/d	n/d	n/d
Nicaragua	2003	15.0	0.6	25/1	11.0	0.7	16/1
Panama	2005	7.4	0.6	12/1	n/d	n/d	n/d
Paraguay	2003	19.6	1.2	16/1	n/d	n/d	n/d
Peru	2003	17.7	3.3	5/1	14.5	2.9	5/1

Sources: Pan American Health Organization. Human Resources Unit.
Merino, C. Datos básicos sobre formación y distribución de personal de salud. Ecuador 1981–2001.
Peru, Ministerio de Salud, Instituto de Desarrollo de Recursos Humanos. Situación y desafío de los recursos humanos en salud. Lima: IDREH; OPS/OMS; 2005.
Bolivia, Ministerio de Salud. Indicadores de recursos humanos de 2001.
Guatemala, Ministerio de Salud, Inventario de recursos humanos. Informes nacionales, 2005.
Panama, Ministerio de Salud. Inventario de recursos humanos del sector público en salud. Available at: http://www.observatoriorh.org.

gentina, Nicaragua, Panama, and Paraguay) the difference between areas is higher. There is a large contrast between Nicaragua, where some parts of the country have 25 times more physicians and 16 times more nurses than others, and Colombia, which presents the greatest homogeneity in the distribution of health personnel.

Migration of Health Personnel

The migration of health human resources is a highly complex phenomenon, whose visibility grows as health personnel migrate within a country and between countries. This phenomenon is related to market failures in the countries of origin and tends to siphon off younger and more qualified personnel who can join the receiving labor market more easily.

There are two arrangements under which professionals work outside their country of origin: (a) permanent migration, particularly of nurses from the Caribbean to the developed countries, mainly the United States and Canada; and (b) temporary migration of physicians and other health workers from Cuba to different parts of the Region.

In some countries, health personnel migration makes a significant contribution to the health workforce. In Venezuela, the Barrio Adentro Program uses more than 25,000 Cuban cooperants in the field of health. In Chile, migration of health personnel from Ecuador, Peru, and Colombia contributes contingents of professionals to municipal primary care services. Some Caribbean countries, such as Haiti and Saint Lucia, have significantly increased the availability of physicians with the return of students who received their medical training in Cuba.

A study conducted in the United States, the United Kingdom, Canada, and Australia (*27*) indicates that between 25% and 28% of the physicians who practice in those countries graduated elsewhere, and between 40% and 75% of those professionals come from low-income countries. Physicians from the Americas practicing in the four countries studied included 1,589 Jamaican physicians (70% of those practicing in their own country), 1,067 Haitians (55%), 3,262 Dominicans (21%), and variable figures for Peruvian, Bolivian, Guatemalan, Panamanian, Costa Rican, and Colombian physicians, who represent between 4% and 5% of those who remain in their own countries. The case of Haiti is eloquent, because although it has the fewest physicians per capita in the Region, 55% of its doctors have emigrated to one or another of the four countries in question—not even counting other possible destinations. The study omitted countries with fewer than 1,000 physicians, which is why the English-speaking Caribbean (except Jamaica) does not appear, a fact that is interesting if we consider that up to 35% of positions are vacant in some countries in that subregion.

The study in question notes that Canada and Mexico experience the largest emigration of health human resources, which is related to the proximity of both countries to the labor market of the United States, which currently has 170,000 nursing vacancies that are expected to grow to 260,000 by 2010 (this deficit corresponds to 90% of the nurses in Latin America and the Caribbean). Annual demand for residents in medical specialties in the United States is 6,000 higher than the number of physicians who graduate from its medical schools, and therefore the positions are covered by doctors from abroad, many of whom acquire permanent residency in the country (*28*).

To understand the process of migration of health personnel it is necessary to consider the influence of agencies that facilitate that migration and which are generally hired by the health services of the countries seeking foreign workers to recruit nurses or doctors who are willing to emigrate. Some training programs for physicians contribute indirectly to migration of their graduates, and

333

Migration of Health Workers in Peru and Ecuador

According to a study on the migration of health human resources in the Andean area, there are 16,000 Peruvian doctors and 17,000 Peruvian nurses working outside the country. According to the Immigration Directorate, émigré physicians grew in number from 1,060 in 1992 to 1,667 in 2004, while nurses held steady at 1,400. The destinations of Peruvian nurses are Italy, followed by the United States and Spain (Investigación de migración de los recursos humanos de salud en el Área Andina).

A study conducted in Ecuador suggested that 10% of health professionals who had graduated in the three previous years had left the country. More doctors emigrate than nurses, and men emigrate more frequently than women. More graduates of private universities leave the country (26% compared to 7%). The United States is the most frequent destination for young Ecuadoran professionals, followed by Mexico and Chile. Stable and well-paying work and good training opportunities are the prime factors that keep young professionals in a country (María Cristina Merino de Rojas. Migración de médicos y enfermeras recién graduados, en ciudades seleccionadas de Ecuador. Observatorio de Recursos Humanos en Salud, Ecuador. Available at www.opsecu.org/orhs-ecuador.)

---

there is evidence that some medical schools offer programs that are not aligned with national health problems or with available technologies, which leads to dissatisfaction with existing opportunities and is a factor that increases the emigration of health personnel.

Although many countries recognize that the migration of health personnel is a major problem, few efforts are being made to obtain better information about it. In the survey of 28 countries of the Region mentioned earlier, just three felt that they knew enough about trends in internal and external migration of the main health professionals (26).

International Agreements on Migration of Health Personnel

Just three of the 28 countries consulted report having signed international agreements regulating the most frequent movements of health professionals to or from the country (26).

Those countries, which belong to the Commonwealth, have reached an agreement to stop recruiting nurses from the other member countries, but at the same time, the English-speaking Caribbean countries need to recruit physicians from outside. MERCOSUR is moving toward regulating the migration of health professionals in that subregion.

Relationships between Health Workers and Health Institutions

Changes in the Nature of Employment and Contracting Systems

It has already been pointed out that data from population surveys and censuses in 13 countries of the Region with 2.4 million health workers indicate that women account for between 65% and 70%, but that senior positions in public and private institutions are mainly filled by men (29, 30). These studies note that in

2002, the general unemployment rate was 6.2%. In the countries considered, the percentage of women employed ranged from 49% to 70% in the public sector and from 64% to 76% in the private sector. The percentage of unemployed women was significantly higher than the percentage for men (31).

Holding more than one job is a widespread phenomenon and is linked to the increase in the number of part-time jobs and low wages, which force workers to obtain income from a variety of sources. In many countries of the Region a "dual" labor market has grown up that combines the better salaries and working conditions in the private sector with the better social security and other benefits in the public sector. Working at more than one job is more prevalent in Argentina, Brazil, Uruguay, and Peru, and less so in Chile, Panama, and El Salvador. In the case of Peru, a study found that 71% of physicians had two or more jobs. In Uruguay, according to studies conducted in the last 20 years, each doctor holds an average of 2.6 positions. Considerably fewer nurses work at more than one job, which is explained by the longer number of hours each works. In Uruguay, nurses held an average of 1.34 jobs, which is half the figure for physicians.

Diversity in Labor Systems

New technologies, a reduction in the length of hospital stays, and the increase in ambulatory services and home care have an impact on employment in the health sector, where the number of hospital posts tends to fall and the number of posts in the primary care system rises. Thus, in contrast with what happens in other areas, the overall health workforce continues to grow. The most salient effect of sector reforms has not been a reduction in health personnel but an increase in the flexibility of labor relations, through the adoption of alternative forms of subcontracting, often temporary, with private companies, nongovernmental organizations, workers' cooperatives, or other workers' associations (32).

Different Latin American and international studies and sources of information report deterioration in the labor situation of health workers in recent years (*33*). Labor markets in general and health labor markets in particular have seen growth in salaried and part time work, either because protection has been reduced, because what is made to look like autonomous work is really salaried work, or because labor relations are fleeting.

The tendency to reduce protection for health workers has sharpened in many countries (including Argentina, Brazil, and Peru). This reduction assumes the coexistence of different modes of contracting and therefore different protection for workers who perform similar tasks, which raises concerns about the possible effect on the quality of care.

Outsourcing or subcontracting in health initially focused on general services (cleaning, meals, maintenance, and security). Today, however, it includes professional services that are recruited under contracts with medical cooperatives, home-care nurse organizations, rehabilitation services, and others. A study in Brazil indicated that 49% of labor in hospitals with 150 to 300 beds was subcontracted, and the figure for hospitals with more than 300 beds was 38% (*34*). The budget for contracting out in the Costa Rican Social Security Fund has increased year after year for just under a decade.

The deterioration in working conditions, which takes the form of longer working hours, an increase in the intensity of work, or the breakup of health teams, constitutes a set of problems that affect health management and hamper the attainment of institutional objectives. Deterioration in working conditions has an impact on workers, turning occupational health into a real concern for health authorities in many countries of the Region.

Given that the greater flexibility in labor relations has not brought the expected benefits and is creating unforeseen difficulties, many countries are beginning to develop policies to reverse temporary employment in the field of health. In Peru, where there was strong growth in the number of fixed-term contracts for non-personal services (a labor sector that grew by 430% in eight years), a large contingent of physicians and other health workers has recently been appointed permanently. In Brazil, as well, where a large part of the personnel recruited in the municipalities after implementing the Unified Health System (SUS) was hired on temporary contracts (*35*), policies are being applied to reverse this trend in labor conditions for health workers.

Decentralization in Health Human Resources Management

In the last decade, many countries began to decentralize health services management, which led to radical changes in personnel administration in the public sector. A survey administered in 18 countries of the Region showed that the delegation of powers for decentralized human resource management took place in 16 of them, with variations in the degree of decentralization, autonomy, or both (*36*). In general, these processes were not accompanied by strengthening regulatory capacity on the na-

tional level and did not always involve the transfer of financing or the enhancement of skills for decentralized human resource management. Brazil is an exception, since decentralization included transfers of financing and regulatory capacity was delegated, while the national level paid particular attention to health human resources policy formulation and planning.

Health Positions and Career Paths

Dissatisfaction is growing with the forms of labor relations in the health sector. Seventy-five percent of the countries of the Region consulted in 2005 consider that the systems used for contracting, incentives, and evaluation of health personnel do not promote identification by workers with the mission of providing good health services (*26*). Some of the Latin American and Caribbean countries are discussing regulations that would place labor relations in a more well-defined framework. Establishment of a health career path is being considered as a response to the lack of identification of health workers with their function and as a suitable tool for improving the quality of the labor relationship.

Differences persist in nomenclature and the content of the regulations governing public health personnel management. The phrase "health career path" is generally used, but there is also mention of human resource regulations or laws, a health personnel statute, a medical law or "plan of health positions and salaries." In some cases these regulations are exhaustive and in others they are generic; some are intended to be approved in a national law, while others take the form of internal statutes of the ministry of health that do not cover the entire sector (Table 13) (*33*).

Qualifications, Recruitment, and Careers of Health Managers

Many countries of the Region do not have health human resource management systems that are differentiated from the general systems applicable to public servants, which leads to serious problems since they do not reflect real working conditions in the

TABLE 13. The health career path in 19 countries of the Americas.

	Countries	Number
Exists	Brazil, Chile, and the Dominican Republic	3
Being regulated	Colombia	1
Under discussion	Bolivia, Ecuador, Nicaragua, Paraguay, and Uruguay	5
None	Argentina, Costa Rica, El Salvador, Guatemala, Haiti, Honduras, Mexico, Panama, Peru, and Venezuela	10
Total		19

Source: Pan American Health Organization. Human Resources Program.

" *The future of health in the Americas rests on the full development of adequate health services in each country and not on any international agency.* "

Fred Lowe Soper, 1954

field of health. The decentralization processes carried out, the need to reduce costs in an increasingly complex and costly technological structure, and the changes in the make-up of personnel, on the one hand, and sharpening labor conflicts on the other, pose new challenges for the management of health human resources.

Of the countries consulted in 2005, 65% consider that the systems for manager selection and training do not facilitate development of the skills of management teams and do not encourage workers to provide good health services (*37*). However, in the period under consideration some countries have improved the process of selecting service directors and almost all have provided training for health managers. Chile introduced a system to select senior public managers through public competitions and stepped up efforts to establish health management teams. Mexico introduced a career professional service which involves competitions for managers and the establishment of a series of training strategies intended to develop managerial skills in health services.

Management and Regulation of Health Personnel Conflicts

During 2004, labor conflicts in the health sector took the form of 64 national strikes in 10 countries for an increase of 73% in labor conflicts over the previous year. The strikes were called by 31 organizations (12 workers' organizations, 10 physicians' organizations, six nurses' and midwives' organizations, and three organizations of other health professionals). Of all the strikes occurring in the Region, 56% took place in three countries, and the principal demand of 81% of them was an increase in salaries and health sector budgets (*38*).

In some countries the right to strike is regulated differently for public services that are essential for the community, including health care, with a view to guaranteeing the inalienable right of citizens to those services. Regulations attempt to make the general interest compatible with workers' interests, guaranteeing the maintenance of services, and therefore they establish restrictions or limitations on the right to strike.

Training for Health Workers

Reforms in the countries of the Region highlighted the need to have suitable personnel to implement them. The demand for new skills and the modification of the occupational profiles of large groups of health workers led to large-scale training programs and the adoption of new management styles for educational programs and projects. This created an active training market.

An evaluation of 15 training projects carried out in eight countries of the Region (*39*) showed that the sums earmarked to provide training for health personnel differed by country. National projects cost between US$ 700,000 and US$ 350 million, with the educational component representing between 2.8% and 6.5% of the project total. An evaluation of those components shows that although they improved the skills and abilities of health personnel and led to favorable changes in services, they did not contribute to the development of human resource policies. The projects did not improve institutional capacity for managing human resource development, nor did they remedy the phenomena of temporary work or the high mobility of sector workers. Investments in health personnel training, which had been significant in the previous decade in nearly all the countries of the Region, have fallen recently.

Interaction between Professional Training Institutions and Health Services

Programs and Experiences with In-Service Education

There are many experiences in the Region that reflect the interrelations between the institutions that train health professionals and the health services and ministries or departments of health. These interactions have increased recently and have continued to become consolidated. Chile established the National Health Teaching Committee (CONDAS), and in Brazil consolidation of the Human Resources Observatory network made room for cooperation between the managers of the Unified Health System (SUS) and the academic world. Good progress was also made in Bolivia, Costa Rica, Ecuador, Guatemala, Mexico, and Paraguay. Cuba is a special case, since the process of training health personnel is carried out inside the health services, which function simultaneously as professional training centers.

Reforms to study plans geared to primary health care. Most countries of the Region have a supply of professional training but the profiles of graduates differ significantly from health services demand and population needs, which is aggravated by the weakness of the mechanisms required to keep health personnel permanently up to date. Despite unanimous agreement on the importance of establishing systems based on primary health care, there is a relative shortage of professionals trained in family health. The contents of the basic study plans for health professionals and technicians do not emphasize primary care, although it occupies a prominent place in training for nurses.

The different proportions of physicians and nurses in the countries of the Region reflect different strategies to address health problems, with physicians generally being the dominant group. However, there are significant experiences in training primary level health teams, such as those in Cuba, where the doctor and the nurse form the basic professional team. There are undergraduate, professional, and specialized professional services in Bolivia, Costa Rica, Ecuador, El Salvador, Guatemala, Honduras, Mexico, Nicaragua, Panama, Peru, and Venezuela, where doctors, nurses, midwives, and dentists are assigned to provide health care in rural and marginal urban areas, and Brazil has the Family Health Program, whose teams are composed of physicians, nurses, and community health agents (*40*).

Regulations for refocusing training on primary health care. Greater flexibility in training for health professionals has led to the proliferation of private centers which, combined with the absence or weakness of regulatory mechanisms to guarantee the quality of training, means that graduates do not always have the skills necessary to exercise their profession. Of the countries consulted, 90% consider that the government's general regulation of educational content is inadequate and that incentives to promote the design of training plans for health professionals tailored to national realities are insufficient (*26*).

Recently progress has been made in the Region in educational regulation. For example, Colombia issued a decree to guarantee the quality of professional training; Peru established requisites for compulsory undergraduate training for faculties or schools of medicine; and accreditation processes are being developed in Bolivia for several careers in the public system. The Central American System for Accrediting Academic Programs led by the Central American Higher University Council (CSUCA) stands out as a subregional initiative in the field of health education regulation.

FUNCTIONS OF HEALTH SYSTEMS: TRENDS AND CURRENT SITUATION

The Health Sector and the Health System

The health sector is defined as a set of values, standards, and institutions, and the players who produce, distribute, and consume health goods and services, whose main objectives are to promote the health of individuals or population groups. It is assumed that the activities performed by these players and institutions are targeted to disease prevention and control, the delivery of personal and non-personal health services to the population, scientific research on health, training for health care personnel, and the dissemination of information to the public at large.

This definition fits into a conceptual framework that includes: (1) the concept of health adopted by WHO in its 1946 Constitution as "a state of complete physical, mental, and social well-being, and not merely the absence of disease or infirmity," including their determining and conditioning factors; (2) recognition that each country organizes its own health system; (3) relations between the health sector and other social and economic sectors; (4) a dynamic vision of the sector that takes ac-

count of changes in institutions and their members and in the economic context in which they carry out their activities, and their set of values, knowledge, skills, organization, resources, technologies, interests, and power imbalances; and (5) the functional analysis of the system of health services and the implications for action. Therefore, the health sector covers all actions that contribute to better health, including health-related economic and productive activities (*41*).

Health systems have been described in different ways. Although it is essential to define their limits, it should be remembered that health systems act as mediators and coordinators, in a political, economic, and technical framework at a given historical time. Consequently, the definition, limits, and objectives of a health system are specific to each country, reflecting its own values and principles.

PAHO describes three notions of what a health system comprises.[10] In the narrowest sense, a health system is limited to carrying out the activities under the direct control of the ministry of health, which therefore excludes many other public or private initiatives taken outside that institution. In some countries, the above includes traditional public health activities and the partial supply of personal medical services, but does not include all the interventions necessary to improve health and can even exclude the personal medical services provided by other government institutions, nongovernmental organizations, or the private sector. The second notion of the health system covers individual medical services and health services directed to the collectivity, but does not include intersectoral actions to improve health. Accordingly, it would consider traditional public health interventions, such as the dissemination of health information, to be part of the health system, but not intersectoral activities of an environmental nature, such as sanitation and drinking water supplies. The third definition considers all measures whose main purpose is to improve health status, including intersectoral actions such as the establishment of regulations to reduce deaths caused by traffic accidents.

More recently, WHO defined the health system as comprising all the organizations, individuals, and actions whose prime purpose is to improve, maintain, or restore health. This covers actions to influence the health determinants and to improve the health situation. Under WHO's definition, in addition to health establishments, home health care, private suppliers, campaigns to control disease vectors, health insurers, etc., the health system also extends to actions that affect health performed by other sectors (*42*).

---

[10]Based on PAHO/WHO: Critical issues in health systems performance assessment (general information document), Washington, D.C., 2001; Health systems performance assessment and improvement in the Region of the Americas. PAHO/WHO: Washington D.C., 2001; and Reunión Consultiva Regional de las Américas sobre la evaluación del desempeño de los sistemas de salud. Revista Panamericana de Salud Pública 2001; 10 (1).

The selection of one or another of these definitions is directly linked to the concept of government responsibility for health. However, despite the different definitions of the health system and the health sector, it is clear that there has been a gradual fusion of the two concepts. Today, they both denote that the field of action in health requires nondelegable interventions by the government to act on the health determinants, including social, economic, and productive factors that have an impact on health outcomes, and the interventions agreed on by different sectors and agents to influence those outcomes.

Conceptual Differences in the Operational Scope of Health Systems

In recent years, the debate on conceptual and methodological approaches to analyzing and understanding health systems has intensified. Approaches have been taken that study systems by their financial and service-provision models, which can be either public or private, a classification that has contributed progressively to the debate. Another related approach focuses on supply and demand, and involves government participation.

One of the most important aspects of the discussion of the role of government in the health system centers on the definition of the functions of the health system, the powers that go with each function, and its relationship to the structure of the health system. The traditional taxonomy of national health systems was mainly based on the type of ownership that prevails in the system—public or private—and included the responsibility borne by each with respect to the financing and delivery of services. Today, owing to the growing complexity of health systems, differentiated relations have developed among the government, the public sector, financing/insurance schemes, and the private sector. Therefore, the old taxonomy is no longer useful and a new typology has been developed based on the functions of the health system (43), which makes it possible to analyze the health system in terms of its capacity to integrate the population or institutions. With regard to the population, integration refers to the level of access enjoyed by different groups to system institutions. Integration of institutions refers to the organizational and functional arrangements developed to effectively perform the functions of the health system.

Publication of the World Health Report 2000 (4) prompted a broad international discussion that focused on defining the central functions of health systems and evaluating their performance. The report suggested that the key functions of health systems include: service delivery, resource generation, financing (including collecting, pooling, and purchasing), and stewardship. The report argued as well that the fundamental objective of the functions of the proposed system was to achieve optimum levels of health and eliminate inequalities in access. The performance objectives or indicators include good health, responsiveness, and fair financial contribution. This position leads to the need to de-fine priorities and rationalize the distribution of essential public health services using cost-efficiency and social acceptance criteria. In this context, individuals are visualized as service providers, professionals, taxpayers, or consumers, but not as citizens entitled to receive social benefits in health care. Therefore, if that framework is used, it is necessary to spell out the responsibilities that governments will have in the field of health (44).

Based on an analysis of the processes of reform and reorganization of health systems under way in the countries of the Region, PAHO/WHO uses a classification that considers three basic functions of health systems: stewardship, financing/insurance, and the delivery of health services.

General Trends in Health Reforms in Latin America and the Caribbean That Have Influenced the Traditional Functions of Health Systems

Trends in Stewardship

Historically, in public subsystems and national health systems, the ministries of health have focused on regulatory functions and service delivery. However, health sector reforms strongly promoted decentralization of both the government and the health sector which, coupled with the rise of new public and private players in the sector, has led to a marked tendency to reduce traditional responsibilities related to the delivery of health services and increase activities in functions related to sector stewardship. Monitoring and evaluation of the sector reforms carried out in the Americas between 2000 and 2003 highlighted regional trends that have had direct repercussions on the capacity of countries to exercise stewardship over health (45–47).

As a product of the growing move toward separation of the functions of the health system, such as financing, insurance, and service delivery, the trends in reforms that have had the main repercussions include, first of all, segmentation, and second, fragmentation. Also, they have influenced the imbalances observed in decentralization processes and the rise of new public and private players in the health sector, marked by a gradual increase in the participation of private insurers. As a result, the countries of the Region seek to strengthen the stewardship role played by ministries of health in the sector and to consolidate leadership of the sector as a whole in order to have the necessary powers to act as health advocates and negotiate with other sectors that have an impact on health (48).

Trends in Financing and Insurance

Change in the composition of financing. In the Region there are wide variations in the composition (public/private mix) of health financing. It has already been mentioned that the countries with the highest public health expenditure as a percentage of GDP generally have national health insurance systems with universal or near universal coverage, reaching 64% in Bolivia,

78.8% in Costa Rica, 84.1% in Canada, and 86.8% in Cuba, according to the World Bank's 2006 World Development Report.

On average, private spending on health (the purchase of health goods and services) accounts for 52% of national expenditure on health in the countries of the Region.[11] As mentioned in the section on national expenditure on health, to a large extent, the increase in private expenditure on health reflects an increase in direct household spending and growth in private insurers and pre-paid medical plans, with the latter rising since the late 1980s and early 1990s to represent 27% of total private expenditure on health in 1995. Private expenditures have stabilized since then at that level, or approximately 1.2% of GDP.

A second factor that explains the increase in out-of-pocket spending are the shortfalls in the coverage provided by public systems. The poorest population quintiles have limited access to social security because many of them are agricultural or informal sector workers, and they also have limited access to public services per se. Some governments allocate most of their funds to the secondary and tertiary levels of care and to predominantly urban areas, which means that public subsidies can disproportionately favor the urban population and the wealthier quintiles.

Differences in the distribution of public expenditure. National expenditure on health care as a percentage of the national economy varies greatly. The wide differences suggest that although per capita income plays an important role in the percentage of GDP earmarked for health care, other factors could also be having a large impact. For example, the fact that countries spend relatively more or less of their GDP on health appears to be influenced more by national policy decisions regarding universal access and coverage and, to a lesser extent, by the way in which national health systems are organized and financed. For example, in countries with large numbers of poor and where out-of-pocket spending is the main means of financing health care, national expenditure tends to be low. The inverse ratio between the income levels of countries and the distributive impact of public spending on health—which is generally progressive in countries with higher income levels and regressive in countries with lower levels—has already been mentioned. This suggests that in this second group, health policies are either not directed to equity or are not duly monitored to ensure that the neediest population benefits.

Inequities are even greater when the differences in per capita expenditure per beneficiary in public insurance programs are compared. A positive redistributive effect was observed in countries where these costs represent 2.5% of GDP or more (Argen-

tina, Chile, Colombia, and Jamaica), while a negative redistributive effect was observed in countries where they represent about 1% of GDP or less (Ecuador and Guatemala). There is a great deal of room to improve the use of government financing and spending instruments to achieve greater equity in financing and access. Data presented in other sections of this chapter suggest that the governments of Latin America and the Caribbean, particularly the low-income countries, have the potential to make more effective use of existing fiscal instruments to address the challenges in health and equity.

Social health protection as a marginal issue. In recent years, private insurance and pre-paid plans have become important mechanisms for private health care financing in many of the countries of the Region. The rapid growth in the size of these items is the most important factor explaining the recent trends in national health expenditure.

The size of the markets for private insurance and pre-paid plans appears to have been determined by the relative importance of the public health services system, both with regard to the coverage and scope of services, and to the existence or absence of policies that favor the rise of these markets and regulate their operation. The presence of large national or transnational corporations also appears to be a relevant factor in explaining the different relative sizes of the private insurance and pre-paid health plans markets. In Peru, for example, the existence of large private employers who offer health benefits has contributed to the rise of insurance companies as well as to the increase in the supply of high-complexity private health services.

However, the lack of coverage of public health services does not appear to be sufficient for growth of the private health insurance market. In the case of Mexico, that market is relatively undeveloped despite the shortcomings in public health system coverage. On the other hand, even in countries with nearly universal social security systems, such as Argentina, Costa Rica, and Uruguay, large companies provide their employees with complementary health insurance to reduce waiting times in public services, provide access to "better quality care," or both.

The growing importance of private spending on health in the form of private insurance or pre-paid plans is transforming health care markets in the Region. This trend poses a large challenge for health policies, particularly with regard to the design of regulations to ensure efficiency in the operation of those markets and to address inequities in access to health care. Owing to the lack of adequate regulation or the limited enforcement of existing regulations, many people with private health insurance use health services that are subsidized by the government—for example, public hospitals, to keep their premiums low or reduce the cost of their policies. Private insurers can opt to include only a limited number of medical services in their benefits packages, on the assumption that the more costly procedures, which are also generally infrequent, will be subsidized by public hospitals.

---

[11] This calculation includes private consumer spending that may have been financed directly by households through out-of-pocket spending or indirectly through health insurance, prepaid plans, or transfers from other sectors of the economy.

Trends in Health Services Delivery

In the Region, health services continue to face large challenges (49). Access to health care is not universal, and in many cases it is virtually nonexistent for the social groups with the greatest need of it. The supply of health services does not always reflect the expectations, social values, and cultural preferences of the population. In many cases, the delivery of services is ineffective and technical quality is poor. Also, the resources available are not always used adequately, which leads to inefficiencies in the services and drives up costs. In some cases, financing of services is insufficient and unsustainable (41).

As a result of sector reforms or changes in health systems, new patterns of care have been introduced, and in countries where the insurance market is strong the supply of services is now better aligned with demand. In Chile, for example, services are geared to more comprehensive, family-based care, with stress on primary care at family health centers rather than at private physicians' offices, and training that seeks to increase the responsiveness of ambulatory services. In Mexico, the creation of the Seguro Popular de Salud has modified the care model of the Secretariat of Health by clarifying that user benefits are a right, while simultaneously subsidizing the cost of services, limiting patient contributions to a co-payment. In the United States, reforms have been recently made in the Medicare system to extend the benefits to cover medications, whose high cost is a major factor in national health expenditure and a substantial financial burden for pensioners.

Other countries are making changes to respond to different national priorities. Nicaragua, for example, has modified the delivery of services to reflect its epidemiological transition and, like other countries, it has made changes in the three levels of care. The first level has been modified to respond to vulnerable populations, placing stress on gender and geographic distribution, and defining criteria for targeting and exemptions from payment for services. In Brazil, ambulatory services and home care have been stepped up through a variety of strategies that range from modifying the basic care model to preparing plans for the regionalization of public services, joining the efforts that other countries have been making in these areas.

Several countries have given priority in health care to vulnerable groups. In Paraguay, for example, the management of service programs is being centralized in a General Programs Office in order to give priority to mother and child care and focus on rural and indigenous populations. Bolivia and Colombia have programs targeted to vulnerable groups, such as mothers and infants, children under 5, indigenous populations, the elderly, and groups at epidemiological risk. In Cuba, more effective and innovative services have been introduced, such as ambulatory surgery, shorter hospital convalescences, and monitoring through homecare. In Cuba and, to a lesser extent, in Central America, referral and counter-referral services have been enhanced, as has the assessment of services based on quantitative and qualitative indicators, which permits problems to be better identified and timely and proper decisions to be made. Most of the countries have expressed a commitment to providing good quality services suited to the needs of the public but problems often remain in allocating the necessary resources or organizing the services necessary to attain this goal.

With respect to the management model, many countries report that they have made general changes to it. In Panama, the main change has been active participation by the management council in the administration of San Miguel Arcángel General Hospital and the creation of a national health coordinator (CONSALUD), which is a private body of public interest constituted by the Ministry of Health and the Insurance Fund, to finance and purchase health care services from not-for-profit suppliers around the country. Cuba has experienced a sweeping transformation in its care model, which has served to strengthen the community level, promote exchanges of information, and step up the regulatory function of the Ministry of Public Health. This has improved control and implementation of programs in the provinces and provided the main players with the know-how to identify priority problems in the sector and design solutions.

Management commitments and contracts have been introduced between the different levels of the public health system in several countries. In Guatemala, the central Ministry of Health authorities and the regional managers have made a commitment to expand coverage and reduce the incidence of certain diseases. Management commitments have been signed in Nicaragua and Bolivia, and Bolivia has introduced them as part of its mother and child insurance. In 2000, some Bolivian districts began to sign agreements of this kind with autonomous hospitals, even though the regulatory framework for these mechanisms had not yet been defined.

Some countries are also taking steps to remove legislative obstacles to the purchase and sale of services by third parties. In Argentina, regulations to support the decentralization of hospitals have provided a legal framework for the purchase and sale of health services. This legislation permits hospitals to reach agreements with social security services and other entities, obtain payments from users with the ability to pay and from third-party payers, and operate as a services network. The Social Security Administration has begun a study to determine the feasibility of subcontracting certain support services out to third parties, such as meals and laundry. In Chile, the legal and institutional possibility also exists of buying from third parties and selling them services through the public system. In general, this applies to maintenance services and specialized institutions, and to jurisdictions administered by the social groups.

Despite the changes in management models described above, very few countries are considering privatizing public services. Argentina, for example, has found that decentralization of hospital management has provided hospital managers with greater administrative flexibility and allowed the local authorities to privatize some services. El Salvador and Guatemala have examined the possibility of having public services privately managed. On the other hand, Canada, Chile, Costa Rica, Cuba, Honduras, Nicaragua,

Paraguay, and Uruguay have not handed over the operation of any public service to the private sector. Among the changes being introduced, several countries have reported the establishment of procedures to accredit health services. El Salvador, for example, is reviewing accreditation requirements in centers of higher education in order to improve the quality of the professionals who are being trained. In 2000, the Dominican Republic established the National Quality Committee to standardize processes and create protocols to improve service delivery. Argentina has introduced new procedures for the authorization, accreditation, and classification of health services, professional certification and recertification, health control, and the supervision and evaluation of the quality of medical care and health services. However, it is difficult to evaluate how well those procedures are complied with, since the provinces are responsible for these functions. In the Andean subregion, Peru, Bolivia, and Colombia have institutionalized accreditation processes on different service levels.

In addition to defining procedures for accreditation and service delivery, several countries have reported the creation of programs in the ministries of health to improve quality. Trinidad and Tobago has established a Quality Management Directorate to organize a system that will help to improve the quality of care. The directorate includes a system for the accreditation of services on the primary and tertiary levels, and the development of a system of clinical audits. It has also begun to define a plan to bolster the evaluation of health technology and management capacity. In Honduras, the new health agenda includes initiatives related to technical quality and perceived quality. Costa Rica has incorporated similar initiatives that focus on user satisfaction.

Few countries have reported the establishment of programs to evaluate health technologies. In Colombia, the Office of Science and Technology Development of the Ministry of Health has improved its evaluation of technology, including standards for imported technology. In Cuba, the National Technology Evaluation Department was established in 1996 to determine the incidence and viability of health technology in existing systems and identify the equipment that needed to be incorporated. Other national bodies have also been established to evaluate and monitor health technology during the implementation phase.

As for decentralization, many countries of the Region have completed it while others are making progress in applying decentralization policies in the government in general and in health systems. However, health administrative structures continue to be highly centralized. In Guyana and Suriname, administrative levels are being reviewed prior to decentralizing health services, but these efforts are not necessarily linked to other decentralization initiatives in the public administration. Chile decentralized its National Health Service in 1980, dividing it into 26 services and transferring responsibilities for primary care to the municipalities, while the planning and management functions, responsibilities, and resources for decisionmaking remained on the central level. However, in many cases, decentralization of the health system is still incipient. Bolivia, for example, passed the Decentralization and Public Participation Law in 1994, which transferred health infrastructure and equipment from the central level to the municipalities, but, to date, the Ministry of Health continues to administer the sector's human resources.

In many countries, responsibilities, authority, and resources have been transferred to the subnational level, i.e. to regions, provinces, or departments, and in others they have been transferred to the municipal level. In Jamaica and Trinidad and Tobago, decentralization is being implemented by establishing regional health authorities, which manage the provision of health services, although the management of resources continues to be centralized. In Brazil, a new tool for regulating decentralization established an operating standard for health care, which expands the primary responsibilities of the municipalities, defines the process of regionalization of care, creates mechanisms to fortify the managerial capacity of the Unified Health System (SUS), and updates authorization criteria in the states and municipalities. Despite the existence of knowledge, methods, and instruments, activities for promotion, prevention, and recovery continue to suffer from lack of coordination in sector planning.

STEWARDSHIP FUNCTION

Conceptual and Methodological Development of the Stewardship Function, 2001–2005

One of the critical problems faced by the countries of the Region is institutional weakness, a factor that has repercussions on the real possibilities of economic development. In today's context, redefinition of institutional roles and strengthening of the functions of the state that cannot be delegated—such as citizen security, public health, and the social security of vulnerable or excluded groups—have become priorities. Consequently, the countries are attempting to build up and consolidate their capacity to supervise the health system and to have on hand the expertise to promote health and negotiate with other sectors that interact with the health system (48).

It has not been easy to arrive at an operational definition of stewardship in the field of health, since this concept often overlaps with the concept of governance. According to WHO, the government has the capacity and obligation to take responsibility for the health and well-being of its citizens and to direct the health system as a whole, and this governance responsibility should be exercised in three fundamental aspects: providing vision and direction for the health system, collecting and using intelligence, and exerting influence through regulation and other means. WHO also stresses that the degree of capacity and performance by the government in exercising governance over the health system will have a decisive effect on all outcomes (50, 51).

PAHO/WHO uses the phrase "stewardship of the health system" to refer to governance of the system. Accordingly, and in response to Resolution CD40.R12 (52) on stewardship by the ministries of health in sector reform processes, in the period

2001–2005 PAHO/WHO addressed the process of developing the concept and practice of health stewardship as a priority and an intrinsic aspect of the process of modernization of the State. An in-depth debate and exchange of ideas on the conceptualization, sphere of action, and mechanisms for strengthening stewardship capacity in health ensued.[12] Today, the stewardship function in health policy is considered to be the exercise of substantive responsibilities and competencies that are incumbent on the government and that cannot be delegated. That stewardship is exercised by the national health authority (50, 51, 53).

The Stewardship Function and Strengthening Health Systems

The main public depositaries of the health authority are the ministries of health and, in that capacity, they are the primary institutions responsible for exercising the stewardship function. A growing trend has been observed in the Region not to concentrate all tasks in a single institution as in the past, but to create diverse and complementary institutional mechanisms that carry out their different functions in a specialized fashion and with clearly differentiated powers.[13] Structural variations are apparent in the composition of the health authority, depending on whether the country is a federation or a unitary state and on the institutional organization of the health sector (5, 54). However, to consolidate the function of the health authority, its responsibilities and operations need to be restructured and adapted to the new realities which, in turn, will demand a shift from actions that fundamentally involve implementation to actions that are predominantly intended to organize and coordinate a host of actors (55).

Conceptual Framework of the Stewardship Function in Health

While aware that different taxonomies can be adopted regarding the stewardship function, PAHO defined six large areas of responsibility and institutional competencies, which cover the

dimensions of the stewardship function: leadership, regulation, insurance, financing, provision of services, and essential public health functions (Figure 2). Depending on the degree of decentralization in the sector and the separation of functions adopted in the institutional organization of each country, these dimensions will be located at a given level of the health authority (national, subnational, or local) and sometimes responsibilities will be shared by two or more levels.

Effective Health Leadership

Sector leadership constitutes one of the three dimensions of the stewardship function that is the exclusive responsibility of the national health authority (41). Leadership is more relevant when the objectives require significant changes in the existing situation (56). In such cases, the strategies will generate power shares that mobilize the support required to bring them about and increase operating capacity. The health authority will need to develop or build up its capacity to effectively guide sector institutions and mobilize institutions and social groups to support national health policy through: (1) an analysis of the health situation, including the definition of priorities and objectives; (2) the formulation, dissemination, monitoring, and evaluation of health policies, plans, and strategies; (3) the mobilization of players and resources; (4) health promotion and social participation and control in health; (5) the harmonization of international technical cooperation; (6) political and technical participation in national and subregional organizations; and (7) the evaluation of health system performance, including measurement of the goals achieved and the resources used.

In this context, the countries of the Region that exhibit good leadership share some common attributes (57), among them: (1) political support, which is fundamental for effective leadership; (2) the availability of reliable and timely information, which is indispensable for establishing health priorities and objectives; (3) the formulation of health policies and strategies, which should be complemented by their evaluation; (4) awareness-raising among sector players regarding the importance of the leadership function, which facilitates the consolidation of the health authority as lead agency; (5) mobilization of interested players and participation by civil society in health promotion, which are often the keys to success; and (6) participation of the health authority in negotiation, coordination, and evaluation processes with donor agencies to assure that international cooperation in health is effective, responds to the needs identified, and proves sustainable.

Effective Health Regulation and Supervision

Regulation and supervision are necessary to guarantee the government function of organizing relations in the production and distribution of health resources, goods, and services. For a health ministry or department to fully exercise its regulatory function, it must enjoy political and social representativeness,

---

[12] See Pan American Health Organization. Informe Final. Reunión de expertos: desarrollo de la capacidad institucional de la autoridad sanitaria para ejercer la rectoría sectorial. Washington DC 18–20 junio 2001, and Informe Final. Reunión de expertos en rectoría del sector salud en procesos de reforma. Washington DC 14–15 June 2004. Pan American Health Organization. Marco conceptual e instrumento metodológico: función rectora de la autoridad sanitaria nacional: desempeño y fortalecimiento. Edición Especial No. 17: Washington DC: OPS, 2006. http://www.lachealthsys.org/documents/433-funcionrectoradelaautoridadsanitarianacionaldesempenoyfortalecimiento-ES.pdf

[13] At the 40th Meeting of the PAHO Directing Council (1997), the Member States discussed and ratified the dimensions of sector stewardship in health, which include six large areas of institutional responsibility and competencies that are incumbent on the health authority: steering, regulation, insurance, financing, provision of services, and essential public health functions. PAHO/WHO, 40th Directing Council of the Pan American Health Organization, Resolution CD40.R12: Steering role of the ministries of health in the processes of the health sector reform, 1997.

FIGURE 2. Functions of the stewardship role.

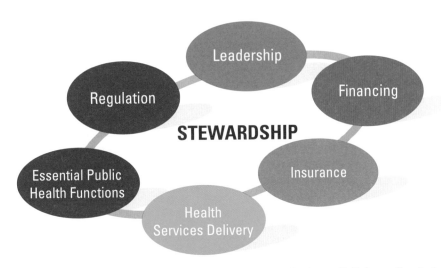

Source: Pan American Health Organization; United States Agency for International Development. Health Systems Strengthening in Latin America and the Caribbean.

solvency, and technical authority, and perform its tasks transparently, subject to scrutiny of its decisions by society (*57*). Regulation in the broadest sense is a tool for supervision that the government uses in combination with other tools to achieve its political objectives and, as a principle, rule, or other type of norm, it conditions and governs the behavior of citizens and of organizations or institutions.

Supervision and control are fundamentally technical activities that are intended to verify concrete compliance with the regulations and require professional specialization and arms-length dealings with the bodies that are supervised. Exercise of supervision is heavily dependent on human and technical resources and the powers that the law confers on the institutions that are called on to perform it. Supervision that translates into the application of sanctions should be subject to review by the courts to guarantee due process and prevent abuses or capricious behavior by the supervisor (*58*). The countries of the Region that exhibit good regulation share some common attributes: (1) the legal framework that supports the health authority in its functions is consistent with the governance it wishes to exercise over the sector as lead agency; (2) the normative function complements supervision; and (3) the professionals who carry out the supervisory function are duly trained for that task (*57*).

Financing Function

The separation of functions that is typical of sector reform in the Region is based on three main financing mechanisms. The first is the creation of autonomous national funds, separate from the ministries of health, that pool public contributions from general taxes, from specific health services institutions, where they

exist, and from employee and employer contributions in the event that the contributive social security regimes in health are merged with general government health allocations. This can be linked to a public insurance plan or to multiple insurance plans that may be public or private. The second mechanism is related to an increase in the percentage of public financing collected by the intermediate and local levels of government from their own taxes or transfers for health activities from the central government. The third is related to a growing share in the composition of overall sector financing in some countries of the Region of private health insurance and certain types of pre-paid services that are funded directly by the beneficiaries, their employers, or both, and that, as a minimum, complement mandatory government plans. Combining these three financing mechanisms in countries that have made attempts to surmount the segmentation of insurance and service delivery caused by differentiated financing mechanisms represents new challenges and duties for the ministries of health in managing sector financing (*41*).

Insurance Function

With regard to insurance, governments have the responsibility of effectively overseeing social protection of health, guaranteeing access to a basic health services plan for all citizens, or through specific plans targeted to special population groups. This demands stronger institutional capacity in the ministries or departments of health to define the content of the basic benefits plans that it is mandatory to offer persons covered by the publicly operated social security system(s). It is also necessary to define the population groups and territories that will be covered by the set of benefits and to protect the rights of users and publicize them. Last, public and private compliance with the services must be regulated and controlled to ensure that no beneficiary of mandatory social health plans is excluded on account of risks related to age or preexisting pathology. Mechanisms must also exist for purchasing or delivering the services included in guaranteed-coverage plans.

Health Services Delivery Function

The trends toward decentralization and a reduction in government intervention in the provision of health services through different mechanisms that enable participation by many social players (public, autonomous, private, and nongovernmental solidarity organizations) have a practical influence on harmonization of the provision of public health services. This has turned the ministries or departments of health more into coordinators of the management and delivery of services by public institutions than direct administrators of services. The function of harmonizing the provision of health services is therefore particularly important in systems in which many public and private players exist, whose activities must be channeled for the purpose of achieving common goals. That function means that the health authority must have the capacity to promote complementarity among different providers and user groups to extend health care coverage in an equitable and efficient manner.

Actions to Strengthen the Stewardship Function in Latin America and the Caribbean

Building Capacity to Regulate and Oversee the Pharmaceutical Sector: The Case of Brazil

Brazil is the first developing country that has implemented a national program to distribute antiretroviral medicines. The program is supported by the country's general policy on drugs, which proposes to "ensure public access to safe, effective, and good quality medicines at the lowest possible cost" (57). The national health authority carries out two types of drug regulation: technical and financial. Technical regulation introduces health standards to assure the quality and safety of drugs, using mechanisms such as licensing, inspection, and surveillance. Financial regulation is intended to introduce policies to reduce the influence of the pharmaceutical industry on the market and to increase consumer access to pharmaceutical products. The tools it uses include price controls, market monitoring, the development of policies on access, and policies to promote the use of generic drugs. Although the accessibility of medicines has always been high on the public agenda, its importance has increased with the AIDS epidemic, and price controls came to play a predominant role in financial regulation.

Building the Leadership Capacity of the Health Authority: The Case of Chile

The health reform process in Chile, which was launched in 2000, brought about a dramatic change in both the public and private health systems, with the objective of providing the population with more and better access to health services, reducing waiting times, expanding the network of establishments, and eliminating financial barriers. This reform process included two fundamental actions that led to the strengthening of the health authority in the leadership area. The first action was to prioritize the concept of leadership and its linkage with a series of proposals that have come to form the foundation of the Chilean health sector. The second was the promotion by the health authority of active participation by civil society in identifying problems, and planning and implementing actions in the field. The reform proposal was based on five main issues, each of which was dealt with in its own draft legislation. The first bill that was passed by congress was called the Health Authority Act, whose purpose was to redesign the regulatory agency. As a result, the health reform process in Chile has been exemplary in introducing legal, institutional, and operational changes to steer the sector toward achieving the main goals of the reform: to improve health effectiveness, equity, and solidarity, and boost efficiency in sector management.

Building the Leadership Capacity of the Ministry of Health: The Case of Costa Rica

Costa Rica is a country that has historically attached priority to public health. Its commitment to universal health care coverage, coupled with sustained investments in the sector and the provision of basic social services, meant that in the 1990s the country had one of the best health situations in the Region, comparable in many respects with the industrialized countries. However, Costa Rica was not exempt from the economic crisis that afflicted the Region in earlier decades. The problems of the fiscal deficit and foreign and domestic debt as well as excessive centralization, inefficiency, and bureaucratic growth in the government apparatus led to a reduction in government financing for the health sector (59) which, in turn, affected the quality of health services, their coverage, and investment levels in the sector. Nonetheless, owing to its commitment to public health, the country opted to focus health sector reform on strengthening the public health system (60).

At the start of the 1990s, a national debate began on the options for addressing the problems affecting the Ministry of Health and the Costa Rican Social Security Fund (CCSS). In 1994, major structural reforms got under way in the organization, financing, and provision of health services, while always maintaining the basic principles of universal coverage and public financing of the CCSS. A leadership and institution-building project for the Ministry of Health was designed, whose objective is to support the ministry in effectively exercising stewardship and transferring activities related to direct care for individuals to the CCSS. Actions focused on separating the functions of delivery and financing (taken over by the CCSS) from the functions of regulation and leadership (the responsibility of the Ministry of Health) to eliminate unnecessary duplication of human resources and infrastructure. The redefinition of institutional functions in the health system as a result of the reform demanded greater capacity in the Ministry of Health to carry out its stewardship function: leading the sector, regulating health goods and services, measuring how well the essential public health functions are performed, modulating financing for health care, supervising insurance, and harmonizing the delivery of services. Much has been achieved since the start of the project in 1994. By 2002, the ministry had made good headway in reorganizing its operations in order to respond to growing demands that required effective exercise of sector stewardship.

Challenges

The countries of the Region are making major efforts to bolster the stewardship function of the health authorities. However, each of them, in light of its situation and possibilities, needs to perform a self-evaluation to analyze its capacity to exercise the leadership function and define actions to improve it. They should keep in mind the following lessons learned from national experiences: (1) the establishment of health priorities and objectives requires reliable and timely information; (2) the formulation of health policies and strategies should be complemented with evaluation; (3) the legal framework that supports the health authority in the exercise of its functions should be consistent with the governance that it strives to exert over the sector in its capacity as lead agency; (4) for regulation to be effective, the regulatory function should be complemented with oversight; (5) for international cooperation in health to be effective, respond to the needs detected, and be sustainable, the health authority should be involved in its negotiation, coordination, and evaluation; and (6) qualified human resources must be available to exercise the stewardship functions.

In short, the great challenge lies in entrenching stewardship as a function of government and its senior authorities and directing institution-building efforts toward enhancing the functions of planning, financing, allocation, and development of resources, public management, and knowledge.

THE PROVISION OF HEALTH CARE SERVICES AS A FUNCTION OF THE HEALTH SYSTEM

Delivery of high quality, efficient, and equitable health services and giving the population access to them is one of three main functions of the health system. This function is probably the one most readily identified, because it embodies the purpose of all health care systems and because its degree of implementation directly affects the ability to maintain health and prevent disease at the individual and community levels. The health care services function is also highly visible since it is embodied in health care organizations, the work of health care professionals, and the interventions and health technology that each society has made available to satisfy this basic human need.

The Governments of the Americas have stressed that vital and health statistics are essential in all phases of program planning and of evaluating the activities carried out by health services and the social effects achieved.

Abraham Horwitz, 1966

Health care services include both personal and public health services, that is, services that respond to individual and collective needs, covering the whole spectrum of care and ranging from health promotion and disease prevention to curative and palliative treatment, rehabilitation, and long-term care. Health care services also encompass physical, mental, dental, and vision services.

Levels of Health Care Services

Health services are classified according to the level of care as primary, secondary, or tertiary. These levels of care are defined by the type of services provided, the degree of complexity, and the capacity to treat various types of health problems and conditions. The designation of primary, secondary, or tertiary often characterizes the infrastructure of the health services system, in particular, health care facilities such as hospitals and clinics. In this context, primary care refers only to a level of care and not to the broader set of values, principles, and essential elements of a health system, as previously discussed in the primary health care strategy.

Emergency care cuts across all levels of care. Yet, it is perhaps the least developed in most countries of the Region, and very few countries have established special programs to strengthen emergency care. In Brazil, for example, the mobile emergency care service units were established in 2003 as part of the unified health care system. As of 2006, the Ministry of Health had established 94 of these mobile units, which are providing services in 647 municipalities. Chile has been expanding its prehospitalization emergency care services, which consist of rescue units of various complexities and a local emergency center supervised by an emergency care physician. In Cuba, 121 Intensive Care Areas (AIMs) have been established since 2004 to provide emergency care services to the population in areas of difficult access to health services or too far from hospital-based emergency care. Each AIM provides 24-hour service and is staffed by emergency care physicians and nursing personnel.

Access to Health Care Services

"Access" can be understood as the ability to obtain care when needed. "Accessibility" refers to the degree to which health services are acceptable to the population and respond to its needs. It is ultimately manifested by the utilization of health services by particular population groups which, *a priori*, can be assumed to

345

be disadvantaged (*61*). Accessibility is affected by the characteristics of the delivery system, of individuals, and of communities (*62*). Access to a regular source of care—a primary care provider or specific site—makes it more likely that individuals will receive a greater number of appropriate health services and, in turn, experience better health outcomes (*63*). Changes in the health situation, as discussed elsewhere in this publication, will require changes in health care services so that they emphasize promotion and prevention rather than just curative care, address chronic as well as acute illnesses, and respond to growing health problems such as substance abuse and violence, among others.

The evaluation and promotion of equitable access to necessary health services is an essential public health function (*5*). A study and survey of decisionmakers in the area of primary health care undertaken in 16 countries in Latin America and the Caribbean found that strategies to increase coverage and access to primary care are some of the most common elements of health care reform efforts in the Region (*64*). These strategies include increasing the total number of primary care facilities, targeting the delivery of a set of basic services to populations with limited access and/or to vulnerable groups such as mothers and children or indigenous populations, as has been the case in Brazil, Costa Rica, Ecuador, Honduras, Jamaica, Mexico, Nicaragua, and Panama, among other countries.

For instance, one of the mechanisms used in Brazil to expand coverage and reduce inequalities is the Basic Health Services Program (PAB). This strategy transfers funds for basic health care services to municipalities for the implementation of previously established activities and for meeting performance goals. The municipalities are responsible for guaranteeing the population access to a package of basic health services, and they receive support from the Ministry of Health to do so. In Mexico, the Opportunities Program includes a set of integrated health care interventions directed to improving the health, nutrition, and educational level of families residing in rural areas, with special emphasis on vulnerable populations. Services are provided free of charge and include a minimum package of essential health services, nutritional interventions for children, improved self care at the level of families and communities through health communication and health education strategies, increased supply of services to satisfy growing demands, and subsidies for families to increase food consumption (*65*).

Despite similar efforts in several countries, only 28% of decisionmakers surveyed in a 2004 regional study considered that primary care services provided adequate coverage and did not leave significant population groups without access to services. According to an exploratory study sponsored by PAHO, only a few countries in the Region have reached rates equivalent to universal coverage (e.g., Canada, Chile, Costa Rica, and Cuba). This same study also reports that approximately 27% of the population in Latin America and the Caribbean do not have permanent access to basic health services, 30% do not have access to care due to finan-

cial barriers, and 21% do not have access due to geographic barriers (*66*).

Quality of Health Care Services

The efforts to define quality of care span many decades. One of the most well known definitions of quality is the one proposed by Donabedian, who described quality of care as "the application of medical science and technology in a way that maximizes its benefits to health without correspondingly increasing its risks. The degree of quality is, therefore, the extent to which the care provided is expected to achieve the most favorable balance of risks and benefits" (*67, 68*). Donabedian also recognized that quality of care has both a technical and an interpersonal component (*69*).

More recently, the Institute of Medicine (IOM) of the United States defined quality as "the degree to which health services for individuals and populations increase the likelihood of desired health outcomes and are consistent with current professional knowledge." High-quality health care services are defined as safe, effective, patient-centered, and timely (*70, 71*).

Safe care refers to services that avoid causing injuries to patients from care that is intended to help them. Effective care refers to providing medical practices or procedures to individuals and communities based on available scientific knowledge to all those who could benefit from them and refraining from providing these services to those not likely to benefit (i.e., avoiding underuse and overuse). Patient-centered care establishes a partnership between practitioners and patients to ensure that health care decisions respect patients' wants, needs, and preferences. As such, it should lead to higher satisfaction among users. This partnership also ensures that patients and their families have the education and support they require to make decisions and participate in their own care. Instead of focusing on disease or organ systems, patient-centered care takes into account the psychosocial and cultural dimensions of illness as well as the family and community context. Timely care refers not only to minimizing unnecessary delays in getting care, but also to the need to provide coordinated care across providers and facilities, and across the spectrum of care ranging from preventive to palliative care.

Quality assurance and improvement with respect to personal and public health services is one of 11 essential public health functions. According to a regional study published by PAHO in 2002, it was among the least developed (*55*). Several countries in the Region have defined and implemented procedures for the accreditation of health care facilities, with the United States and Canada leading in this area. Several countries in Latin America also have developed accreditation programs, including Argentina, Belize, Bolivia, Brazil, Colombia, Costa Rica, the Dominican Republic, El Salvador, Honduras, Jamaica, Peru, Suriname, and Trinidad and Tobago (*72*). The degree of implementation of these accreditation programs varies by country, and almost all of them focus on hospitals.

Equity and Efficiency in the Delivery of Health Care Services

In the context of quality, equity is a crosscutting aspect of health services and refers to the distribution of quality health care services across population groups based on need rather than other criteria not inherently linked to health, such as ethnicity, geographic location, socioeconomic status, or insurance coverage. Universal coverage and equal access to care are the foundation of an equitable health system, as discussed elsewhere in this publication. The second crosscutting aspect of high-quality health services is efficiency in the allocation of resources and the delivery of services to reduce waste and obtain the best possible value for the resources used (73).

Development of High-Performing Health Care Delivery Systems

Challenges to Developing High-Performing Health Care Delivery Models

Most countries in the Region face a set of common challenges with respect to the performance of health care delivery systems. These include the rapid increase in the cost of services, insufficient health care services, inequitable access to services, deficiencies in technical efficiency, low level or lack of evidence with respect to the effectiveness and cost effectiveness of most services provided, insufficient quality of services, and low levels of consumer satisfaction and social participation in health.

An analysis of the situation with respect to hospital care, specifically, shows the following (66):

- An overemphasis on highly specialized care and the use of costly health care technologies.
- A concentration of health care facilities in metropolitan urban areas.
- A growing gap between the demand and supply of services.
- An imbalance in the distribution of patients between public and private sector hospitals based on financing schemes, whereby the public system usually cares for the more costly cases while private hospitals pre-select patients and limit access to more costly procedures.
- A lack of sufficiently developed management systems.
- A lack of quality control systems linked to hospital procedures, particularly for medium- and high-complexity procedures.

In addition, most health care delivery models have tended to emphasize personal care services rather than public health services; curative care rather than preventive care; and services centered on a specific disease episode or a visit, rather than on treating the person as a whole and establishing a care partnership, in the context of family and community. Furthermore, services are generally characterized by a lack of continuity of care due to the lack of access to a regular source of care, and the lack of an integrated and coordinated network of services.

Emerging Trends in Health Care Delivery Models

In general, changes in health services delivery at the level of primary care have focused on providing a better fit between the delivery of services and the population's needs and demands for health care, with an emphasis on ambulatory care, and increasing access and equity. Stepped up efforts in this direction should help to address some of the deficiencies noted above.

Although we cannot refer to a single dominant model of health care services delivery, there are a number of common trends, particularly at the primary care level (64). Their relative importance and level of implementation varies across countries in the Region. One of the most evident trends has been the shift from hospital-based inpatient care to specialized ambulatory care including increased use of ambulatory or same-day surgery, day hospitals, and home health care, to reduce costly hospital stays. This trend is most evident in higher-income countries such as the United States and Canada, because it often requires complex technologies, costly investments, and retraining of personnel. However, it is increasingly evident in other countries in the Region. In Panama, for example, the public health insurance system provides home care for patients requiring care for chronic conditions. In Chile, one of the strategies has been to develop new ways to deliver specialized ambulatory care independently of hospitals, such as the use of health care referral centers for the more common specialties and diagnostic and treatment centers for more complex ambulatory care.

An increased focus on health care at the level of the family, rather than on individual care, is also evident in Brazil, Chile, and Cuba. This approach tends to favor integrated care rather than a select set of services and has stimulated the use of a team approach to care where nurses and auxiliary personnel are integral members, rather than the more traditional hierarchical model where most or all of the decisionmaking power resides with physicians. Although 58% of primary care decisionmakers surveyed in 16 Latin American and Caribbean countries reported the existence of family health policies or programs, about the same proportion reported that these only reach half of the country's population or less (64).

An emphasis on health promotion and prevention, rather than solely curative and rehabilitative care, is another common trend in new health delivery models implemented in several countries in the Region. The relative emphasis on health promotion and disease prevention is greater for lower- than higher-income countries, most likely due to efforts to expand coverage through preventive services (64).

Taking health care services to places where users live, work, and study, rather than having users always go to seek services at health care facilities, is another strategy to increase access used in health care delivery models. School-based health care programs for students have been established in high- as well as low-income countries. In the United States, over 1,000 schools (mostly high schools) have health centers (*74*). In Nicaragua, school-based health care was established in several schools in 2001 as part of a pilot program. As of 2006, four schools had health centers. The program has also enhanced the coordination between schools and municipalities to increase coverage of child immunizations and improve child nutrition and oral health.

Another common way to increase access to integrated care is the establishment of primary care teams with assigned populations. In Cuba, each primary care team (including one family physician and nurse) is assigned about 120 families, and the team must live in the same neighborhood as their assigned population. The physician's office and residence are often in the same building. The teams provide care in the office, but they also conduct home visits and field visits. Schools and work sites often have their own health care centers (*75*).

Mobile clinics and/or mobile health care teams are not necessarily a new trend but continue to be used in many countries in the Region particularly for areas of low population density or hard-to-reach areas where health care facilities and personnel are not available on a permanent basis. For example, in Panama, this is the primary objective of the so-called itinerant health caravans.

The Goal: Integrated Health Care Services

Integrated systems are among the most recently proposed models of health care delivery. These refer to inter-organizational health care networks that articulate clinical, functional, normative, and systemic dimensions coordinating health services over space (from the home to diverse types of health care facilities) and time (for an episode of illness and over the life cycle). An integrated delivery system has the necessary resources and capabilities to address the majority of health problems of a population at various stages of the life cycle (*76*). Integration of services is sometimes described as being horizontal or vertical in nature, but truly integrated services require both. This means having a horizontal component articulating facilities and services at the same level of care (e.g., hospitals, health centers) and a vertical component integrating services and the corresponding service providers along the continuum of care (e.g., home health care agencies, physicians' offices, hospitals, nursing homes, hospices).

From the patient's perspective, the following are characteristics of an integrated health services delivery system (*76*):

- The existence of an integrated health information system including medical records, so that patients do not have to repeat their medical history each time they seek care; the patient's medical record would also include information on utilization of services and procedures.
- No unnecessary duplication of diagnostic and laboratory procedures.

- Easy and timely access to a health care provider at the primary care level.
- Access to various levels of care with the capacity to resolve the specific set of health problems.
- Information on treatment options and participation in decisionmaking as equal partners with health care providers.
- Regular follow-up care to prevent problems with any chronic conditions.
- Health counseling and support for appropriate self-management of chronic conditions and self-care to increase individuals' autonomy and their informed use of the health care system.

Experiences with integrated health service models in the Region are growing, but few have been studied and evaluated. In El Salvador, the first level of care has been completely redefined through the definition of basic integrated health care systems (SIBASIs), designed according to the principles of a primary health care strategy, with a high level of participation of all relevant social institutions. The SIBASIs constitute the basic operational level of the health care system, and their structure includes health care facilities at the primary care level linked to facilities at the secondary and tertiary levels and organized into coordinated networks designed to respond to the population's health care needs. Legislation approved in 2006 defines the regional authorities as the technical and administrative level responsible for the management of resources assigned for the SIBASIs. It also establishes a referral system that will enable continuity and coordinated integrated care.

Many integrated health care models have been implemented on an experimental or pilot basis for restricted geographic areas and populations, commonly at the local or regional level. For example, in Peru, EsSalud (the public health insurance system) sponsored a pilot program in several polyclinics to apply and examine implementation of new strategies for the integration of services. These included conducting a needs assessment and diagnosis of the health situation of defined population groups, establishing a triage system according to population groups, increasing the hours of operation, redistribution and reorganization of physical resources, improved information systems, establishing quality-improvement processes including benchmarking, and incorporating several primary care facilities into the polyclinic (the report on the pilot project focuses on the experiences of a polyclinic that provides primary, secondary, and tertiary medical care, including emergency services) (*77*). Lessons learned include the importance of identifying and adapting best practices to improve the supply and integration of services, the need for a new organizational culture to support changes based on the establishment of good communication channels between managers and health providers to increase buy-in, and informing users about the changes in health services delivery to decrease potential resistance to change.

Effects of High-Performing Health Care Delivery Models
on Health Outcomes

Only a few studies have been carried out that show an association between changes in health delivery models—specifically primary care services—and health outcomes. In Costa Rica, comprehensive reform at the level of primary care included increasing access, focusing first on the most deprived areas (access increased by 15% in those health care districts), reorganizing health professionals into multidisciplinary primary care teams, and assigning responsibility for a particular geographic area and population to each primary care team or EBAIS. For every five years of primary health care reform, child mortality was reduced by 13% and adult mortality was reduced by 4%, independent of other health determinants (*78*). Equity in access to care was also improved (*79*).

In the case of Brazil, the Family Health Program also includes multidisciplinary health teams responsible for providing care to an assigned population. Depending on the availability of resources, dentists, social workers, and psychologists may be members of the team or instead be incorporated into support networks for a number of teams. The objectives of the program, initiated in 1994, are to extend access to basic health promotion, prevention, and treatment through low-cost and highly effective health services. By 2004, enrollment multiplied from one million to over 60 million, and the program was in operation in over three fourths of municipalities (*66*). The implementation of this program has been linked to reductions in infant mortality, as was the case with similar programs in Costa Rica and Mexico.

Challenges in the Organization and Management
of Health Care Services

Although the Americas Region is very diverse with health systems and health care services of various types and complexities, a number of challenges are shared by many countries with regard to the organization and management of health care services, including:

- Insufficient knowledge of the health situation and needs of the population served, including vulnerable populations, particularly in cases where there is not an assigned population.
- Weak or nonexistent articulation between the primary care level and other levels of care through effective referral mechanisms and information systems.
- Centralization of management and decisionmaking.
- Unclear distinctions between health care delivery and health care financing and insurance functions.
- Management of services based on inputs and resources, rather than processes and results.
- Social participation generally limited to consultative processes rather than direct participation in the management of services.

It is also important to note that the organization and management of health care services must be defined, taking into account basic ethical principles (*80*). These principles include justice, or equity in access to and receipt of high-quality care; respect for persons as reflected in a person- and family-centered care approach with a high level of community participation; beneficence, or the provision of high-quality effective services based on evidence; and nonmaleficence, or the provision of services through systems that assure safe care that avoids injury to patients and the overuse of ineffective health care services, which can cause harm.

Trends in the Management of Health Care Services

Table 14 below shows the results of a survey of 36 policymakers and 46 health care executives regarding the most commonly used management models for hospitals, specialized ambulatory care facilities, and services networks in 15 countries of Latin America and the Caribbean, including Argentina, Bahamas, Brazil, Bolivia, Colombia, Costa Rica, Cuba, Chile, Dominican Republic, Honduras, Mexico, Nicaragua, Peru, Saint Lucia, and Trinidad and Tobago (*72*). The most common models are direct public administration, cooperatives of health care professionals, and private management models, whether for-profit or not-for-profit. Among those surveyed, 10% to 14% stated that these management models do not adequately respond to health care needs, and another 70% responded that they only do so to a partial extent.

The same survey identified the following emerging trends in hospital and specialized ambulatory health services (*66*):

- Greater flexibility in the management of human resources.
- Transformations in the organization of hospital services.
- Changes in financing mechanisms for hospital services.
- Increase of managed care.
- Economic evaluations and health technology assessment.
- Evidence-based health care.
- Increased sharing of best practices regarding diagnosis and treatment.
- Greater management of services from a technical perspective, rather than just a financial or human resource perspective.

Colombia, Cuba, and Mexico are among the few countries in Latin America to have established a health technology assessment program. For instance, in Mexico, the National Center of Technological Excellence (CENETEC) has developed a database of health technologies that includes information on efficacy, safety, cost-effectiveness, and compliance with technical standards and is used for purchasing and assigning medical equipment. The database includes 22 practice guidelines, 31 technological guidelines, 125 documents on technical specifications, eight medical equipment guidelines, six consumer information publications, and various reports on technology assessment and biomedical engineering (*81*). In Colombia, the Ministry of Health's Office of Science

349

TABLE 14. Management models by type of health care facility or network.

Type of facility or network	Management model
Hospital	Direct public management Privatized or outsourced management Cooperatives of medical professionals Private for-profit
Specialized ambulatory care	Direct public management Indirect public organization Privatized or outsourced management Cooperatives of medical professionals Private for-profit
Health care services networks	Direct public management Cooperatives of medical professionals Private for-profit

Source: Organización Panamericana de la Salud. Estudio regional sobre asistencia hospitalaria y ambulatoria especializada en América Latina y el Caribe, 2004.

and Technology Development has improved health technology assessment and defined standards for importing and evaluating health technology. Cuba has a National Office of Technology Assessment to determine the impact of health technology in existing systems and to identify new medical equipment that may be acquired (72).

Policymakers and administrators made suggestions to accelerate the development of appropriate management models and improve management of care, including (66):

- Decentralizing the administration of public hospitals and increasing autonomy.
- Decentralizing health care services in general.
- Reviewing the system of financing to eliminate economic barriers confronted by public facilities when trying to provide services at the minimal level of quality required for appropriate functioning of the system.
- Reinforcing coordination across institutions to form networks of integrated services and giving priority to services delivered through networks.
- Defining quality criteria and implementing quality assurance and quality improvement programs.
- Defining and establishing incentives and other mechanisms to motivate health care personnel.
- Training and continuing education of technical and administrative personnel.

Decentralization of health care services management and delivery continues to be one of the main components of health care reform efforts in many countries in the Region. Brazil is one of the countries where decentralization has been the most expansive. The Unified Health System or SUS was established in 1990. It is based on the goals of universal and equitable access to care through a regionalized system of health care services organized by level of complexity under the direction of municipal, state, and federal level authorities. The decentralization of health care services is one of its most important strategies. Decentralization of services has been accompanied by increased regulatory capacity and is ruled by a new agreement approved in February 2006 by the Tripartite Inter-managerial Committee and the National Health Council, which establishes a new framework for management of the system at all levels of government.

Capacity-Building for Optimal Management of Health Care Services

Capacity is traditionally defined as the ability of individuals, organizations, and systems of care to perform their main functions. It is most often used to refer to financial support, medical equipment and facilities, human resource development, and technical skills. However, capacity building is a continuous process of developing and strengthening the knowledge and skills needed to manage health care. These skills include the ability to: conduct needs assessments and identify gaps in access to and delivery of care; define a plan to reduce these gaps through capacity building and the definition of specific strategies and actions; and monitor and evaluate processes and the results obtained (82).

With respect to this last area, and regarding the use of outcome indicators of health care services, the survey of Latin American and Caribbean policymakers, hospital administrators, and managers of various ambulatory care facilities described previously (66) found the following:

- 59% of respondents reported that these facilities conduct analyses of the results of health services, mostly with respect to financial indicators.
- 63% reported that facilities measured the rate of hospital-related infections (one of the key indicators of patient safety).
- 71% reported that facilities use quality indicators, but only 57% reported the use of consumer surveys with respect to satisfaction and/or experiences with care, and only 46% regularly review guidelines for care.
- 63% reported using indicators of the productivity of health care personnel, and 52% use indicators of the use of material resources (such as equipment) and medicines.

Experiences at the international level have shown that key factors for capacity building in management include: recognizing the importance of developing the necessary skills to manage change; ensuring the skills necessary for basic management of services, acknowledging the importance of organizational culture when promoting change at this level; recognizing the presence of potential barriers external to the health services delivery system such as the political, legislative, and regulatory structure; and the need to build capacity in stages and not try to institute change all at once.

Health Care Services Monitoring and Performance Measurement

The basis for the effective management of health care services is the availability of timely and accurate information for analysis, reporting, monitoring, and performance measurement. A management information system that is flexible, periodically reviewed and updated, properly financed, and sustainable is essential for decisionmaking. Such a system provides managers with information for strategic planning, as well as routine management of health care services. Other design principles for an effective management information system (*83*) include linking it to specific evidence-based goals for improvement and including measures to evaluate progress with respect to key attributes of health care services at any level of the system: access, quality (safety, effectiveness, person centeredness, timeliness, and coordination of care), equity, and efficiency.

A number of countries in the Region have embarked on processes to foster effectiveness, efficiency, and equity in the delivery and management of health services by implementing methods and tools to monitor the resource flows associated with health care delivery and evaluate institutional performance with respect to previously defined standards for both process and outcome measures. The use of methods that generate information for the analysis of productivity, performance, and resource utilization is essential for meeting institutional goals, negotiating contracts for the provision of services, increasing accountability, monitoring institutional performance, and improving management practices (*84*).

In Ecuador, regular tracking of process indicators has enabled program managers to monitor the effects of legislation implemented to provide free maternity care and infant care services on the quality of care. Several process indicators of quality showed significant improvement after only nine months. For example, the proportion of births where a set of standardized guidelines were followed (e.g., maternal blood pressure and fetal heart rate monitoring) increased from 44.5% in 2003 to 83.6% in 2004 (*85*).

In the Bahamas, the Department of Public Health has initiated a pilot implementation of a new public health information system at four sites. The system is an automated, integrated client health records and reporting system that supports implementation, tracking, and reporting of public health interventions, as well as follow-up and case management at the individual level.

A number of countries in Latin America and the Caribbean have implemented management information systems for use in health care facilities. In Mexico, for example, more than 100 hospitals have implemented a management information system. Modules for resource generation and costs are the most extensively developed, including costing of 1,800 hospital-based procedures and cost-recovery programs. In one department in Colombia, a management information system was piloted successfully in 2004 in three hospitals, and the system is expanding its use to 36 hospitals in another department. The system has been particularly useful to public hospitals, which in Colombia must negotiate and manage contracts for services with insurance or managed care companies as well as county and department level health authorities. Chile implemented a management information system in 2003, which was later expanded to seven hospitals where it has additionally been used to negotiate budgets based on the costs and complexity of the production of various services.

Emerging Trends in Health Care Services

Certain key developments in health care services that can expand access to care are still mostly in the beginning stages. These include for instance the use of information and communication technology, increased globalization and trade in health services, research on mapping the human genome, and new treatments, medicines, and health care technologies.

In rural or hard-to-reach areas, information and communication technologies facilitate the increase of access to specialists and services that are more complex. When properly used, telehealth can reduce barriers in access to care due to geographic obstacles, inadequate distribution of health providers, costs, and lack of supervision and support of health workers at the primary care level (*86*). For example, in rural areas of the United States, telehealth is used by primary care providers to consult with specialists on specific cases in the presence of the patients. Information technology can also be used to increase access to diagnostic services by radiologists, using specialized scanners to transmit the images to radiologists who analyze the images at other locations. This type of technology can provide continuing education to health care providers of all types. In Mexico in 2006, 18 health care facilities in four states had trained personnel who could provide telemedicine services. Eight other federal facilities also provided telemedicine services as well as continuing education using the same type of technologies.

MEDICINES AND HEALTH CARE TECHNOLOGIES

Medicines

Pharmaceutical Policies

Pharmaceutical policies, with their harmoniously interrelated components of access, quality, and rational use, form part of health care or health insurance system policies, designed to maintain comprehensiveness in structural, financial, and managerial aspects and, above all, to attain the health goals established by the countries. The formulation and implementation of pharmaceutical policies involves health, industrial, and science and technology

FIGURE 3. Interrelated aspects in the formulation of drug policies.

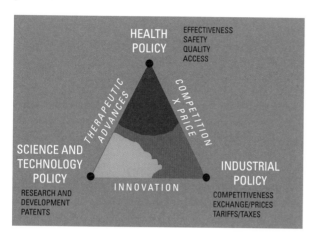

Source: Adapted from Tobar F. Políticas para mejorar el acceso a los medicamentos. Boletín Fármacos, julio 2002; 5(3).

aspects. This triad can be represented by a triangle with industrial policy, science and technology policy, and health policy on the vertices (Figure 3) (*87*).

From the standpoint of industrial policy, the goal is domestic and international competitiveness to consolidate the supply. From the standpoint of science and technology policy, interest centers on research and development and on technological improvement of pharmaceutical forms. From the standpoint of health policy, in addition to ensuring public access to medicines, oversight of the quality of the products, their safety, and therapeutic performance is also called for. Health concerns share the need with industrial policy to promote competition through prices, and with science and technology they share the concern for promoting therapeutic advances. In turn, the latter shares with industrial policy the promotion of innovation and quality.

From the standpoint of health policy, medicines are primarily a social good, while from the viewpoints of industrial policy and innovation, they are a consumer good. Since reality is more complex than this, a pharmaceutical policy can be centered on different aspects as determined by national priorities.

After the different trends that lined up on the vertices of the triangle over the last three decades, today a better balance appears to exist. Some countries have stronger structures that include regulatory agencies. This is true of Brazil and Argentina, which are playing an acknowledged leadership role, attempting to guide pharmaceutical policies toward striking balances at different points inside the triangle rather than on the vertices. Other countries are making efforts to identify spaces that will permit them to move toward the center of the triangle with certain innovations, although for the time being they are more involved in regulation than implementation. Ecuador, for example, approved a law on generic drugs in 2000 which spans the entire cycle, from

production to consumption, and which, in addition to requiring the use of cheaper drugs in the public sector, also requires that 20% of the production of all laboratories be generic and establishes higher drugstore profit margins on sales of generic drugs (*88*). Through growth in government procurement, several countries of the Region (including Bolivia, Chile, the Dominican Republic, Jamaica, Peru, and Uruguay) spurred an increased supply of competitive products.

In the countries, these measures can form part of official comprehensive pharmaceutical policies or can stem from decisions on specific policy components. According to the most recent WHO report (*89*), of 27 countries in the Region that responded to a survey on the pharmaceutical situation in 2003, 16 reported that they had a national drug policy and in nine the policy was official.

The Pharmaceutical Market

The market for medications is one of the fastest growing in the world. In the last five years alone, it grew by more than 50%.[14] The United States is the market leader in the Region and in the world with US$ 190 billion in invoicing in 2005–2006.[15] It is followed in the Americas by Canada with US$ 13 billion (*89*). Together, the two countries account for 50% of the world market, and they doubled their sales in the last six years. The pharmaceutical market has also grown steadily in Latin America and the Caribbean since 2002 and is expected to maintain the pace until the end of the present decade (*90*). The region represents 8% of the world market. In 2006, the three countries with the highest sales were Brazil (US$ 8.1 billion), Mexico (US$ 7.8 billion), and Argentina (US$ 2.1 billion) (*91*).

As in the other regions, the share of competing products (also called multiple-source or generic) is growing. This means that larger numbers of units are being sold, given that this segment charges much lower prices. Of the countries of the Region, 80% have rules to promote prescriptions that include the common international denomination in the public sector, but just 33% have done so in the private sector (*92*). Argentina is one of the most advanced in this area, where 78% of prescriptions include the generic name (*93*).

Supply and demand. The pharmaceutical industry is extensively globalized today. International companies are rapidly increasing their share of the Latin American market. In Argentina, national producers have a larger market share (50% of laboratories), followed by Chile with 43%, Uruguay with 26%, Brazil with 25%, and Mexico with 12% (*94*). The deregulation of the econ-

---

[14] In 2000, the world market was US$ 356 billion, and in 2005 it was US$ 602 billion. Source: International Medical Statistics (IMS) Health Total Market Estimates and Global Pharma Forecasts (includes IMS audited and unaudited markets).

[15] The data presented are from IMS and correspond to the period between July 2005 and June 2006. Taxes and retailer profit margins are not included.

omy introduced in the last decade encouraged multinationals to concentrate their production in the largest countries of the Region. Since then, interregional trade has been on the rise. Participation by Europe and the United States has been declining as a share of the Region's imports, particularly when volumes rather than prices are considered.

No country is completely self-sufficient. The United States is the world's largest producer of drugs, but it is also the largest importer and has a negative balance of trade in this item. All the countries import materials and, for finished products, dependence is proportionate to the level of industrial development. For example, in Brazil, imports account for 19% of the market (95), 30% in Argentina (96), 40% in Peru,[16] 50% in Uruguay (97), and 80% in Ecuador (98). Demand for drugs is highly concentrated, and more than 80% of world production is consumed in the 12 most highly developed countries.

More than half of the Region's inhabitants have difficulties in obtaining essential medicines. According to the WHO survey, in 60% of the countries of the Region access to essential medicines in 2003 was below 80% (92). Prices are the main barrier, although access also depends on income. When prices are adjusted for purchasing power parity, Uruguay, the country with the lowest average prices, turns out to be the most expensive (99). Another barrier has been attributed to the fact that the very fast pace of innovation in the industry is not responsive to the problems that prevail in less-developed countries and areas (100). Estimates suggest that just 3% of expenditure on research and development in the pharmaceutical industry goes to produce drugs to fight those diseases, which account for 90% of the global burden of disease in the developing world (101).

Financing. According to IMS projections for 2006, Latin American countries spend more than US$ 22 billion (almost US$ 40 per capita/year) on medicines. Drugs are financed from three main sources: household expenditure (out-of-pocket); insurance plans (public, mutual, and private) which generally finance 100% of the drugs needed by their members during hospitalization but a smaller portion for ambulatory patients; and government expenditure to supply drugs for public health services.

Two-thirds of financing for medicines in Latin America comes from households, and the other two sources combined pay for just one-third. This introduces strong regressiveness, since lower income groups use more than 70% of their health expenditures to buy drugs (102). Social insurance and public insurance (which are spreading in the Region) still only offer partial coverage, and Costa Rica alone is comparable with European or Australian social security.

---

[16] In 2006, the National Statistics and Information Institute of Peru estimated that the market was about US$ 462.5 million, and imports were US$ 185.5 million. See also, M.I Terra, G Bittencourt et al. Estudios de Competitividad Sectoriales. Industria Manufacturera. Departamento de Economía. Facultad de Ciencias Sociales. UDELAR. Documento No 23/05. Montevideo, Uruguay.

> " *The challenge of achieving the goal of health for all will require the unflagging commitment of governments, the allocation of required resources, and the reform and restructuring of health systems in order to obtain maximum equity, efficiency, and effectiveness.* "
>
> Héctor Acuña, 1983

The larger the share of public financing, the greater the access and the lower the average price. In Chile, government procurement increased with the AUGE system (universal access with explicit guarantees) and comes close to 30% of total expenditure; in Brazil, the Unified Health System (SUS) provides 25% of all the drugs prescribed in the country (103); in Peru, 21% is financed (104), and in Argentina about 15% (105).

Trade and Health

In recent years, the subject of intellectual property rights related to access to medicines has been permanently present on the health agenda. Since 1999, when the World Health Assembly adopted the Revised Drug Strategy Resolution, WHO was given the mandate of cooperating with the Member States in the monitoring and analysis of the implications of international agreements, including trade agreements, for the pharmaceutical sector and public health. Since then, several developing countries have led a movement to permanently track this issue and place it on the agenda of the governments of the Member States. In 2001, 2002, and 2003 specific resolutions were approved related to access to medicines (106–108), with clauses relating to the public health implications of trade agreements, particularly the Trade Related Intellectual Property Rights Agreement (TRIPS) of the World Trade Organization (WTO). These aspects have been included in resolutions related to the response to HIV/AIDS (109).

The Doha Declaration (Ministerial Declaration on TRIPS and Public Health) adopted on 14 November 2001 at the WTO's Fourth Ministerial Conference in Doha, Qatar, represents a historical framework for relations between trade and public health. The declaration reaffirms the flexibility provisions established in the TRIPS Agreement and the right of countries to use those provisions to promote access to medicines.

The bilateral and subregional free trade agreements currently being discussed, negotiated, or implemented by different countries constitute a significant concern in the Americas Region and in other regions, given the impact that their application could have on health, particularly on access to medicines. One of the main reasons for concern is the possibility of imposing more restrictive conditions than were established in earlier agreements, particularly the TRIPS Agreement, and their effects on domestic legislation. These trends are known as TRIPS Plus or WTO Plus. Since treaties of this kind are generally superimposed on domestic legislation, they end up imposing greater restrictions and forcing countries to change their legislation. It is also known that conflicts arise within governments when discussing such agreements. In the past, conflicts of this kind led a number of governments to discuss trade agreements without inviting the health sector to participate. Although this is apparently an everyday problem in the developing countries, it can also be anticipated that the health systems of the industrialized countries will be unable to continue to afford the rising cost of reimbursing patients for new medicines for significant public health problems.

Patents are an instrument of economic policy that may or may not bring benefits to a given country. It has been argued that patents spur investments in science and technology development, producing innovations and benefits for society. However by their very nature, they also create legal monopolies that permit high prices to be charged and hobble market competition.

Harmonization

The Region of the Americas has made great strides in the field of harmonization. The Pan American Network for Drug Regulatory Harmonization (PANDRH) sponsored by PAHO/WHO, which was established in 1999 at the Second Pan American Conference on Drug Regulatory Harmonization, has grown and is increasingly well entrenched as a regional strategy for supporting national and subregional processes. Today, the network has 12 working groups that are coordinated by representatives of the drug regulatory authorities of the different countries of the Region, except the pharmacopoeia group, which is coordinated by the United States Pharmacopoeia (USP). Today, the different groups are composed of 110 professionals from regulatory offices that bring together representatives of industry and academe, 72% of whom are from national regulatory agencies. The working groups have recently extended to technical discussion groups and have incorporated more than 80 additional professionals, all from national regulatory offices.

To date, the network, whose main objective is to contribute to all aspects of the quality, safety, and effectiveness of pharmaceuticals, has produced several tangible products, two of which have already been approved by the conference: the Harmonized Guideline for Good Manufacturing Practices (GMP) Inspection, prepared by the working group on GMP; and Good Clinical Practices: Document of the Americas. Other studies that are ready are: the strategy for implementing bioequivalence studies; common requirements for the registration of medicines; definition and criteria for the classification of medicines; and the series of documents on consignment notes, basic structure, and definitions and indicators to step up the fight against counterfeit medicines.

One of PANDRH's most successful activities has been to design and carry out educational activities on regulations. The network has held some 50 courses on the quality of medicines (good manufacturing practices, good laboratory practices, validation of processes, practical application of high performance liquid chromatography, bioequivalence, and good clinical practices).

National universities in the Region cooperated in these activities, which are mostly national in nature. Through them, more than 1,700 professionals in different countries have been kept abreast of new developments.

Supply of Medicines

National models for obtaining supplies of medicines in the Region are cyclical systems in which the primary functions or processes depend on the efficient execution of a previous function and are supported by it. For example, the selection of medicines is based on an evaluation of needs and drug use, and procurement requirements stem from the decisions made during the selection process.

The list of essential medicines serves as a guide for the public sector in procuring medicines and is used as a primary reference in some countries for reimbursements for drugs financed by private insurance plans. Procurement systems evolve as decentralization of the health system progresses. In the larger countries, such as Brazil and Colombia, the responsibility for procuring most medicines has been transferred to the local level (the health departments or local institutions), while centralized distribution systems or systems administered directly by the ministry of health or an autonomous agency contracted by the public sector for that purpose continue to operate in the smaller countries.

The decentralization process creates certain problems since the health areas at the departmental (or state), municipal, or district levels need to develop the capacity to organize a procurement process that assures that medicines will be available continuously in health facilities. In some cases, decentralization leads to significant increases in the cost of medicines because the economies of scale that result from the consolidation of demand are lost, particularly for more expensive drugs. That is why the countries are considering the possibility of redefining the criteria for differentiating between expensive products that would be procured at the central level through consolidated purchases and inexpensive products that can be purchased at the decentralized level. The centralized procurement systems in the smaller countries are also evolving as they obtain greater managerial independence from the ministry of health; however, the ministry continues to bear prime responsibility for the procurement and distribution of medicines in most countries (86%) (92).

Regardless of the extent of decentralization in distribution systems, all the countries continue to face major challenges in the procurement and regulation of the supply of medicines. Studies on essential drug supply systems in various countries conducted in the last two years by PAHO and the Cooperative of Hospitals of Antioquia (COHAN), a PAHO/WHO Collaborating Center, indicate that national health policies and pharmaceutical policies, and the conditions governing the procurement of medicines established by external financial agencies, do not facilitate the integration of distribution systems. Consequently, procurement processes are often isolated and disconnected, parallel distribution systems exist, and there is overlapping of functions on the district and national levels, with no coordination. Frequently, the products are obtained through isolated procurement mechanisms that fail to consider the importance of implementing and monitoring the system as a whole. In the last instance, this leads to shortages and increased costs, and missed opportunities to use the financing available.

The cost of medicines in the public sector continues to soar. Brazil reports that in 2006 that cost amounted to some 11% of the national health budget, which is more than double the 5% reported in 2002. Furthermore, public sector drug costs are rising exponentially as a result of the proliferation of court cases throughout the Region to defend patients' rights and provide individual patients or groups of patients with expensive medicines that do not appear on the list of essential drugs. To justify the inclusion or exclusion of drugs on official lists and apply the use of those lists more strictly in the public sector, the health sector is examining processes and evaluating the use of health technologies taking a test-based approach (scientific and economic).

PAHO's Strategic Fund, in which 17 countries already participate, is a technical cooperation tool that was established to support the countries in planning and procuring strategic public sector supplies. The Strategic Fund provides technical support for procurements and regulation of the supply, particularly for basic products related to HIV, where procurements are complicated because of the challenges of projecting needs when different lines of treatment exist; the need to determine the status of product patents; and the policies of differentiated pricing that are applied by some manufacturers throughout the Region. The countries that participate in the Strategic Fund are attempting to work together to address similar challenges in the procurement and supply of other expensive complex medicines, including immunosuppressants and cancer drugs.

Rational Use of Medicines

As has been mentioned, major efforts are being made to improve access to medicines, but they have not always been accompanied by a strategy for their rational use. The concept of essential medicines, which will be 30 years old in 2007, is a cornerstone of pharmaceutical policies, and selection of the list is a powerful tool for guaranteeing rational use. In 2003, 22 countries reported that they had a list, with an average of 400 medicines, but ranging from a low of 346 to a high of 618 (*92*). However, these lists were used primarily for public sector procurement and only in a few cases for reimbursements under public or private insurance. Most countries have formal medications and therapeutics committees, but their functions and real impact on effective execution of guidelines, formularies, and selection of medicines vary greatly from country to country. The national therapeutic formularies and standardized treatment guides, although they are sometimes mandatory in institutions, frequently do not form part of medical practice and require great efforts and training, and institutional

coordination to comply with. The La Plata (Argentina) Collaborating Center continues to support regional training in problem-based pharmacotherapy. The course, aimed at instructors, is given each year. In the last five years the Collaborating Center has given courses in Argentina, Brazil, Mexico, Guatemala, and Cuba, where it trained about 200 teachers and 50 physicians and primary care coordinators. The center is also cooperating on a distance course on the rational use of medicines for 5,000 prescribers under the REMEDIAR program (an initiative that provides essential medicines for 15 million people in Argentina).

Brazil has offered a course on problem-based pharmacotherapy in 21 of the country's 27 states, which trained 1,022 professionals, including physicians, dentists, pharmacists, nurses, and veterinarians. Some initiatives have also been designed to educate the community about rational use of medicines, ranging from local campaigns in primary schools in Costa Rica to a Spanish edition of the international course on Promoting Rational Drug Use in the Community, developed by Health Action International in Nicaragua.

Self-medication continues to be a problem in the Region, with consequences related particularly to the use of antibiotics. Over-the-counter sales of antibiotics, combined with a high rate of prescription errors, contributes significantly to drug resistance. An ambulatory survey conducted in 2005 in Nicaragua and Honduras calculated that more than 30% of antibiotics were purchased without prescription and that nearly 50% of antibiotics were wrongly prescribed (*110*). Excessive use of antibiotics in illnesses such as upper respiratory infections has been widely documented even in developed countries like the United States. Chile is one of the countries that has adopted a national strategy to address this problem and has obtained positive results in a reduction of antibiotic use through the introduction of regulatory measures in 1999.

With regard to drug dispensing, since 2002, the Pharmaceutical Forum of the Americas, whose members include national and regional pharmaceutical associations, the International Pharmaceutical Federation, and PAHO, has been carrying out a project in four countries on the pharmaceutical treatment of hypertension (*111*) to obtain pharmacological and non-pharmacological therapeutical results. Activities in each country are coordinated by a national group, whose participants are drawn from universities, medicine information centers, the national pharmaceutical association, the ministry of health, and PAHO/WHO. The forum also launched a project on good pharmaceutical practices that began in Uruguay in 2005.

Vaccines

In the last 10 years, the Latin American and Caribbean countries have increased their dependence on imported vaccines produced outside the Region. New products and their combinations with classical vaccines produced by large consortia forming different types of business partnerships have replaced a large part of national production. With the introduction of the triple viral vaccine (measles, rubella, and mumps), the production of measles vaccine has been stopped. The arrival of the pentavalent vaccine (diphtheria, whooping cough, tetanus, hepatitis B, and *Haemophilus influenzae* type b) meant that DPT was only used as a reinforcement. In some countries, such as Brazil, its use was replaced by nationally produced quadruple DPT-Hib vaccine. Some types of production, such as oral polio vaccine produced in cell cultures in Mexico, are highly likely to be replaced in the short term by inactivated polio vaccine. Smaller productions in Chile, Venezuela, and Colombia have been reduced or totally eliminated.

In the Region, attempts at self-supplying vaccines in the 1990s were affected by the use of new products introduced by immunization programs in most countries. Today, few producers in the Region have the capacity to modernize their technical infrastructure and installations to produce the combined vaccines that are necessary to meet the demands of their immunization programs. Judging from WHO certification, just two products are prequalified for good manufacturing practices: the yellow fever vaccine in Brazil and the hepatitis B vaccine in Cuba. Some products, such as the *Haemophilus influenzae* type b polysaccharide-tetanus protein conjugate in Cuba and the quadruple vaccine (DPT-Hib) in Brazil, are promising efforts, seeking review for prequalification by WHO. The valuable attempts made by the governments of Venezuela, Colombia, and Cuba to reinitiate the production of DPT (Venezuela and Cuba) and yellow fever vaccines (Colombia) with the development of new production plants that meet current standards for complying with good manufacturing practices are worth mentioning.

As an alternative for continuing with competitive production, some producers are associating with international manufacturers outside the Region. For example in Brazil, BioManguinhos (which produces Hib and triple viral vaccines) and the Instituto Butantan (which produces seasonal influenza vaccines) have established partnerships with European pharmaceutical consortia.

Vaccine Regulation

The national regulatory authorities (NRAs) are the main agencies responsible for guaranteeing the quality of vaccines used in the countries and to that end they need to work in permanent cooperation with the immunization programs. PAHO conducts a continuous training program in the basic functions of the NRAs in the area of vaccines, to guarantee compliance with the six basic functions (licensing, good manufacturing practices, lot release, laboratory testing, clinical evaluation, and post-marketing surveillance) required by WHO for the NRAs in vaccine-producing countries and in at least two functions for the NRAs in countries that purchase products through United Nations agencies.

An additional challenge for the NRAs in Latin America has been the growth in the market for new vaccines whose clinical development and licensing processes do not take place in the country of biological production. Traditionally, licensing in the country of origin (in general a developed country) was a quality assurance for NRAs in the Region. However, with new products that are not a necessity in the country of origin, first licensing is granted by the NRA that buys the product for the first time, meaning that it assumes responsibility for comprehensive evaluation of the vaccine, including the analysis and interpretation of the first clinical trials obtained during its development. This holds true for the new vaccines against rotavirus and the human papilloma virus, which have been made available to the Latin American and Caribbean countries.

To support the NRAs in the challenge posed by the arrival of the new vaccines, PAHO's Essential Medicines, Vaccines and Health Technologies Unit has organized a series of courses and workshops to present alternatives for evaluating the information, which are included in the common technical document (dossier) and offer training materials for the authorities to generate the technical experience needed for comprehensive evaluation of the new products, including the production process, quality control, stability and preclinical tests, and clinical trials. Evaluation of the effectiveness of the new products constitutes an additional element in the task of the NRAs, for which the introduction of these new biologicals poses a challenge but also an opportunity for joint and individual growth in knowledge and experience in the important function of vaccine regulation.

Imaging and Radiotherapy Services

Imaging Services

Conventional diagnostic radiology (basic and specialized), interventional radiology, echography, and diagnostic and therapeutic nuclear medicine are currently playing an essential function in clinical health care processes (*112*). These diagnostic imaging services cover a wide range of clinical applications, from the diagnosis and monitoring of very common diseases and situations with a high incidence, such as respiratory diseases, traumas, digestive disorders, control of pregnancy and breast disorders, etc., to more complex diseases such as tumors, AIDS, central nervous system conditions, or cardiovascular diseases (*113*). Image formation technologies continue to be a rapidly changing field and are revolutionizing each medical specialty. This is partly due to the high level of innovation demonstrated by the companies that manufacture the equipment.

Progress in communications technology over the last decade has directly influenced health sciences in the field of telemedicine and, in particular, teleradiology. In the United States, teleradiology billings have grown exponentially over the last five years. Teleradiology involves applications available through communications networks—a virtual world in which the connection between the place where the images are generated and the place where they are interpreted is based more on business models and the Internet than on the person who is on duty when the image needs to be read (*114*). These advances can be very useful in places where there is a shortage of radiologists to interpret the images, such as in the Caribbean, the Amazon, or remote areas such as Easter Island. However, although introduction of this technology is being explored in different parts of Latin America and the Caribbean, no successful case has been reported, which is undoubtedly due to the lack of adequate and stable communications infrastructure and the shortage of financial resources to make the initial investments and maintain the network.

Another example of technological progress is the increased use of interventional radiology in recent years. It is now possible to treat different diseases using cannulae or embolization media (*115*), which permits patients to be treated as outpatients instead of requiring long hospital stays. Governments and the public around the world have quickly come to appreciate the benefits of interventional radiology, and therefore there is considerable pressure from the public and the media to expand the spectrum of these procedures. As a result, the practice of interventional radiology has spread broadly in countries that offer all health care levels in a relatively short time.

Digital radiology, which uses devices to store photostimulable phosphorus, was introduced into clinical practice in the 1980s. It is another imaging area that has seen surprising changes and whose use has gradually increased in Latin America and the Caribbean. New types of digital imaging formation devices are being introduced on the market (*116*).

In the area of computerized tomography, first with the introduction of explorations with helical and more recently with multislice techniques, examination times per patient have been shortened considerably. It is now possible to perform more examinations in a given time, expand the scope of certain examinations, and introduce certain new techniques and examinations, for example in cardiology. The new image formation devices hold great promise for diagnosing a variety of cardiovascular anomalies.

The United Nations Scientific Committee on the Effects of Atomic Radiation (UNSCEAR) periodically examines the world status of radiology services. At present, UNSCEAR is preparing a report that will be presented to the United Nations General Assembly in 2007. PAHO is cooperating with this activity in the Americas. The last report presented to the General Assembly and officially published dates from 2000 (*117*).

In most countries of the Region, the level of access to radiology services is far lower than in the industrialized countries. While the annual frequency of radiological studies exceeds 1,000 per 1,000 population in the latter group, in health care level 2 countries (including 22 countries of the Region) the value is around 150, and in level 3 countries (five countries) it is about 20. Apart from being scarce, access to radiology services is inequitable, since most of these services are provided in health centers in the big cities, and so a large part of the rural population has no access

to them. Their high cost also makes them inaccessible to poor urban populations.

The clinical efficiency of these services hinges on the quality of care provided. The existence of well-trained professionals and implementation of quality assurance programs are essential for achieving the main objective, which is an accurate diagnosis. A multicenter study conducted by PAHO in Argentina, Bolivia, Colombia, Cuba, and Mexico demonstrated that there is a direct relationship between the accuracy of radiological interpretation and the quality of radiographic images. In all cases, radiologists from the participating institutions and a panel of external experts reached coinciding diagnoses when they examined good-quality images but there were discrepancies when the images were poor. In turn, the quality of the images was directly related to the training of radiology technicians, the quality of film processing, and the condition of the film/screen combination. The study concludes that stress should be placed on ongoing training for technicians and on procuring and maintaining equipment and accessories, particularly negatoscopes, intensifier screens, and developer machines on account of the influence they have on the quality of the images and therefore on accurate diagnoses (*118*). The clinical advantages of imaging services are enormous; however, in practice these services can represent an unnecessary cost for health care systems in the countries of the Region if the quality is unacceptable (*113*).

Radiotherapy Services

Radiotherapy is used today for the treatment of many kinds of tumors, and is frequently administered in combination with surgery or chemotherapy or both. The goal of radiotherapy is to achieve cytotoxic levels of irradiation at well-defined target volumes, minimizing to the extent possible the exposure of healthy surrounding tissues. Internationally, it is believed that radiotherapy will continue to be key for the treatment of cancer in the coming decades. Its curative function is particularly important for tumors of the head and neck, cervix-uterus, breast, and prostate, to say nothing of its palliative function and effectiveness in relation to the cost of all these diseases. In comparison with other types of therapy, the costs per patient treated are relatively low if the equipment is used optimally.

Malignant neoplasms are the second-leading case of death in the Region (*119*). Recent reports from specialized agencies suggest that the population will continue to grow and will gradually age in Latin America and the Caribbean (*120*). WHO has called attention to the significant increase expected in the number of cancer patients in the developing countries in the near future and, aware of this problem, in 2005 the 58th World Health Assembly approved a resolution on cancer prevention and control that recognizes the importance of radiotherapy in managing and treating this disease (*121*).

Radiotherapy is applied using one of two methods: teletherapy in which a beam of radiation outside the body is targeted to tissue;

"Equity and efficiency are two of the basic requirements of a health service system."

Carlyle Guerra de Macedo, 1989

and brachytherapy in which radioactive sources are placed in a natural body cavity or inserted directly into a tumor. The therapeutic external radiation beams most commonly used are produced by two types of machines: cobalt units that contain radioactive sources of Co-60, which are the most widely used in Latin America and the Caribbean, and linear accelerators, which are more common in the industrialized countries and which are gradually being introduced in Latin American and Caribbean countries.

According to the database of the Directory of Radiotherapy Centers (DIRAC) kept by the International Atomic Energy Agency (IAEA/WHO) (122), in 2005, the industrialized countries had an average of 6.4 high energy radiotherapy units per 1 million population, while the average in Latin America and the Caribbean was 1.4 per 1 million population, and there are countries whose average is far below that figure, such as Peru, Nicaragua, El Salvador, Guatemala, and Haiti, and others where these services are virtually nonexistent, such as many Caribbean countries. As for the human resources compiled in DIRAC, the data for the industrialized countries indicate there are 9 radiotherapists and 5 medical physicists for 1 million population, compared to 1.6 and 0.7 per 1 million in Latin America and the Caribbean, while in the field of technology, 86% of teletherapy units are linear accelerators in the former, with the figure falling to 42% in Latin America and the Caribbean. Also, most of the technology and clinical techniques in use date back to the 1960s and 1970s which reduces their therapeutic impact on different diseases. As a consequence, while the industrialized countries cure approximately half of their cancer patients and at least half of the patients diagnosed require radiotherapy, in many Latin American and Caribbean countries neither the technology nor appropriate human resources are available to provide such services (123) and in some cases access to them is very limited or nonexistent.

According to the GLOBOCAN 2002 database of the International Center for Cancer Research (IARC), a WHO agency (124), the annual incidence of cancer in Latin America and the Caribbean is about 833,000 cases, in other words, fewer than 200 cases per 100,000 population. The figure appears to reflect underestimations if it is compared with the numerical data available in some of the Region's ministries of health and is far below the figure for the more industrialized countries of nearly 500 cases per 100,000 population.

Many factors influence the effectiveness and safety of radiotherapy treatments, such as accurate diagnosis and the stage of the disease, good therapeutic decisions, the precise location of the tumor, and the planning and delivery of treatment. This com-

plexity points to the need to introduce quality assurance programs to improve the effectiveness and safety of treatments. Given the limited therapeutic capacity described above and taking the estimate of 833,000 new cases a year as valid, calculations indicate that in Latin America and the Caribbean at least 120,000 patients will die each year who could potentially have been cured if they had had access to radiotherapy services that operated properly under national cancer control programs.

Planning and Management of Imaging and Radiotherapy Diagnostic Services

The costs of these services, considering both the initial investment and operating costs, make careful planning and management of their development necessary, but the latter are not always adequate in the Region, which means that the services are less effective than desirable. Frequently, the costs of procuring and maintaining equipment are much higher than in the industrialized countries, and geographic distribution and use times are not optimum. All these aspects become more critical with the incorporation of more complex and costly methods, such as computerized tomography, magnetic resonance imaging, linear accelerators, and high-dose brachytherapy.

The developing countries face different challenges in adopting health technologies, since most of the medical devices are designed for use in the industrialized countries. As a result, close to 30% of complex equipment goes unused, while the equipment that operates is out of service between 25% and 35% of the time owing to poor maintenance capacity. One fundamental reason is inefficient management of the technologies, including planning, procurement, and subsequent operation (125).

For management purposes, it is crucial to differentiate between equipment and service: a magnetic resonance machine is not a magnetic imaging service, and a linear accelerator is not a radiotherapy service. One of the common mistakes made by some health managers when they incorporate complex technology is failing to consider in the planning process many of the elements necessary for the operation of the services prior to incorporating the technology. Decisionmakers often focus on the equipment rather than on the service, despite the fact that the service is the main thing for health care.

Aware of this problem, some ministries of health, for example those in Argentina, Costa Rica, El Salvador, Guatemala, Venezuela, and Uruguay, have asked PAHO for technical cooperation in introducing and placing these technologies in service more effectively and adequately. The financial and health costs of technology problems are significant in countries like Argentina, Brazil, Colombia, Dominica, Haiti, Honduras, Panama, Paraguay, and Venezuela, where equipment costing millions of dollars that has been bought or donated has never been put into service or is significantly underused. The causes of these problems are many, but the common denominator is the lack of analysis of the situation by experts prior to buying equipment. It should be kept in mind in particular that private or institutional donors frequently do not have sufficient technical capacity to carry out the processes of incorporating equipment satisfactorily.

Protection against Radiation Risks

The advantages and risks of using radiation in medical, industrial, or research applications are well known. The high potential risk for health that their use implies makes it necessary to take special precautions to protect patients, workers, the public, and the environment from radiation. International organizations with mandates in this field, including PAHO, agreed by consensus on the International Basic Safety Standards for Protection against Ionizing Radiation and for the Safety of Radiation Sources (BSS) (126), at the 24th Pan American Sanitary Conference (Resolution CSP24.R9) (127), which include among the technical requisites the need to implement a broad program of quality assurance in medical exposure to radiation, with the participation of qualified experts in the corresponding disciplines, keeping in mind the principles established by WHO and PAHO and counting on national regulatory authorities.

Today, the world is going through a period of major technological changes in the fields of imaging and radiotherapy, and the impact of these changes on the doses of radiation that the future population of the world will receive is very difficult to predict. Facility in acquiring images through new technologies could lead to unnecessary exposure of patients to radiation, unless timely measures are adopted. This, coupled with the increase in the amount of equipment, will have significant repercussions on the doses of radiation that the public receives, making it important for regulatory authorities to continue evaluating protection and safety in medical radiology.

After the recommendations of an international conference on radiological protection of patients held in 2001, the International Atomic Energy Agency, WHO, PAHO, and UNSCEAR prepared an International Action Plan for the Radiological Protection of Patients (128) which includes a strategy to help the countries oversee medical exposure doses. It is hoped that implementation of this plan—which has already established activities for 2006/2008—will modify the growing trend toward medical exposure in the future.

As for regulatory capacity, just 21 countries of the Region have authorities with specific mandates in this sphere and where they exist, in many cases their technical capacity and resources are too limited to satisfactorily carry out the functions established in the national regulations adapted from the BSS. Where regulations exist, the competent authority is located in the ministry of health, in other government agencies, or divided between the two. In all events, exposure to medical radiation should be regulated by the ministries of health. The weakness and scant involvement by the health authorities in this area are of concern in many countries and jeopardize the safety of patients, and even their lives (129, 130).

Failure to manage spent radioactive sources is common in Latin American and Caribbean countries. Closely related to this and to the environmental impact that this waste can have, radioactive waste needs to be properly managed, including its preparation and safe storage. A number of radiological accidents have occurred in the Region, some of which have caused deaths (131). This circumstance, coupled with the current international situation in which terrorists might use radioactive materials and the scant response capacity to radiological emergencies, demands improvements in preparedness and response in this field.

It should be underlined that WHO has started up an international project on the health risks of electromagnetic fields. In the Region there is growing public concern over these risks, while standards and technical knowledge in this sphere vary widely from country to country (132).

Blood Services

Voluntary blood donation continues to be weak in the Region. The 2002 edition of this publication listed Aruba, Bermuda, Canada, Cuba, Curaçao, Saint Lucia, and the United States as countries with universal voluntary donors; the Cayman Islands, Suriname, and Uruguay reached that goal in 2004. Bolivia, Dominican Republic, Honduras, Panama, Paraguay, and Peru officially report paying blood donors, but the exchange of money between the patients' relatives and blood donors is common in all those countries where forced replacement donation is imposed by hospital-based blood banks. Despite the fact that 2 million prospective donors were deferred in 2004, when about 8 million units of blood were collected in the Caribbean and Latin America, 150,000 units were discarded because the donors carried one or more of the markers for transfusion-transmitted infections, a figure that represents at least US $ 7.5 million in collection and testing supplies. More importantly, the lack of voluntary blood donors results in insufficient blood components and hampers universal screening of blood. In 2004, 16 of the 39 countries with data reported testing all the blood collected for transfusions, compared with 14 in 2000, but the Region as a whole has not achieved 100% coverage of screening for any of the basic markers of infections (Tables 15 and 16), which was the goal set in the Strategic and Programmatic Orientations of the Pan American Health Organization for 1999-2002. Tests to detect hepatitis C, *Trypanosoma cruzi*, and human T-lymphotropic virus type 2 (HTLV-II) pose the biggest challenge.

The other goal set in the Strategic and Programmatic Orientations for 1999–2002, that all blood banks must participate in quality programs, has not been achieved either. Almost half of the blood banks do not participate in external evaluation of performance, and incorrect results are common among those who do. The excessive number of blood banks, mostly associated with hospitals, limits the implementation of quality programs and contributes to the poor efficiency of national systems. Overall,

TABLE 15. Blood services: blood collection and screening for infectious markers, countries of Latin America, 2003 and 2004.

Country	Year	No. of blood banks	No of units collected	HIV	HBsAg	VHC	Syphilis	Trypanosoma cruzi
Argentina	2003	578	780,440	100	100	99	100	100
	2004	578	751,412	100	100	99	100	100
Bolivia	2003	38	38,621	94	93	82	95	80
	2004	25	40,910	99	99	93	99	83
Brazil	2003	367	2,931,813	100	100	100	100	100
	2004	562	3,044,493	100	100	100	100	100
Chile	2003	55	173,814	100	100	100	100	67
	2004	52	186,292	100	100	100	100	68
Colombia	2003	142	495,004	99	99	99	99	99
	2004	123	502,065	99	99	99	100	99
Costa Rica	2003	24	48,625	100	100	100	100	93
	2004	31	54,258	100	100	100	100	100
Cuba	2003	44	589,106	100	100	100	100	...
	2004	47	528,026	100	100	100	100	...
Dominican Republic	2003	81	77,115	100	100	100	100	...
	2004	66	61,745	99	99	99	99	...
Ecuador	2003	33	79,204	100	100	100	100	100
	2004	39	98,695	100	100	100	100	100
El Salvador	2003	32	76,142	100	100	100	100	100
	2004	32	79,368	100	100	100	100	100
Guatemala	2003	48	68,626	99	99	99	99	99
	2004	46	60,638	99	99	100	99	99
Honduras	2003	28	48,783	100	100	100	100	100
	2004	29	47,679	99	99	100	99	99
Mexico	2003	540	1,136,047	100	100	100	100	33
	2004	536	1,225,688	96	96	96	90	32
Nicaragua	2003	24	46,558	100	100	76	100	94
	2004	24	49,416	100	100	85	100	100
Panama	2003	23	46,176	100	100	100	100	95
	2004	25	44,323	100	100	100	100	86
Paraguay	2003	49	29,718	97	96	96	95	96
	2004	45	41,846	99	99	99	99	99
Peru	2003	92	145,665	99	96	99	94	96
	2004	172	183,489	74	74	74	74	75
Uruguay	2003	41	99,675	100	100	100	100	100
	2004	67	96,993	100	100	100	100	100
Venezuela	2003	270	342,526	100	100	100	100	100
	2004	270	380,724	100	100	100	100	100

Sources: Pan American Health Organization. Blood Transfusion Medicine in the Caribbean and Latin American Countries 2000–2003. Washington, DC: PAHO, 2005. Pan American Health Organization. Technical Documents. Policies and Regulations.THS/EV-2005/005. Washington, DC: OPS; 2006.

blood banks collect and process an average of 1,600 units of blood per year. Incorrect identification of potentially infected donors is more common in smaller blood banks, especially in those that use rapid tests for screening. Furthermore, because hospital-based blood banks tend to collect and process blood in unsystematic ways, sharing blood units among them is virtually nonexistent—a situation that in 2004 prompted discarding about 175,000 outdated blood units with an estimated processing cost of US $ 8,750 million. Countries with the lowest availability of blood tend to discard more blood units.

Clinical and Public Health Laboratories

Of the estimated 40,000 laboratories in the Region, 98% are clinical diagnostic laboratories and 2% are public health laboratories. Most clinical laboratories belong to the private sector, and the public health laboratories generally come under the ministries of health. In most countries, a national reference laboratory heads a network of public health laboratories that may or may not be linked to a hospital, as part of the surveillance system. Apart from these activities, which are carried out in coordination with epidemiology departments, the public health laboratories

TABLE 16. Blood services: blood collection and screening for infectious markers, countries of the Caribbean, 2003 and 2004.

Country	Year	No. of blood banks	No of units collected	HIV	HBsAg	VHC	Syphilis	HTLVI/II
Anguilla	2003	1	124	100	100	...	100	...
	2004	1	78	100	100	...	100	...
Antigua and Barbuda	2003	2	1,330	100	100	...	100	...
	2004	2	1,227	100	100	11	100	...
Aruba	2003	2	2,651	100	100	100	100	100
Bahamas	2003	3	5,134	100	100	100	100	100
	2004	3	5,521	100	100	100	100	100
Belize	2003	7	2,883	100	100	...	100	...
	2004	7	2,978	100	100	...	100	...
Bermuda	2003	1	2.277	100	100	100	100	...
British Virgin Islands	2003	1	318	100	100	52	100	...
	2004	1	343	100	100	100	100	...
Cayman Islands	2003	2	731	100	100	100	100	100
	2004	2	702	100	100	100	100	100
Curaçao	2003	1	6,066	100	100	100	100	100
	2004	1	6,595	100	100	100	100	100
Dominica	2004	1	804	100	100	...	100	100
Grenada	2003	1	808	100	100	100	100	100
	2004	1	703	100	100	100	100	100
Guyana	2003	5	4,250	100	100	100	100	...
	2004	5	4,887	100	100	100	100	...
Haiti	2003	5	8,711	100	100	89	100	...
	2004	8	9,513	100	100	93	100	...
Jamaica	2003	10	26,092	100	100	100	100	100
	2004	10	23,600	100	100	100	100	100
Montserrat	2003	1	66	100	100	...	100	...
	2004	1	83	100	100	...	100	...
Saint Kitts and Nevis	2003	1	420	100	100	...	100	...
	2004	1	347	100	100	...	100	...
Saint Lucia	2003	2	1,653	100	100	100	100	100
	2004	3	1,782	100	100	100	100	100
Saint Vincent and the Grenadines	2003	1	939	100	100	100	100	100
	2004	1	942	100	100	100	100	100
Suriname	2003	1	6,240	100	100	100	100	100
	2004	1	7,696	100	100	100	100	100
Turks and Caicos Islands	2003	2	211	100	100	60	100	...

Sources: Pan American Health Organization. Blood Transfusion Medicine in the Caribean and Latin American Countries 2000–2003. Washington, DC: PAHO, 2005. Pan American Health Organization. Technical Documents. Policies and Regulations.THS/EV-2005/005. Washington, DC: OPS; 2006.

can perform tests as part of the licensing and control of medicines. Each country's reference laboratory has the authority for standardization, regulation, training, planning, supervision, evaluation, investigation, and dissemination of information.

Public health institutions, and laboratory services in particular, are essential for the surveillance of diseases and play a central role in the epidemic investigation chain. However, problems frequently exist in the Region with regard to organization, management, and financial resources. The common denominator for the shortcomings is that the information produced is not always of good quality. These factors mean that the decisionmaking process and the design of interventions are limited and that public health

laboratories are unable to carry out their essential role in the health system.

These developments, apart from other factors related to the context and development of the disciplines involved, have been forging a clearer concept of the public health function that a laboratory should perform. The function includes the sustainable implementation of a quality management system in the networks of laboratories; close linkage with epidemiological surveillance of diseases, whose reporting is mandatory, and the International Health Regulations; the indispensable integration of actions to respond to outbreaks and emergencies; and support for epidemiological research.

❝*The effective management of information is critical to stopping the spread of new pandemics, whether infectious or noninfectious in origin.*❞

George A.O. Alleyne, 1998

Publication of the *Laboratory Quality Assurance Manual on General Concepts for Public Health Laboratories* in 2002, based on ISO 9001, launched the introduction of the quality system in public health reference institutions in the Region and led to restructuring of laboratory networks in Bolivia, Colombia, Dominican Republic, Ecuador, Honduras, Panama, Paraguay, and Uruguay. Two regional workshops, one on laboratory management aspects and the other on quality management systems, attended by public health reference laboratory directors, consolidated the feasibility of the process.

To consolidate the linkage between laboratories and epidemiology and step up surveillance for infectious diseases in the Region, two subregional meetings were held in Central America and South America on basic concepts in epidemiology and data analysis in the laboratory. Under agreements reached at the annual meetings of the Central American Network for the Prevention and Control of Emerging and Reemerging Diseases (RECACER) in 2002 and 2003, a model questionnaire was prepared to evaluate the response capacity of national laboratory networks to contain epidemic events. This tool was used in the processes of restructuring the national laboratory networks in the countries in question.

The most recent natural disasters in the Region—El Niño and hurricanes Mitch and George in Central America and the Dominican Republic; Stan and Katrina in Cuba, Mexico, and the United States; the earthquake in El Salvador; volcanic eruptions in Ecuador and Colombia; landslides in Venezuela; floods in Haiti, Guyana, Guatemala, Argentina, and Colombia, etc.—highlighted the need to integrate the public health laboratories into health sector contingency plans and revealed the importance of having diagnostic confirmation of highly lethal transmissible diseases and having basic tests for management of the injured and the timely provision of safe blood.

Efforts were directed to integrating the laboratory component into the surveillance system by defining seven essential functions of public health laboratories: (1) public health referral; (2) strengthening of the surveillance system; (3) integrated information management; (4) development of policies and regulations; (5) ongoing training and education; (6) research promotion and development; and (7) communications and strategic partnerships. In advance of technical and managerial training for laboratory directors, the methodology was harmonized in Central America by preparing consensual manuals of procedures for acute diarrheas, acute respiratory infections, bacterial meningitis, dengue, leptospirosis, measles, hantavirus, anthrax, and tuberculosis, and on the regional level the process of external evaluation of performance was broadened with support from the National Tropical Disease Center (CENETROP) in Santa Cruz, Bolivia, the regional program for monitoring and surveillance of resistance to antibiotics, and the system of networks for the surveillance of bacterial agents that cause pneumonia and meningitis (Regional Vaccine System—SIREVA II), in 20 countries.

As for clinical diagnostic laboratories, with the cooperation of the Latin American Confederation of Clinical Biochemistry (COLABIOCLI), the regulations on laboratory certification were reviewed and updated in Costa Rica, Ecuador, Guatemala, Honduras, Nicaragua, and Panama. Sustainable programs were established for external evaluation of clinical biochemistry performance targeted to public and private laboratories in seven countries. Also, through the United Kingdom International External Quality Assessment Scheme (UK-IEQAS) an external evaluation of performance in clinical chemistry, hematology, and parasitology was conducted in 20 countries: Argentina, Bahamas, Barbados, Belize, Brazil, Chile, Colombia, Costa Rica, Cuba, Dominican Republic, Ecuador, El Salvador, Honduras, Jamaica, Mexico, Nicaragua, Paraguay, Suriname, Uruguay, and Venezuela.

SCIENTIFIC INFORMATION ON HEALTH: ACCESS AND UTILIZATION

As an activity to produce new knowledge to benefit society, research and its products are a classical example of a public good.[17] In recent years, access to scientific information and its use have become crucially important in a new global scenario where governments, users, and interested parties are required to demonstrate greater accountability and transparency in the management of resources. This reality extends to the agencies and organizations that operate social programs, since citizen dissatisfaction with them if they fail to attain their goals is often expressed at the ballot box. Therefore, reliable data and scientific information are needed to establish health priorities and to monitor and evaluate the performance of systems versus the goals or expected outcomes.

In the area of health systems, research is one of the 11 essential public health functions and one of the least developed in the Region over the last decade (5). However, significant initiatives were promoted to establish and strengthen mechanisms for oversight and governance in health research. Some of them, such as the Latin American and Caribbean Center on Health Sciences Information (BIREME), have been catalysts for regional progress in networks to promote solidarity and equity (networks of health li-

---

[17] Health research studies how social, economic, technological, and behavioral factors and other aspects related to the structure and organization of systems affect access to health care, the quality and cost of care, and the health and well-being of individuals, families, and communities. The main goals are not simply to learn but to identify the most effective ways to organize, finance, and deliver more effective, equitable, and safe care. (Source: AcademyHealth, June 2000; Agency for Healthcare Research and Quality, February 2002).

braries, resources, and information centers). For example, the LILACS (Latin American and Caribbean Literature on Health Sciences) database, which is more than 25 years old, collects and registers the content of peer-reviewed scientific journals published in the Region, most of which do not appear in international databases. The SciELO (Scientific Electronic Library Online) network was developed later with the participation of national science and technology agencies. Its objective is to raise the visibility and quality of scientific journals in the Region, improve access to them, and establish indicators for evaluating their use and impact. In 1998, the Virtual Health Library (VHL) was created, which received contributions from several national and thematic initiatives and brings together a broad range of health information sources. The VHL is active in many countries of the Region, where it is developed to different degrees, but follows a common model and responds to national conditions and needs.

During the World Summit on the Information Society which was held in two phases, the first in 2003 and the second in 2005 (133), a call was made to promote universal access to scientific knowledge that affects the development and well-being of peoples. It also advocated the incorporation of new formats to facilitate the use of research results and the democratization of knowledge (134). However, one essential factor is still missing for efficiently targeting efforts and avoiding duplication of work: good situation analysis indicators and resources for research are not available in the Latin American and Caribbean countries.

Trends in Scientific Production in Latin America and the Caribbean: 2000–2005

As for the development of indicators to study scientific production in health in the Region, mention should be made of publications of systematic reviews and clinical trials that reflect the results of studies that are frequently used to synthesize and dis-

seminate new knowledge for informed decisionmaking in health, and which are specially indexed. Publications of this kind account for almost 4.6% of all the documents indexed between 2000 and 2005 in the MEDLINE database and 0.8% of those registered in LILACS (Table 17).

To analyze the publication of systematic reviews and clinical trials by country, we used the country of publication of the journals in LILACS and MEDLINE, considering that the index is not organized by country of affiliation (Table 18). In the studies published in Latin American journals indexed in MEDLINE (0.51% of the total indexed in that database) Argentina, Brazil, and Mexico stand out with 83% of the total. In LILACS, Argentina, Brazil, and Colombia contributed 76% of the Latin American total for the period.

As there is no registry of the production of new knowledge and information is not widely available, indirect indicators were used for the production of new knowledge in health, such as the number of original scientific studies published in indexed journals. In the period 2000–2005, MEDLINE registered 66,322 publications by authors from 37 countries of the Region (Table 19). Latin America and the Caribbean's share in the MEDLINE database averaged 2% of world production.

LILACS lists authors from 23 countries who produced 92,794 publications in the same period (Table 20). LILACS began to identify the countries of affiliation of authors in 2000 and considers all authors, unlike MEDLINE which focuses on the first-named author. Seven countries contributed 94% of Latin American and Caribbean scientific publications appearing in both databases: Argentina, Brazil, Chile, Colombia, Cuba, Mexico, and Venezuela.

If registration in the most representative international databases is taken as a quality indicator, it can be inferred that there has been a gradual improvement in the quality of scientific journals in recent years (Table 21—see the footnote to the table). In MEDLINE, the total number of Latin American journals indexed

TABLE 17. Clinical trials and systematic reviews indexed in LILACS and MEDLINE, 2000–2005.

Types of articles	Total	2000	2001	2002	2003	2004	2005
LILACS							
CT+SR	994	163	172	177	189	185	108
Other types	116,141	21,909	20,260	20,876	20,386	18,212	14,498
Total registered	117,135	22,072	20,432	21,053	20,575	18,397	14,606
% total	0.8	0.7	0.8	0.8	0.9	1.0	0.7
MEDLINE							
CT+SR	150,879	21,151	22,130	23,666	25,796	28,313	29,823
Other types	3,158,544	468,630	496,441	516,260	541,243	565,310	570,660
Total registered	3,309,423	489,781	518,571	539,926	567,039	593,623	600,483
% total	4.6	4.3	4.3	4.4	4.5	4.8	5.0

CT = clinical trials; SR = systematic reviews

Sources: MEDLINE; Virtual Health Library; Latin American and Caribbean Literature on Health Sciences (LILACS), October 2006.

TABLE 18. Clinical trials and systematic reviews published in Latin American and Caribbean journals indexed in MEDLINE and LILACS, 2000–2005.

Country	Total		2000		2001		2002		2003		2004		2005	
	MEDLINE	LILACS	MEDLINE	LILACS	MEDLINE	LILACS	MEDLINE	LILACS	MEDLINE	LILACS	MEDLINE	LILACS	MEDLINE	LILACS
Argentina	61	94	6	17	9	12	10	16	13	17	12	19	11	13
Bolivia	0	12	0	1	0	0	0	4	0	5	0	1	0	1
Brazil	417	457	47	68	59	65	64	76	63	96	85	100	99	52
Chile	59	60	14	6	5	10	5	8	7	11	15	16	13	9
Colombia	9	203	0	30	0	48	0	40	6	39	0	24	3	22
Costa Rica	1	4	1	0	0	0	1	1	0	1	0	2	0	0
Cuba	6	20	0	4	0	6	1	1	3	2	1	4	0	3
Ecuador	0	1	0	0	0	1	0	0	0	0	0	0	0	0
Guatemala	0	1	0	1	0	0	0	0	0	0	0	0	0	0
Jamaica	15	6	6	4	1	1	1	0	1	0	0	0	6	1
Mexico	166	47	26	17	20	12	32	13	30	4	25	1	33	0
Nicaragua	0	13	0	1	0	4	0	1	0	1	0	5	0	1
Panama	1	0	0	0	1	0	0	0	0	0	0	0	0	0
Paraguay	0	1	0	0	0	0	0	1	0	0	0	0	0	0
Peru	8	9	0	2	2	3	0	0	2	2	1	0	3	2
Puerto Rico	11	6	2	1	0	1	0	0	2	0	3	3	4	1
United States (PAHO)	0	5	0	3	0	0	0	0	0	0	0	1	0	0
Uruguay	0	2	0	1	0	0	0	0	0	1	0	0	0	0
Venezuela	20	53	2	7	6	9	2	15	3	10	5	9	2	3
Total LILACS		994		163		172		177		189		185		108
Latin American and Caribbean representation in MEDLINE	774		104		103		116		130		147		174	
World total in MEDLINE	150,879		21,151		22,130		23,666		25,796		28,313		29,823	
% Latin America and Caribbean in MEDLINE	0.5		0.5		0.5		0.5		0.5		0.5		0.6	

Source: MEDLINE; Virtual Health Library, October 2006.

TABLE 19. Latin American and Caribbean publications in MEDLINE by country of affiliation of the first-named author, 2000–2005.

MEDLINE	Publications	2000	2001	2002	2003	2004	2005
World total (2000–2005)	3,150,403	483,885	500,961	517,481	544,402	564,440	539,234
Latin American and Caribbean total	66,322	8,978	9,833	11,229	12,174	13,282	10,826
Percentage of world total	2.1	1.9	2.0	2.2	2.2	2.4	2.0
Total by country							
Antigua	3	1	1	—	—	—	1
Argentina	9,642	1,496	1,648	1,747	1,658	1,707	1,386
Bahamas	20	3	2	5	6	1	3
Barbados	89	13	14	16	16	19	11
Belize	3	—	—	—	2	—	1
Bolivia	63	14	9	19	8	8	5
Brazil	33,329	4,107	4,574	5,545	6,281	7,015	5,807
Chile	3,913	577	576	657	723	753	627
Colombia	1,407	171	176	265	253	285	257
Costa Rica	343	40	84	59	67	40	53
Cuba	1,445	226	252	219	278	291	179
Dominica	5	—	2	—	1	2	—
Dominican Republic	20	6	3	2	4	3	2
Ecuador	179	24	19	29	43	34	30
El Salvador	22	2	3	6	1	4	6
French Guiana	65	6	12	8	10	16	13
Grenada	120	39	15	17	12	21	16
Guadeloupe	50	19	11	4	7	7	2
Guatemala	87	10	16	21	14	15	11
Guyana	5	1	1	2	—	1	—
Haiti	39	5	2	8	5	9	10
Honduras	23	2	2	3	4	5	7
Jamaica	377	65	106	67	34	60	45
Martinique	36	7	11	4	2	8	4
Mexico	10,896	1,533	1,647	1,863	1,992	2,164	1,697
Netherlands Antilles	30	4	4	4	5	8	5
Nicaragua	39	5	2	7	5	11	9
Panama	316	32	46	47	56	80	55
Paraguay	41	6	7	6	9	8	5
Peru	484	54	75	72	95	102	86
Puerto Rico	540	47	75	60	105	160	93
Saint Lucia	1	—	—	1	—	—	—
Suriname	26	1	5	2	3	5	10
Trinidad and Tobago	210	40	38	40	35	30	27
Uruguay	749	112	112	113	132	140	140
U.S. Virgin Islands	5	2	2	—	1	—	—
Venezuela	1,700	308	281	311	307	270	223

Sources: MEDLINE; Virtual Health Library, June 2006.

rose from 45 (2000) to 66 (2005). In the databases of Thomson Scientific (a company that manages the registry previously known as ISI), the health journals indexed increased in number from 21 (2000) to 32 (2005). The percentage of journals from the Region is still very small compared to the total indexed in international databases. They represent 1.3% in MEDLINE, 0.4% in the Science Citation Index, and 1.9% in EMBASE.

One of the objectives for developing the LILACS database was to index journals published in the countries of the Region and to work with the journals to unify standards and raise the visibility of regional publications. All the journals indexed in LILACS are chosen by national selection committees and must comply with minimum requirements for frequency, regularity, and peer review. Some 1,500 journals on health are published in the Region and 738 of them were selected for inclusion in LILACS. These journals are published in 19 Latin American and Caribbean countries and by PAHO (Table 21). SciELO's selection criteria (http://www.scielo. org/scielo_org_en.htm) are stricter than those of LILACS and comparable with the main international databases. SciELO includes journals from 11 Latin American and Caribbean countries,

TABLE 20. Latin American and Caribbean publications in LILACS, by country of affiliation of the authors, 2000–2005.

LILACS (2000–2005)	Publications	2000	2001	2002	2003	2004	2005
Total in the database	92,794	16,558	16,221	16,195	16,849	15,203	11,768
Total with country identified	77,353	12,251	12,999	13,365	13,984	12,986	11,768
Total Latin America and the Caribbean	73,927	12,073	12,709	12,958	13,499	12,503	10,185
Total with country unknown	16,697	4,307	3,222	2,830	2,865	2,217	1,256
Total by country							
Argentina	6,331	1,142	1,211	1,071	1,133	1,017	757
Barbados	19	2	7	3	2	5	—
Bolivia	270	36	47	53	71	48	15
Brazil	44,716	6,496	6,690	7,830	8,294	8,166	7,240
Chile	7,423	1,399	1,413	1,243	1,270	1,288	810
Colombia	3,943	651	667	831	782	470	542
Costa Rica	320	75	52	76	73	32	12
Cuba	3,186	334	368	614	765	709	396
Dominican Republic	5	—	1	—	—	2	2
Ecuador	186	27	29	45	46	31	8
El Salvador	5	—	—	2	1	1	1
Guatemala	98	25	29	18	15	9	2
Guyana	1	—	1	—	—	—	—
Honduras	140	17	19	42	30	30	2
Jamaica	292	36	66	49	42	67	32
Mexico	3,535	1,160	1,401	369	273	188	144
Nicaragua	7	1	—	1	1	2	2
Panama	22	4	3	2	5	4	4
Paraguay	65	12	11	12	19	7	4
Peru	474	86	80	69	110	80	49
Trinidad and Tobago	54	9	17	17	6	3	2
Uruguay	373	39	89	51	87	58	49
Venezuela	3,196	629	612	678	618	438	221

Source: Latin American and Caribbean Literature on Health Sciences (LILACS), June 2006.

Spain, and Portugal. Of the 345 journals in SciELO from Latin American countries, 51% are in the health area.

Thirteen countries are represented in MEDLINE, eight in the Science Citation Index, four in the Social Sciences Citation Index, and eight in EMBASE. The scientific production of Bolivia, Dominican Republic, Guatemala, Honduras, and Paraguay is reported only in LILACS. The number of health journals from Latin America and the Caribbean appearing in the main databases for the Americas and the intersections between the different databases are shown in Figure 4.

Current Situation and Initiatives

There are various information inputs that help to strengthen and improve different aspects of research for the development of public health. The following are worth noting: the Virtual Health Library (VHL), SciELO, ScienTI, CRICS, and RICTSAL.

The Virtual Health Library (VHL) (www.virtualhealthlibrary.org)

This is a decentralized, dynamic collection of information sources selected on the basis of quality criteria and available on the Internet. Its objective is to offer equitable access to scientific and technological information on health. In November 2006, the regional portal brought together 101 national and thematic portals and 10 institutional portals.

SciELO (www.scielo.org)

This is a model of cooperative electronic publication of scientific journals on the Internet, adopted by a number of Ibero-American countries to raise their visibility and increase access to the Region's scientific production. Access can be had to the full texts of the journals indexed in SciELO from numerous databases, directories, and known search engines, such as MEDLINE, Web of Science, Cross Ref, Google, and the Directory of Open Access Journals (DOAJ). In 2005, the set of collections in the SciELO network had about 7 million visitors a month. SciELO Brazil received more than 3 million, and SciELO Chile had more than 1 million monthly visits.

International Network of Information and Knowledge Sources for Sciences, Technology and Innovation Management (ScienTI) (www.scienti.net)

This is a public network of information and knowledge sources, whose objective is to contribute to the management of

TABLE 21. Indexing of Latin American and Caribbean journals in databases.

Country of publication	Journals indexed in databases					
	LILACS (2006)	SciELO (2006)	MEDLINE (2006)	ISI/SCIE (2005)	ISI/SSCI (2005)	EMBASE (2005)
Argentina	120	5	7	3	0	10
Bolivia	9	0	0	0	0	0
Brazil	289	85	31	12	2	46
Chile	66	18	3	4	0	4
Colombia	59	8	2	0	1	3
Costa Rica	12	9	1	1	0	0
Cuba	34	19	1	0	0	2
Dominican Republic	1	0	0	0	0	0
Ecuador	14	0	0	1	0	0
Guatemala	4	0	0	0	0	0
Honduras	1	0	0	0	0	0
Jamaica	2	0	1	1	0	1
Mexico	51	4	12	1	3	21
Panama	0	0	1	0	0	0
Paraguay	4	0	0	0	0	0
Peru	11	11	1	0	0	0
Puerto Rico	2	0	2	0	0	0
United States (PAHO)	3	1	1	0	1	0
Uruguay	10	6	0	0	0	0
Venezuela	46	9	3	2	0	4
Total Latin America and the Caribbean	738	175	66	25	7	91
Total indexed titles	738	198	4,959	6,088	1,747	4,872
Percentage Latin America and the Caribbean	100	88.4	1.3	0.4	0.4	1.9

Sources: Lists of journals indexed in the different databases.

LILACS: Latin American and Caribbean Literature on Health Sciences. List of titles indexed in LILACS, October 2006. Available at: http://ccs.bvsalud.org/serial/list-base.php?lang=pt&graphic=yes&base%5B%5D=&base%5B%5D=LILACS&country=AL_C&orderby=country&Submit=pesquisar.

SciELO: Scientific Electronic Library Online. List of health titles indexed in SciELO, October 2006. Available at: http://ccs.bvsalud.org/serial/list-base.php?lang=pt&graphic=yes&base%5B%5D=&base%5B%5D=SciELO&country=AL_C&orderby=country&Submit=pesquisar.

MEDLINE-MEDLARS Online. List of journals indexed in MEDLINE 2006, published by the US National Library of Medicine, January 2006. Available at: http://www.nlm.nih.gov/tsd/serials/lji.html.

ISI/SCIE: Science Citation Index Expanded, Thomson Scientific (ex ISI). Science Citation Index Expanded 2005, Thomson Scientific, March 2005. Available at: http://scientific.thomson.com/media/pdfs/sourcepub-journals/wos_scie_a5021_final.pdf.

ISI/SSCI: Social Sciences Citation Index, Thomson Scientific (ex ISI). Web page Science Social Sciences Citation Index 2005, published by Thomson Scientific, March 2005. Available at: http://scientific.thomson.com/media/pdfs/sourcepub-journals/wos_ssci_a5022_final.pdf.

EMBASE: Excerpta Medica Database. EMBASE list of journals indexed in 2005, published by Elsevier, June 2005 (printed version).

scientific, technological, and innovative activities. In is integrated with the Virtual Health Library. ScienTI is an expression of international cooperation among national science and technology organizations, international science and technology cooperation organizations, research and development groups in information and knowledge systems, and sponsoring institutions. It also offers indicators on research in the Region and allows access to directories of researchers and research groups and institutions. In 2006, network participants included Portugal and 11 countries of the Region.

Regional Congress on Health Sciences Information (CRICS) (www.bireme.br)

CRICS was launched in 1992 and is held every two years to evaluate regional and international progress in the areas of scientific and technical information management, scientific communications, bibliotechnology, and information technologies and their applications in national research, education, and health care systems in Latin America and the Caribbean. The Seventh Congress (CRICS 7) was held in Brazil in 2005 and was attended by more than 1,200 participants from 73 countries and experts in

FIGURE 4. Participation of Latin American and Caribbean health journals in the main databases, 2006.

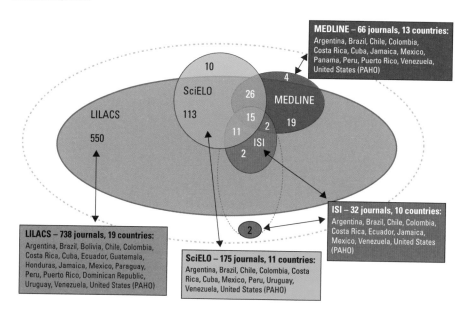

MEDLINE – 66 journals, 13 countries: Argentina, Brazil, Chile, Colombia, Costa Rica, Cuba, Jamaica, Mexico, Panama, Peru, Puerto Rico, Venezuela, United States (PAHO)

LILACS – 738 journals, 19 countries: Argentina, Brazil, Bolivia, Chile, Colombia, Costa Rica, Cuba, Ecuador, Guatemala, Honduras, Jamaica, Mexico, Paraguay, Peru, Puerto Rico, Dominican Republic, Uruguay, Venezuela, United States (PAHO)

SciELO – 175 journals, 11 countries: Argentina, Brazil, Chile, Colombia, Costa Rica, Cuba, Mexico, Peru, Uruguay, Venezuela, United States (PAHO)

ISI – 32 journals, 10 countries: Argentina, Brazil, Chile, Colombia, Costa Rica, Ecuador, Jamaica, Mexico, Venezuela, United States (PAHO)

Source: Latin American and Caribbean Center on Health Sciences Information, 2006.

different fields, including librarians and specialists in scientific dissemination, health professionals, health sector managers, editors of scientific journals, and researchers. The congress's recommendations are reflected in the documents Salvador Declaration: Commitment to Equity (*135*) and Salvador Declaration on Open Access: The Viewpoint of Developing Countries (*136*). These documents state that universal access to information and knowledge is an essential condition for promoting the health and quality of life of individuals and communities.

Network of Science and Technology Health Indicators (RICTSAL)

RICTSAL was launched in Buenos Aires in September 2004, with representatives of science and technology institutions and the ministries of health of Argentina, Brazil, Chile, Colombia, Costa Rica, Mexico, and Uruguay, jointly with PAHO and the Network of Science and Technology Indicators (RICYT). RICTSAL's mission is to promote, in a framework of international cooperation, the conceptual development of tools for the measurement and analysis of science, technology, and innovation in the field of health in the Americas, in order to learn more about them and support decisionmaking.

Outlook and Needs

Although different initiatives and networks are devoted to synthesizing knowledge and developing capacity, the commitment, participation, backing, and leadership of the regulatory

and health authorities (national science and technology institutions) is indispensable if those efforts are to respond effectively to the needs of each country, and if progress in health research is to be monitored and regulated.

The Ministerial Summit on Health Research was held in November 2004 in Mexico. The Mexico Declaration on Health Research (*137*) drafted there received the backing of the ministers of health and heads of delegations of the 58 WHO Member Countries. The declaration urges the countries, the scientific community, and international organizations to implement strategies and activities to step up research to improve the health and development outcomes of the population.

In response to the Mexico Declaration, initiatives have been promoted to provide training and develop human resources for health research, increase the production and systematic use of the results of research on public health, strengthen the leadership and governance of health research, and promote the development of databases and registries to monitor the status of research and learn about what resources are available (*138, 139, 140*). Strategies are also being implemented to prioritize research on public health and spur investments in this field. This will require coordination of the work of numerous initiatives, such as those promoted by the Council on Health Research for Development (COHRED: http://cohred.org), the Global Forum for Health Research: (http://www.globalforumhealth.org), and the Alliance for Health Policy and Systems Research (http://www.alliance hpsr.org), among others. The development of registries and indicators of scientific production is also being encouraged. The current trend is to promote the development of government policies to lend sustainability to research for equity and development.

Investments have been promoted in research on neglected topics of local interest, including aspects such as research on health systems, evaluation of the massification of interventions, and conditions that require multisector approaches (for example, prevention of traffic accidents, burns, drownings, gunshot wounds, and interventions to reduce violence). The World Alliance for Patient Safety (http://www.who.int/patientsafety) is developing working networks whose main goal is to create a culture of patient safety.

On other fronts, universal access to the results of research used to guide health policies and care is being promoted. WHO has promoted the development of an open portal that integrates the registries of clinical trials (http://www.who.int/ictrp). Networking is also being promoted under existing initiatives to spur the use of research results such as the Cochrane Collaboration (http://www.cochrane.org). In the last decade, major agreements were reached to facilitate access to biomedical and health publications for developing countries including the Health InterNetwork Access to Research Initiative (HINARI) (http://www.who.int/hinari).

The strategy of bringing together different initiatives, networks, and working groups in the Region has made it possible to identify synergies, minimize duplication of work, promote cooperation, and develop solidarity among countries to join forces to develop and bolster capacity, for the larger purpose of achieving successful and sustainable initiatives. By way of example, some of the initiatives and networks that have been working steadily in the Americas are mentioned below:

- The Latin American Network of Clinical Epidemiology (LatINCLEN) (http://www.latinclen.org) is oriented to training and research in clinical epidemiology, biostatistics, social sciences, and health economics.
- The Ibero-American Cochrane Network (http://www.cochrane.es) promotes research synthesis and meta-analysis, indexation of "grey" publications, development of new methodologies for secondary research, and offers a compilation of syntheses of scientific literature.
- The Latin American Forum of Research Ethics Committees (http://www.flaceis.org) offers a locus for dialogue to develop and strengthen research ethics.
- The Latin American Association of Schools of Public Health (ALAESP http://www.alaesp.sld.cu).
- The Latin American Social Sciences Faculty (http://www.flacso.org).

Scientific information is necessary but not sufficient for better health decisions to boost the effectiveness of interventions that will add to the gains in health and quality of life. Other key factors that require consideration and that mold decisionmaking

> *It is estimated that between 25% and 30% of the total population of the Region has no access to health care, despite the fact that universal declarations signed by most countries and the national laws of many more guarantee universal access to such care. Health reform processes have made uneven progress on this issue. In many cases, a significant gap exists between the state of development of national social protection systems and the legal framework that supports them.*
>
> Mirta Roses, 2005

processes and their results include sociocultural situations, the values of the decisionmakers, and the resources available. Other aspects should also be gradually dealt with to ensure that decisionmaking processes, practices, and policies are sufficiently well grounded in scientific evidence, such as the variability in information use patterns, the ability to appropriate knowledge, and decisions to react to new knowledge (*141*). The development of new communications technologies has spectacularly changed the panorama for the use of scientific information and has brought new solutions and new challenges in its wake.

In a short time, society has passed from restricted access to knowledge to a situation of great contrasts, since in some places limitations persist, while in others individuals feel overwhelmed by the amount of information and have difficulty in establishing the limits of a study and mastering the store of information and knowledge necessary to carry it out. These new challenges have led to the application of methodologies to synthesize knowledge and evaluate scientific literature critically, the establishment of standards for publishing and sharing information, the development of registries of basic data and scientific production, the incorporation of new information skills into human resource training, and much more. But the countries are still facing a changing scenario, and it is crucial to integrate initiatives to respond effectively to these challenges and have available basic information for a good situational analysis and the design of strategic responses.

RENEWING PRIMARY HEALTH CARE IN THE AMERICAS

The World Health Organization championed primary health care even before 1978, when it adopted the approach as central to the achievement of the goal of "health for all." Since that time, the world—and primary health care with it—has changed dramatically. The purpose of renewing primary health care is to revitalize countries' capacity to mount a coordinated, effective, and sustainable strategy to tackle existing health problems, prepare for new health challenges, and improve equity. The goal of such an endeavor is to obtain sustainable health gains for all.

Several reasons warrant the adoption of a renewed approach to primary health care. These include: new epidemiological challenges; the need to correct weaknesses and reduce inconsistencies that characterize some widely divergent approaches to primary health care; the development of new tools, knowledge, and best practices that can increase the effectiveness of primary health care; a growing recognition that primary health care can strengthen society's ability to reduce inequities in health; and an expanding consensus that primary health care represents a powerful approach to address the causes of poor health and inequality.

The Context for Primary Health Care

A thorough examination of primary health care is timely, as most of the countries in the Americas have undergone dramatic changes over the past three decades. These changes include democratization and consolidation of democracy, redefinition of the role of the state, economic liberalization, and health and social services reforms, including the expansion of the role of the private sector in areas that were traditionally the responsibility of the public sector. Although not always successful, health sector reforms have been aimed at achieving goals of streamlining health care financing, decentralizing authority for planning and implementation, and, more recently, have sought to improve the quality of care and enhance equity (142). In most countries, these reforms have taken place against the backdrop of widespread poverty, increasing inequality, social exclusion, political instability, and environmental deterioration (143, 144). Furthermore, the effects of globalization have increased the degree of interdependence of nations as well as their vulnerability to external forces; significant demographic and epidemiological trends have shifted the burden of disease; while new forms of political, social, and economic arrangements as well as technological developments are being introduced.

A renewed approach to primary health care is essential to meet internationally agreed-upon development goals. Some of the most relevant include those contained in the United Nations Millennium Declaration, which address the fundamental determinants of health as articulated by the WHO Commission on Social Determinants of Health and ensure health as a human right, as is established in some national constitutions and articulated by civil society groups. In addition to renewing and reinterpreting the approach and practice of primary health care to address the challenges of the 21st century, the renewal of primary health care will require building upon the legacy of Alma-Ata and the primary health care movement, and taking full advantage of lessons learned and best practices built up in more than a quarter-century of experience.

The Region of the Americas boasts a rich intellectual tradition of researching the causes and consequences of health disparities (145). Regardless of how equity is defined, few would deny that health disparities among the people of the Americas are inequitable. A recent analysis found that "despite a sizable reduction in infant mortality, levels of inequality among countries have remained almost constant between 1955 and 1995" (146). The results are similar when examining the situation within countries where sizeable gaps exist for a variety of health indicators, including maternal mortality (indigenous versus non-indigenous women), access to health services (between urban and rural populations), and life expectancy (between racial and ethnic groups) (147).

In our Region, income-related disparities are associated with poorer health performance and in some cases, their effects threaten to reverse the progress already made in many countries (148, 149, 150). Thus, reducing or eliminating inequities in health warrants the development and implementation of health and development strategies truly fueled by social values and able to address the causes as well as the consequences of inequities. Four main approaches have been employed to raise the levels of equity in health: (1) increasing or improving the provision of health services for those in greatest need (151, 152); (2) restructuring health financing mechanisms to aid the disadvantaged (153, 154, 155); (3) developing programs to aid the poor in obtaining basic goods such as housing, water, food, or income (156); and (4) altering broader social and economic structures to influence more distal determinants of health inequities (157). Research on various aspects of health equity has been part of the published literature for more than three decades, yet the evidence to determine the most effective strategies in any given circumstance remains insufficient (158).

Renewing primary health care means more than simply adjusting the original approach to current realities; rather, it requires a critical examination of its meaning and purpose. Overall, perceptions about the role of primary health care in social and health system development fall broadly into four categories (see Table 22). A study conducted in 2003, which included over 200 decisionmakers from 16 Latin American and Caribbean countries, confirmed the relevance of the primary health care approach for the respondents. Yet, the study also showed that disagreements and misconceptions about primary health care still exist, even within the same country (64) (see Table 23). Regardless of the predominant approach applied, the majority of informants interviewed (75%) saw primary health care as a valuable approach that requires redefinition and reinvigoration. Most respondents believed that such a redefinition requires new implementation strategies, including changes to primary health care organization and financing, human resources development, health policy formulation, health management and administration, and greater government transparency. They added that this process should involve partnerships among providers, communities, governments, international agencies, and international networks to set health priorities, create incentives for applied research and

TABLE 22. Approaches to primary health care.

Approach	Definition or concept of primary health care (PHC)	Emphasis
Selective PHC	Involves a limited number of high-impact services to address some of the most prevalent health problems in developing countries. One of the main programs that included services of this kind was known as GOBI (growth monitoring, oral rehydration techniques, breast-feeding, and immunization) and also as GOBI-FFF when food supplementation, female literacy, and family planning were added.	Specific set of health service activities for the poor.
Primary care	Refers to the gateway to the health system and the site for continuous health care for the majority of the population. This is the most common concept of PHC in Europe and other industrialized countries. More narrowly defined, this approach is directly related to the availability of general or family physicians.	Health system level of care.
Alma-Ata Comprehensive PHC	The Alma-Ata Declaration states that: "Primary health care is essential health care based on practical, scientifically sound and socially acceptable methods and technology made universally accessible to individuals and families in the community through their full participation and at a cost that the community and country can afford to maintain … It forms an integral part both of the country's health system … and of the overall social and economic development of the community. It is the first level of contact of individuals, the family and community … bringing health care as close as possible to where people live and work, and constitutes the first element of a continuing health care process."	Strategy for organizing health care systems and society to promote health.
Health and human rights	Conceives of health as a human right and underlines the need to respond to the broader social and political determinants of health. It differs on account of its greater stress on the social and political implications of the Alma-Ata Declaration, rather than on account of its principles. It maintains that if the social and political content of Alma-Ata is to improve equity in health care, it should be more oriented to the development of "inclusive, dynamic, transparent policies supported by legislation and financial commitments" rather than to specific aspects of disease.	A philosophy that cuts across the health and social sectors.

Sources: Walsh JA, Warren KS. Selective primary health care: an interim strategy for disease control in developing countries. N Engl J Med 301(18):967–974; 1979.

Institute of Medicine. Defining primary care: an interim report. Washington, DC: National Academy Press; 1994.

WHO. Primary Health Care: Report of the International Conference on Primary Health Care. Alma-Ata USSR. 6–12 September, 1978. Geneva: WHO; 1978.

Tarimo E, Webster EG. Primary health care concepts and challenges in a changing world. Alma-Ata revisited (Current Concerns ARA paper number 7, document WHO/ARA/CC/97.1). Geneva: WHO; 1997.

People's Health Movement, editor. Health for All Now! Revive Alma-Ata! The Alma-Ata Anniversary Pack. Unnikrishnan, Bangalore (India): People's Health Movement, 2003.

Movement PsH, editor. The medicalization of health care and the challenge of health for all. People's Health Assembly; 2000 December 2000; Dhaka, Bangladesh.

Vuori H. Primary health care in Europe: problems and solutions. Community Medicine 1984;6:221–31.

Vuori H. The role of the schools of public health in the development of primary health care. Health Policy 1985;4(3):221–30.

human resource development, encourage cost-effectiveness in resource allocation, advocate for increased resources, and promote healthy public policies.

The 44th PAHO Directing Council in September 2003 approved a resolution calling for Member States to adopt a series of recommendations to strengthen primary health care. The following year and in response to the above mandates, PAHO/WHO created a working group on primary health care to advise on the organization of future strategic and programmatic orientations of the primary health care approach. Its first meeting was held in June 2004, in Washington DC, and the second took place in San José, Costa Rica, in October of that year.

To discuss the draft position paper, national consultations took place in 21 countries: Argentina, Bolivia, Brazil, Chile, Colombia, Costa Rica, Cuba, Dominican Republic, Ecuador, El Salvador, Guatemala, Guyana, Jamaica, Mexico, Nicaragua, Panama, Para-

TABLE 23. Key informant perceptions of primary health care roles.

To what extent do you agree with the following statements?	Percentage agreement or total agreement	No.
PHC is the first level of care.	80	160
PHC is the gateway to the health system.	71	152
PHC is viewed in different ways by different health care providers.	67	188
PHC is a combination of approaches.	62	158
PHC is low-technology care.	55	187
PHC is a health service for the poor.	52	173
PHC is a strategy for socioeconomic development.	51	154
PHC is viewed differently in different parts of the country.	44	184

Source: Pan American Health Organization. Revisión de las políticas de atención primaria de salud en América Latina y el Caribe. Washington, DC: OPS; 2003.

guay, Peru, Suriname, Trinidad and Tobago, and Venezuela. The technical recommendations produced by the Regional Consultation held in Montevideo, Uruguay, became part of the position paper and of the Regional Declaration on Primary Health Care (Declaration of Montevideo), fully endorsed by the 46th Directing Council of PAHO in September 2005.

Since approval of the Declaration of Montevideo, several countries have renewed or reinvigorated their efforts to incorporate the core values, principles, and elements of the primary health care strategy into the development of their national health systems. PAHO/WHO has continued to provide technical cooperation for the countries on the matter and has stepped up efforts to disseminate the renewed primary health care approach within the Region. Its efforts have centered on streamlining the primary health care strategy in all of its technical cooperation activities and areas of work.

Building Primary Health Care-Based Health Systems

The renewal of primary health care must be an integral part of health systems development, and an overarching and enabling approach to the organization and operation of the health system, where the right to the highest attainable level of health is its main goal. Furthermore, a primary health care-based system maximizes equity and solidarity and contributes to sustained population health gains. Such a system is guided by the principles of responsiveness, quality orientation, government accountability, social justice, sustainability, participation, and intersectorality.

A primary health care-based health system is composed of a core set of functional and structural elements that guarantee universal coverage and access to equity-enhancing services that are acceptable to the population. It provides comprehensive, integrated, and appropriate care over time, emphasizes prevention and promotion, and ensures first-contact care. The essential base for planning and action are the families and the communities where the system operates. A primary health care-based health

system requires a sound legal, institutional, and organizational foundation as well as adequate and sustainable human, financial, and technological resources. It employs optimal management practices at all levels to ensure quality, efficiency, and effectiveness, and it develops active mechanisms to maximize individual and collective participation in health. A primary health care-based health system develops and is a catalyst in intersectoral actions that address determinants of health and equity.

The essence of the renewed definition of primary health care is the same as in the Alma-Ata Declaration. The new definition has a whole-system perspective, however—one that applies to all countries without distinction and includes all relevant sectors (public, private, and nonprofit). It differentiates values, principles, and elements; highlights equity and solidarity; and incorporates new principles such as sustainability and a quality orientation. The renewed definition discards the notion of primary health care as a pre-established set of services, since these should be customized to local needs. Similarly, it dispels the notion of primary health care as defined by specific types of health personnel, since primary health care teams ought to be defined according to needs, cultural preferences, evidence, and available resources. Moreover, it specifies organizational and functional elements that can be measured and evaluated, and which form a logical and cohesive approach for firmly grounding health systems on the primary health care approach. Renewed primary health care intends to guide the transformation of health systems so that they achieve their goals while being flexible enough to change and adapt over time to meet new challenges. It recognizes that primary health care is more than just the provision of health services and that success depends on other health system functions and other social processes.

Due to the great variation in national economic resources, political circumstances, administrative capacities, and historical development of the health sector, each country will need to design its own strategy for primary health care renewal. Figure 5 presents the proposed values, principles, and elements of a pri-

FIGURE 5. Core values, principles, and elements in a primary health care-based health system.

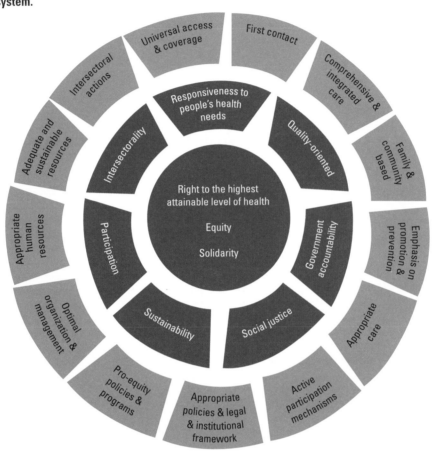

Source: Pan American Health Organization. Renewing Primary Health Care in the Americas. A position paper. Washington, DC: OPS; 2007.

mary health care-based system, Table 24 shows their definitions, and Table 25 the essential elements of a primary health care-based health system.

The Way Forward

An approach to renewing primary health care will encompass: (1) completing primary health care implementation where it has fallen short (the unfinished health agenda) by guaranteeing all citizens the right to health and universal access, actively promoting equity in health care, as well as improvements in and a better distribution of health and quality-of-life indicators; (2) strengthening primary health care to address new challenges by improving citizen and community satisfaction with services and providers, maximizing the quality of care and management, and strengthening the policy environment and institutional structure necessary for the successful fulfillment of all health system functions; and (3) lo-

cating primary health care in the broader agenda of equity and human development by linking primary health care renewal with efforts (such as the Millennium Declaration) to strengthen health systems, promoting sustainable improvements in community participation and intersectoral collaboration, and investing in human resource development. Success will mean learning from experiences, developing advocacy strategies, and articulating the expected roles and responsibilities of countries, international organizations, and civil society groups involved in the renewal process.

Interest in primary health care has been renewed throughout the world. Various organizations have recognized that strengthening health systems is a prerequisite for assuring economic growth, advancing social equity, improving health, and providing treatments to combat ravaging diseases such as HIV/AIDS. Yet, much work remains to convince the key actors that primary health care is the logical and appropriate locus for collaboration, investment, and action. The time for action is now.

TABLE 24. Core values and principles of a primary health care-based health system.

Values	Definition
Right to the highest possible level of health care	The constitutions of many countries and different international agreements (including the Constitution of the World Health Organization) refer to the rights of citizens and the responsibilities of governments and other legally defined players and lay the judicial and legal groundwork to enable citizens to protest when their entitlements are not complied with.
Equity	Counters unfair differences in health status, access to health care, and healthy environments, and in the treatment received in the social services and health care systems.
Solidarity	The extent to which people in a society undertake to work together for the common good to define and achieve a common goal. In local and national governments, this value takes the form of voluntary associations and other forms of participation in civic life.

Principles	
Responsiveness to health care needs of the population	Health care systems should focus on people in order to meet their needs to the fullest extent possible. This implies that PHC should meet the health care requirements of the population based on available evidence, while promoting respect for individual preferences and needs, without considering socioeconomic, cultural, racial, or ethnic status, gender, or other factors.
Quality orientation	In addition to responding to the needs of the population, services should anticipate them and treat every one with dignity and respect, while providing the best possible treatment for their health problems. This means equipping health professionals with fundamental clinical knowledge and with the tools necessary for their continual professional development, and having adequate procedures for evaluating the efficiency, effectiveness, and safety of preventive and curative interventions, assigning resources properly, and having an appropriate incentive system.
Government responsibility and accountability	This principle assures that the government complies with or is forced to comply with social rights and that citizens are protected from encroachment on those rights. It requires the development of specific regulatory and legal policies and procedures to permit citizens to demand their rights if they are not respected. This principle should be applied to all the functions of the health system, regardless of the type of provider (public, private, or nonprofit). It requires continuous monitoring and improvement of the performance of the health system, which should be transparent and subject to social control.
Social justice	The government's activities should be evaluated on how well they assure the well-being of all citizens, particularly the most vulnerable groups.
Sustainability	Requires the use of strategic planning and the creation of lasting commitments. Investments should be sufficient to meet the public's current health care requirements while planning to meet tomorrow's challenges.
Participation	Individuals should be involved in decision-making on the allocation of resources, the establishment of priorities, and in processes to facilitate accountability. Individuals should be capable of making free and informed decisions to improve their health and that of their families. Social participation in health care is one of the facets of general civic participation that permits the health system to reflect social values and is a means of social control over public and private actions that affect society.
Intersectorality	The health sector should work together with other sectors and players to assure the alignment of public policies and programs, maximizing their potential contribution to health and human development.

Source: Pan American Health Organization. Renewing Primary Health Care in the Americas. A position paper. Washington DC: OPS; 2007.

TABLE 25. Essential elements of a primary health care-based health system.

Universal access and coverage	Financing and organizational provisions should cover the entire population, eliminating barriers to access, reflecting needs, preferences, and local cultures, protecting people from financial risks, and meeting the objectives of equity.
First contact	Primary care should operate as the gateway to the health and social services system for all new patients and as the place where the majority of problems are resolved. A health system based on primary care strengthens this type of attention by operating as the first level of care, although some of its functions extend beyond that level.
Comprehensive, integrated, and continuous care over time	The range of services available should be adequate for providing and integrating health promotion, disease prevention, early diagnosis, curative and palliative care, rehabilitation, and support to enable patients to manage on their own.
Family and community orientation	Primary care takes a public health approach that uses community and family information to assess risks and prioritize interventions. Families and communities are the first rung on the ladder of planning and interventions.
Emphasis on disease prevention and health promotion	Primary care involves health promotion, public health, and regulatory and policy approaches, in order to improve labor conditions and safety, reduce environmental risks, and coordinate population-based health promotion with other sectors.
Appropriate care	A health system based on primary care does not focus on care of an organ or a disease, but rather its activities focus on individuals as whole persons during their life cycle. It assures that interventions are pertinent, effective, efficient, and safe and that they are based on the best clinical evidence available.
Active participation mechanisms	Actions that help to ensure transparency and accountability on all levels, including empowering people to better manage their own health and encouraging communities to become active participants in establishing health priorities and in system management, evaluation, and regulation.
Solid legal, political, and institutional framework	Part of the leadership function of the health system consists of identifying, empowering, and coordinating the players, actions, procedures, and legal and financing systems that enable the PHC system to carry out all its specific functions transparently, subject to control by society and free of corruption.
Policies and programs that favor equity	Activities to overcome the negative impact of social inequity on health and assure that everyone is treated with dignity and respect. Should incorporate both horizontal and vertical equity.
Optimum organization and administration	Practices to enable innovation to continuously improve the organization and supply of safe care, which should comply with quality levels, offer satisfactory working conditions for health personnel, and respond flexibly to people's needs.
Adequate human resources	Health care providers, community workers, administrators, and auxiliary personnel should possess an adequate mix of skills and knowledge. They should also be able to rely on a productive work environment, training to maximize interdisciplinary teams, and incentives to treat people with dignity and respect. This requires strategic planning, long-term investments, and coordination of national and international human resource policies.
Adequate and sustainable material resources	Resources should be sufficient to provide universal coverage and access based on the best available data and analysis of the health situation.
Intersectoral actions	Primary care, the health system, and other sectors should work together to promote health and human development addressing health determinants through linkage with the public education system, the workplace, economic and urban development programs, agricultural development and marketing programs, potable water and sewage services, etc.

Source: Pan American Health Organization, Health Systems Strengthening Area, Health Policies and Systems Development Unit.

References

1. Dye TR. Understanding public policy. 9th edition. Upper Saddle River: Prentice Hall; 1998.

2. Lasswell H. Politics: Who Gets What, When, How. New York: Meridian Books; 1958.

3. Sojo C, Pérez Sainz, JP. Reinventar lo social en América Latina. In: Desarrollo social en América Latina: temas y desafíos para las políticas públicas. Costa Rica: Facultad Latinoamericana de Ciencias Sociales; 2002.

4. World Health Organization. World Health Report 2000. Health Systems—Improving Performance. Geneva: WHO; 2000.

5. Pan American Health Organization. Public Health in the Americas: New Concepts, Analysis of Performance, and Basis for Action. Washington, DC: PAHO; 2002 (Scientific and Technical Publication No. 589).

6. Esping-Andersen G. The Three Worlds of Welfare Capitalism. Princeton: Princeton University Press; 1990.

7. Pan American Health Organization; Swedish International Development Cooperation Agency. Exclusion in Health in Latin America and the Caribbean. Washington, DC: PAHO; 2004.

8. Economic Commission for Latin America and the Caribbean. Shaping the Future of Social Protection: Access, Financing and Solidarity. Montevideo: ECLAC; 2006.

9. Mesa-Lago C. Las reformas de salud en América Latina y el Caribe: su impacto en los principios de la seguridad social. Santiago de Chile: CEPAL; 2005.

10. Medici A. Las reformas incompletas de salud en América Latina: algunos elementos de su economía política. Bienestar y Política Social. 2006;2(1)1–26.

11. Comisión Interamericana de la Seguridad Social. Reformas de los esquemas de la seguridad social. Informe de la seguridad social en América Latina 2004.

12. Fleury S. ¿Universal, dual o plural? Modelos y dilemas de atención de la salud en América Latina: Chile, Brasil y Colombia. In: Molina C, Núñez J, eds. Servicios de salud en América Latina y Asia. Washington, DC: Banco Interamericano de Desarrollo; 2001. pp. 3–39.

13. Pan American Health Organization; International Labor Organization. ILO/PAHO Joint Initiative on the Extension of Social Protection in Health. Washington, DC: PAHO/ILO; 2005.

14. Pan American Health Organization; Swedish International Development Cooperation Agency. Methodological guide for the characterization of exclusion in health. Washington, DC: PAHO; 2001.

15. World Health Organization. World Health Assembly Resolution WHA58.33. Geneva: WHO; 2005.

16. Pan American Health Organization. Twenty-sixth Pan American Sanitary Conference Resolution CSP 26.R19. Washington, DC: PAHO; 2002.

17. Pan American Health Organization. Major trends in health legislation in the English-speaking Caribbean 2001–2005. Washington, DC: PAHO; 2006. Available from: http://www.paho.org/English/DPM/SHD/HP/health-legislation-trends.htm.

18. Pan American Health Organization. Major trends in health legislation in Canada 2001–2005. Washington, DC: PAHO; 2006. Available from: http://www.paho.org/English/DPM/SHD/HP/health-legislation-trends.htm.

19. Pan American Health Organization. Major trends in health legislation in the United States of America 2001–2005. Washington, DC: PAHO, 2006. Available from: http://www.paho.org/English/DPM/SHD/HP/health-legislation-trends.htm.

20. Joint Learning Initiative. Human resources for health: overcoming the crisis. Cambridge: Harvard University Press; 2004.

21. Anand S, Baernighausen T. Human resources and health outcomes. Lancet. 2004; 364(9445):1603–9.

22. Pan American Health Organization. Development and Strengthening of Human Resources Management in the Health Sector. (CD43/9). XLIII Directing Council. Washington, DC: PAHO; 2001. Available from: http://www.paho.org/english/gov/cd/cd43_09-e.pdf.

23. Pan American Health Organization. Observatory of Human Resources in Health. (CD45/9). XLV Directing Council. Washington, DC: PAHO; 2004. Available from: http://www.paho.org/English/GOV/CD/cd45-09-e.pdf.

24. Macinko J, Guanais F, Marinho de Souza MF. Evaluation of the impact of the family health program on infant mortality in Brazil, 1990–2002. J. Epidemiol. Community Health. 2006;60:13–19.

25. Pan American Health Organization. Toronto Call to Action, 2006–2015. Towards a Decade of Human Resources in Health. Regional Meeting of the Observatory of Human Resources in Health. Washington, DC: PAHO; 2005.

26. Pan American Health Organization. Regional consultation on the critical challenges for human resources in health in the Americas. Regional Meeting of the Observatory of Human Resources in Health. Critical Challenges for Human Resources in Health: A Regional View. Toronto, Canada, 4–7 October 2005.

27. Mullan F. The metrics of the physician brain drain. N Engl J Med. 2005;353: 1810–18.

28. Chen LC, Boufford JI. Fatal flows: Doctors on the move. N Engl J Med. Oct 2005;353(17):1850–52.

29. Pautassi LC. Equidad de género y calidad en el empleo: Las trabajadoras y los trabajadores en salud en la Argentina. Santiago de Chile: CEPAL; 2001. Available from: http://www.observatoriorh.org/esp/pdfs/lcl1506e.pdf.

30. Standing H, Baume E. Equity, equal opportunities, gender and organization performance. Workshop on Global Health Workforce Strategy, Annecy, France, 9–12 December 2000.

Geneva: WHO; 2001. Available from: http://www.observatoriorh.org/eng/pdfs/equity%20gender.pdf.

31. Pan American Health Organization. Human Resources for Health in the Americas: Strengthening the Foundation. Washington, DC: PAHO; 2006.

32. Nogueira R, Passos, Santana J. Paranaguá 2003. Human resource management and public sector reforms: trends and origins of a new approach. Discussion paper. Brasilia; 2002.

33. Organización Panamericana de la Salud. Desafíos de la gestión de los recursos humanos en salud 2005–2015. Washington, DC: OPS; 2006.

34. Cherchiglia M. Terceirização nos serviços de saúde: Alguns aspectos conceptuais, legais e pragmáticos. In: Lima JC, Santana JP. Especialização em desenvolvimento de recursos humanos em saúde, CADRHU. Natal: PAHO/WHO; 1999. pp. 367–385.

35. Brazil, Conselho Nacional de Secretários de Saúde. Situação de vinculo do trabalho nas secretarias estaduais de saúde, Ministério da Saúde, Coordenação Geral de Desenvolvimento de Recursos Humanos para o SUS. CONASS; 1999.

36. Arroyo J. Sobre las transiciones y contra-transiciones en el desarrollo de capacidades en el campo de recursos humanos en salud. Seminario Regional de Responsables de Políticas de Recursos Humanos en la Región de las Américas. Construyendo capacidad institucional para el desarrollo de políticas de recursos humanos. Reunión de Consulta Regional de la OMS, Varadero, Cuba, 7–11 de octubre de 2002.

37. Rigoli F, Rocha C, Foster A. Critical challenges for human resources in health: a regional view. Revista Latino-Amer de Enfermagem. Jan/Feb 2006;14(1):7–16. Available from: http://www.scielo.br/pdf/rlae/v14n1/en_v14n1a02.pdf.

38. Scavino J. Panorama de organizaciones de profesionales y trabajadores de la salud en las Américas. Serie Desarrollo de Recursos Humanos 35. Washington, DC: OPS; 2004. Available from: http://www.observatoriorh.org/esp/publicaciones.html.

39. Davini MC, Nervi L, Roschke MA. Capacitación del personal de los servicios de salud, proyectos relacionados con los procesos de reforma sectorial. Serie Observatorio N° 3. 2002. Available from: http: //observatorio_ rh.tripod.com/observatorio-rh/id10.html.

40. Organización Panamericana de la Salud. El servicio social de medicina en América Latina. Situación actual y perspectivas. Informe de taller regional. Washington, DC: OPS; 1997.

41. Organización Panamericana de la Salud. Lineamientos metodológicos para el análisis sectorial en salud: una herramienta para la formulación de políticas. Serie Iniciativa Regional de Reforma del Sector Salud en América Latina y el Caribe, Edición especial N° 9. Washington, DC: OPS; 2004. Available from: http://www.lachealthsys.org/documents/lineamientosmetodologicosanalisissectorialensaluduna herramientaparalaformulacion-ES.pdf.

42. World Health Organization. WHO's health system strengthening strategy. Geneva: WHO; 2006.

43. Londoño JL, Frenk J. Structured pluralism: towards an innovative model for health system reform in Latin America. Health Policy. 1997 Jul;41(1):1–36.

44. Brazil, Oswaldo Cruz Foundation; Ministry of Health. Report of the workshop on health systems performance: the world health report 2000. Rio de Janeiro, 14–15 December 2000.

45. Organización Panamericana de la Salud. Análisis de las reformas del sector salud en la subregión de Centroamérica y la República Dominicana, 2ª edición. Washington, DC: OPS, 2002. Available from: http://www.lachealthsys.org/esp/index.php?option=com_content&task=view&id=55&Itemid=30.

46. Organización Panamericana de la Salud. Análisis de las reformas del sector salud en los países de la Región Andina. Iniciativa Regional de Reforma del Sector Salud en América Latina y el Caribe. Edición especial N° 11. Washington, DC: OPS; 2002. Available from: http://www.lachealthsys.org/esp/index.php?option=com_content&task=view&id=57&Itemid=30.

47. Pan American Health Organization. Analysis of Health Sector Reform in English-Speaking Caribbean. Washington, DC: PAHO; 2002. Available from: http://www.lachealthsys.org/documents/events/belize/AnalysisHSREnglishSpeakingCaribbean.pdf.

48. Roses M. Steering role of the Ministries of Health: challenges for the 21st century. Keynote address at the Hospital Governance Workshop for Ministers of Health and Permanent Secretaries of the Organization of Eastern Caribbean States, Bridgetown, Barbados, 5–6 November 2003.

49. Pan American Health Organization. Analysis of health sector reform: region of the Americas. Latin America and Caribbean Health Sector Reform Initiative Series No. 12. Washington, DC: PAHO; 2004.

50. World Health Organization. Report on the WHO meeting of experts on the stewardship function of health systems. Meeting on the stewardship function in health systems. (HFS/FAR/STW/00.1). Geneva, Switzerland, 10–11 September 2001.

51. Travis P, Egger D, Davies P, Mechbal A. Towards better stewardship: concepts and critical issues. Geneva: WHO; 2002. Available from: http://www.who.int/healthinfo/paper48.pdf.

52. Pan American Health Organization. Steering Role of the Ministries of Health in the Process of Health Sector Reform. XL Directing Council, Resolution CD40.13. Washington, DC: PAHO; 1997.

53. Saltman RB, Ferroussier-Davis O. The concept of stewardship in health policy. Bull World Health Organ. 2000;78:732–39.

54. Correa JL. Proyecto de autoridad sanitaria. Comunidad virtual de gobernabilidad y liderazgo. Available from: http://www.gobernabilidad.cl/modules.php?name=News&file=article&sid=441.

55. Organización Panamericana de la Salud. Marco conceptual e instrumento metodológico. Función rectora de la autoridad sanitaria nacional: desempeño y fortalecimiento. Edición especial N° 17. Washington, DC: OPS; 2006. Available from: http://www.lachealthsys.org/documents/433-funcion rectoradelaautoridadsanitarianacionaldesempenoy fortalecimiento-ES.pdf.

56. Organización Panamericana de la Salud. Desarrollo de la capacidad de conducción sectorial en salud. Una propuesta operacional. Serie Organización y Gestión de Sistemas y Servicios de Salud N° 6. Washington, DC: OPS; 1998. Available from: http://bvs.insp.mx/articulos/2/10/05122000.pdf.

57. Organización Panamericana de la Salud. La función rectora de la autoridad sanitaria nacional en acción: lecciones aprendidas. Serie Iniciativa Regional de Reforma del Sector Salud en América Latina y el Caribe, Edición especial N° 18. Washington, DC: OPS; 2007. Available from: http://www. lachealthsys.org/esp/index.php?option=com_content&task=view&id=101&Itemid=54.

58. Pan American Health Organization. Essential public health functions. XLII Directing Council, Resolution CD42.R14. Washington, DC: PAHO; 2000.

59. Costa Rica, Ministerio de Salud. Análisis sectorial de salud de Costa Rica. San José: MINSA, 2002. Available from: http://www.lachealthsys.org/documents/analisissectorial desaluddecostaricapartei-ES.pdf.

60. Clark M. Health sector reform in Costa Rica: Reinforcing a public system. Washington, DC; 2002.

61. Institute of Medicine. Guidance for the national healthcare disparities report. Washington, DC: National Academy Press; 2002.

62. Aday LA. At risk in America: the health and health care needs of vulnerable populations in the United States. 2nd ed. New York: John Wiley & Sons Inc.; 2001.

63. Institute of Medicine. Care without coverage: too little, too late. Washington, DC: National Academy Press; 2002.

64. Pan American Health Organization. Review of the policies of primary health care in Latin America and the Caribbean. Final report. Vol 1. (THS/OS/04/1). Washington, DC: PAHO; 2003.

65. Mexico, Secretaría de Salud. Press note No. 2006-103, February 2006. Available from: http://www.salud.gob.mx.

66. Pan American Health Organization. Regional study on the hospital and ambulatorial assistance specialized in Latin America and Caribbean. (THS/OS/04/2). Washington, DC: PAHO; 2004.

67. Donabedian A. Explorations in quality assessment and monitoring: the definition of quality and approaches to its assessment. Vol. II. The criteria and standards of quality. Ann Arbor: Health Administration Press; 1982.

68. Donabedian, A. Evaluating the quality of medical care. Milbank Memorial Fund Quarterly. 1966;(44):166–203.

69. Donabedian A. The criteria and standards of quality. Ann Arbor: Health Administration Press; 1982.

70. Institute of Medicine. Envisioning the national health care quality report. Washington, DC: National Academy Press; 2001.

71. Institute of Medicine. Crossing the quality chasm. Washington, DC: National Academy Press; 2001.

72. Pan American Health Organization. Analysis of health sector reform: region of the Americas. Latin America and Caribbean Health Sector Reform Initiative Series No. 12. Washington, DC: PAHO; 2004.

73. European Observatory on Health Systems and Policies. Glossary. Available from: http://www.euro.who.int/observatory/Glossary/TopPage. Accessed 3 June 2006.

74. National Assembly of School Based Health Care. Available from: http://www.nasbhc.org/. Accessed 6 September 2006.

75. Torre Montejo E. Salud para todos es posible. 1ª edición. La Habana: Sociedad Cubana de Salud Pública; 2005. Available from: http://www.undp.org.cu/pub_otros.html. Accessed 6 September 2006.

76. Hartz ZMA, Contandriopoulos AP. Integralidade da atenção e integração de serviços de saúde: desafios para avaliar a implantação de um sistema sem muros. Cadernos de Saúde Pública. 2004;20 Sup 2:S331–S336.

77. EsSalud. Atención integral en salud: implementación de la atención integral en salud en el policlínico Hermana María Donrose Sutmoller. Lima: EsSalud; 2004.

78. Rosero-Bixby L. Evaluación del impacto de la reforma del sector de la salud en Costa Rica mediante un estudio cuasi-experimental. Rev Panam Salud Pública. 2004;15(2):94–103.

79. Rosero-Bixby L. Spatial access to health care in Costa Rica and its equity: A GIS-based study. Soc Sci Med. 2004;58:1271–84.

80. Beauchamp TL, Childress JF. Principles of Biomedical Ethics. 5th edition. New York: Oxford University Press; 2001.

81. Mexico, Secretaría de Salud. Available from: http://www.salud.gob.mx: 8080/JSPCenetec/web_consulta/html/institucion/terminos.html.

82. Milen A. What do we know about capacity building? An overview of existing knowledge and good practice. Geneva: WHO; 2001. Available from: http://www.unescobkk.org/fileadmin/user_upload/aims/capacity_building.pdf. Accessed 6 September 2006.

83. Institute of Medicine. Performance measurement: accelerating improvement. Washington, DC: National Academy Press; 2006.

84. World Health Organization. Issues in health information 3: integrating equity into health information systems. Unpub-

lished. 2006. Available from: http://www.who.int/entity/healthmetrics/library/issue_3_05apr.doc. Accessed 8 September 2006.

85. Hermida J. Asegurando la calidad en salud: estrategias claves y tendencias en América Latina. [Presentation]. Antigua (Guatemala): OPS; 2004.

86. World Organization of Family Doctors. Rural information technology exchange. Using information technology to improve rural health care. Available from: http://www.globalfamilydoctor.com/aboutWonca/working_groups/write/itpolicy/ITPoli.htm. Accessed 6 September 2006.

87. Tobar F. Políticas para mejorar el acceso a los medicamentos. Bol Fárm. julio 2002;5(3). Sección Ventana Abierta.

88. República del Ecuador. (2000) Ley de Producción, Importación, Comercialización y Expendio de Medicamentos Genéricos de Uso Humano. Registro oficial 59. 17 de abril de 2000.

89. Pan American Health Organization, Center for Pharmaceutical Policies, National School of Public Health. Pharmaceutical situation in Latin America and the Caribbean. Structure and processes. Rio de Janeiro: NAF/ENSP; 2006.

90. IMS Health. Latin America: overcoming economic challenges. Available from: http://www.imshealth.com/web/content/0,3148,64576068_63872702_70260998_71226846,00.html.

91. IMS Health. Global Pharmaceutical Perspectives 2005. Total Market Estimates and Global Pharma Forecasts. 2005.

92. Pan American Health Organization, Center for Pharmaceutical Policies, National School of Public. Pharmaceutical situation in Latin America and the Caribbean. Structure and processes. Rio de Janeiro: NAF/ENSP; 2006.

93. Tobar F. Mitos sobre los medicamentos en Argentina: una mirada económica. Bol Fárm. enero 2006;9(1).

94. Unión Industrial Argentina Cadena Farmacéutica. Quinto Foro Federal de la Industria Región Pampeana. Jornada de trabajo. 26–27 May 2006.

95. Frenkel J. O mercado farmacêutico brasileiro: a sua evolução recente, mercados e preços. Campinas: Instituto de Economia da Unicamp; 1999.

96. Argentina, Ministerio de Salud y Ambiente. La industria de medicamentos en Argentina: un análisis de la producción, el consumo y el intercambio comercial. Diagnóstico y perspectivas. Buenos Aires: Ministerio de Salud y Ambiente; 2006.

97. Uruguay, Asociación de Laboratorios Nacionales. La industria de medicamentos en Uruguay, 2006.

98. Consorcio Care Ecuador; Johns Hopkins University, Bloomberg School of Public Health. Evaluación de la situación actual de la utilización y disponibilidad de medicamentos, con recomendaciones para conseguir una repartición más efectiva. Quito: Proyecto Modersa; 2006. Unpublished.

99. Brazil, Ministério do Planejamento, Orçamento e Gestão; Instituto Brasileiro de Geografia e Estatística; Programa de Comparación Internacional. Primeros resultados del Programa de Comparación Internacional en América del Sur. Consumo de los hogares en 2005. Available from: http://siteresources.worldbank.org/ICPINT/Resources/PCI_spn_28junho06.pdf.

100. World Health Organization. Medicines strategy: countries at the core 2004–2007. Geneva: WHO; 2004. Available from: http://whqlibdoc.who.int/hq/2004/WHO_EDM_2004.5.pdf.

101. Hale and healthy. The Economist. 14 April 2005. pp. 69–70.

102. Inter-American Development Bank. Sustaining development for all: expanding access to economic activity and social services. Washington, DC: IDB; 2006. pp. 157–158.

103. Centro de Informaciones y Estudios del Uruguay. El impacto de las políticas de medicamentos genéricos sobre el mercado de medicamentos en tres países del MERCOSUR. (CEALCI 07/05). Montevideo: CIESU; 2005.

104. Miranda Montero JJ. El mercado de medicamentos en el Perú. ¿libre o regulado? Lima: Instituto de Estudios Peruanos; 2004. p. 21.

105. Falbo R. Estudio sobre el gasto en medicamentos en Argentina. Buenos Aires: Ministerio de Salud y Ambiente; 2003.

106. World Health Organization. WHO medicines strategy. World Health Assembly Resolution WHA54.11. Geneva: WHO; 2001. Available from: http://policy.who.int/cgi-bin/om_isapi.dll?infobase=wharec-e&softpage=Browse_Frame_Pg42. Accessed 8 Februrary 2007.

107. World Health Organization. Ensuring accessibility of essential medicines. World Health Assembly Resolution WHA55.14. Geneva: WHO; 2002. Available from: http://policy.who.int/cgi-bin/om_isapi.dll?infobase=WHA&jump= WHA55.14&softpage=Browse_Frame_Pg42#JUMPDEST_WHA55.14. Accessed 8 February 2007.

108. World Health Organization. Intellectual property rights, innovation and public health. World Health Assembly Resolution WHA56.27. Geneva: WHO; 2003. Available from: http://policy.who.int/cgi-bin/om_isapi.dll?infobase=wharec-e&softpage=Browse_Frame_Pg42. Accessed 8 February 2007.

109. World Health Organization. Scaling up treatment and care within a coordinated and comprehensive response to HIV/AIDS. World Health Assembly Resolution WHA57.14. Geneva: WHO; 2004. Available from: http://policy.who.int/cgi-bin/om_isapi.dll?infobase=wharec-e&softpage=Browse_Frame_Pg42. Accessed 8 February 2007.

110. Organización Panamericana de la Salud, Tecnología y Prestación de Servicios de Salud. Estudio de utilización de antibióticos en hogares de Nicaragua y Honduras. [Report excerpt]. Washington, DC: OPS; 2006.

111. Pan American Health Organization. Pharmaceutical Care to Hypertensive Patients. Pharmaceutical Forum of the Ameri-

cas. Available from: http://www.paho.org/Spanish/AD/THS/EV/FFA-proyecto-2004.pdf. Accessed 7 February 2007.

112. Pan American Health Organization. Organization, development, quality control and radiation protection in radiological services—imaging and radiation therapy. Washington, DC: PAHO; 1997.

113. Jiménez P, Borrás C, Fleitas I. Accreditation of diagnostic imaging services in developing countries. Rev Panam Salud Pública. 2006;20(2/3):104–12.

114. Hayes JC. Teleradiology: New players, high stakes create capital opportunity. Diagnostic Imaging Journal. November 2006:66–81.

115. World Health Organization. Efficacy and radiation safety in interventional radiology. Chapter 1. Geneva: WHO; 2000.

116. Feig SA. Screening mammography: a successful public health initiative. Rev Panam Salud Pública. 2006;20(2/3): 125–33.

117. United Nations Scientific Committee on the Effects of Atomic Radiation. Sources and effects of ionizing radiation. UNSCEAR 2000 report to the General Assembly, with scientific annexes. Vienna: UNSCEAR; 2000.

118. Fleitas I, Caspani CC, Borrás C, Plazas MC, Miranda AA, Brandan ME, et al. La calidad de los servicios de radiología en cinco países latinoamericanos. Rev Panam Salud Pública. 2006;20(2/3):113–24.

119. Pan American Health Organization. Health Situation in the Americas. Basic Indicators. Washington, DC: PAHO, 2006.

120. United Nations, Department of Economic and Social Affairs. World Population Prospects. The 2004 Revision. New York: United Nations; 2005.

121. World Health Organization. Cancer prevention and control. World Health Assembly. (WHA58.22). Geneva: WHO; 2005.

122. International Atomic Energy Agency, Directory of Radiotherapy Centers. Available from: http://www-naweb.iaea.org/nahu/dirac/default.shtm. Accessed 1 December 2006.

123. Castellanos ME. Las nuevas tecnologías: necesidades y retos en radioterapia en América Latina. Rev Panam Salud Pública. 2006;20(2/3):143–50.

124. International Agency for Research on Cancer. Available from: http://www.iarc.fr/index.html. Accessed 1 December 2006.

125. World Bank. Proceedings: International Forum for Promoting Safe and Affordable Medical Technology in Developing Countries. Washington, DC; 2003.

126. Food and Agriculture Organization of the United Nations; International Atomic Energy Agency; International Labor Organization; Nuclear Energy Agency of the Organization for Economic Cooperation and Development; Pan American Health Organization; World Health Organization. International basic safety standards for protection against ionizing radiation and for the safety of radiation sources. (Safety Series 115). Vienna: IAEA; 1997.

127. Pan American Health Organization. Twenty-fourth Pan American Sanitary Conference Resolution CSP24.R9. Washington DC: PAHO; 1994. Available from: http://www.paho.org/Spanish/GOV/CSP/ftcsp_24.htm. Accessed 1 December 2006.

128. International Atomic Energy Agency. International Action Plan for the Radiological Protection of Patients. Available from: http://www-ns.iaea.org/downloads/rw/radiation-safety/PatientProtActionPlangov2002-36gc46-12.pdf. Accessed 1 December 2006.

129. Borrás C. Overexposure of radiation therapy patients in Panama: problem recognition and follow-up measures. Rev Panam Salud Pública. 2006;20(2/3);173–87.

130. International Atomic Energy Agency. Accidental Overexposure of Radiotherapy Patients in San José, Costa Rica. Vienna: IAEA; 1998.

131. International Atomic Energy Agency. The Radiological Accident in Goiania. Vienna: IAEA; 1988.

132. Skvarca J, Aguirre A. Normas y estándares aplicables a los campos electromagnéticos de radiofrecuencias en América Latina: guía para los límites de exposición y los protocolos de medición. Rev Panam Salud Pública. 2006; 20(2/3): 205–212.

133. United Nations, International Telecommunication Union. World Summit on the Information Society. Geneva 2003 and Tunis 2005. Available from: http://www.itu.int/wsis/index.html. Accessed 13 December 2006.

134. European Organization for Nuclear Research. The Role of Science in the Information Society [conference]. Geneva, 8–9 December 2003. Available from: http://rsis.web.cern.ch/rsis/00Themes/01Health/Health.html. Accessed 13 December 2006.

135. Declaration of Salvador: Commitment to Equity. Ninth World Congress on Health Information and Libraries, Salvador da Bahía, Brazil, 20–23 September 2005. Available from: http://www.icml9.org/channel.php?lang=en&channel=91&content=438. Accessed 13 December 2006.

136. Salvador Declaration on Open Access: the developing world perspective. Ninth World Congress on Health Information and Libraries, Salvador da Bahía, Brazil, 20–23 September 2005. Available from: http://www.icml9.org/channel.php?lang=en&channel=91&content=439. Accessed 13 December 2006.

137. World Health Organization. Ministerial Summit on Health Research. Report by the Secretariat. (EB115/30). 2005. Available from: http://www.who.int/gb/ebwha/pdf_files/EB115/B115_30-en.pdf. Accessed 13 December 2006.

138. Krleža-Jeric K, Chan A, Dickersin K, Sim I, Grimshaw J, Gluud C. Principios del registro internacional de protocolos y resultados de ensayos clínicos a base de intervenciones de salud en seres humanos: Declaración de Ottawa (part 1). Rev Panam Salud Pública. 2006;19(6):413–16.

139. Cuervo LG, Valdés A, Clark ML. El registro internacional de ensayos clínicos. Rev Panam Salud Pública 2006;19(6): 363–70. Available from: http://www.revista.paho.org/?a_ID=510.

140. World Health Organization. International Clinical Trials Registry. Available from: http://www.who.int/ictrp/en/. Accessed 13 December 2006.

141. Hanney SR, Gonzalez-Block MA, Buxton MJ, Kogan M. The utilization of health research in policy making: concepts, examples and methods of assessment. Health Research Policy and Systems. 2003;1:2.

142. Infante A, de Mata I, López-Acuña A. Reforma de los sistemas de salud en América Latina y el Caribe: Situación y tendencias. Rev Panam Salud Pública. 2000;8(1/2):13–20.

143. Londoño J, Szekely M. Persistent poverty and excess inequality: Latin America 1970–1995. J Appl Econ. 2000;3(1): 93–134.

144. Szekely M. The 1990s in Latin America: another decade of persistent inequality, but with somewhat lower poverty. Working Paper 454. Washington, DC: IDB; 2001.

145. Almeida-Filho N, Kawachi I, Filho AP, Dachs JN. Research on health inequalities in Latin America and the Caribbean: bibliometric analysis (1971–2000) and descriptive content analysis (1971–1995). Am J Public Health. 2003;93(12): 2037–43.

146. Schneider MC, Castillo-Salgado C, Loyola-Elizondo E, Bacallao J, Mujica OJ, Vidaurre M, et al. Trends in infant mortality inequalities in the Americas: 1955–1995. J Epidemiol Community Health 2002;56(7):538–41.

147. Pan American Health Organization. Health in the Americas. Washington, DC: PAHO; 2002.

148. Iyer S, Monteiro MF. The risk of child and adolescent mortality among vulnerable populations in Rio de Janeiro, Brazil. J Biosoc Sci. 2004;36(5):523–46.

149. Vega J, Dieter Holstein R, Delgado I, Perez J, Carrasco S, Marshall G, et al. Chile: socioeconomic differentials and mortality in a middle-income nation. In: Evans T, Whitehead M, Diderichsen F, Bhuiya A, Wirth M, editors. Challenging inequities in health: from ethics to action. Oxford: Oxford University Press; 2001.

150. Barraza-Llorens M, Bertozzi S, González-Pier E, Gutiérrez JP. Addressing inequity in health and health care in Mexico. Health Aff. 2002;21(3):47–56.

151. Politzer RM, Yoon J, Shi L, Hughes RG, Regan J, Gaston MH. Inequality in America: the contribution of health centers in reducing and eliminating disparities in access to care. Med Care Res Rev. 2001;58(2):234–48.

152. Gwatkin DR, Bhuiya A, Victora CG. Making health systems more equitable. Lancet. 2004;364(9441):1273–80.

153. Gilson L, Kalyalya D, Kuchler F, Lake S, Oranga H, Ouendo M. The equity impacts of community financing activities in three African countries. Int J Health Plann Manage. 2000; 15(4):291–317.

154. Gilson L, McIntyre D. Removing user fees for primary care: necessary, but not enough by itself. Equinet Newsletter 2004;42.

155. Giraldo JFO, Palacio DH, García LEF. Resource distribution for the Basic Care Plan with equity approach, Bogotá 2002. Rev Saúde Pública 2003;37(5):640–43.

156. Morris SS, Olinto P, Flores R, Nilson EA, Figueiro AC. Conditional cash transfers are associated with a small reduction in the rate of weight gain of preschool children in northeast Brazil. J Nutr. 2004;134(9):2336–41.

157. Atiku J. Fertility reduction programmes should accompany land reforms. Afr Women Health. 1994;2(3):16–20.

158. Macinko J, Starfield B. Annotated bibliography on equity in health, 1980–2001. Int J Equity Health. 2002;1(1):1.

Chapter 5
HEALTH AND INTERNATIONAL COOPERATION

The global commitment to work towards a world with enhanced social equity and reduced poverty that informs the Millennium Development Goals (MDGs) likewise drives the international cooperation agenda. In the Americas, international cooperation takes the forms of overseas development assistance, public/private partnerships, technical cooperation among countries, and subregional integration initiatives.

Official development assistance (ODA)—comprised of grants and loans from developed countries to developing countries that target the latter's economic development and welfare—is increasingly channeled toward sub-Saharan Africa and Southeast Asia (two-thirds of all ODA in 2005), with proportionately diminished assistance for Latin America and the Caribbean (less than one-tenth of all ODA in 2005). The volume of aid per capita shows comparable differences: in 2004, per capita ODA to Africa reached US$ 34, while it was US$ 13 for Latin America and the Caribbean. Actual aid flows to individual countries depend on how each is classified: low income and lower-middle income countries receive most ODA. In general, that portion of ODA that goes to health—basic health care, disease prevention and control, family planning, and health sector infrastructure, management, and administration—has been increasing. Of total ODA for health disbursed between 2002 and 2004, 17% (US$ 402.6 million) went to Latin America and the Caribbean—three-fourths of it furnished by bilateral agencies—mainly to combat sexually transmitted infections and to effect policies related to health, the population, and primary health care. A major portion of multilateral assistance for health aid to Latin America and the Caribbean came from development banks—the World Bank, Inter-American Development Bank, Andean Development Corporation, Caribbean Development Bank, and Central American Bank for Economic Integration. Philanthropic foundations and nongovernmental organizations (NGOs) contributed another significant portion of health aid to the region. Ideally, official development assistance targets each country's health priorities based on the "global burden of disease" indicator—an estimate of the magnitude of diseases, injuries, and risk factors as measured by disability-adjusted life years (DALYs); the aim is for health-related ODA to be consistent with health priorities. Notwithstanding, in Latin America and the Caribbean, the relationship between disease burden and allocated funding has been discrepant; for example, while noncommunicable diseases account for 60% of the burden, those diseases receive only 27% of ODA for health.

Public/private partnerships, a new form of health cooperation that brings together diverse stakeholders, have been on the increase over the past decade. The leading source of health aid since it was set up in 2002—the Global Fund to Fight AIDS, Tuberculosis, and Malaria brings together donor and recipient countries, NGOs, businesses, foundations, international development organizations, and impacted communities to fight three of the world's most devastating diseases; in Latin America and the Caribbean, that agenda has meant an allocation by the Global Fund of US$ 466 million. The Global Alliance for Vaccines and Immunization has raised nearly US$ 3.3 billion, has provided vaccination coverage to millions of previously uncovered children, and has averted an estimated 1.7 premature deaths worldwide. The Onchocerciasis Elimination Program for the Americas—a collaboration among Merck Sharp and Dohme, NGOs such as the Carter Center, the Centers for Disease Control and Prevention, endemic countries, and others—aims to eliminate the disease as a public health problem and interrupt its transmission by 2007. Finally, a major objective of numerous public/private partnerships has been cooperation in managing natural disasters in the Americas, for which more than US$ 21 million were raised between 2000 and 2005.

Technical cooperation among countries—a horizontal, reciprocal process in which two or more countries work together to build individual and collective capacity through cooperative exchanges of knowledge, skills, resources, and technology—includes more than 200 health projects approved by the Pan American Health Organization (PAHO) since 1998 in areas such as disease control, risk management, environmental health, family and community health, health care services, disaster mitigation and risk management, and humanitarian aid.

To assure the greater effectiveness of development assistance, ever more emphasis is being placed on "harmonization" (encouraging donors to dovetail their various efforts), "alignment" (assuring that donors' and recipient countries' priorities are in line with one another), and a United Nations reform process that targets the coordination of various U.N. agencies' operations in developing countries. A major initiative to address the hemispheric health challenges is the adoption by all the countries of the Region of the Health Agenda for the Americas, 2008–2017.

To enhance their political and economic advantages, countries in the Americas with common histories, cultures, and, in some cases, borders have formed regional integration processes. While their priority is trade, these processes have also laid the groundwork for social and health-related cooperation. In the Southern Cone, the main regional integration scheme, MERCOSUR, is exploring the harmonization of health regulations. The Andean Community of Nations has a health sector integration process, the Hipólito Unánue Agreement, that bolsters individual and joint country efforts to improve their people's health. The Central American Integration System has established an Alliance for Sustainable Development and holds meetings of health ministers known as RESSCAD that incorporate a wide range of health sector institutions, including social security and water supply and sanitation agencies. The Caribbean Community has established a Caribbean Cooperation in Health Initiative that prioritizes strengthening health systems, developing human resources, and addressing family health, food and nutrition, noncommunicable and communicable diseases, mental health, and environmental health issues. The North American Free Trade Agreement between Canada, Mexico, and the United States includes provisions for cooperation in health among the three countries.

OFFICIAL DEVELOPMENT ASSISTANCE

Official development assistance (ODA) has become an increasingly important tool in furtherance of the MDGs (1). The Development Assistance Committee (DAC) of the Organization for Economic Cooperation and Development (OECD) defines ODA as nonreimbursable grants and subsidized loans to developing countries and territories on the DAC list of ODA recipients.

By definition, ODA must be furnished by the official sector of a donor country and geared to promoting the recipient country's economic development and welfare. Loans must have a grant element of at least 25%. The DAC's Credit Report System (CRS) and aggregate annual statistics (2) record and closely monitor trends in ODA. Both furnish data on aid commitments and disbursements by the 22 member countries of the DAC[1] and are the main source of data for this section of the chapter. ODA recipients are countries included on the list of developing nations first published by the DAC in 1962 to establish a comprehensive reporting system for ODA and other contributions by DAC member countries to developing countries. According to the DAC, the lists are published for statistical purposes only and are not designed to furnish guidance with respect to the geographic distribution of aid flows or country eligibility. Between 1993 and 2005, the DAC list was divided into two parts, with Part I of the list showing all

countries and territories receiving ODA, which were referred to as developing countries. In 2005, the DAC decided to maintain a single list of ODA recipients, eliminating Part II altogether. The current DAC list includes four groups of countries eligible for ODA; namely, the least developed countries, low income countries, lower-middle income countries, and upper-middle income countries, with countries classified according to their per capita gross national income.

The Elusive 0.7% of GNP Aid Target

ODA flows reached a record US$ 106.5 billion in 2005, equivalent to 0.33% of the GNP of DAC member countries, up from 0.26% of the GNP of the same group of countries in 2004 (3). Projections based on aid commitments by DAC member countries put the volume of ODA at US$ 130 billion by the year 2010, nearly double the figure for the year 2000. Thus, only 0.33% of GNP was devoted to ODA in 2005 and, according to projections, ODA flows in the year 2010 will represent 0.35% of the GNP of DAC member countries. Figure 1 shows ODA trends over the past decade and a half and projections through 2010.

In 1970, the U.N. General Assembly recommended that each industrialized country step up its official assistance to developing countries and "exert its best efforts to reach a minimum net amount of 0.7 per cent of its gross national product at market prices by the middle of the decade" (4). The recommendation to the effect that donor countries allocate at least 0.7% of their GNP to ODA was reaffirmed at recent world summits of heads of state and government, the Millennium Summit in 2000, the In-

---

[1]The member countries of the DAC are Australia, Austria, Belgium, Canada, Denmark, Finland, France, Germany, Greece, Ireland, Italy, Japan, Luxemburg, the Netherlands, New Zealand, Norway, Portugal, Spain, Sweden, Switzerland, the United Kingdom, and the United States.

Classification of International Cooperation

There is no standard or universally accepted classification system for international cooperation. The conceptual framework for development aid varies according to the experiences, background, interests, and priorities of the countries and organizations involved. Thus, rather than having the discipline of a science, existing classification schemes are simply an empirical grouping of the different types of cooperation offered and received by participating countries.

Cooperation is defined as **bilateral** when originating in an agreement between two countries and their respective official financial or technical agencies. Government agencies channeling funding to developing countries are known as **bilateral agencies.** Cooperation is defined as multilateral when the relationship is between a country and **multilateral international organizations** (e.g., development banks, United Nations agencies). Cooperation is defined as **horizontal** (also known as **technical cooperation among countries, or TCC**) when the main players are two or more developing countries and it involves bilateral and multilateral relations among governments, institutions, corporations, individuals, and nongovernmental organizations (NGOs) in two or more developing countries. **Nongovernmental** cooperation refers to aid furnished by NGOs, philanthropic foundations, or other private organizations.

Source: Berro M, Barreiro A, Cruz A. América Latina y la cooperación internacional. Montevideo: Instituto de Comunicación y Desarrollo; 1997.

ternational Conference on Financing for Development (Monterrey, 2002), and the 2005 U.N. General Assembly High-Level Dialogue on Financing for Development. Only five countries have surpassed this target: Denmark, Luxemburg, the Netherlands, Norway, and Sweden (2).

ODA for Latin America and the Caribbean

In 2005, there were 150 ODA recipients in different parts of the world, but with a somewhat irregular pattern of ODA distribu-

tion. From a geographic standpoint, the top priorities for ODA in 2005 were sub-Saharan Africa and Southeast Asia, with 66% of all ODA going to these two regions and a mere 9% being allocated to Latin America and the Caribbean. A look at trends over the period 1998–2004 shows a steady increase in aid flows to Africa and a relatively stable or diminishing flow of aid to Latin America and the Caribbean (Figure 2).

There are three ways of measuring ODA. One is in total U.S. dollars; a second is as a share of GNP; and a third is in terms of aid per capita, which shows the volume of aid received by a given

FIGURE 1. Official development assistance, 1990–2005 and estimates through the year 2010.

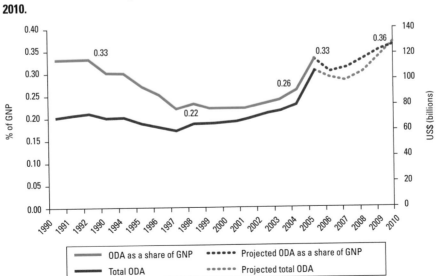

Source: Organization for Economic Cooperation and Development. Adapted from DAC members' net ODA 1990–2005 and DAC Secretariat simulation of net ODA in 2006 and 2010. Available at http://www.oecd.org/dataoecd/57/30/3530618.pdf.

FIGURE 2. Official development assistance, by region, in constant 2004 US dollars.

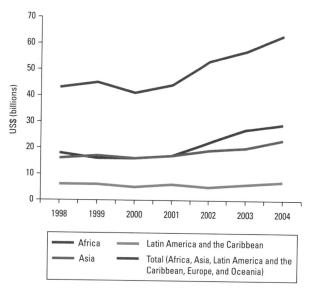

Source: Organization for Economic Cooperation and Development. Online CRS database on aid activities and DAC online database on annual aggregates (http://www.oecd.org/dac/stats/idsonline).

FIGURE 3. Official development assistance per capita, by region, 1998–2004.

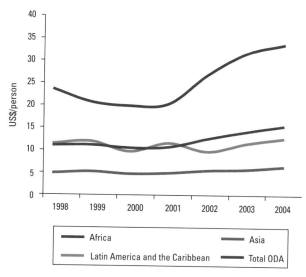

Source: Organization for Economic Cooperation and Development. Online CRS database on aid activities and DAC online database on annual aggregates (http://www.oecd.org/dac/stats/idsonline).

region or country per person and helps to standardize aid measurements by adjusting for the population factor. For example, the level of total ODA went from US$ 10 per capita in the year 2000 to nearly US$ 15 per capita in 2004. However, a breakdown by region puts the level of ODA to Africa at US$ 34 per capita in 2004, compared with US$ 13 per capita for Latin America and the Caribbean, which is below the global average, albeit above the figure for Asia, which was US$ 6 per capita. While the Asian and Latin American regions rank second and third among ODA re-

cipients in total U.S. dollars, in terms of aid flow per capita, they rank third and second, respectively (Figure 3).

Within Latin America and the Caribbean, most ODA has gone to low and lower-middle income countries which, in 2004, took in US$ 27 and US$ 14, respectively, in aid per capita. The level of aid for upper-middle income countries in Latin America and the Caribbean (US$ 2 per capita in 2004) is below the region-wide average and below the figure for aid flows to both low and lower-middle income countries (Figure 4).

Classification of World Economies

According to the World Bank classification of world economies, low income countries are those with a gross national income (GNI) per capita at or below US$ 905. Countries with a GNI per capita of between US$ 906 and US$ 3,595 are classified as lower-middle income countries, and countries with a GNI per capita of between US$ 3,596 and US$ 11,115 are classified as upper-middle income countries. High income countries have a GNI per capita of over US$ 11,115. The only country in Latin America and the Caribbean classified as a low income country is Haiti, while Antigua and Barbuda, Aruba, Bahamas, Barbados, Bermuda, the Netherlands Antilles, and Trinidad and Tobago are classified as high income economies.

Argentina, Belize, Brazil, Chile, Costa Rica, Dominica, Grenada, Mexico, Panama, Saint Kitts and Nevis, Saint Lucia, Saint Vincent and the Grenadines, Uruguay, and Venezuela are classified as upper-middle income economies. All other Latin American and Caribbean nations—Bolivia, Colombia, Cuba, the Dominican Republic, Ecuador, El Salvador, Guatemala, Guyana, Honduras, Jamaica, Nicaragua, Paraguay, Peru, and Suriname—are classified as lower-middle income countries.

Source: World Bank. Data and statistics, country classification.

FIGURE 4. Official development assistance per capita to Latin America and the Caribbean, by income level, 1998–2004.

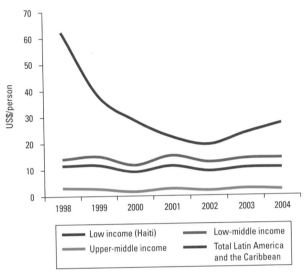

Source: Organization for Economic Cooperation and Development. Online CRS database on aid activities and DAC online database on annual aggregates (http://www.oecd.org/dac/stats/idsonline).

In general, aid is the main component of foreign capital flows to low-income countries (representing 2.8% of their GNP), while middle-income countries have a much larger flow of private capital, with aid representing only 0.2% of their GNP (*5*).

Official Development Assistance for Health

ODA for health is the portion of assistance going to the health sector into such areas as basic health; basic health care; basic health infrastructure; control of infectious diseases; general health; medical services; training and research; health policy administration and management; population; population policy administration and management; reproductive health and health care; family planning; the control of sexually transmitted infections (STIs), including HIV/AIDS; and health and population (*2*).

According to recent OECD data, ODA for health grew at an average annual rate of 5.4% during the 1990–2005 period (*6*). The share of bilateral versus multilateral aid held steady over the 1996–2004 period, with two-thirds of health aid in the form of bilateral aid and one-third in the form of multilateral aid. Bilateral aid commitments for health by DAC member countries over the 1973–2003 period totaled US$ 66 billion, with another US$ 18 billion in loan commitments by development banks coming to the health sector during that same period.

The United States has been the leading bilateral donor for health aid in absolute terms, although Ireland has furnished the most health funding in relative terms (35% of health aid for the 2002–2004 period). The volume of multilateral aid has increased since 1999, and particularly since 2002 with the establishment of

the Global Fund to Fight AIDS, Tuberculosis, and Malaria, which furnished some US$ 3.7 billion in aid over the 2002–2006 period.

Worldwide disbursements of ODA for health during the 2002–2004 period totaled US$ 8.58 billion, of which 45% went to Africa and 17% was allocated to Latin America and the Caribbean (US$ 402.6 million). These funds were used mainly to combat STIs, including HIV/AIDS, and for the implementation of health and population and primary health care policies (*7*).

However, aid to Latin America and the Caribbean for the control of STDs and HIV/AIDS accounted for only 7% of worldwide ODA for health (Figure 5). In contrast, funding for medical services and training and research in the region accounted for 14% of worldwide health-related ODA allocated to this area. A breakdown of ODA flows over the 1990–2004 period by sector shows a slight upward trend in aid to the health and population sector, whose share of the total went from 4% in 1990 to 7% in 2004 (Table 1).

ODA for Health in Latin America and the Caribbean

Health funding accounted for 13% of total worldwide ODA for the 2002–2004 period (*6*), up from 8.7% for the period 1996–1998. The 11% share of total ODA allocated to the Latin American and Caribbean region in 1998 had declined to 8.7% by 2004. While there is clearly an upward trend in worldwide aid for health, the level of aid going to Latin America and the Caribbean is declining, which took in US$ 402.6 million in health aid over the period 2002–2004 from bilateral, multilateral, and private sources (*7*) (Figure 6).

Bilateral agencies furnished 75% of all health aid for Latin America and the Caribbean over the period 2002–2004. The five leading donor countries were the United States, Japan, Spain, France, and Canada, with France and Canada earmarking the largest share of aid funding for the health sector and allocating at least 10% of all health aid to Latin America and the Caribbean (Table 2). The largest donor of cooperation funding for health in Latin America and the Caribbean in absolute terms was the United States, which furnished more than US$ 135 million.

Multilateral organizations furnished 22% of all health aid for Latin America and the Caribbean over the period 2002–2004, with 8% of all health aid disbursements for the Latin American and Caribbean region by multilateral organizations during this period made by development banks, in the form of reimbursable financial cooperation. The *World Bank Group* provided more than US$ 5.3 billion in assistance for Latin America and the Caribbean in fiscal year 2004 (*8*), including US$ 5 billion in the form of International Bank for Reconstruction and Development loans and US$ 338 million in International Development Association credits. As of June 2004, its ongoing project portfolio in Latin America and the Caribbean totaled US$ 19.3 billion. In fiscal year 2003, the World Bank channeled 27% of its loans (US$ 1.57 billion) into the funding of health projects and crucial social services in Latin American and Caribbean nations. World Bank-financed health-related projects have buttressed policies in Latin

FIGURE 5. Official development assistance for health to Latin America and the Caribbean, amounts and percentage, by sector, 2002–2004.

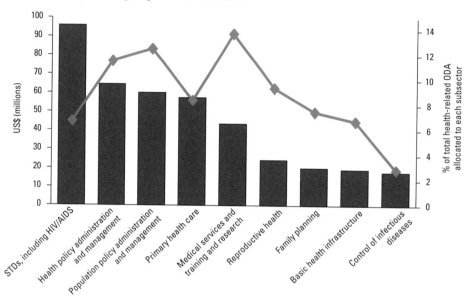

Source: Organization for Economic Cooperation and Development. Online CRS database on aid activities and DAC online database on annual aggregates (http://www.oecd.org/dac/stats/idsonline).

American and Caribbean countries designed to improve health and nutritional conditions and population outcomes for the poor.

The volume of *Inter-American Development Bank* lending in 2005 topped US$ 7 billion (*9*), up 17% from the previous year. Loan disbursements increased by nearly 20%, totaling US$ 5.3 billion.

The *Central American Bank for Economic Integration* approved a total of US$ 2.45 billion in loans during 2004 and 2005, with US$ 2.43 billion in disbursements (*10*), representing a quarter of the value of all loans approved and disbursed in the entire history of the Bank and making it the main source of multilateral development financing for Central America. There were important breakthroughs in 2005 in the Bank's three strategic areas of globalization, integration, and poverty alleviation (*11*), with large numbers of loans being approved for the social sectors, including

health. The Bank furnished US$ 13.6 million in nonreimbursable cooperation funding in 2004 and 2005 in support of various projects, including fire prevention and training programs and rehabilitation for burned children in Central America and initiatives designed to strengthen social integration.

The *Andean Development Corporation* approved approximately US$ 43 billion in financing in 2005 (*12*), with more than US$ 30 billion in disbursements and a total loan and capital investment portfolio of over US$ 8 billion. In its 35 years of operation, the Corporation has become the leading source of multilateral financing for Andean Community nations and an important alternative source of financing for its other shareholders.

The *Caribbean Development Bank* approved 15 loans in 2005 (*13*) totaling US$ 146 million and another US$ 14 million in

TABLE 1. Official development assistance to Latin America and the Caribbean, by sector, 1990–2004.

Sector	1990–1992	1993–1995	1996–1998	1999–2001	2002–2004
Education	4%	3%	6%	7%	8%
Health and population	4%	8%	8%	6%	7%
Water supply and sanitation	5%	9%	9%	7%	4%
Other social sectors	22%	23%	21%	35%	38%
Economic infrastructure	21%	13%	14%	8%	5%
Production	13%	11%	12%	8%	10%
Multisector	12%	14%	8%	12%	11%
Other	19%	19%	22%	17%	17%
Total	100%	100%	100%	100%	100%

Source: Organization for Economic Cooperation and Development. Online CRS database on aid activities and DAC online database on annual aggregates (http://www.oecd.org/dac/stats/idsonline).

FIGURE 6. Official development assistance for health to Latin America and the Caribbean, by type of source, 2002–2004.

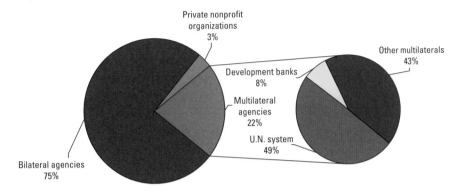

Private nonprofit
organizations
3%

Other multilaterals
43%

Development banks
8%

Multilateral
agencies
22%

U.N. system
49%

Bilateral agencies
75%

Total ODA for health: US$ 402.6 million

Source: Organization for Economic Cooperation and Development. Online CRS database on aid activities and DAC online database on annual aggregates (http://www.oecd.org/dac/stats/idsonline).

grants for member countries of the Caribbean Community. Approximately 12% of all financing approved by the Bank was for the health and disaster mitigation and risk management sectors.

Private organizations (philanthropic foundations and NGOs) supplied 3% of all health aid for Latin America and the Caribbean during the 2002–2004 period. According to independent reports on private aid flows (*10*), some 68,000 corporate, community, or independent foundations made US$ 33.6 billion in grants to countries around the world in 2005, 5.5% above the level of funding furnished by these same sources in 2004. The Latin American and Caribbean region and Africa rank third and fourth among recipients of philanthropic foundation funding, after the Asian Pacific and Eastern Europe. U.S. foundations contributed US$ 3.2 billion in 2002, US$ 3.0 billion in 2003, and US$ 2.8 billion in 2004.

Foundations around the world allocated approximately US$ 3.4 billion to health projects in 2004, which translates into an annual growth rate of 1.3% for the 2001–2004 period. This increase in funding was attributable to a US$ 750 million contribution by the Bill & Melinda Gates Foundation to the GAVI Alliance (formerly known as the Global Alliance for Vaccines and Immunization). The Bill & Melinda Gates Foundation made 112 grants for health totaling US$ 1.2 billion in 2004.

The Pan American Health and Education Foundation (PAHEF) is an especially important philanthropic foundation for the Region of the Americas. PAHEF administers health-related grants and presents international awards recognizing excellence in inter-American health, community service, health literature, veterinary public health, and bioethics.

TABLE 2. Health aid for Latin America and the Caribbean, by funding source, 2002–2004.

Donor	Health aid (US$ million)	Share of total health aid (%)	Aid to all sectors (US$ million)
United States	135.2	33.6	1776.0
Japan	44.0	10.9	944.0
GFATM	37.2	9.3	37.2
Spain	34.5	8.6	537.4
UNFPA	33.0	8.2	33.0
France	24.7	6.1	243.5
Canada	13.0	3.2	131.1
Netherlands	11.4	2.8	265.8
Germany	10.5	2.6	737.2
Switzerland	9.8	2.4	124.7
Other sources	49.3	12.3	624.2
All donors	402.6	100	5,454.1

GFATM: Global Fund to Fight AIDS, Tuberculosis and Malaria.
UNFPA: United Nations Population Fund.
Source: Organization for Economic Cooperation and Development. Online CRS database on aid activities and DAC online database on annual aggregates (http://www.oecd.org/dac/stats/idsonline).

"Over the past decade, the most important accomplishment in the field of public health in the Americas has been the rapid increase in international collaboration to solve health problems in the hemisphere and the sustained improvement in the coordination of activities of the various official entities participating in this work."

Fred Soper, 1958

Global Burden of Disease and Official Development Assistance for Health

The purpose of ODA for health is to help developing countries meet their health goals as a way of promoting the population's development and well-being. These health goals are set based on each country's health priorities, generally using health situation indicators showing the types of diseases and injuries responsible for the deterioration in human health.

The use of health measurements based on health-adjusted life expectancy estimates has become increasingly common in the last 30 years. Generically, when such measurements are based on a population approach, they are referred to as synthetic or summary measures of population health. One of the most useful such measures is the global burden of disease, a new indicator used to estimate and compare the magnitude of diseases, injuries, and risk factors in different parts of the world through a joint assessment of their lethal and nonlethal effects, referred to as disability-adjusted life years, or DALYS. By looking at flows of health aid within the framework of national health priorities, it is possible to establish their degree of consistency with these priorities.

The OECD has already highlighted discrepancies between health priorities as reflected by the burden of disease and health-related ODA (14). According to a 2002 World Health Organization (WHO) study on the global burden of disease (15), although HIV/AIDS accounted for only 2.3% of the total global burden of disease in Latin America and the Caribbean, 25% of all health aid received by Latin America and the Caribbean during the 2002–2004 period was allocated to combating HIV/AIDS. Likewise, even though non-communicable chronic diseases accounted for 60% of the total burden of disease during the same period, this health category was allocated only 36% of all health aid (Figure 7). Finally, injuries accounted for 16% of the burden of ill health but were allocated only 10% of aid funding.

Figure 7 also provides similar information at the country level for Bolivia, Guyana, Haiti, Honduras and Nicaragua, the five leading recipients of health-related ODA in the Latin America and Caribbean region. These five countries all qualify for the World Bank/International Monetary Fund Highly Indebted Poor Countries (HIPC) initiative, a debt relief program assisting numerous countries around the world.

PUBLIC/PRIVATE PARTNERSHIPS: A NEW FORM OF HEALTH COOPERATION

While ODA is channeled through official government agencies in donor and recipient countries, over the past few years, an effort has been made to strengthen different types of partnerships between the public and private sectors. More than 70 health partnerships were formed over the 1995–2005 period involving many different types of stakeholders and achieving important gains (16).

The Global Fund to Fight AIDS, Tuberculosis, and Malaria (GFATM) has been a leading source of health aid funding since its inception in 2002. The Global Fund is a public/private partnership, whose board of directors consists of representatives of the governments of donor and recipient countries, NGOs, businesses, foundations, and impacted communities, as well as of key international development partners, including WHO, the Joint United Nations Program on HIV/AIDS, and the World Bank. The Global Fund was created specifically for purposes of radically increasing funding for combating three of the world's most devastating diseases and steering this funding into areas with the greatest needs. As a partnership of different governments, civil society, the private sector, and impacted communities, the Global Fund is an innovative approach to international health financing.

In five rounds of grant-making between 2002 and mid-2006, the Global Fund approved 350 program grants in 131 countries for a total of US$ 4.9 billion, with the largest share of funding going to Africa (Figure 8).

The Latin American and Caribbean region has been allocated a US$ 466 million share of all funding supplied by the Global Fund since its formation (17). Figure 9 shows grants and disbursements for Latin America and the Caribbean in all proposal rounds by the Global Fund.

The Global Fund is the main donor for HIV/AIDS prevention and control interventions in Latin America and the Caribbean, with a total of 22 programs with approved GFATM funding for a five-year period. This funding was an important factor in meeting the target set by heads of state at the Special Summit of the Americas in Monterrey, Mexico (2004), which was to provide at least 600,000 individuals in the Americas living with HIV/AIDS with access to antiretroviral therapy by the year 2005. By the end of June of that year, there were an estimated 622,275 individuals in the Americas receiving treatment. Over the 2002–2005 period, 108,415 new courses of therapy were started in Latin America and the Caribbean, and the number of individuals receiving treatment grew from 196,000 to 304,415. Data for the sixth funding round published in November 2006 showed 85 new programs in 62 countries worldwide totaling US$ 846 million, with four Latin American and Caribbean nations (Cuba, Guatemala, Paraguay, and Peru) receiving US$ 48 million in funding.

FIGURE 7. Global burden of disease and official development assistance in Latin America and the Caribbean and in Bolivia, Guyana, Haiti, Honduras, and Nicaragua, 2002–2004.

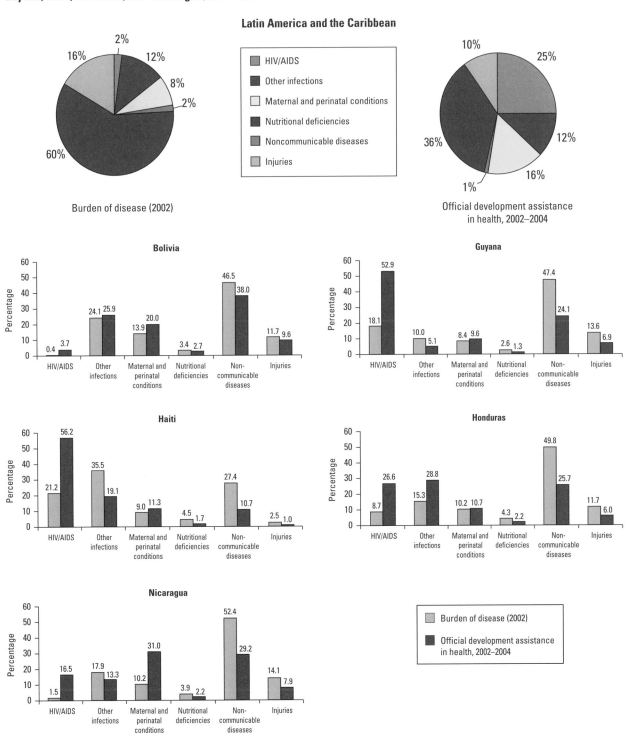

Latin America and the Caribbean

Legend:
- HIV/AIDS
- Other infections
- Maternal and perinatal conditions
- Nutritional deficiencies
- Noncommunicable diseases
- Injuries

Burden of disease (2002)

Official development assistance in health, 2002–2004

Bolivia

Guyana

Haiti

Honduras

Nicaragua

Legend:
- Burden of disease (2002)
- Official development assistance in health, 2002–2004

Source: Organization for Economic Cooperation and Development. Online CRS database on aid activities and DAC online database on annual aggregates (http://www.oecd.org/dac/stats/idsonline).

FIGURE 8. Aid disbursements by the Global Fund to Fight AIDS, Tuberculosis, and Malaria, by region, 2002–mid-2006.

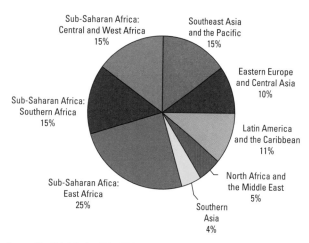

Source: The Global Fund to Fight AIDS, Tuberculosis and Malaria. Funds committed and disbursed. (http://www.theglobalfund.org)

The Global Alliance for Vaccines and Immunization (now known as the *GAVI Alliance)* was formed in 2000 to help the poorest countries provide enough vaccines to immunize their entire child populations. This public/private partnership builds on the strengths of various immunization partners, including governments, the United Nations Children's Fund (UNICEF), PAHO/WHO, Bill & Melinda Gates Foundation, World Bank, vaccine manufacturers, NGOs, and research centers. As of 2005, the Alliance had raised nearly US$ 3.3 billion in traditional financing from governments and private donors and collected more than

FIGURE 9. Amounts approved and disbursed by the Global Fund to Fight AIDS, Tuberculosis, and Malaria, Latin America and Caribbean region, 2002–mid-2006.

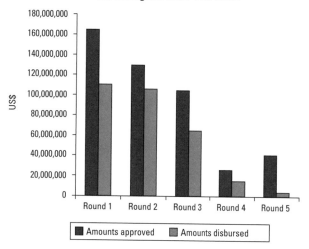

Source: The Global Fund to Fight AIDS, Tuberculosis and Malaria. Funds committed and disbursed. (http://www.theglobalfund.org)

half this sum (*18*). As of the end of that same year, GAVI had successfully vaccinated millions of children previously without access to this coverage, administering the combination diphtheria-pertussis-tetanus vaccine to close to 13 million children and vaccinating 90 million children against hepatitis B, approximately 14 million children against *Haemophilus influenzae* type b, and some 14 million children against yellow fever. Estimates put the number of premature deaths prevented through the assistance furnished by GAVI as of the end of 2005 at over 1.7 million. Some of these deaths would have involved infants, while others (deaths from vaccine-preventable diseases such as hepatitis B) would have cut short the lives of adults during their most productive years.

The Onchocerciasis Elimination Program for the Americas (OEPA) is the product of a decision made in 1987 by the international pharmaceutical firm of Merck Sharp & Dohme to provide supplies of the drug ivermectin to onchocerciasis control programs free of charge. The OEPA was created in 1991 as a multinational partnership of various types of entities, endemic countries, NGOs, the U.S. Centers for Disease Control and Prevention, academic institutions, lending agencies, and PAHO. The OEPA is supported by the River Blindness Foundation and the Carter Center in the United States. It has marshaled the necessary political, economic, and technical support to work towards the goal of eliminating all morbidity from onchocerciasis from the Region of the Americas by the year 2007 through the mass distribution of ivermectin (*19*). The goal of the OEPA is to interrupt the transmission of river blindness in six endemic countries in the Region of the Americas: Brazil, Colombia, Ecuador, Guatemala, Mexico, and Venezuela. In 2002, national programs in these countries administered 749,182 ivermectin treatments, reaching 65%–85% of the affected population.

The Western Hemisphere countries stepped up their *cooperation in the management of natural disasters* over the 2001–2005 period, including national disaster programs in the health sector, by forging better working relations with various international organizations such as UNICEF, the United Nations Development Program (UNDP), and the United Nations Office for the Coordination of Humanitarian Affairs; NGOs such as the International Federation of Red Cross and Red Crescent Societies, the International Committee of the Red Cross, and Doctors Without Borders; and donor countries, particularly Canada, the United Kingdom, and the United States.

A total of US$ 21,195,085 in funding was raised over the 2000–2005 period from various donors to meet Region-wide needs for controlling and mitigating the effects of emergencies and disasters in the Americas. This was achieved by strengthening alliances and partnerships with bilateral and multilateral cooperation agencies and private organizations, with 85% of this aid coming from bilateral cooperation agencies. The United Kingdom furnished the largest volume of funding through the Department for International Development, its official cooperation agency, followed by the European Commission's Humanitarian Aid Office. The five leading recipients of this assistance dur-

FIGURE 10. Emergency and disaster management aid to Latin America and the Caribbean, 2000–2005.

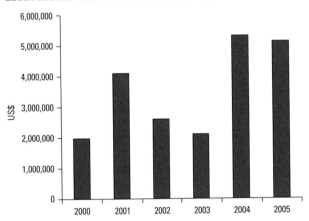

Source: Pan American Health Organization (PAHO), Emergency Preparedness and Disaster Relief.

ing 2000–2005 were Colombia, El Salvador, Guatemala, Haiti, and Nicaragua. The volume of disaster aid going to Latin America and the Caribbean increased from nearly US$ 2 million in 2000 to more than US$ 5 million in 2005 (Figure 10).

TECHNICAL COOPERATION AMONG COUNTRIES

As the supply of cooperation funding in the form of ODA for Latin America and the Caribbean has dwindled, the developing countries have looked for new types of cooperation to complement ODA, such as Technical Cooperation among Countries (TCC). TCC is, basically, a process in which two or more countries work together to build individual or collective capacity through cooperative exchanges of knowledge, skills, resources, and technology. The main characteristic of TCC is the sharing of specialized skills and successful experiences in health among countries in a more horizontal, reciprocal, and comprehensive relationship than that of classic official development assistance, which tends to be unidirectional. TCC, also known as horizontal cooperation or South-South cooperation, was originally designed to complement ODA and help offset the dwindling supply of cooperation resources from traditional donors who, with worldwide pressure from economic reforms and current political phenomena, have changed their aid priorities in terms of both the geographic regions targeted and the issues addressed.

Unlike the case of ODA, in which aid flows are monitored by the OECD through a detailed database, there is no single source of consolidated, standardized data on TCC.

PAHO, in particular, approved a total of 175 TCC projects over the 1998–2003 period, or 51 projects (29%) in the two-year 1998–1999 period, 56 projects (32%) in the two-year 2000–2001 period, and 68 projects (39%) in the two-year 2002–2003 period. The five countries in the Americas qualifying for the HIPC initiative—Bolivia, Guyana, Haiti, Honduras, and Nicaragua—are all actively participating in TCC projects sponsored by PAHO. Of a total of 44 projects approved in the two-year 2004–2005 period, 18 (41%) involved one of these five countries (*20*).

More than half of all available TCC resources from PAHO during the 1998–2003 period went to the Andean area and Central America, helping to promote the active exchanges of skills and experiences among the countries in these subregions in areas such as disease control and risk management, environmental health, family and community health, health care services, intersectoral action, disaster mitigation and risk management, and humanitarian aid (*21*).

TCC Project Helps to Improve Health Conditions of South American Chaco Residents

The Chaco is a remote region with an inhospitable climate spanning parts of Argentina, Bolivia, and Paraguay. Its inhabitants are various ethnic and indigenous groups whose rights to health and an adequate standard of living have long been overlooked. In 2000, the residents of the Chaco joined efforts to improve their living conditions, using a health approach as the principal integrating focus.

The Confederation of Indigenous Peoples of the South American Chaco Region (COPICHAS) mounted a project over the 2000–2003 period, with assistance from PAHO/WHO, whose goal was to develop and strengthen the Confederation's institutional capacity to implement strategies and carry out programs to improve health conditions and the quality of life of Chaco residents. The main components of the project were geared to strengthening communications among the different indigenous groups of the area, training the local leadership in social project management, and capacity-building for analysis of health situation and living conditions. Project outcomes include the establishment by COPICHAS of an organizational infrastructure for mounting long-term, sustainable cooperation initiatives in conjunction with other indigenous organizations.

HARMONIZATION, ALIGNMENT, AND COORDINATION OF INTERNATIONAL COOPERATION RESOURCES FOR HEALTH

One of the main challenges in terms of international cooperation for health in the Americas is the need to achieve harmonization, alignment, and the most effective coordination of resources possible.

The leading multilateral development banks, international organizations, bilateral agencies, and representatives of recipient countries gathered in Rome in February 2003 for the First High-Level Forum on Harmonization. The Paris Declaration on the effectiveness of development assistance, approved by delegates to the Second High-Level Forum in March 2005, made a change in the aid effectiveness program, turning the general consensus forged in Rome into more specific commitments to step up harmonization, alignment, and coordination efforts, and established mechanisms for monitoring progress in this direction (22).

The Rome Declaration (23) spelled out the commitment of its signatories to ensure that harmonization efforts were tailored to circumstances in recipient countries and that development assistance was aligned with the priorities of the partner/recipient country and in keeping with the good practices agreed upon by the international community at that meeting.

The participants in the Second High-Level Forum in 2005 evaluated progress in this area. In addition to representatives of all bilateral and multilateral cooperation agencies active in the Region of the Americas, the meeting was also attended by representatives of Bolivia, Guatemala, Guyana, Honduras, Jamaica, and Nicaragua.

As new modalities of technical cooperation, alignment and harmonization are clearly the new trend in assistance provision. "Harmonization" refers to donor efforts to synchronize their respective operations, while "alignment" is the synchronization of donor priorities with priorities in the recipient country, which are given precedence. The main goal of aid alignment and harmonization efforts is to build leadership in recipient countries and country ownership of the goals of the foreign assistance and to avoid duplication of efforts and structures for the delivery and monitoring of such aid, which not only increases the transaction cost of aid, but places more of a burden on the recipient country.

The harmonization and alignment agenda includes all types and modalities of aid and is designed, among other things, to ensure that a larger share of aid is delivered through mechanisms promoting program-based approaches such as budget support and sector-wide approaches (SWAPs), in which all major funding allocated to a particular sector goes to support a single spending program and policy and the government is the sole implementation and distribution agency for these funds.

In the Americas, discussions of initiatives such as the Poverty Reduction Strategy and SWAPs as part of the aid alignment and harmonization process are beginning to pick up momentum. An evaluation of budget support as an aid disbursement mechanism in 2001 revealed what were clearly positive outcomes in five of the seven countries studied: Burkina Faso, Malawi, Mozambique, Nicaragua, Rwanda, Uganda, and Vietnam (24).

In the Americas, Bolivia, Brazil, the Dominican Republic, Ecuador, Guyana, Honduras, Jamaica, Mexico, and Nicaragua have all mounted aid harmonization and alignment efforts (25) tracked as a part of monitoring activities by the World Bank. However, though such processes are already underway in the countries of Latin America and the Caribbean, efforts in this respect in the health sector remain somewhat limited to date.

Along these same lines, the United Nations reform process is designed to improve the efficiency and effectiveness of the operations of various U.N. agencies in developing countries. The United Nations Development Group is using two tools to achieve its goals in this reform process: Common Country Assessments and the United Nations Development Assistance Framework, both of which are designed to better synchronize inter-agency operations in developing countries, while at the same time serving as an opportunity to promote intersectoral action in the Americas.

THE FUTURE OF INTERNATIONAL COOPERATION IN THE AMERICAS

The most important challenge for Latin America and the Caribbean with respect to ODA is, at the very least, to sustain the share of aid for health in the Americas at its current level in the face of the priority accorded other parts of the world in recent years.

On one hand, the number of Latin American and Caribbean nations eligible for official bilateral aid from donor countries is steadily decreasing with the reported progress in the indicators of poverty and well-being used by such countries, despite the persisting gaps and inequities in this region. Moreover, there is an urgent need to make the use of ODA resources more effective by aligning aid flows with country interests and priorities and by better synchronizing the operations of the different bilateral and multilateral agencies and organizations supporting work in the health sector in these countries.

Without question, one of the greatest challenges facing the Americas is the implementation of the Health Agenda for the Americas 2008–2017 endorsed by the Governments of Western Hemisphere countries as a framework for joint action by national and international stakeholders with an interest in helping to improve the health of the peoples of this Region over the next decade.

TCC is an option for addressing the likely rollback in future financial aid to the Americas. The countries of this Region have developed adequate and, in some cases, mutually complementary capacities and skills for the attainment of health and development goals in Latin America and the Caribbean. Nevertheless, it is important that such projects take a long-range view. Exchanges within the framework of TCC activities need to be viewed as the first step in a longer-term, sustainable process that will require time and additional funding as well as the establishment of mechanisms to help countries define the expected outcomes of TCC activities, bearing in mind their long-term impact, including corresponding monitoring and evaluation methods and procedures.

More specifically, the Americas have gained a considerable amount of experience in disaster management, with international cooperation playing a pivotal role in strengthening disaster mitigation, preparedness, and response systems. The Region has learned to share its experience and capabilities with other parts of the world, surmounting geographic barriers and establishing a virtuous cycle global cooperation in coping with disasters. In the wake of natural disasters such as the powerful earthquake striking Bam, Iran, in 2003; the devastating Indian Ocean tsunami of 2004; and the major earthquake hitting Pakistan and India in 2005, experts from various Latin American and Caribbean nations quickly responded with invaluable assistance and solidarity, thereby providing a model for efficient and effective international cooperation.

"International organizations in general need to accept the fact that they confront fundamental demands for change. The prospects for such change are under way, including the implementation of a series of new approaches for the 1990s. These approaches encourage subregional initiatives by groups of countries, favor closer relation between national priorities and initiatives and technical cooperation efforts, press for realizing the full potential of available national resources, support decentralization and regionalization of national health systems, and favor concentrating efforts on the most critical areas in need. Beyond that, we are also pressing for acknowledgment of the major impact that political decisions have on health activities, for application of the "health for all" principles and primary care strategy, for integration of health into the socioeconomic process, and for better application of science and technology to meet people's basic needs."

Carlyle Guerra de Macedo, 1990

HEALTH AND INTEGRATION PROCESSES IN THE AMERICAS

Today's world is shaped by two parallel, mutually complementary phenomena: globalization and regional integration. On the one hand, globalization promotes interdependence by placing all countries in a single arena in which they are forced to compete for markets and capital while, on the other hand, regionalization seeks to create integration blocs of countries with a shared history and culture and, in some cases, common borders to improve their development opportunities and options in a globalizing environment.

Regional integration processes in the Americas are principally motivated by political and economic goals, with countries seeking to protect their autonomy and identity while at the same time positioning themselves in a stimulating albeit hostile and competitive globalized environment. Regional integration processes in the Americas have their own development dynamics, with periods of stagnation and development, in which trade issues are given top priority. However, such processes have all helped lay the groundwork for progress in social areas, including those related to health.

Integration in the Southern Cone

The Southern Cone countries of South America—Argentina, Brazil, Chile, Paraguay, and Uruguay—are members of several subregional integration or cooperation blocs simultaneously and have forged subregional alliances in the area of health, which in some cases have been incorporated into economic integration processes.

The Southern Cone is a heterogeneous subregion in terms of its social, economic, demographic, epidemiological, and health situation characteristics and the responsiveness of its health systems, which vary not only from one country to another, but within different geographic areas of the same country. In terms of population, Brazil is the largest nation, with more than 186 million inhabitants, while Uruguay accounts for the smallest share of the subregion's population, with more than 3 million inhabitants. Brazil (21.8%) and Uruguay (19.6%) have the highest population densities, while Paraguay (15.1%) and Argentina (13.9%) have the lowest population densities. Looking at the population's age structure, Paraguay (at 70.5%), with its more youthful population, and Uruguay (at 60%), with the steady growth in its older adult population, have the highest dependency ratios of the five Southern Cone countries. All of the countries have a predominantly urban population, with the sole exception of Paraguay. According to population data for 2005, Argentina (at 26.4%) and Uruguay (at 24.3%) were two of the four Latin American and Caribbean countries (along with Cuba and Chile) with the smallest share of youths under the age of 15 (26).

The Southern Cone has a fairly small indigenous population. In Brazil, 52.2% of the indigenous population lives in urban areas, compared with a mere 8.4% of the indigenous population of Paraguay. There are large differences in national averages for the Southern Cone countries in terms of per capita income, as well as in the income ratios for the top and bottom 20% of their respective populations (26).

MERCOSUR is the principal regional integration process for the Southern Cone countries, all of which hold either full or associate membership status. These countries are also members of the Union of South American Nations. Brazil is a member of the

Amazon Cooperation Treaty Organization, while Chile is a member of the Andean Health Agency-Hipólito Unánue Agreement on Health.

MERCOSUR is the customs union (a free trade area with a common trade policy) for Argentina, Brazil, Paraguay, and Uruguay. Thus far, Chile (1996), Bolivia (1997), and Peru (2003), and Colombia, Ecuador, and Venezuela became associate members (2004), with Venezuela later becoming a full member (2006).

MERCOSUR has three decision-making bodies: the Common Market Council, the Common Market Group, and the MERCOSUR Trade Commission, which is a technical body. There are 15 Working Subgroups for the coordination of macroeconomic and sector policies, including groups on the Environment, Agriculture, Labor Issues, Employment and Social Security, and Health. MERCOSUR also includes other advisory bodies, such as the Joint Parliamentary Commission, the Economic and Social Consultative Forum, and the Commission of Permanent Representatives to MERCOSUR. Its Secretariat is permanently headquartered in Montevideo, Uruguay.

Meetings of MERCOSUR health ministers deal with the harmonization of health policies, while Working Subgroup 11 (Health) deals with the harmonization of health regulations. As an integration process, the health challenges addressed by MERCOSUR all have to do with sustaining ongoing efforts to harmonize regulations as the basis for free trade in health products. The main needs are to improve the institutional performance of regulatory agencies and the harmonization of corresponding regulations, including provisions relating to good manufacturing practices and quality control for the pharmaceutical industry, blood and blood products, medical supplies, household health supplies and chemicals, information and epidemiological information processing systems, and technology evaluation, among others. According to the MERCOSUR agenda, the focus of this subregional integration and cooperation process is on access to timely information; organ, tissue, and cell donation and transplants; implementation of the International Health Regulations; a health surveillance system for dengue and other diseases; improving health conditions in border communities; developing an integrated policy for controlling the HIV and STD epidemics; sexual and reproductive health; an integrated tobacco control policy, oversight in the management of natural disasters and incidents with hazardous materials; an environmental and occupational health policy; public health research; and equitable access to knowledge as a health-related regional public good within the framework of MERCOSUR.

Integration in the Andean Area

The Andean area consists of Bolivia, Chile, Colombia, Ecuador, Peru, and Venezuela. Colombia has the largest population (with 41,242,948 inhabitants), and Bolivia has the smallest population (with 9,182,000 inhabitants). Ecuador has the highest population density, while Bolivia has the lowest population density. A look at the age structure of the Andean area's population shows Bolivia with the highest dependency ratio due to its large child population and steadily growing older adult population.

Bolivia and Ecuador and, to a lesser extent, Peru have primarily rural populations. These same countries have a large indigenous population, generally concentrated in sparsely populated rural areas.

International migration is one of the most complicated and challenging phenomena for the Andean area countries, where patterns of migration in terms of points of origin and destination are constantly changing. However, there are certain more or less typical interregional and intra-regional migratory movements. In general, the main type of migration is labor-related, tied to the deep-seated economic imbalances between the area countries. Another major cause of migration is the displacement of entire groups as a result of political violence and internal strife, such as in the case of Colombia. The Office of the United Nations High Commissioner for Refugees estimates the number of internally displaced persons in Andean area countries at somewhere between 2 and 3.3 million, many of whom seek refuge in other area countries.

The integration movement in this area began in 1969, culminating with the official establishment of the **Andean Community of Nations** in 1996, whose General Secretariat is headquartered in Lima, Peru. The Andean Community currently consists of Bolivia, Colombia, Ecuador, and Peru, with Argentina, Brazil, Chile, Paraguay, and Uruguay serving as associate members.

The counterpart of the Community's political and trade integration process in the health sector is the Meeting of Andean Area Health Ministers (REMSAA, for its Spanish acronym) of signatory countries to the Hipólito Unánue Agreement for Cooperation in Health in Andean Area Countries. This agreement, officially referred to as the Andean Health Agency-Hipólito Unánue Agreement (ORAS-CONHU, for its Spanish acronym) since 2002, is designed to synchronize and bolster individual and joint efforts by member countries to improve their population's health. It coordinates and promotes activities geared to improving health conditions in member countries, giving top priority to cooperation mechanisms fostering the development of subregional systems and methodologies. To this end, it coordinates efforts in furtherance of this goal with those of other subregional, regional, and international organizations. The governing body for the ORAS-CONHU is REMSAA.

REMSAA has made some progress in improving access to drugs, and the Subregional Technical Commission for a Drug Access Policy has developed a work plan for carrying on joint negotiations with respect to HIV/AIDS medications.

To address border health issues, ORAS-CONHU is implementing the PAMAFRO Project aimed at controlling malaria in border zones of the Andean countries, and, specifically, lowering the disease's incidence in the highest-incidence areas. The project has received funding from the Global Fund to Fight AIDS, Tuberculosis, and Malaria and technical cooperation and logistical assistance from PAHO/WHO, as the product of an initiative among Andean area ministers of health and coordinated efforts by Ecuador, Colombia, Peru, and Venezuela (27).

Malaria and dengue are still major public health problems in all Andean area countries with the exception of Chile. In the case of malaria, the magnitude of the problem is further compounded by the resistance of *Plasmodium falciparum* to cloroquine and other antimalarial drugs. All four dengue virus serotypes are in circulation in the Andean area, producing outbreaks of dengue hemorrhagic fever in the past few years. While human rabies transmitted by dog bites is in the process of being eliminated, there are still bat-transmitted wild rabies outbreaks in the Amazon region, affecting mainly resident indigenous communities. The HIV/AIDS epidemic is still concentrated among high-risk population groups. Its prevalence rate in adults aged 15–49 is 0.5%, compared with rates of over 10% among men who have sex with men, with a large margin of fluctuation according to the city and population group in question. The principal transmission mode is through sexual contact, although in Chile, parenteral transmission by intravenous drug users is also an important mode of transmission. Stepped-up trade and free trade agreements have created a need for the incorporation of plant and animal health regulations into existing food safety legislation, as well as for the establishment of laboratory networks to inspect and certify the quality of food products earmarked for domestic consumption and export.

Integration in Central America

The Central American area includes the countries of Belize, Costa Rica, the Dominican Republic, El Salvador, Guatemala, Honduras, Nicaragua, and Panama, with a population of approximately 50 million inhabitants. As far as its cultural diversity is concerned, Guatemala puts the share of its indigenous and/or native population at 48%, compared with 19% for Belize, 10% for Panama, 8% for Nicaragua, 7% for Honduras, 2% for Costa Rica, and an estimated 11% for El Salvador in 2006 (26). According to a UNDP report, there are a total of approximately 6,100,000 members of indigenous groups in this subregion (which account for 12% of the total population of Central America and the Dominican Republic) (28). This same source reported a total of 506,753 immigrants in all Central American countries combined in 2001, with close to 70% coming from within the Central American subregion, and 59% of the immigrants going to Costa Rica and 16% to Panama.

There were roughly 1,300,000 emigrants from Central American countries in or around 1990, whose main country of destination was the United States. By the year 2000, this figure had jumped to close to 1,800,000.

There are large divides between the rich and poor in Central America in terms of their means and opportunities. The wealthiest 20% of the population of El Salvador, Guatemala, Honduras, and Panama has 20–25 times more income than the poorest 20%. The wealthiest 20% of the population of Costa Rica and the Dominican Republic has 10–12 times more income than the poorest 20%. Nicaragua has the largest income gap, which could potentially cause a regression in health and development indicators (26).

All area countries are part of the **Central American Integration System (SICA)**, in which the Dominican Republic is an associate state and the other countries are member states. The Central American countries have been involved in integration processes for more than 40 years, achieving a number of major breakthroughs in the 1990s. The Tegucigalpa Protocol of 1991 created and implemented a new institutional framework based on SICA and established a basic program platform known as the Alliance for Sustainable Development.

The SICA General Secretariat is permanently headquartered in San Salvador, El Salvador, although several SICA entities are based in other countries. The Central American Parliament, for example, is based in Guatemala City, and the Central American Court of Justice is located in Managua, Nicaragua. ICA's top decision-making body is the Meeting of Heads of State and Government of its member countries. Other SICA bodies include the Executive Council of Foreign Ministers and Ministerial-Level Sectoral Councils, including the Council of Health Ministers. SICA also includes intersectoral bodies, such as the Meeting of Ministers of Agriculture, the Environment, and Health. It has a Consultative Committee and a Social Integration Secretariat, which operates as a specialized sectoral body. Other institutions include the Nutrition Institute of Central America and Panama, the Central American Higher University Council, the Regional Coordinating Committee for Water Supply and Sanitation Agencies, and the Regional International Organization for Plant Protection and Animal Health.

There have been Meetings of Central American Health Ministers since 1956. Since 1985, these meetings have been referred to as Meetings of the Health Sector of Central America and the Dominican Republic (RESSCAD) to reflect their expansion to include other health sector agencies and institutions, such as social security and water supply and sanitation agencies. The Dominican Republic became a full-fledged member in 2000 after attending the meetings as an observer for more than a decade. PAHO/WHO serves as the technical secretariat for RESSCAD under the provisions of Article 3 of the RESSCAD Regulations approved at the XVI RESSCAD Meeting held in 2000.

Other integration bodies helping to further the social agenda include the Central American Bank for Economic Integration; the Central American Public Administration Institute; the Central American Institute for Industrial Research and Technology; the Coordination Center for the Prevention of Natural Disasters in Central America; the Regional Water Resources Commission; the

"While new and reemerging diseases represent a threat, there are other worries too. Natural disasters, chemical and nuclear accidents, climate change and its consequences, and bioterrorism all have the potential to affect international public health security. However, the same forces of globalization that allow pathogens to move freely around the world, can also be used to build multinational partnerships to help us expand access to drugs and vaccines, improve public health infrastructure in developing countries, and launch better public health workforce education programs worldwide."

Mirta Roses, 2007

Permanent Central American Commission for the Eradication of Illegal Drug and Psychotropic Substance Production, Trafficking, Consumption, and Use; and the International Organization for Plant Protection and Animal Health.

In addition, there are a number of ad hoc intergovernmental secretariats, such as the Central American Council of Social Security Agencies, the Central American Electricity Board, the Central American Council for Sports and Recreation, the Central American Commission on Housing and Human Settlements, and the Science and Technology Commission of Central America and Panama.

Integration in the Caribbean

The Caribbean subregion includes the nations of Antigua and Barbuda, the Bahamas, Barbados, Belize, Dominica, Grenada, Guyana, Jamaica, Saint Kitts and Nevis, Saint Lucia, Saint Vincent and the Grenadines, Suriname, and Trinidad and Tobago; the British overseas territories of Anguilla, Bermuda, the British Virgin Islands, the Cayman Islands, Montserrat, and the Turks and Caicos Islands; the French overseas departments of French Guiana, Guadalupe, and Martinique; and the Netherlands Antilles autonomous territories of Bonaire, Curaçao, Saba, Saint Eustatius, and Saint Maarten.

The subregion is made up of small islands and mainland states with areas of anywhere from 13 km^2 (Saba) to 214,970 km^2 (Guyana) and populations ranging in size from approximately 1,400 inhabitants (Saba) to as many as 2,651,000 inhabitants (Jamaica). This multilingual, multiethnic, multicultural area is marked by wide gaps in socioeconomic development levels, health conditions, health needs, and available resources.

The framework for technical cooperation in this subregion is somewhat complex. The Caribbean countries are members of various subregional integration processes, some of which also include Latin American countries, such as the Amazon Cooperation Treaty Organization and the Association of Caribbean States (ACS). Moreover, all independent countries have bilateral agree-

ments and relations with other countries, some with Cuba and others with multilateral financial institutions such as the World Bank and the International Monetary Fund. The GFATM, the President's Emergency Plan for AIDS Relief (a U.S. Government initiative created in 2003), and the William J. Clinton Foundation also fund health projects in this subregion. There are a number of powerful NGOs, trade associations, and private enterprises operating at the subregional and country levels marshalling resources that in many cases outstrip the volume of government funding. United Nations and Inter-American System agencies and organizations are also cooperation partners in this subregion.

The main subregional cooperation agency is the **Caribbean Community (CARICOM)**, whose Secretariat headquarters are located in Georgetown, Guyana. The PAHO/WHO Office of Caribbean Program Coordination entered into an agreement with CARICOM in 1978 and is also involved in cooperation initiatives with the Organization of Eastern Caribbean States and the ACS. The Caribbean Epidemiology Center and the Caribbean Food and Nutrition Institute are specialized PAHO/WHO centers and CARICOM regional health institutions. Other health institutions within the CARICOM system include the Caribbean Environmental Health Institute, the Caribbean Health Research Council, and the Caribbean Drug Research and Testing Laboratory.

The Eastern Caribbean Cooperation Strategy for 2006–2009 crafted in 2005 by PAHO/WHO established the following five strategic directions: enabling the health systems to ensure equitable access and improve quality of services; strengthening public health leadership; reducing preventable mortality, avoidable morbidity, and disability in priority health areas; reducing vulnerability and threats to health arising from environmental and economic causes, including natural and other hazards; and enabling optimal use of global, regional, and subregional collective agreements for national health development (*29*).

The main health challenges for this subregion are reflected in the priorities set by CARICOM's strategic framework for cooperation in health known as the Caribbean Cooperation in Health (CCH) Initiative. The priorities for Phase II (1999–2003) of the Initiative were strengthened health systems, human resources development, family health, food and nutrition, chronic noncommunicable diseases, communicable diseases, mental health, and environmental health. Health promotion was viewed as a cross-cutting strategy. Among other things, the Nassau Declaration of 2001 by CARICOM Heads of Government endorsed CCH Phase II commitments as "the framework under which all regional and subregional, national, and institutional sector plans for health will be considered" and focused on HIV/AIDS, chronic noncommunicable diseases, and mental health as work priorities (*30*). A subsequent evaluation of Phase II of the CCH Initiative conducted at the request of the Heads of Government highlighted a number of achievements, along with a few weaknesses. Phase III, covering the period 2007–2015, whose design is nearly finalized, will address the findings of the Phase II evaluation.

Integration in North America

In January 1994, the **North American Free Trade Agreement** **(NAFTA)** was established among Canada, Mexico, and the United States. The NAFTA Secretariat headquarters are located in Ottawa, Mexico City, and Washington, D.C.

The three nations of North America, while they do share some similarities, are for the most part very different in social, economic, demographic, and epidemiological terms, as well as health conditions and the response capacity of health care systems. The population of the North American subregion is approximately 442 million (49% of the total population of the Region of the Americas as a whole). In each of the three countries, the majority of the population resides in urban areas; only 21% are rural inhabitants. Mexico has the highest crude birth rate (19.6 per 1,000 population), compared to 13.9 per 1,000 population in the United States and 10.1 per 1,000 population in Canada. The average dependency ratio is 49.9% for the three countries as a whole, with Mexico having the highest rate (56%) (*26*).

The North American subregion has a high migration rate and number of border crossings. Along the U.S.-Mexico border alone, there are an estimated 400 million border crossings a year (*31*). According to the International Organization for Migration, in 2006 approximately 450,000 undocumented persons emigrated from Mexico to other parts of the world, principally the United States and Canada (*32*). According to U.S. immigration authorities, there are an estimated 11 million undocumented persons currently residing in this country, with 6 million of these coming from Mexico (*33*).

Trade between the three NAFTA partners has grown considerably over the past dozen years, standing at US$ 297 billion in 1993 and US$ 810 in 2005. One indication of the commercial interdependence between the three countries is the fact that Canada and Mexico have become the first and second largest markets, respectively, for the United States. Furthermore, Mexico has tripled the volume of its agricultural exports to the United States, which stood at US$ 3.6 billion in 1993 and US$ 9.3 billon in 2005 (*34*).

During the signing of NAFTA, the three partners also signed the North American Agreement on Labor Cooperation and the North American Agreement on Environmental Cooperation. The Commission on Labor Cooperation and the Commission for Environmental Cooperation were established for the implementation of the respective agreements. Additionally, Mexico and the United States established the Border Environmental Cooperation Commission and the North American Development Bank.

In a 2006 publication, the Commission for Environmental Cooperation analyzed data obtained from national pollutant release and transfer registers in North America and emphasizes the reporting of chemical carcinogens, developmental toxicants, and neurotoxicants. Although data were available only for the United States and Canada, the report discusses in specific terms the potential impact of these substances on the health of children in North America (*35*).

Even while NAFTA's primary focus is on economic integration, various health-related aspects are addressed through its aforementioned labor and environmental agreements. PAHO has collaborated with the Commission for Environmental Cooperation in the provision of technical assistance in environmental health issues and in consensus-building within the context of the International Health Regulations, whose latest revision (2005) was unanimously adopted by WHO member countries at the World Health Assembly in May of that year and which entered into force in June 2007.

Additionally, PAHO maintains a permanent presence along the Mexico-United States border through its Field Office located in El Paso, Texas. Established in 1942 at the request of the two Governments, the Office coordinates and oversees a variety of health-related technical cooperation activities along the border area, interacting with the federal government officials of Mexico and the United States, as well as the political leaders of the area's 10 border states (Arizona, California, New Mexico, and Texas in the United States and Baja California, Chihuahua, Coahuila, Nuevo León, Sonora, y Tamaulipas in Mexico) and with their respective public health authorities. The Field Office's work focuses on developing and implementing effective responses to the unique health situation characterizing this multicultural and multilingual geographic area and building a consensus among government and public health authorities at the local, state, and federal levels regarding the need for collective, well-integrated health promotion and prevention programs. Among its priorities are the development of information systems enabling the comparability of core health data and improved informational exchanges, surveillance and control of such communicable diseases as tuberculosis and HIV/AIDS, and, more recently, situation and risk factor analysis of various chronic noncommunicable diseases, particularly diabetes.

References

1. Organization for Economic Cooperation and Development. OECD Journal on Development. Development Cooperation Report 2005. Vol. 7 No. 1. Paris: OECD; 2006.

2. Organization for Economic Cooperation and Development. Online CRS database on aid activities and DAC online database on annual aggregates. Available at: http://www.oecd .org/dac/stats/idsonline. Accessed on 30 September 2006.

3. Organization for Economic Cooperation and Development. Aid flows top 100 billion in 2005. Available at: http://www .oecd.org. Accessed on 30 September 2006.

4. Asamblea General de las Naciones Unidas. Vigésimo quinto período de sesiones. Resolución de la Asamblea General 2626 (XXV) del 24 de octubre de 1970. Estrategia Internacional del Desarrollo para el Segundo Decenio de las Naciones Unidas para el Desarrollo.

5. Radelet S. A primer for foreign aid. Working paper No. 92. Washington, DC: Center for Global Development; 2006.

6. Organization for Economic Cooperation and Development. Recent trends in official development assistance to health. Paris: OECD; 2006. Available at: http://www.oecd.org/dataoecd/1/11/37461859.pdf. Accessed on 30 September 2006.

7. Organization for Economic Cooperation and Development. Aid to health—disbursement—pivot tables. January 2006. Available at: http://www.oecd.org.

8. World Bank. 2005 Annual Report. Washington, DC: World Bank; 2006.

9. Inter-American Development Bank. 2005 Annual Report. Washington, DC: IDB; 2006.

10. Banco Centroamericano de Integración Económica. XLIV Memoria anual de labores 2005. Tegucigalpa: BCIE; 2006.

11. Banco Centroamericano de Integración Económica. Tendencias y perspectivas económicas de Centroamérica. Tegucigalpa: BCIE; 2006.

12. Corporación Andina de Fomento. Informe anual 2005. Caracas: CAF; 2006.

13. Caribbean Development Bank. 2005 Annual Report. Wildey (Barbados): CDB; 2006.

14. MacKeller L. OECD Development Centre Working paper No. 244. Priorities in global assistance for health, AIDS and population (HAP). Paris: OECD; 2005.

15. World Health Organization. Health statistics; Burden of disease project [Web page]. Available at: http://www.who.int/healthinfo. Accessed on 30 September 2006.

16. Bill & Melinda Gates Foundation; McKinsey & Company. Global Health Partnerships: Assessing Country Consequences. Washington, DC: McKinsey & Company; 2005.

17. The Global Fund to Fight AIDS, Tuberculosis, and Malaria. Funds committed and disbursed [Web page]. Available at: http://www.theglobalfund.org. Accessed on 30 September 2006.

18. GAVI Alliance. A brief description of the GAVI Alliance and Fund [Web page]. Available at: http://www.gavialliance.org. Accessed on 3 September 2006.

19. World Health Organization. Onchocerciasis Elimination Program for the Americas (OEPA) [Web page]. Available at: http://www.who.int. Accessed on 30 September 2006.

20. Pan American Health Organization. 47th Directing Council. Performance Assessment Report of the Biennal Program Budget of the Pan American Health Organization, 2004–2005. (CD47/10). Washington, DC: PAHO; 2006.

21. Pan American Health Organization. 136th Session of the Executive Committee. Technical Cooperation among Countries in the Region. (CE136/11, Rev.1). Washington, DC: PAHO; 2005.

22. Pan American Health Organization. 40th Session of the Subcommittee on Planning and Programming. PAHO Framework for Resource Mobilization. (SPP40/4). Washington, DC: PAHO; 2006.

23. World Bank. Rome Declaration on Harmonization. Available at: http://www.worldbank.org/harmonization. Accessed on 30 September 2006.

24. Seco S, Martínez J. An overview of sector-wide approaches (SWAPs) in health. Are they appropriate for aid-dependant Latin American countries? London: DFID Health Systems Resource Centre; 2001.

25. Dos Santos J. Harmonization and alignment for achieving greater aid effectiveness. Available information on country level activities [Web page]. Available at: http://www.aidharmonization.org. Accessed on 30 September 2006.

26. Pan American Health Organization. Health situation in the Americas. Basic indicators 2006. Washington, DC: PAHO; 2006.

27. Organismo Andino de Salud-Convenio Hipólito Unánue. [Information]. Available at: http://www.orasconhu.org. Accessed on 23 August 2006.

28. Programa de las Naciones Unidas para el Desarrollo. Segundo informe sobre desarrollo humano en Centroamérica y Panamá. ASDI; PNUD; 2003.

29. Pan American Health Organization. Eastern Caribbean Cooperation Strategy. 2006–2009. Office of the Caribbean Program Coordinator; 2005.

30. Caribbean Community Secretariat. Nassau Declaration on Health 2001: The Health of the Region is the Wealth of the Region. Nassau: CARICOM; 2001.

31. United States, U.S. Customs and Border Protection. Office of Field Operations Strategic Plan Fiscal Year 2007–2011. Securing America's borders at ports of entry; 2006.

32. International Organization for Migration. Mexico: Facts and Figures. Available at: http://iom.int/jahia/page484.html. Accessed on 25 June 2007.

33. Hoefer M, Rytina N, Campbell C. Estimates of the unauthorized immigrant population residing in the United States: January 2005. Population estimates. August 2006. Office of Immigration Statistics. U.S. Department of Homeland Security. Available at: www.uscis.gov/graphics/shared/statistics/publications/ILL_PE_2005.pdf.

34. United States, Executive Office of the President, Office of the United States Trade Representative. Trade Facts; March 2006.

35. Commission for Environmental Cooperation. Toxic Chemicals and Children's Health in North America: A Call for Efforts to Determine the Sources, Levels of Exposure, and Risks that Industrial Chemicals Pose to Children's Health; May 2006. Available at: http://www.cec.org/pubs_docs/documents/index.cfm?varlan=english&ID=1965. Accessed on 17 July 2007.

Chapter 6
PROSPECTS FOR
REGIONAL HEALTH

The countries of the Americas have made significant progress in reducing mortality and morbidity over the past several decades, although inequities persist among and within countries. Both that progress and those inequities are occurring in circumstances of constant flux. Going forward, continuation of that progress and remediation of those inequities will depend on myriad, dynamic factors and trends and on how individuals, populations, governments, and the international community address them.

Trends that Condition the Future of Health

Health in the Americas over the coming years and decades will take shape as current trends unfold. Three macro trends will prevail, namely those related to the socioeconomic context, the health situation, and the health system response, which explains the structure of the contents—general context, health conditions, and sector response—in both the regional and country volumes of this publication.

Socioeconomic Trends. As has been described in the preceding pages, a range of socioeconomic trends—namely those related to the economy, the population, education, the environment, health access, and international aid—impacts the health of the population of the Region. Although the per-capita gross domestic product in Latin America and the Caribbean grew by over 4% from 2001 to 2005 and the numbers of poor are decreasing, 40% of the population (205 million) continue to live in poverty and over 15% (79 million) in extreme poverty. Income and its distribution greatly influence health status.

While the Region's population growth has slowed, an ever-larger portion of that population is over 60. Health systems will need to take account of an aging population's health profile and the implications it will have for the nature and delivery of health services. A second major demographic factor influencing health is urbanization which, albeit enabling people greater access to social services, also tends to promote unhealthy behaviors—among them, poor nutrition, drug and alcohol abuse, alienation, and violence.

Progress in education in the Americas—while still compromised by inequities in terms of gender, ethnic group, and geographic location—has been characterized by major gains in the past couple of decades. About 94% of the population is literate, and some 95% of boys and girls alike are enrolled in primary education.

Latin America and the Caribbean have attained high overall coverage rates of water supply (91%) and sanitation (77%), although rural areas tend to have less coverage. The major environmental challenges stem from air, water, and soil contamination, the risks of industrialization and unplanned development, and the destructive impact of disasters.

Millions of people in the Region lack health insurance coverage (218 million) and access to health services (over 100 million). This exclusion from health is the result of poverty, marginalization, and various forms of discrimination and stigmatization, which in turn relate to language, informal employment, un- and underemployment, geographic isolation, lack of education and access to information.

A final socioeconomic trend relates to official development aid. Much of that aid is now either going to other regions of the world, resulting in a reduced share for the Americas, or, in the case of bilateral assistance, is targeting specific countries rather than general regional development.

Health Situation Trends. Communicable diseases—such as malaria, dengue, tuberculosis, HIV/AIDS, and zoonoses—continue to represent major threats to the health of the population of Latin America and the Caribbean, and certain "neglected" diseases—among them, filariasis, leptospirosis, and Chagas' disease—disproportionately afflict the region's poor. Increasingly, however, the leading causes of death and illness in all of the countries of the Americas are noncommunicable chronic diseases—especially cardiovascular diseases, cancer, and diabetes—together with violence, trauma, occupational diseases, and mental illness.

While health indicators have generally improved over the recent past, in large measure as the result of primary care interventions, health inequalities persist. Indigenous groups, women, the poor and uneducated, rural inhabitants, and the elderly are less healthy than other groups in society.

Health System Trends. Among the most prevalent trends characterizing health systems in the Region are the segmentation of services, the inadequacy of health financing policies, the poor allocation of health resources, and the emphasis on terciary and individual health care at the expense of primary and public care. Health sector reforms that began in the 1990s actually weakened the position of health ministries, rendering them less able to assume sector leadership and to perform their essential health functions.

National health expenditures in Latin America and the Caribbean represented less than 7% of the region's gross domestic product (about US$500/capita/year) and comprised two main rubrics: public health expenditures (mostly for government services) and private expenditures (including out-of-pocket expenditures for goods and services).

The health workforce poses a number of problems: in many countries, too few health workers are available for the population's needs (less than 25 health workers per 10,000 population, which is considered the minimal coverage); those health workers are unevenly distributed; and they have not been adequately trained and developed to meet the health needs of the population. Moreover, meeting those needs in the future will require targeted policies and capital investments in science and technology applied to health.

Response to Regional Trends: The Health Agenda for the Americas, 2008–2017

As they have many times for over a century, and faced today with the trends and challenges described in the foregoing paragraphs, the countries of the Americas have united once again in their commitment to work together to improve the health of people throughout the Region. Toward that end, they have collectively crafted a "Health Agenda for the Americas, 2008–2017" based on "expected trends and challenges in the decade, and focusing on concrete improvements in the health of the peoples of the Americas." Approved by delegations of the countries of the Americas to the World Health Assembly (Geneva, May 2007) and launched at the General Assembly of the Organization of American States (Panama City, June 2007), the Health Agenda is a "high-level political instrument" that establishes specific regional public health goals in eight principal "areas of action," the combined aim of which is to reduce inequalities among and inequities within countries.[1] Those areas of action are summarized below:

1. Strengthening the national health authority. Health authorities should secure broad commitment to, and high-level political will in support of, development of the population's health, for which they need to assure proper governance, effective leadership, and transparent accountability. Towards those ends, national health authorities ought to pursue a number of critical strategies, namely they should: assume the steering role in health; perform essential public health functions; enlist the participation of other sectors, society at large, and communities, with clear delineation of the various parties' respective roles; strengthen primary health care approaches and address the social determinants of health;

---

[1]The full version of the Health Agenda is available at http://www.paho.org/English/DD/PIN/Health_Agenda.pdf.

A Tradition of Regional Health Plans

Among their other major functions, governments set goals for the improvement of their populations' health and, in the context of those goals, assess health conditions and gaps. At any given juncture in a country's history, such an assessment will invariably point to progress both made and pending. In the Americas, countries have worked together for over a century to deal collectively with national and regional health challenges, and for over a half-century their efforts have crystallized in regional health plans. Those health plans are, by definition, blueprints for hemispheric and national action to enhance the health and well-being of the peoples of the Americas.

In 1961, with the Charter of Punta del Este and especially the **Ten-Year Public Health Program** of the Alliance for Progress, countries in the Region, at the highest political level, agree for the first time on a continental program to advance health. That program sets forth the goal "to increase life expectancy at birth by a minimum of five years, and to increase the ability to learn and produce, by improving individual and public health." Toward that end, the program recommends the preparation of national plans and the formulation of a general health policy.

In 1972, the Ministers of Health of the Americas, taking up where the Charter of Punta del Este left off, devise a new **Ten-Year Health Plan for the Americas** that declares health a universal right, recognizes the importance of social participation in decisionmaking, and sets as the principal new goal the extension of health services to unserved and underserved populations "to make it feasible to attain total coverage of the population by the health service system in all the countries of the Region"—thus adumbrating what would become the global aspiration of health for all.

As they had at the outset of the previous two decades, at the beginning of the 1980s the countries of the Region set out to evaluate gains and shortfalls in realizing past health plans for the Americas and to cast a new plan in light of intervening experience. By 1980, most of the countries had defined or confirmed their national strategies to achieve the goal of health for all, in consonance with the Declaration of Alma-Ata iterated in 1978 by the International Conference on Primary Health Care and subsequently adopted by the World Health Assembly in 1979. Those national strategies become the basis for formulating **Regional Strategies for Health for All by the Year 2000.** In the 1990s, there follow a series of regional plans of action and strategic orientations and program priorities.

In the context of that legacy, the **Health Agenda for the Americas, 2008–2017,** is the latest in a series of expressions of the collective will of the countries of the Region.

arrange for legal frameworks that enable proper management of the health system; base decisionmaking on validated evidence; establish reliable information systems for financial management, budgeting, and accounting; and advocate a central role for health as part of the hemispheric development agenda.

2. Tackling health determinants. Education, employment, income, and other social factors directly impact health. It follows that gains in health do not depend entirely on the efforts of the health sector; rather, improving the population's health demands action along a number of social fronts and collaboration among many other institutions and sectors—education, agriculture, law enforcement, transportation, and the like. It will be important to assure that national development plans address health determinants and allocate resources to overcome the problems of social exclusion, exposure to risks and violence, unplanned urbanization, and the effects of climate change. Countries will want to maintain and augment health promotion campaigns—especially targeting mothers, children, and families—through proper nutrition and breastfeeding, vaccination, and respiratory and infectious disease prevention and control.

3. Increasing social protection and access to quality health services. At present, labor-market uncertainty in the countries of the Region is compromising family incomes and, by extension, social security and access to health care. For families that lack protection, expenditures for health services can be catastrophic. Governments should endorse public policies that protect all their citizens; that assure the population's access to necessary health care services, drugs, and technologies; that deliver comprehensive, effective, and efficient services using referrals and cross-referrals, evidence-based practices, and family/community models of care centered on promoting health and preventing disease; and that regulate private-sector health care so that it contributes to attaining national goals for public health.

4. Diminishing health inequalities among countries and health inequities within them. Although regional indicators show that significant gains have been made in the population's health in recent decades, major inequalities persist among countries and profound inequities prevail within them. Those systematically deprived of the benefits of social inclusion—the poor, people with little or no education, rural inhabitants, indigenous peoples and other ethnic groups, women, and the elderly, among others—experience worse levels of health or are exposed to greater health risks and have less access to health services. Governments need to provide health interventions that respond to the special needs of each group: culturally acceptable health services for indigenous groups that respect their rights as citizens; sexual and reproductive health services for women, from conception through care of the newborn; integrated care of adolescents and young adults that address their development needs, mental health, and tendencies towards risky behaviors; maintenance of the quality of life of the elderly and their participation in self-care; and assurance of health policy and program parity for males and females. International development assistance should target funding activities that contribute to reducing inequities in health.

5. Reducing the risk and burden of disease. In every country in the Americas, the epidemiological profile is changing—changes projected to intensify in the years to come—and the health sector needs to adapt its policies and programs accordingly. The prevention and control of communicable diseases continue to be important, and intensive efforts should aim to control and eliminate the "neglected" diseases that tend to disproportionately afflict the poor. At the same time, countries will need to address the leading causes of illness and death: noncommunicable diseases—diabetes, cerebro- and cardiovascular diseases, cancer, etc.—and external causes such as traffic injuries, homicides, and other forms of violence. Toward that end, individuals, the health and education sectors, the media, and society at large should actively promote healthy lifestyles and behavior—principal among them, the availability of healthier foods, better dietary habits, greater physical activity, and the cessation of smoking.

6. Strengthening the management and development of health workers. The countries of the Region, including the more developed ones, as well as areas within all of them, are experiencing critical shortages of doctors and nurses. To meet the increasing and changing needs for health workers, governments should base their health workforce policies and plans on evidence regarding those needs; seek equitable distribution of health workers to assure the availability of their services to the most needy; promote working conditions to stem the emigration of health workers; improve health personnel management, and link health worker training to the needs of health services.

7. Harnessing knowledge, science, and technology. Research enables countries to better understand the relationship between health determinants and their consequences and to select interventions that are appropriate and effective. The design of health policies and the conduct of health programs should be based on the evidence of state-of-the-art research. Countries should bolster investigation into the nature and scope of social determinants of health, strengthen research on traditional and complementary medicines, monitor adherence to bioethical principles, and ensure the equitable application of scientific and technological advances.

8. Strengthening health security. Individual and collective security throughout the Americas is threatened when pandemics and natural and man-made disasters strike. Migratory movements and unsafe food-trade practices can accelerate disease transmission. Governments must prepare for health emergencies and outbreaks and be ready to provide relief when they occur. To prevent and control the spread of disease within and beyond their borders, countries should assure compliance with the latest iteration of the International Health Regulations. Joint efforts between the health and agriculture sectors should target preventing and controlling zoonotic diseases, including preparations for a potential avian influenza pandemic. And countries should collaborate with international organizations to respond rapidly and effectively to circumstances that threaten health security.

Perspectives Regarding Action in Health

In their presentation to the international community of the Health Agenda, the Ministers and Secretaries of Health of the countries of the Americas urged "all Governments, civil society, and the international community which contribute to technical cooperation and development financing, to consider this Agenda as a guide and inspiration when developing public policies and implementing actions for health in pursuit of the well-being of the population of the Americas." In support of that declaration, the Secretariat of the Pan American Health Organization invited a select group of international public health experts to offer their guidance with respect to both the future of health in the Americas and the implementation of the Health Agenda. Specifically, the experts were asked: *"What orientation would you give policy- and decisionmakers regarding implementation of the Health Agenda for the Americas and what prospects for change would you recommend that they take into account?"* What follows are the responses to that twofold question from distinguished leaders with profound experience in international health: George A.O. Alleyne, Stephen Blount and Jay McAuliffe, Paolo Buss, Nils Kastberg, Gustavo Kourí, Sylvie Stachenko, Muthu Subramanian, Ricardo Uauy, and Marijke Velzeboer-Salcedo. Those responses broach a wide array of themes, from epidemiological priorities, to population- and age-group considerations, to health sector and health workforce challenges. Three main themes recur—the need to redress inequities in health, the importance of intersectoral and international cooperation, and the role of information, knowledge, science, and technology in advancing health—and underscore the richness of these perspectives on the future of health in the Americas; those themes are highlighted throughout this chapter ("Recurrent Themes").

COMMENTS OF DR. GEORGE A.O. ALLEYNE

In providing policy- and decisionmakers orientation regarding implementation of the Health Agenda for the Americas and prospects for change that they should take into account, I will assume that these individuals represent the same "type" of person, so I will not distinguish between them in my response, referring to them generally as "policymakers"; moreover, I will assume that these are policymakers in the health sector. My response comprises six principal "orientations."

Appreciate the nature of public policy and the role of policymakers. The policy change process needs to be approached with a clear understanding of the political process. As Michael Reich points out in "The Politics of Reforming Health Policies":

The first skill is to assess the political intentions and actions of stakeholders. Stakeholders include individuals, groups, and organizations that have an interest in a policy and the potential to influence related decisions. . . . In general, political strategies are needed to address four factors that determine the political feasibility of policy change. The four factors are: players, power, position, and perception.

All too frequently policymakers in health are naïve in their belief that, because their cause is noble, their proposals will be instantaneously accepted. Thus, the first orientation that is critical for policymakers, especially new ones, is to be aware of how public policy is formed and of the various stakeholders involved. They must avoid at all costs trying to replace the often very competent technical staff they have at their disposal. One of the grave problems encountered in the health sector is that of the erstwhile health professional who has become a policymaker in the public sector without appreciating that his or her role has changed. Recognition of the basic difference between public policy in general and healthy public policy is a must. It is fine to be able to direct policy in a narrow field of health, but—to the extent that health is determined by many factors outside the traditional health sector—it is important to be clear that healthy public policy, which is critical for achieving much of the Health Agenda, needs a specific set of tools and understanding. The policymaker has to understand that healthy public policy comprises technical, ethical, and political inputs and that all of those inputs must be managed. The tendency in the health sector is to focus exclusively on technical aspects and to ignore the others. No health agenda, no matter how laudable, no matter how technically sound and socially desirable, has any chance of success without a keen appreciation of the nature of public policy and the role of policymakers—factors which, unfortunately, the health organizations that craft such agendas tend not to emphasize sufficiently.

Acquire the tools to articulate a case for health vis-à-vis other sectors. The Health Agenda speaks definitively to health in-

equities, the social determinants of health, and the need for the policymaker to make the case that these inequities and determinants merit attention. The first and most important task, however, is to be able to articulate clearly the value of health to all other sectors and thus to society as a whole. The Health Agenda addresses health almost exclusively in terms of the good that health is, which is undoubtedly true. If, however, health policymakers are to argue a case for the appropriate allocation to health, they have to do so not only on the basis of the intrinsic importance of health, but on that of the contribution of the population's health to all other aspects of national development. It is now abundantly clear that we have hitherto underestimated the value of health to economic welfare. While advocacy of the need to increase social protection and government responsibility for it is ethically correct, as important, if not more so, is the argument that the provision of social protection helps persons and families to avoid falling into a poverty trap or to escape from it—both of which are of critical economic and political significance. More than anecdotal evidence attests to the inadequacy of health sector presentations in fora where decisions are made about resource allocation. This lack of persuasiveness on the part of the health sector results directly in the chronically low allocation to health in the Americas. Thus, the policymaker has to have the tools to argue for the instrumental value of health, and, unless that argument is compellingly made, the Health Agenda will not be adequately resourced and therefore will not fulfill its expectations. We now have the tools to be able to make the case for the role of health in human development, and organizations that advocate for the Health Agenda have a responsibility to arm the health policymaker with those tools.

The policymaker can demonstrate the benefit to be derived from appropriate health interventions, comparing interventions that have the same denominator; for instance, cessation of smoking could be assessed in terms of cost per disability-adjusted life year (DALY) averted or of some measure of health, in the same way that coronary bypass surgery could be, since they both would use the same denominator. In order to compare health interventions with interventions in other sectors, however, the policymaker must be able to present data that show the relative cost-benefit of the health and non-health activity or program. How, for example, might the health policymaker argue to support noncommunicable disease control in the face of competing arguments to build new roads?

In making the vague plea for intersectoral collaboration, which is indeed necessary to address many of the components in the Health Agenda, the policymaker is often placed in the position of a mendicant rather than that of an equal partner seeking the contribution of other sectors to healthy public policy. Noncommunicable diseases, which are highlighted in the Health Agenda, represent an excellent example of the need for healthy public policy and intersectoral collaboration. The tools for the primary prevention and control of many, if not most, of these diseases lie outside the traditional health sector; as examples, the imposition of tobacco taxes is usually not in the hands of the health policymaker, and the solutions to an array of health problems require modifications in trade and agricultural policies. Intersectoral involvement in health promotion can only be achieved if the case is made that health has a value beyond the intrinsic or constitutive.

Emphasize information as a key resource. It is critical that very careful attention be paid to the collection of appropriate data and, on the basis of those data, the generation of information. The need for data and information will confront the policymaker at every turn, and, indeed, the case for health as set out above can only be made on the basis of reliable data that are collected regularly: the value of the data increases when they are collected on a regular basis with some established periodicity. Evidence now exists of the cost-effectiveness of information as an intervention to ensure good health outcomes. Any serious call for an end to inequities must first be based on a demonstration of inequalities, and the policymaker must understand the difference between these two concepts. The Health Agenda emphasizes health determinants and health inequities and calls for governments to address them. And yet any satisfactory program to address inequity depends on a prior determination of inequalities, their genesis, and their modifiable contributing or risk factors. A call for an end to inequity is hollow without the ability to collect the relevant data and to monitor the results of whatever interventions are applied to modifiable risk factors. The policymaker must be oriented to understand the difference between vertical and horizontal equity—i.e., treating everyone the same or targeting those most in need—as the approaches to redress them are very different. In any case, every approach depends on a good system of knowing what is "upon the people" and of dealing with that knowledge accordingly.

Establish priorities. If every problem is addressed at the same time and with the same degree of urgency or priority, chaos will result. It will soon be obvious to the policymaker that change takes place only in response to specific interventions, so it must be clear who is responsible for introducing and monitoring those interventions. The interventions available within the health sector for addressing health determinants, diminishing health inequities, and reducing the risk and burden of disease are of two types—those that address specific problems and those that strengthen the health system—and approaches to both types have their place within the Health Agenda. The policymaker should not, however, get drawn into useless discussion about the relative importance of addressing disease-specific interventions versus applying measures to strengthen the health system. The essential public health functions model shows clearly the need for a dual approach.

Excellent tools are now available to determine the priorities to be addressed in both disease prevention and control and health system governance and toward that end cost-effectiveness analy-

sis can be of critical importance. Thus, for example, the policymaker will be able to determine the opportunity costs of not utilizing a cost-effective intervention to address a disease problem that seriously affects the population. In addition, it will be possible to determine which interventions or programs are of such low cost-effectiveness that their use and continuity should be seriously scrutinized and justified. Notwithstanding, it must be stressed that cost-effectiveness analysis, albeit an essential tool for the policymaker, will be but one of the factors to be taken into account when choosing among priorities. Unfortunately, the policymaker will have to face the reality that for some of the population's health conditions, such as mental health problems, few cost-effective interventions are currently available at the personal level and virtually none are at the population level.

Be realistic and avoid fantasy. The policymaker will often be confronted with very attractive schemes designed by very well meaning persons who do not appreciate the nature of emerging social forces, such as globalization and the growing inequality of power and markets. The area of human resources and the health workforce is one such. In this very critical area, a heavy dose of realism is in order regarding a number of issues, included among them that of migration. It is time the health community realized that it is impossible to stop persons from moving freely; by the same token, it is unrealistic to think that developed countries will desist from importing trained health workers or that this traffic can be regulated internationally. More realistic would be an approach that deals with factors over which the policymaker has some control. In like manner, a good measure of realism is needed when confronting the laudable, but often unrealistic aspirations that tend to characterize health agendas in general.

Be patient. With regard to the prospects for change that policymakers should take into account, I would urge patience, as the changes that will affect implementation of the Health Agenda are likely to be incremental and evolutionary rather than abrupt. A major change will surely be the growing power and influence of nongovernmental actors within and outside of the state; public health policymakers will have to seek actively a *modus vivendi* with the other nongovernmental state actors. The government or the public sector cannot carry out all the activities necessary for the Health Agenda. The health sector policymaker will need considerable patience and negotiating skill to deal with these new actors. Finally, the policymaker will also need patience in interacting with the changing international architecture, given the growing number of agencies having an interest in health. The local solution is for the policymaker to have the patience and courage to insist on the primacy of the local plan and to convince others to comply with it. The steering role of the policymaker in health will not be restricted to any given agency, rather it extends to all the actors in health at the national level.

In closing, I would merely like to add to this series of orientations an expression of my every hope that the Health Agenda succeeds, as will be evidenced by measurable improvement in the health of the peoples of the Americas.

Dr. George Alleyne
Director Emeritus, Pan American Sanitary Bureau
Special United Nations Envoy for HIV/AIDS
in the Caribbean
Chancellor, University of the West Indies
Chairman, Caribbean Commission on Health
and Development

COMMENTS OF DRS. STEPHEN BLOUNT AND JAY MCAULIFFE*

A fundamental challenge for national health policy- and decisionmakers charged with implementing the Health Agenda for the Americas, 2008–2017, is to effectively transform the proposed "areas of action" into real action. As a starting point, each country will need to establish its own implementation plan. It will also need to regularly apply an objective, user-friendly, and transparent monitoring tool for each area of action—an approach that will document the status quo at the outset and the degree of progress achieved subsequently. The same tool should be used to motivate the appropriate institutions to take the continued actions needed.

Cross-cutting issues. Ministries of Health (MOHs) should seek *engagement and partnerships* with other health-related organizations in areas of overlapping interest. While MOHs are best positioned to exercise leadership in the health sector, they are unlikely to possess all the resources needed to be able to fully respond to all of the areas of action. Other governmental agencies, academic institutions, nongovernmental organizations, and businesses in the private sector can assist the MOH in these areas. It requires, however, a commitment from the MOH to support such partnerships, a full understanding by the partner institution of the desired outcomes and a commitment to them, and a set of agreed-upon, well-established terms for the collaboration.

Tackling health determinants. While the health sector is limited in its ability to address many determinants of health, such as poverty and education, environmental determinants have a tremendous impact on health in many developing countries and present opportunities for being modified. Collaborations with other sectors—water and sanitation, education, agriculture, and environmental regulation, to name a few—should be encouraged as a means of achieving *healthy environments.*

Harnessing knowledge, science, and technology. To fully understand the health problems that most need to be addressed and the most effective methods for doing so requires establishing an institutional culture within the public health sector that values and demands high-quality information and that develops the capacity to generate it—that is, the pursuit of *applied epidemiology and research.* Policymakers must have staff who can review the health literature and translate the most current research findings into appropriate guidance for country decisionmakers' use in orienting program plans and implementing health activities. Establishing field epidemiology training programs has been one successful strategy for Ministries of Health to increase their capacity to collect high-quality data and transform them into information and knowledge that are applied to existing program needs. These programs have conducted prompt investigations of disease outbreaks, which are needed to understand such crises and to define the most effective measures to control them. While collection of vital statistics and surveillance data has long been a routine function of Ministries of Health, the incorporation of operational research into their practice is limited and needs to be expanded. As the public health sector increasingly embarks on initiatives to address noncommunicable diseases, establishing an evidence base founded on sound research will be important to the success of new strategies that seek to influence health-related behaviors critical to the advances needed in this area. Research must be used to guide the formulation of health communications and health marketing and to assess the results achieved.

Planning for the assessment and expanded use of new and effective *technologies* in the public health sector is critical; examples include new vaccines, rapid diagnostic kits, geographic information systems, and information technology tools. Decisionmakers in the public health sector must stay abreast of the development of new technologies and be innovative in finding opportunities to apply them to more effectively address priority health problems.

Strengthening solidarity and health security. To deal with public health threats and emergencies, an institutional capacity to effectively implement *risk communication* and *social mobilization* interventions is critical. Principles for these interventions and the methods for carrying them out must be incorporated into public health security plans. Whether in response to crises resulting from pandemic influenza, severe outbreaks of unknown etiology, or natural disasters, countries need to have an established capacity to perform risk communication and social mobilization functions when the moment arrives.

In times of crisis, *regional networks* can serve important needs, and their development should be promoted. The network of field epidemiology training programs of Central America is a good case in point: it has assisted individual countries in their response to major natural disasters (e.g., El Salvador's recent earthquake), toxic exposures (e.g., Panama's experience with medica-

* The authors would like to acknowledge the contributions to this text of various colleagues at the United States Centers for Disease Control and Prevention.

407

tions contaminated with diethylene glycol, DEG), and the need to strengthen capacity to respond to an influenza pandemic.

Reducing the risk and burden of disease. The Health Agenda for the Americas appropriately recognizes the need to increase efforts to target *noncommunicable diseases* (NCDs). Promoting healthy behaviors and lifestyles contributing to the prevention of NCDs is essential; the public must be advanced from its current stage of awareness of NCDs to a stage of action that modifies behaviors. Countries must strengthen operational research and guidelines for practice in health communication and marketing that assist in identifying the public's needs and preferences for information, products, and resources that support adoption of healthier behaviors. Regular monitoring of the prevalence of key risk behaviors should be adopted to assess the effectiveness of prevention activities.

Policy- and decisionmakers need to give greater emphasis to *injuries* as a public health problem and to extend the focus on this concept beyond "traffic accidents." WHO estimates for 2002 in Latin America and the Caribbean show that disability-adjusted life year (DALY) rates for injuries typically represent 10-20% of total DALY rates. Recommendations for surveillance systems are available that will provide basic descriptive data regarding injuries and can lead to the identification of opportunities for effective interventions. Collaboration with other sectors—such as transportation and justice—will enhance data collection and the development of interventions.

Care should be taken to assure that the existing commitment to combat *communicable diseases* not diminish. In the case of neglected diseases such as onchocerciasis and lymphatic filariasis, which have programs for elimination in place, countries' commitments need to be reaffirmed and efforts consolidated to achieve this objective. Successful strategies, such as the large-scale distribution of donated ivermectin for lymphatic filariasis, should be widely disseminated. Neglected diseases, which generally affect the most vulnerable or marginalized segments of the population, deserve priority attention to achieve better health equity.

The success of *immunization* programs in the Americas—smallpox and polio eradication, measles elimination, current efforts to eliminate rubella—lays the foundation for the introduction of new vaccines and for the evolution from child to family immunization programs. Supplementary vaccination activities, such as PAHO's Vaccination Week in the Americas, must be supported to reduce inequities and ensure protection for those who lack ready access to health care. Integration of other services during immunization campaigns should be considered when feasible.

Strengthening the management and development of health workers. To develop the skills and knowledge of the public health and health care *workforce*, approaches are needed to make education and training accessible in resource- and time-constrained environments. New ways to provide information and skill-based training to health workers where they live and work will enable them to remain in the communities where they are most needed. The expectation of expanded information and communication technologies, together with other innovations, will play a role in providing opportunities for education and training in health and public health fields to broader audiences.

Public health training should be at the core of efforts to improve the management of public health systems—especially in new program areas—and emerging threats. A priority objective for such training should be to support workers who are developing the scientific basis for new interventions and who have responsibility for managing such programs.

Stephen B. Blount, M.D., M.P.H.
Director, Coordinating Office for Global Health
Centers for Disease Control and Prevention
Health and Human Services
United States of America
Atlanta, Georgia
and
Jay McAuliffe, M.D., M.P.H.
Acting Chief, Geographic and
Program Coordination Branch
Division of Global Preparedness and
Program Coordination (proposed)
Coordinating Office for Global Health
Centers for Disease Control and Prevention
Health and Human Services
United States of America
Atlanta, Georgia

COMMENTS OF DR. PAOLO BUSS

Any vision of the future of health in the Americas should not focus solely on efforts to strengthen health systems and to improve the quality of health care services. At best, such a focus would perpetuate the regional health situation as it stands, or perhaps something merely somewhat better. Our focus has to be on the central issue underlying the most disturbing problems that confront our countries: the inability of almost one-half of the inhabitants of Latin America and the Caribbean to attain the benefits of human development and, thus, their relegation to an existence of unacceptable inequities.

In Latin America and the Caribbean, progress toward poverty reduction has proceeded at a relatively slow pace, with some 60% of the proposed period (1990–2015) having elapsed and hardly more than 30% of the targeted reduction attained. In the country in the Region that I know best, Brazil, progress has been much greater, with almost 80% of the goal attained, in large measure because effective social projects have been carried out and health

---

RECURRENT THEME

Redressing inequities in health and the right to health

Our focus has to be on the central issue underlying the most disturbing problems that confront our countries: the inability of almost one-half of the inhabitants of Latin America and the Caribbean to attain the benefits of human development and, thus, their relegation to an existence of unacceptable inequities.

—Paolo Buss

. . . the concept undergirding everything related to the development of health is that the entire population should have access to health—regardless of economic status, type of employment, race, place of residence, or the like.

—Gustavo Kourí

Policymakers will want to assure that commensurate attention is given to achieving greater health equity among those population groups [afrodescendents and indigenous populations] compared to that prevailing among the rest of the population. . . . We should stress 'coverage' to indicate the need that health services go beyond 'access' and generate demand to ensure coverage.

—Nils Arne Kastberg

The policymaker must be oriented to understand the difference between vertical and horizontal equity—i.e., treating everyone the same or targeting those most in need—as the approaches to redress them are very different. In any case, every approach depends on a good system of knowing what is "upon the people" and of dealing with that knowledge accordingly.

—George Alleyne

Greater inequality will surely result, unless the regulatory framework presently in place is reexamined to take into account the situation of countries that have serious limitations in resources—limitations that today prohibit their access to the new diagnostic and therapeutic tools that the future will bring.

—Ricardo Uauy

Implementation of the Agenda should focus on two objectives: (1) improving the health and well-being of people; and (2) reducing avoidable inequities in health and health care by addressing basic determinants and prerequisites of health.

—Muthu Subramanian

As regards efforts to diminish health inequities among and within countries, UNIFEM strongly concurs with the Agenda's distinction of sexual and reproductive health as a priority issue in the Americas.

—Marijke Velzeboer-Salcedo

---

service coverage has expanded. Notwithstanding, that progress has been compromised by the persistence in the country of large gaps in income, which weaken the bonds of social integration and lower the levels of social capital and political participation.

In that context, and bearing in mind the Millennium Development Goals, it is worth noting that, although three of the eight goals relate to health, the first of them is the eradication of extreme poverty and hunger, without which it is doubtful that progress will be made towards any of the other goals. As a reflection of that association, the World Health Organization recently called attention to the fact that the poorest countries in the world will have difficulty attaining the MDGs and that in many of them progress, as measured by the respective indicators, has stalled.

In recent decades, the focus on improving health conditions has centered on health system reform, the aim being to assure a social dividend and to contain the increasing costs imposed by economic sectors. It has become obvious, however, that this strictly sectoral approach is insufficient to achieve the universality, accessibility, and inclusivity in health to which the entire population is entitled.

The health sector crisis is not necessarily a reflection of its irremediable failure or its irreversible deterioration. Rather, the problem lies in a general inability to overcome the status quo, with decisionmakers limiting themselves to their conventional perspective and resisting any involvement in new, potentially more powerful orientations. At the same time, globalization is having significant negative effects that restrict the free political determination of nation states, leading to a form of colonialism that subordinates our countries' development to the influences of foreign trends and policies.

Meanwhile, from a more positive point of view, the gradual acceptance of the concept of social determinants of health and the corresponding increase in health promotion activities will enable more opportunities to improve the quality of life of many population groups in the Region. Among the factors that have the greatest influence on their health is a broad array of social and economic conditions: poverty, injustice, lack of education, lack of social protection, poor nutrition, social exclusion and discrimination, gender discrimination, inadequate housing, urban decay, lack of potable water, violence, and the absence or inadequacy of health care services. The political reorientation of most of the governments in South America should result in greater sensitivity to these conditions and could lead to measures to redress them.

In that context, two important initiatives merit mentioning that could mitigate the negative conditions noted above. Both of these initiatives are based on a renewal of the concept of health as a public good—the objective of public policies crafted with the concerted participation of different segments of the population—as contrasted with the concept of health as a private good, produced in the form of medical care for individuals and governed by the dictates of the marketplace, a concept that informed many of the health reforms carried out in the Region, particularly during the 1990s. The first of these initiatives is social participation, which, as it has spread throughout the Region, has reinforced the value of empowering society as a whole. The second initiative targets the development of effective intersectoral coordination, as a governmental strategy for more cohesive and forceful action based on an open, inclusive dialogue among the social and economic sectors. Both initiatives could contribute to overcoming social constraints in Latin America and the Caribbean, by enabling a new approach to governance wherein all of society, and not just the political powers that be, promotes a collective approach to common, shared objectives.

Allow me to refer, again, to experiences in my country by drawing attention to examples of well-managed interventions, although I am sure that similar examples are underway, with similarly successful outcomes, in other Latin American and Caribbean countries. In Brazil, social participation has made great strides, thanks to a wide network of Municipal Health Councils (Conselhos Mu-

nicipais de Saúde) that have been integrated in a tripartite scheme along with state and national jurisdictions. Also effective have been the family health program, which today covers 60% of the population and which aims to reach half of the remaining population by the end of this decade, and the HIV/AIDS control program, which has emphasized prevention of the disease, production and free distribution of available medicines to all patients, and comprehensive epidemiological surveillance—an approach that is being adopted in a number of other countries. Finally, immunization and breastfeeding programs have expanded with great results, as have the human milk banks that are widely used in the country.

At the international level, in regional integration summits, the countries of Latin America and the Caribbean can resist global governance and achieve, in a context of regional solidarity, conditions that support local policies; they can join forces to break with the protectionism of more powerful countries; and can cooperate amongst eachother to achieve greater self-sufficiency in confronting the demands of human development in general and of health in particular. Convergence of the interests of foreign policy and of health could have a tremendous impact on development, as exemplified by the Framework Convention on Tobacco Control; implementation of the International Health Regulations; the Global Strategy on Diet, Physical Activity, and Health; the probable adoption of the WHO resolution on Intellectual Property Rights; and the development of science and technology in the health field.

Similarly, at the international level, recent promotion of the Decade of Human Resources in Health has served as an important catalyst for implementation, at the international and national levels, of a series of measures that aim to balance the problem of insufficient or poor distribution of health professionals, as well as to reorient the preparation of those professionals to the real needs of the population. The fruits of that initiative are already beginning to have an impact on programs that introduce new theoretical contents in academic training, that diversify the fields of practice of students, and that promote new teaching approaches. These experiences will no doubt influence health actions in our Region and throughout the world. In that respect as well, the program supported by the Inter-American Development Bank to train a critical mass of nursing auxiliaries is noteworthy: a large-scale training methodology has resulted in the addition of 350,000 workers to the health system, and the methodology is now being considered for the training of mid-level technicians.

As these initiatives proceed apace, we will continue to have to live with a number of problems, as the Region still is undergoing an epidemiological transition characterized by the coexistence of the problems of underdevelopment with those of the developed world.

It follows that we will continue to have to depend on large pharmaceutical companies for the procurement of a wide variety of medicines and supplies, as we have not reached the extent of development in research and technology that would permit us a certain independence—not only in the production of existing medicines but in the production of new drugs that will accompany advances in science. The scant importance that the countries give to intersectoral coordination means that in most of them the health sector is not able to influence technological development.

We will continue to confront increasing problems that result from global warming, especially in the Caribbean and Central America, although the effects of this phenomenon are spreading to other areas. Nonetheless, we can do little beyond recognizing that the cause of global warming stems from environmental degradation not in our countries but in the developed world. No less important is the growing threat of urban violence in Latin America and the Caribbean caused predominantly by drug trafficking and accidents—problems that in some countries have reached alarming proportions.

Meanwhile, we continue to be committed to thwarting the negative influences on the health of our populations and to combating poverty and social exclusion, violence, and environmental degradation. We are likewise committed to a concerted multisectoral approach and to broader social participation, in the hope that, together, we can achieve a brighter future for Latin America and the Caribbean, with greater health and a better quality of life.

Dr. Paolo Buss
President
Oswaldo Cruz Foundation
Rio de Janeiro, Brazil

COMMENTS OF DR. NILS ARNE KASTBERG

UNICEF is pleased with this Health Agenda for the Americas, and with its alignment with the goals of the Millennium Declaration and its strong value focus on human rights, universality, access, and inclusion; on Pan American solidarity; on equity in health; and on participation. And UNICEF particularly welcomes the significant references to children and adolescents in the Agenda. We consider that the work of the Ministries of Health and of the Pan American Health Organization is of fundamental importance for the well-being of children and their mothers in the Region. Within that overall positive perspective, we would like to provide the following complementary orientation to that provided in the Health Strategy to policy- and decisionmakers who will be implementing this Agenda.

Making the MDGs a reality at the local level to address disparities in health. The Health Agenda underscores the importance of alignment with the Millennium Declaration and emphasizes the inequalities that need to be addressed. It will be important, therefore, to establish benchmarks and monitor progress towards achievement of the MDGs—not just as national averages but as expressions of the reality at the local level. The importance of developing measures that disaggregate data in order for public health services to monitor progress and results for the MDGs at the local level is well illustrated by the example in the Agenda, whereby 40% of the municipalities in Latin America and the Caribbean do not reach the immunization goal of routinely vaccinating 95% of children under 1 year of age. The disaggregation of data could help Health Ministries to more forcefully advocate for resources to strengthen health services in the areas where health outcomes are weakest.

Providing the "people context." Policy- and decisionmakers in the health sector will want to give particular attention to the "people context" so that efforts to prevent unhealthy trends can be strengthened. Included among other fundamental considerations of the human geography are: the number of pregnancies and children born, the high number of teenage pregnancies, the number and percentage of children suffering from chronic undernutrition, and the like.

Addressing violence. It will be important to give special consideration to the involvement of health in the early detection of intrafamiliar violence and to the drama health services face when interacting with other state services responsible for protecting women and children, but who do not live up to their responsibility. The link between violence, sexual abuse, and incest is evidenced by the startling figure that 20% of pregnancies are now among adolescents, and most of those pregnancies are unwanted. PAHO and WHO have been been instrumental in contributing to the United Nations Study on Violence against Children, presented to the General Assembly on 11 October 2006. That study estimates that in Latin America and the Caribbean 80,000 persons under 18 years of age die every year as a result of intrafamiliar violence. It is critical that attention continue to be given to the reporting of these cases, to follow-up actions that services other than health need to take, to the traumatic situation this presents for health staff to have to witness day after day, often without assistance from other sector services. Increasingly in certain urban settings of the Region, the leading cause of hospitalization of adolescents is injuries caused by violence. Policy- and decisionmakers must make sure that violence of this nature, observed during the day-to-day work of health services, is systematically captured and monitored and that the necessary follow-up action is taken.

Trends in the health system response: mobilization for health promotion. Policymakers would benefit from familiarity with examples in countries of the Region of successful health promotion. The UNICEF Brazil Office considers that the 27,000 health promotion teams in that country reach some 70 million people—an excellent example of mobilization for health. The Vaccination of the Americas campaign promoted by PAHO and supported by UNICEF is another example of mobilization for disease prevention that has reached countless heretofore unreached individuals. Young people could be recruited for health promotion efforts, as another strategy for broadcasting messages that give greater emphasis to preventive, rather than curative, services.

Afrodescendents and indigenous populations in Latin America. Afrodescendents in Latin America, who represent some 150 million persons, face similar differences in health indicators in relation to the average population, as do indigenous populations, who number between 40 and 50 million persons. Policymakers will want to assure that commensurate attention is given to achieving greater health equity among these population groups and compared to that prevailing among the rest of population.

Chronic undernutrition and the young mother. Chronic undernutrition was not one of the 48 MDG indicators for MDG1b, Hunger. Through United Nations interagency work and in the 2005 joint United Nations report to the Americas on MDGs, coordinated by ECLAC, the United Nations Regional Directors Team for Latin America and the Caribbean concluded that the chronic undernutrition indicator was the most relevant indicator for our Region to measure progress on MDG1b. In implementing the Health Agenda for the Americas, UNICEF would thus recommend that this issue be given particular attention. We consider that greater focus on the adolescent mother—especially during the nine months before birth and the nine to 36 months after birth— is critical to a number of key health promotion, early detection, and health problem prevention measures. Policymakers will want to make sure that this issue is tackled, to support national programs already underway that target eradicating chronic undernutrition, and to seek national intersectoral action, including access to potable water and sanitation in rural areas, as many countries still have a large proportion of rural populations without access to those services. By 2017 chronic undernutrition should have been eradicated from the Americas.

Specific suggestions. It is important to emphasize in regard to HIV/AIDS, the feminization of the pandemic in many countries, the transmission to young women, the need to attain universal access and coverage in the Region, including through pan-American solidarity, the need to reduce mother-to-child transmission to as close to zero as possible. With regard to community involvement in health services, as the Director of PAHO has so appropriately indicated on many occasions, we should stress "coverage" to indicate the need that health services go beyond "access," and generate demand to ensure coverage. The theme of pan-American solidarity suggests that, in addition to collaboration on common targets, it is important that countries recognize the issue of access

to health across borders, the provision of health staff across borders, and the increase in south-south collaboration beyond the Americas.

Again, UNICEF would like to congratulate PAHO for advancing this Agenda, and will continue to be a close partner in mobilizing society for better health in the Americas!

Dr. Nils Arne Kastberg
Regional Director
United Nations Children's Fund
Latin America and the Caribbean Regional Office

COMMENTS OF DR. GUSTAVO KOURÍ

The Health Agenda for the Americas, 2008–2017, sets a direction going forward for health throughout the hemisphere. In contemplating the future of health in the Region, it should prove useful to consider the example of Cuba, where the concept undergirding everything related to the development of health is that the entire population should have access to health—regardless of economic status, type of employment, race, place of residence, or the like. In effect, a public health system should be accessible, universal, free, and a force for solidarity. Crucial to realizing those conditions is political will, without which nothing can be achieved.

At the same time, the public health system should have in place excellent services that enable the conduct of high-level, costly studies that will benefit patients. Too often, the quality of public health services is very low, and only in private services can certain studies be carried out.

Public health is based on a preventive rather than a curative principle. Conversely, the private sector requires a lot of patients in order to be profitable; consequently, its thrust is curative, because if the private system doesn't have patients, it collapses. The problem, as is evident from the Health Agenda for the Americas, is complex. Modifications to the health sector have failed in the Americas, where many of the public health systems have been privatized.

Cuba has a system that is unique in the Americas, and possibly in the world. In addition to having the health indicators of a developed country, it provides cooperation to some 70 countries, where more than 30,000 of its health workers are helping the most needy population groups in those countries. The principle informing Cuba's health system is not to give away what it cannot use, but, rather, to share what it has.

In addition, because many countries are elaborating comprehensive health plans that include the development of human capital for health, Cuba, as a demonstration of its solidarity with other countries, has established the Latin American Medical School (*Escuela Latinoamericana de Medicina* or ELAM), which is preparing thousands of students from Latin America, other continents, and even the United States of America. Along similar lines of solidarity, the country works with others to confront epidemics, as is happening in the most recent cases of collaboration, namely with the control of malaria in Gambia and Jamaica.

In its commitment to scientific and technological development, Cuba has produced a number of vaccines, such as that for meningitis B, the country's vaccine being the first in the world against this group of meningoccus; the vaccine against hepatitis B, which has had a tremendous impact on national public health; DPT, which no longer is of commercial interest; the first synthetic vaccine produced in the world, against *Haemophilus influenzae* b; and other vaccines that are being used in the country's health system and which have resulted in vaccine-preventable diseases having little impact on morbidity and mortality in the country, where the population is immunized against 13 diseases. A vaccine has even been developed for cholera, a disease that doesn't exist in Cuba but that does represent a public health threat in other countries, where the vaccine will be made available.

Cuba has made important contributions to the scientific understanding of poliomyelitis, dengue, HIV/AIDS, tuberculosis, and other communicable diseases.

In summary, these gains have been achieved because health is considered a human right, the full and absolute responsibility of the state, and cannot be treated like a marketable good. Moreover, health should be coupled with the development of science and a likewise universal and free education, as health and education go hand in hand.

Dr. Gustavo Kourí
Instituto "Pedro Kourí"
Havana, Cuba

COMMENTS OF DR. SYLVIE STACHENKO

Given what is known about the underlying determinants of both communicable and noncommunicable diseases, and given the clear relationship between health and economic and human development, three high-level orientations to the Health Agenda for the Americas, 2008–2017 are that:

1. Investment in health at the population level implicates the engagement of health and non-health sectors and public and private entities in collaborative relationships;
2. The health of populations and the health system are national assets that serve and underpin other sectors, that investment in health at the levels of the population as well as among individuals can give returns on investment that contribute to economic policy goals within countries and subregionally in the Americas, particularly when investments target populations experiencing relative inequity in health status; and

3. Dealing with the global industry, whose products and practices can compromise the population's health, requires global instruments for health protection.

The evidence is strong that strategic and coordinated investments by various non-health sectors, acting within their traditional domains, can achieve health goals at the same time as the respective non-health sector goals are attained, amounting to protection and improvement in the health of populations.

As for proposals for change, whole-of-government approaches with corresponding executive level whole-of-government governance mechanisms to coordinate action on the underlying determinants of health are the means by which the health of populations and human development become the responsibility of multiple public sectors. Policy- and decisionmakers in the health sector need to seek out the opportunities to engage their national counterparts in other public sectors to, first, raise awareness and, second, instill in non-health sectors the responsibility they hold for disease and for health.

Within the whole-of-government coordinating mechanisms, the role of public health practitioners as the cross-sector stewards of the population's health needs to be elevated, with a corresponding increase in government expenditure for the population/public health components of health systems, and an understanding that non-health sector policy proposals are to be assessed in terms of their potential impact on health status and on the underlying determinants of illness and health disparities.

Given the global nature of certain industries whose products and practices are known to contribute to or cause disease, and given that countries in the Americas have dramatically different, if any, capacities and levers at hand to influence these global industries on which their populations may be dependent, cross-national and subregional initiatives and instruments are needed for industry practices to change for the simultaneous benefit of populations in multiple countries.

Policy- and decisionmakers in public health need to engage with their counterparts in other countries to use their collective voice to draw attention to their common issues and to leverage broader support from the public at large, from national and international agencies and nongovernmental organizations and from sympathetic non-health sectors to create the critical mass of public and political pressure for specific global industries to change their practices and products, such that populations are protected and, where possible, corporate goals are met simultaneously—creating win-win situations.

Dr. Sylvie Stachenko
Deputy Chief Public Health Officer and
Director, WHO Collaborating Centre on
Chronic Noncommunicable Diseases Policy
Public Health Agency of Canada
Ottawa, Ontario

COMMENTS OF DR. MUTHU SUBRAMANIAN

Over the past three decades, since the Global Strategy for Health for All by the Year 2000 was launched in 1977, the Region of the Americas has made significant progress toward improving peoples' health in all the countries of the hemisphere. Relying on primary health care (PHC), inequalities in health levels between and within countries have been reduced and access to all elements of PHC has increased, although the pace of that progress has not been uniform among countries nor among population groups within them. The historical focus on mortality to reflect health status and health policy achievements has led to the assignment of a low priority to non-life threatening diseases, which in turn has resulted in a large part of the gains in life expectancy being accompanied by greater illness and disability; that is, life expectancy in the Region has increased much faster than "healthy life expectancy," understood to mean the number of years that an individual can be expected to live in good health. Generally speaking, the principles underlying the Global Strategy and the primary health care approach have proved their relevance and validity in improving peoples' health and reducing disparities in health levels, although their actual impact has fallen short of their potential. The collective experience gained with implementation of the Strategy and application of the PHC approach to achieve better health for all has contributed to conceptual and operational aspects of public health practice at national, regional, and global levels. Concerns have arisen with the widening disparities—common sources of social tension and unrest—in health status and health care access within countries and with the gap between life expectancies and healthy life expectancies. In that context, effective implementation of the Health Agenda for the Americas, 2008–2017 should ensure that the increases in life span of individuals are accompanied by freedom from additional years of suffering, pain, and disability—thus making longer life a prize, not a penalty.

Orientation for implementation of the Agenda. To attain the health outcomes set forth in the Health Agenda, the orientation of policy- and decisionmakers should be to shift away from the emphasis on health care: the focus should be to give all the peoples of the Region a positive sense of health and enable them to make full use of their physical, mental, and emotional capacities and, on that basis, to choose priorities and allocate resources. Such a shift in focus will inspire people to think afresh, to undertake new initiatives, and to work together in innovative ways. It will require a trade-off between increasing life expectancies—through mortality-reduction strategies—and increasing healthy years of life lived by, in addition to improving survival chances, preventing premature morbidity and avoidable disability through healthy ways of living and the elimination or reduction of preventable health risks among individuals and in the environment.

Implementation of the Agenda should focus on two objectives:

1. Improving the health and well-being of people, and
2. Reducing avoidable inequities in health and health care by addressing basic determinants and prerequisites of health.

Furthermore, to achieve and sustain positive health for all the peoples of the Region, sustained action will be required to:

- Add years to life by increasing life expectancy and reducing premature deaths,
- Add life to years by increasing years lived free from ill health, reducing or minimizing the adverse effects of illness and disability, and improving the quality of life through healthy lifestyles as well as healthy physical and social environments, and
- Add health to life by reducing disease and disability.

In policy- and decisionmakers' implementation of the Agenda's focus on lifestyles, the environment, and health care, they should assure the involvement of all levels of society and reach out to all partners and sectors that can influence health.

Changing scenarios and resulting challenges. Health development thrives in an environment that recognizes the myriad health benefits to socioeconomic progress and is conducive and receptive to health action being or becoming an integral part of the functions and activities of social and economic sectors. Unlike the political and economic upheavals of the 1980s and 1990s, the 21st century has begun with a favorable environment for health development in the Region, as summarily described in the paragraphs that follow.

Health systems environment. The regionalization of *peace* is gathering momentum: there have been no major wars or inter-country conflicts in the Region during the past decade. A new political landscape, more characterized by *democracy*, has been emerging, particularly in Latin America: 2006 proved to be a year of major political transformations with the emergence of democratically elected leaders in a number of Latin American countries. Greater attention is being paid to bolstering regional integration and consolidating democratic institutions. Increasing emphasis is being given to social spending and to achieving social justice, which should enhance people's participation in development—especially in activities aimed at improving their health and well-being.

The global community is increasingly recognizing that national action to improve people's health has global benefits. The Global Health and Foreign Policy Initiative, launched in 2006, aims to broaden the scope of *foreign policy* to include health; a set of actions for raising priority for health in foreign policy has also been outlined in the Agenda for Action (the Oslo Ministerial Declaration). These initiatives augur well for a smooth implementation of the Health Agenda for the Americas.

RECURRENT THEME

Promoting intersectoral collaboration and international cooperation in health

Policy- and decisionmakers in public health need to engage with their counterparts in other countries to use their collective voice to draw attention to their common issues and to leverage broader support from the public at large, from national and international agencies and nongovernmental organizations and from sympathetic non-health sectors to create the critical mass of public and political pressure for specific global industries to change their practices and products, such that populations are protected and, where possible, corporate goals are met simultaneously—creating win-win situations.

—Sylvie Stachenko

A major change will surely be the growing power and influence of nongovernmental actors within and outside of the state; public health policymakers will have to seek actively a *modus vivendi* with the other nongovernmental state actors. The government or the public sector cannot carry out all the activities necessary for the Health Agenda. The health sector policymaker will need considerable patience and negotiating skill to deal with these new actors. . . . Intersectoral involvement in health promotion can only be achieved if the case is made that health has a value beyond the intrinsic or constitutive.

—George Alleyne

It has become obvious . . . that a strictly health-sector approach is insufficient to achieve the universality, accessibility, and inclusivity in health to which the entire population is entitled. . . . Convergence of the interests of foreign policy and of health could have a tremendous impact of development. . . . We are likewise committed to a concerted multisectoral approach and to broader social participation, in the hope that, together, we can achieve a brighter future for Latin America and the Caribbean, with greater health and a better quality of life.

—Paolo Buss

While Ministries of Health are best positioned to exercise leadership in the health sector, they are unlikely to possess all the resources needed to be able to fully respond to all of the areas of action. Other governmental agencies, academic institutions, nongovernmental organizations, and businesses in the private sector can assist the MOH in these areas. . . . In times of crisis, regional networks can serve important needs, and their development should be promoted.

—Stephen Blount and Jay McAuliffe

The theme of pan-American solidarity suggests that, in addition to collaboration on common targets, it is important that countries recognize the issue of access to health across borders, the provision of health staff across borders, and the increase in south-south collaboration beyond the Americas.

—Nils Arne Kastberg

Health development thrives in an environment that recognizes the myriad health benefits to socioeconomic progress and is conducive and receptive to health action being or becoming an integral part of the functions and activities of social and economic sectors. . . . The implementers of the Health Agenda should address the need to intensify ownership of health and environmental challenges and to assure an awareness of those challenges among the practitioners of disciplines generally less informed of health issues—such as architects, builders, and developers.

—Muthu Subramanian

All those who hold stake in the health of the hemisphere should capitalize on the political will in pro of health expressed repeatedly in countless Presidential summits. . . . It is likely that the collective PAHO membership could best contribute by striking strategic partnerships with other regional or international organizations that operate in the Americas.

—Ricardo Uauy

Decisionmakers [should] be made aware of the important work being carried out among various sectors, institutions, and United Nations agencies, such as the particularly successful interagency collaboration between PAHO and UNIFEM at the regional, subregional, and country level.

—Marijke Velzeboer-Salcedo

In Latin America and the Caribbean, *economic growth* has been solid in recent years and can be expected to continue, albeit perhaps at a slower pace. Domestic demand is becoming a major driver of that growth, with countries' economies less constrained by the vagaries of external demand. Gaps in growth rates among countries have been narrowing lately, resulting in broad-based growth throughout the Region. Greater economic growth is accompanied by decreasing *unemployment*, which has reached its lowest level since the mid-1990s. At the same time, ill-health among the employed is increasingly recognized as a major contributor to less-than-optimal labor productivity. With falling inflation, *real wages* have been increasing as well.

With regard to *literacy*, more than 90% of adults 15 years of age and older in Latin America and the Caribbean are literate, and the gender-gap has been narrowing; among young adults (15–24 years), more than 96% are literate. These young literate people are now making the transition into adulthood in a rapidly changing world with emerging information and communication technologies reshaping their lives and behavior. A priority focus for those implementing the Agenda should be to enable and ensure that these young people practice healthy behavior and that they sustain it over time.

Pre-primary school *enrollment* has become the norm in the Americas. In order not to separate "care" from "education," intensive efforts, such as Early Childhood Care and Education (ECCE), have been made to expand and improve the early childhood foundation, including good health, hygiene, nutrition, and a nurturing and safe environment that supports children's cognitive and socioemotional well-being. A major challenge for the Health Agenda will be to take advantage of this education-health synergy to carry out health action that can enable children and youth to pursue a harmonious health continuum as they develop and prosper as healthy adults.

The *health of the environment*—healthier food, clean water, and a safe environment—proved to be a huge contributor to better health in the 20th century. More recently, health improvements have also been made through initiatives focusing on children's environmental health and on "built environments"—man-made surroundings that provide the setting for human activity, ranging from large-scale civic surroundings to personal places—focusing not so much on urban tenements but on fragmented and sprawling communities that foster car dependency, inactivity, obesity, loneliness, fossil fuel and resource consumption, and, of course, environmental pollution. The implementers of the Health Agenda should address the need to intensify ownership of health and environmental challenges and to assure an awareness of those challenges among the practitioners of disciplines generally less informed of health issues—such as architects, builders, and developers; moreover, with the aging of the population, many of whose members will live into their 80s and 90s, those practitioners should be made aware of the housing design needs of the elderly. Furthermore, over and above the traditional concerns for safe water, attention should be directed to containing "emerging contaminants," such as residues of pharmaceutical and personal-care products that find their way into rivers from sewage treatment plants and by leaching into groundwater from septic systems, possibly causing harm to human beings.

The 2006 chart of progress toward attainment of the Millennium Development Goals shows that the Americas have met, or are advancing towards meeting, the targets set for 2015 with respect to most of the MDGs, the exceptions being "youth unemployment" and "loss of forest cover"; notwithstanding, disparities in achievement levels within the Region exist. Stubborn poverty seems to have been cracked, and both the number and the percentage of the total population of poor have fallen appreciably in the Americas. The Pan American Health Organization has designated five countries in the Region for urgent and intensified support, due to the intolerable nature of their health situation, poverty level, and indebtedness. In 2006, the Inter-American Development Bank agreed to provide additional resources to meet the MDGs, under a debt-relief package. The United Nations Conference on Trade and Development (UNCTAD) is placing emphasis on a "productive capacity" initiative, that singles out health as a crucial element in the poverty reduction strategy for the least-developed countries, such as Haiti.

Strategic advantage should be taken of these many favorable developments by policy- and decisionmakers charged with implementing the Health Agenda for the Americas over the coming decade.

Health care systems. Changes in the *population* in the Americas will have major implications for the planning and training of human resources for health. On the one hand, the elderly population in North America will increase and, by about 2015, will exceed the child population; the working population, however, will continue to grow. On the other hand, in Latin America and the Caribbean the child population is decreasing and is expected to fall below the elderly population by about 2040, around which time the working age population will stop growing. Such a transformation in the population profile will require a balancing of human resources for health to address the changing health care load, with needs for child care decreasing and those for care of the elderly increasing; the health of working adults will also demand greater attention, to ensure that their productivity is not compromised.

The Region is highly *urbanized*, particularly in Latin America and the Caribbean, where in 2005 about 77% lived in cities; the urban proportion is likely to exceed 80% by 2015 and 85% by 2030. In organizing primary health care delivery, those charged with implementing the Health Agenda will need to be cognizant of the challenge of rising urbanization and of a corresponding decrease in rural population growth.

The health care sector. Despite the great promise of the PHC movement, two major constraints have inhibited its effectiveness in improving peoples' health, namely:

1. Greater emphasis has been paid to *financing* health services to achieve increased access than to *allocation of resources* to improve health outcomes. All the countries in the Region have achieved the target of at least 5% of GNP allocated to health, but a sufficient proportion of that increase has not gone to accelerating access to primary health care and to services oriented toward better health outcomes.

2. Insufficient emphasis has been given to reorienting and training *human resources for health*, to bridging clinical and public health practices, and to enabling health professionals to function effectively under the new health paradigm of positive health as defined by the Constitution of WHO—not merely the absence of diseases and disabilities—and further fine-tuned by the health for all goal of ensuring that all citizens of the world can lead a socially and economically productive life. The new paradigm implies not only achieving increases in disability-free life expectancy, but also creating physical, cultural, and policy environments that enable individuals who *already* have disabilities (those born with them) that impose restrictions on their functional capabilities to participate in and contribute to society, thereby making their lives worth living. The new paradigm contrasts the old, fragmented, parochial way of addressing population health issues with a bold approach that deals with the interconnectedness of innate factors—genes, age, and sex—and other influences from the social, economic, and physical environment as well as from individual and community behavior and lifestyles. Guiding principles underlying the wholeness of population health will thus lead to new ways of approaching present, emerging, and future population health issues and transform the way the health care community thinks and works.

Health care delivery. The Region faces remarkable challenges due to epidemiological and demographic changes, and correspondingly radical changes are needed in the existing health care delivery system. Nor can the system insulate itself from global developments, be they of the economy, trade, or related to health emergencies. The ability to deal with those challenges, however, depends on what happens at the local and national levels. The difference that health care delivery makes over the coming decades should stem primarily from greater emphasis on living long *and* leading a healthy life, not on mere survival.

The eight elements of the primary health care package outlined in the Declaration of Alma-Ata should be revisited and revised to reflect the current health situation. Under each of those elements, medical and especially public health evidence-based interventions should be deconstructed and then reconstructed around an integrated PHC delivery framework to improve the health of people, individually and collectively. Such a revised PHC package should be given overriding health priority and proper support by the health system, which may itself require strengthening to ensure health improvement, fair access, effective delivery of appropriate health care, efficiency, sensitivity to individual and community needs, and above all be targeted to attain improved health status. Concepts of sophistication, efficiency, and professionalism must yield to relevance, effectiveness, and acceptability. Advantage should be taken of knowledge and experience gained over the last three decades by the Region and the countries in the application of the PHC approach to health systems development and of recent advances in scientific, technological, biological, and behavioral areas relevant to the enhancement of health.

Knowledge generation and sharing. The coming decades will witness at least three revolutions: a biological and technological revolution, a behavioral revolution, and a revolution in health care delivery. The conditions for generating information related to these revolutions and for sharing scientific knowledge are themselves changing, as a consequence of the increased intensity of communication, the growing interface between disciplines, and the tighter interaction between science and technology. Major economic and social implications and ethical consequences are arising from the closer interconnection among scientific discoveries (such as genetic mutation and cloning and their applications), technological know-how, and commercial exploitation as well as between information *per se* and the communication technologies that disseminate it. People have a "right to well-being" by exercising their "right" to scientific knowledge and research, to information on experiences in applying them, and to the results emanating from them. The challenge lies in empowering people and communities with the capability of comprehending scientific information and its relevance to tackling their health issues so that they can participate meaningfully in improving their own health.

Major contributions to prolong life and improve its quality have been made in the Region over the past decades. Yet, further improvement in population health is possible, and many challenges remain. Better understanding of disease processes and of the determinants of individual and community health as well as incredible advances in medical, biological, technological, and related areas are affording possibilities for a quantum leap in population health. For all its successes and aspirations, however, the Americas will not be free from the ravages of ill-health and suffering until all its people are protected and the health of the entire population is promoted. The Health Agenda for the Americas, 2008–2017 addresses the Region's concerns and, if judiciously implemented, offers the promise of better health for all people throughout the hemisphere in years to come. Are we ready?

Dr. Muthu Subramanian
Former Director, World Health Organization
Princeton, New Jersey

COMMENTS OF DR. RICARDO UAUY

The Health Agenda for the Americas, 2008–2017, sets forth eight areas of action, each of which is both strategically very important in its own right and potentially a significant contributor to the Agenda's desired final outcome—namely improving the health of the peoples of the Americas. It would thus be futile to try to discriminate which of these areas is more important or to suggest that other areas, which may be as important, have been ignored. The paragraphs that follow purport merely to contribute to the agenda-setting process that the countries of the Region, collectively, have undertaken.

The Pan American Health Organization—whose membership comprises all the governments in the Region—is clearly in a position to influence the population's health outcomes in the coming decade. This influence is especially relevant for the worse-off countries: in their case, PAHO's actions are key to their future health; moreover, PAHO has the opportunity to leverage human and material resources in favor of the worse-off countries within the Region. Even the better-off countries could benefit from a proactive Organization that leads the Region by providing technical stewardship with a common perspective.

All those who hold stake in the health of the hemisphere should capitalize on the political will in pro of health expressed repeatedly in countless Presidential summits (of Heads of State of the Americas, Ibero/Hispano-American, South American, Mercosur, Andean countries, and the like). As a recent example of the existing opportunities, beneficial use could be made of the call by the President of Brazil for "hunger zero"—not only for Brazil but for every country in the Region, thus echoing the oft-expressed will of governments of the Region to put an end to hunger and malnutrition. What could be more energizing, more galvanizing than an appeal to eradicate hunger and malnutrition in all its forms, thereby commiting to prevent the deaths of 40,000 children under 5 years of age who today suffer from severe malnutrition and die from preventable infections? Attaining this goal is not an impossible dream: the Region of the Americas has the resources and the skilled professionals to realize it. Other attainable goals arise in the arena of immunizable diseases: just as the member governments of PAHO had their finest moments, in the not-too-distant past, in the eradication of smallpox and poliomyelitis, so too is it now possible for them to contemplate significantly reducing—if not eliminating altogether—measles, tetanus, and diphtheria.

The Health Agenda provides a conceptual framework that integrates these eight areas of action from an overall regional perspective. Together, the countries, through PAHO's Governing Bodies, should clearly present how this perspective can best orient the actions and policies of individual governments. It bears noting that policy options and the political context will, at the end of the day, determine what actually gets done. That said, the Organization's ultimate mandate is to serve the people of the Americas, rather than specific governments. The indisputable fact is that,

over the 10-year period that the Agenda covers, most countries will experience changes in governments and even in the guiding political/policy frameworks that orient their actions. To assure that PAHO's technical cooperation is effective over the long term, the Organization should have a policy framework that transcends a specific political context. PAHO will want to continue engaging technical and community groups that are part of each country's national leadership so as to be able to support member governments in the design, implementation, and evaluation of the actions proposed by the Agenda. Policymakers will want to consider assigning to each "area of action" a clearly stated goal or set of goals and corresponding indicators, so that 10 years from now it will be possible to evaluate the impact of the Agenda.

Each of the eight areas could be a pillar for the Organization's technical cooperation over the next decade. While each area has its own relative merit, it will be important to consider where the greatest strengths of the PAHO community lie and what potential value it can add to each of these areas. In several areas, it is likely that the collective PAHO membership could best contribute by striking strategic partnerships with other regional or international organizations that operate in the Americas. To get beyond the Agenda's lofty goals, good intentions, and, frankly, wishful thinking, national and international health policymakers will want to confront the challenges ahead by giving weight, and meat, to the actions outlined in the Agenda.

The Agenda is well presented in terms of technical background, attempting to cover as comprehensively as possible each of the eight areas. This is clearly a strength, from the standpoint of the analysis. At the same time, however, it should be fully understood that to induce the necessary changes in the present regional health situation, policymakers must assure that effective action is taken.

The concept of aligning the Health Agenda with the MDGs is very good; notwithstanding, the MDGs are clearly insufficient to advance comprehensively the health situation in many of the countries in the Region. PAHO provides an excellent forum for the regional discussion necessary to adapt the MDGs to the regional reality. That discussion among PAHO's member governments could serve to define how each will contribute to improving health and well-being not only in one country but in all those that have insufficient human and material resources to address their problems alone.

What orientations would one give to policy- and decisionmakers on implementing the Health Agenda for the coming decade (2008–2017)? As indicated in the foregoing paragraphs, policy options should be both ambitious and realistic. The need for critical actions should arise from the people themselves. The only sustainable solution to chronic health problems in the Region, which represent the most burdensome group cause of morbidity and mortality in the hemisphere, is one that starts with the community demands for improved health and well-being through the democratic channels of political participation. In turn, communities, through their respective governments, could approach PAHO whenever and wherever the cooperation of the Organization is needed. For its part, PAHO should promote the right to health and more equal access to services; should provide the necessary technical support for advocacy, program design, implementation, and evaluation; and should work with the governments to advance health effectively and efficiently. Most important, the Organization should hold itself and others accountable for its adherence to the stated vision and mission that justify PAHO's very existence.

What prospects for change should be taken into account in looking towards the future of health? The Health Agenda reflects reasonably well the expected regional trends, but it fails to sufficiently emphasize the decline in fertility and the dramatic increase in the proportion of older people that is occurring throughout most of the Region. The need to keep people healthy and well for longer than has heretofore been the case will be an imperative in the coming decades. Industrialized countries have become rich before growing older; in contrast, most of the countries in the Americas are becoming older before attaining the necessary wealth to care appropriately for those with age-related limitations.

Finally, the need to contribute to closing health disparities should consider the fact that science and technology, as they are presently being promoted, are forces that most likely will increase rather than decrease inequality among countries. That greater inequality will surely result, unless the regulatory framework presently in place is reexamined to take into account the situation of countries that have serious limitations in resources—limitations that today prohibit their access to the new diagnostic and therapeutic tools that the future will bring.

Ricardo Uauy, M.D., Ph.D.
Professor of Public Health Nutrition,
Institute of Nutrition and Food Technology,
University of Chile, Santiago, Chile
London School of Hygiene and Tropical Medicine,
London, United Kingdom
President, International Union of Nutritional Sciences

COMMENTS OF DR. MARIJKE VELZEBOER-SALCEDO

The United Nations Development Fund for Women (UNIFEM) congratulates the countries of the Americas for their elaboration of the regional Health Agenda and for explicitly identifying gender equity as one of its guiding principles. An overarching theme of our orientation to policy- and decisionmakers to consider when implementing the Agenda would be that gender equity is central to all its areas of action, in concurrence with the spirit of the Millennium Development Goals:

The Millennium Development Goals acknowledge that women's empowerment and gender equality are prerequisites for devel-

opment, and all the health-related goals require action in this area if they are to be achieved [*emphasis added*]. Women's health is adversely affected by the prevalence among them of poverty, lack of employment, violence and rape, limited power over their sexual and reproductive lives, and lack of influence in decision-making. Expanding access to sexual and reproductive health care is essential. Those working with governments and public health authorities must actively promote a gender perspective in the design and implementation of health policies and programs. Monitoring and evaluation should routinely use sex-disaggregated data.

In that context and with regard to the Agenda's analysis of health trends in the Americas, the exclusion of women is a major issue. It bears noting, as examples of their social exclusion, that a high proportion of women still do not receive trained care at childbirth and do not have access to contraceptive technologies—factors that relate directly to high rates of maternal mortality and adolescent fertility.

One of the principal areas of action set forth in the Health Agenda is strengthening of the national health authority. UNIFEM considers it important, in using the term "participation," to underscore that it should extend to decisionmaking, since the concept of social participation has often been promoted more as a pragmatic instrumental concept for the purpose of rubber-stamping or implementing decisions taken by others. Participation ought to be understood as an exercise in civil rights that influences the processes that affect the common good. In that regard, women should be singled out, since they are, and have always been, more frequently active participants in the execution of community programs, particularly in the health sector, although they continue to be excluded from the formulation, design, and resource allocation phases of those programs.

UNICEF considers that women's empowerment is a key strategy to tackle health determinants—one of the Agenda's eight areas of action. As clarified in the Millennium Declaration, the third MDG, "gender equality and empowerment of women," represents not only an end in itself but also a *sine qua non* for attaining the other seven MDGs. In that context, we applaud the Agenda's specific reference to gender in the section on "tackling health determinants" as a structural determinant of health inequity and suggest that policy- and decisionmakers be made aware of the important work being carried out among various sectors, institutions, and United Nations agencies, such as the particularly successful interagency collaboration between PAHO and UNIFEM at the regional, subregional, and country level.

Implementing the area of action related to harnessing knowledge, science, and technology will require that information for understanding and monitoring health dynamics be routinely disaggregated by sex, age, socioeconomic status, and other socioeconomic variables, in order to identify group-specific needs, assess inequalities, plan responses, and monitor changes. Toward

419

Grounding health in information, knowledge, science, and technology

The need for data and information will confront the policymaker at every turn, and, indeed, the case for health as set out above can only be made on the basis of reliable data that are collected regularly: the value of the data increases when they are collected on a regular basis with some established periodicity.

—George Alleyne

To fully understand the health problems that most need to be addressed and the most effective methods for doing so requires establishing an institutional culture within the public health sector that values and demands high-quality information and that develops the capacity to generate it—that is, the pursuit of applied epidemiology and research.

—Stephen Blount and Jay McAuliffe

. . . health should be coupled with the development of science and a likewise universal and free education, as health and education go hand in hand. ... The public health system should have in place excellent services that enable the conduct of high-level, costly studies that will benefit patients. Too often, the quality of public health services is very low, and only in private services can certain studies be carried out.

—Gustavo Kourí

People have a "right to well-being" by exercising their "right" to scientific knowledge and research, to information on experiences in applying them, and to the results emanating from them. The challenge lies in empowering people and communities with the capability of comprehending scientific information and its relevance to tackling their health issues so that they can participate meaningfully in improving their own health.

—Muthu Subramanian

The disaggregation of data could help Health Ministries to more forcefully advocate for resources to strengthen health services in the areas where health outcomes are weakest.

—Nils Arne Kastberg

Planning for the assessment and expanded use of new and effective technologies in the public health sector is critical; examples include new vaccines, rapid diagnostic kits, geographic information systems, and information technology tools. Decisionmakers in the public health sector must stay abreast of the development of new technologies and be innovative in finding opportunities to apply them to more effectively address priority health problems. . . . The success of immunization programs in the Americas—smallpox and polio eradication, measles elimination, current efforts to eliminate rubella—lays the foundation for the introduction of new vaccines and for the evolution from child to family immunization programs.

—Stephen Blount and Jay McAuliffe

Other attainable goals arise in the arena of immunizable diseases: just as the member governments of PAHO had their finest moments, in the not-too-distant past, in the eradication of smallpox and poliomyelitis, so too is it now possible for them to contemplate significantly reducing—if not eliminating altogether—measles, tetanus, and diphtheria.

—Ricardo Uauy

---

that end and because the availability of gender-sensitive information is indispensable for monitoring progress in gender equality, UNIFEM and PAHO are collaborating on the production and dissemination of basic gender indicators on health and its determinants.

Another area of action focuses on strengthening solidarity and health security. In implementing the Agenda, any effort to deal with violence must take into account the most frequent type of violence, namely that which is gender-based. It is crucial for policy- and decisionmakers to understand that gender-based violence is not only a public health matter but also a human rights issue that affects one out of three women in the Region.

As regards efforts to diminish health inequities among and within countries, UNIFEM strongly concurs with the Agenda's distinction of sexual and reproductive health as a priority issue in the Americas. We would urge, however, that policymakers not limit the scope of this issue to the maternal sphere. Sexual health must also be emphasized, particularly in the context of the individual's power to make free, informed, responsible, and safe decisions, which will, in turn, contribute to lowering the number of unwanted pregnancies, reducing maternal and child mortality rates, reducing gender-based violence and related health complications, and halting the spread of HIV/AIDS.

Increasing social protection and access to quality health services will indeed require effective dialogue among relevant stakeholders. Because of their role in setting health priorities, those stakeholders should broadly include civil society, particularly women's groups. In applying the concept of collective financing, in addition to the consideration of subsidies across generations and income groups, subsidies that cross over the sexes are also important. In the absence of such subsidies, women carry a heavier health care expenditure load than men, because of women's greater need for health services throughout their lives—a greater need that derives mainly, but not exclusively, from their reproductive function. Moreover, because of the cultural centrality of their role as caregivers and homemakers and their predominance in the informal sector of the economy, women are more frequently deprived of the social protection that comes with full-time employment.

In the context of people working for health, another area of action set out in the Agenda, policymakers will want to bear in mind the issue of unpaid care provided at home. Women continue to carry the main responsibility of caregiving at home, and that care, according to international statistics, accounts for more than 80% of all health care. Because this unpaid work tends to be neither recognized nor valued, women are disadvantaged in terms of available time and the social protection associated with paid work. The health care system cannot keep relying as heavily as it has in the past on this unpaid work: on one hand, the demand for services will increase due to the aging of the population and the related increase in chronic diseases; on the other, the available time for unpaid caregiving is diminishing and will continue to do so, as women increasingly enter the labor force. Human resource policies will have to take these trends into account, particularly when decisions are being made regarding the reduction or expansion of public services. These issues are of particular interest to UNIFEM, because of their impact on gender equality and women's autonomy. We have been collaborating with PAHO and ECLAC towards raising public and government awareness in this respect, and, together, we are spearheading the incorporation of unpaid health care in the system of national accounts, with particular reference to satellite accounts.

We thank the Pan American Health Organization for the opportunity to provide an orientation to policy- and decisionmakers at the local, national, and international levels who will have the challenge of realizing the Health Agenda for the Americas over the coming decade. As we are all stakeholders in the pursuit of the Agenda, we in UNIFEM heartily wish for its every success.

Dr. Marijke Velzeboer-Salcedo
Chief, Latin America and Caribbean Section
United Nations Development Fund for Women

The Continuing Regional Commitment: Planning for the Future of Health in the Americas

Inclusion in this edition of *Health in the Americas* of perspectives regarding the future of health and the countries' collective commitment to address its challenges through a common agenda follows a long-standing tradition. Since its inception, the serial publication has stressed the importance of regional health policies and plans for accomplishing health goals throughout the hemisphere. Beginning with the first edition in 1954, every Director of the Pan American Sanitary Bureau has used the publication to link the countries, their regional Organization, and the Secretariat that serves that Organization to the challenge of addressing the future of health in the Americas through collective commitments expressed in regional plans:

The 1954 edition begins with the words of **Fred Lowe Soper** (Director from 1946 to 1958):

> For planning of health programs in the Americas, measurement of the problems is essential. Progress in health work requires basic information regarding the population being served, the health conditions in the countries, and the medical resources and needs. This principle has been recognized by the provisions of the Pan American Sanitary Code and the Constitution of the Pan American Sanitary Organization [*sic*] for the exchange of information regarding the prevention of disease and the preservation of health in the Western Hemisphere. Future progress depends in large part on measurement of the problems by the provision of accurate data for coordinated health planning.

In launching the 1966 edition, **Abraham Horwitz** (Director from 1958 to 1975) notes that:

> The Governments of the Americas have agreed to fulfill within the decade beginning in 1962 a series of objectives to prevent disease, to provide timely treatment and rehabilitation for the sick, and to promote well-being. They have recognized planning as the tool for establishing priorities among the health

problems and for allocating resources accordingly, so as to benefit the largest number of people.

Héctor R. Acuña (Director from 1975 to 1983) situates the 1978 edition at the mid-point of the Ten-Year Health Plan for the Americas:

It seemed particularly appropriate to focus the analysis on the progress achieved in attaining the goals set forth in the Plan. Likewise, attention is drawn to those areas where increased effort will be required by the countries if these goals are to be met.

Carlyle Guerra de Macedo (Director from 1983 to 1995) presents the 1986 edition as documenting:

the progress made by the Member Countries of the Pan American Health Organization toward meeting their collective goal of health for all by the year 2000 . . . and [providing] an overall evaluation of the situation in regard to attainment of that goal by the end of this century.

In his introduction of the 2002 edition, **George A.O. Alleyne** (Director from 1995 to 2003) sets the stage for the pages that followed:

In broad terms, the Region's health situation can be viewed as a reflection of the dual impact of the demographic changes and shifts in epidemiological profiles. It also mirrors the effectiveness of health policies. . . .

For her part, the current Director of the Pan American Health Organization, **Mirta Roses Periago** (2003–), hopes that this 2007 edition will serve as a reminder that:

behind every number and every statistic is the life of a girl, a boy, a woman, or a man living in some corner of the Region [and that] the 2012 edition of this publication will bring news of the countries' great progress in their common covenant to attain better health and longer, fuller, more fruitful lives for all the peoples of the Americas, especially those who thus far have been excluded from the benefits of development.

ACRONYMS

ACT	Amazon Cooperation Treaty Organization
ADC	Andean Development Corporation
AIDIS	Inter-American Association of Sanitary and Environmental Engineering
AIDS	Acquired immunodeficiency syndrome
ALAESP	Latin American and Caribbean Association of Public Health Education
API	Annual parasite index
BCIE	Central American Bank for Economic Integration
BIREME	Latin American and Caribbean Center on Health Sciences Information (PAHO)
BMI	Body mass index
CAN	Andean Community of Nations
CAREC	Caribbean Epidemiology Center (PAHO)
CARICOM	Caribbean Community
CCA	Common Country Assessments (NU)
CDB	Caribbean Development Bank
CDC	Centers for Disease Control and Prevention (USA)
CEHI	Caribbean Environmental Health Institute
CELADE	Latin American and Caribbean Demographic Center (ECLAC)
CEPIS	Pan American Center for Sanitary Engineering and Environmental Sciences (PAHO)
CERSSO	Regional Center for Occupational Safety and Health
CFNI	Caribbean Food and Nutrition Institute (PAHO)
CHRC	Caribbean Health Research Council
CIDA	Canadian International Development Agency
CIOMS	Council for International Organizations of Medical Sciences
COHRED	Council on Health Research for Development
COLABIOCLI	Latin American Confederation of Clinical Biochemistry
COPICHAS	Confederation of Indigenous Peoples of the South American Chaco Region
CPC	Caribbean Program Coordination (PAHO)
CPI	Consumer price index
CRICS	Regional Congress on Health Sciences Information
DAC	Development Assistance Committee (OECD)
DALY	Disability-adjusted life years
DANIDA	Danish International Development Agency
DOTS	Directly observed treatment, short course
EAP	Economically active population
ECLAC	Economic Commission for Latin America and the Caribbean (UN)
EPA	Environmental Protection Agency (USA)
EPI	Expanded Program on Immunization
FAO	Food and Agriculture Organization of the United Nations
FCTC	Framework Convention on Tobacco Control (WHO)
FIOCRUZ	Oswaldo Cruz Foundation
GAVI	Global Alliance for Vaccines and Immunization
GDP	Gross domestic product
GEF	Global Environment Facility
GFATM	Global Fund to Fight AIDS, Tuberculosis, and Malaria
GIVS	Global Immunization Vision and Strategies

GMP	Good manufacturing practices
GNI	Gross national income
GNP	Gross national product
GTZ	German Technical Cooperation Agency
HACCP	Hazard analysis critical control point
HDI	Human development index (UNDP)
HINARI	Health InterNetwork Access to Research Initiative
HIPC	Heavily Indebted Poor Countries Initiative (IMF/World Bank)
HIV	Human immunodeficiency virus
HPSRI	Health-Promoting Schools Regional Initiative
IACHR	Inter-American Commission on Human Rights
IAEA	International Atomic Energy Agency
IAM	Amazon Malaria Initiative
IBRD	International Bank for Reconstruction and Development (World Bank)
IBWC	International Boundary and Water Commission
ICOH	International Commission on Occupational Health
ICPD	International Conference on Population and Development
ICRC	International Committee of the Red Cross
IDA	International Development Association (World Bank)
IDB	Inter-American Development Bank
IFRC	International Federation of Red Cross and Red Crescent Societies
IHR	International Health Regulations
ILO	International Labor Organization
IMCI	Integrated Management of Childhood Illnesses
IMF	International Monetary Fund
INCAP	Institute of Nutrition of Central America and Panama (PAHO)
IOM	International Organization for Migration
IPCC	United Nations Intergovernmental Panel on Climate Change
IRET	Regional Institute for the Study of Toxic Substances
ISCA	Central American Health Initiative
IUHPE	International Union for Health Promotion and Education
JICA	Japan International Cooperation Agency
JMP	Joint Monitoring Program (WHO/UNICEF)
LAMM	Latin American and Caribbean Initiative for Maternal Mortality Reduction
LILACS	Latin American and Caribbean Literature on Health Sciences (PAHO)
MDG	Millennium development goals
MERCOSUR	Southern Common Market
NAFTA	North American Free Trade Agreement
NGO	Nongovernmental organization
OAS	Organization of American States
OCHA	Office for the Coordination of Humanitarian Affairs (NU)
ODA	Official development assistance
OECD	Organisation for Economic Co-operation and Development
OECS	Organization of Eastern Caribbean States
OEPA	Onchocerciasis Elimination Program for the Americas
OIE	World Organization for Animal Health
ORAS-CONHU	Andean Health Agency-Hipólito Unánue Agreement
OREALC	Regional Office for Education in Latin America and the Caribbean (UNESCO)
PAHEF	Pan American Health and Education Foundation
PAHO	Pan American Health Organization

PANAFTOSA	Pan American Foot-and-Mouth Disease Center (PAHO)
PANCAP	Pan Caribbean Partnership Against HIV/AIDS
PANDRH	Pan American Network for Drug Regulatory Harmonization
PASB	Pan American Sanitary Bureau
PHAC	Canadian Public Health Agency
PHEFA	Hemispheric Program for the Eradication of Foot-and-Mouth Disease
PLAGSALUD	Occupational and Environmental Aspects of Exposure to Pesticides in the Central American Isthmus
PPP	Purchasing power parity
RAVREDA	Amazon Network for the Surveillance of Antimalarial Drug Resistance
RBM	Roll Back Malaria
RECACER	Central American Network for the Prevention and Control of Emerging and Reemerging Diseases
RELAB	Latin American Biology Network
RELAC	Latin American and Caribbean Network of Environmental Laboratories
REMSAA	Meeting of Andean Area Health Ministers
REPAMAR	Pan American Environmental Waste Management Network
REPIDISCA	Pan American Network of Information and Documentation in Sanitary
RESSCAD	Meeting of the Health Sector of Central America and the Dominican Republic
RICTSAL	Network of Science and Technology Health Indicators
RICYT	Network of Science and Technology Indicators
RIMSA	Inter-American Meeting at Ministerial Level on Health and Agriculture
SARS	Severe Acute Respiratory Syndrome
SciELO	Scientific Electronic Library Online
ScienTI	International Network of Information and Knowledge Sources for Sciences, Technology and Innovation Management
SICA	Central American Integration System
SIDA	Swedish International Development Cooperation Agency
SIREVA	Regional System of Vaccines (PAHO)
TCC	Technical cooperation among countries
UN	United Nations
UNAIDS	Joint United Nations Program on HIV/AIDS
UNASUR	Union of South American Nations
UNDAF	United Nations Development Assistance Framework
UNDG	United Nations Development Group
UNDP	United Nations Development Programme
UNEP	United Nations Environment Programme
UNESCO	United Nations Educational, Scientific, and Cultural Organization
UNFPA	United Nations Fund for Population Activities
UNGASS	United Nations General Assembly Special Session
UNHCR	United Nations High Commissioner for Refugees
UNICEF	United Nations Children's Fund
UNIFEM	United Nations Development Fund for Women
UNSCEAR	United Nations Scientific Committee on the Effects of Atomic Radiation
VHL	Virtual Health Library
VIVSALUD	Inter-American Healthy Housing Network
VWA	Vaccination week in the Americas
WFP	World Food Program
WHO	World Health Organization
WTO	World Trade Organization